Virtual Reality in the Assessment, Understanding and Treatment of Mental Health Disorders

Virtual Reality in the Assessment, Understanding and Treatment of Mental Health Disorders

Editors

Giuseppe Riva
Silvia Serino

MDPI • Basel • Beijing • Wuhan • Barcelona • Belgrade • Manchester • Tokyo • Cluj • Tianjin

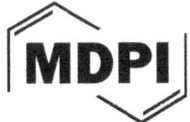

Editors
Giuseppe Riva
Department of Psychology,
Università Cattolica
del Sacro Cuore
Italy

Silvia Serino
MySpace Lab, Department of
Clinical Neurosciences,
University Hospital Lausanne (CHUV)
Switzerland

Editorial Office
MDPI
St. Alban-Anlage 66
4052 Basel, Switzerland

This is a reprint of articles from the Special Issue published online in the open access journal *Journal of Clinical Medicine* (ISSN 2077-0383) (available at: https://www.mdpi.com/journal/jcm/special_issues/Virtual_Reality_Mental_Health_Disorders).

For citation purposes, cite each article independently as indicated on the article page online and as indicated below:

LastName, A.A.; LastName, B.B.; LastName, C.C. Article Title. *Journal Name* **Year**, *Volume Number*, Page Range.

ISBN 978-3-03943-775-7 (Hbk)
ISBN 978-3-03943-776-4 (PDF)

© 2020 by the authors. Articles in this book are Open Access and distributed under the Creative Commons Attribution (CC BY) license, which allows users to download, copy and build upon published articles, as long as the author and publisher are properly credited, which ensures maximum dissemination and a wider impact of our publications.

The book as a whole is distributed by MDPI under the terms and conditions of the Creative Commons license CC BY-NC-ND.

Contents

About the Editors vii

Giuseppe Riva and Silvia Serino
Virtual Reality in the Assessment, Understanding and Treatment of Mental Health Disorders
Reprinted from: *J. Clin. Med.* **2020**, *9*, 3434, doi:10.3390/jcm9113434 1

Federica Scarpina, Silvia Serino, Anouk Keizer, Alice Chirico, Massimo Scacchi, Gianluca Castelnuovo, Alessandro Mauro and Giuseppe Riva
The Effect of a Virtual-Reality Full-Body Illusion on Body Representation in Obesity
Reprinted from: *J. Clin. Med.* **2019**, *8*, 1330, doi:10.3390/jcm8091330 11

Luca Provenzano, Giuseppina Porciello, Sofia Ciccarone, Bigna Lenggenhager, Gaetano Tieri, Matteo Marucci, Federico Dazzi, Camillo Loriedo and Ilaria Bufalari
Characterizing Body Image Distortion and Bodily Self-Plasticity in Anorexia Nervosa via Visuo-Tactile Stimulation in Virtual Reality
Reprinted from: *J. Clin. Med.* **2020**, *9*, 98, doi:10.3390/jcm9010098 27

Gad Drori, Paz Bar-Tal, Yonatan Stern, Yair Zvilichovsky and Roy Salomon
UnReal? Investigating the Sense of Reality and Psychotic Symptoms with Virtual Reality
Reprinted from: *J. Clin. Med.* **2020**, *9*, 1627, doi:10.3390/jcm9061627 45

Mariano Alcañiz Raya, Javier Marín-Morales, Maria Eleonora Minissi, Gonzalo Teruel Garcia, Luis Abad and Irene Alice Chicchi Giglioli
Machine Learning and Virtual Reality on Body Movements' Behaviors to Classify Children with Autism Spectrum Disorder
Reprinted from: *J. Clin. Med.* **2020**, *9*, 1260, doi:10.3390/jcm9051260 61

Marta Matamala-Gomez, Birgit Nierula, Tony Donegan, Mel Slater and Maria V. Sanchez-Vives
Manipulating the Perceived Shape and Color of a Virtual Limb Can Modulate Pain Responses
Reprinted from: *J. Clin. Med.* **2020**, *9*, 291, doi:10.3390/jcm9020291 81

Bruno Porras Garcia, Marta Ferrer Garcia, Agata Olszewska, Lena Yilmaz, Cristina González Ibañez, Mireia Gracia Blanes, Gamze Gültekin, Eduardo Serrano Troncoso and José Gutiérrez Maldonado
Is This My Own Body? Changing the Perceptual and Affective Body Image Experience among College Students Using a New Virtual Reality Embodiment-Based Technique
Reprinted from: *J. Clin. Med.* **2019**, *8*, 925, doi:10.3390/jcm8070925 97

Yonatan Stern, Danny Koren, Renana Moebus, Gabriella Panishev and Roy Salomon
Assessing the Relationship between Sense of Agency, the Bodily-Self and Stress: Four Virtual-Reality Experiments in Healthy Individuals
Reprinted from: *J. Clin. Med.* **2020**, *9*, 2931, doi:10.3390/jcm9092931 111

Wenceslao Peñate, Francisco Rivero, Conrado Viña, Manuel Herrero, Moisés Betancort, Juan De la Fuente, Yolanda Álvarez-Pérez and Ascensión Fumero
The Equivalence between Virtual and Real Feared Stimuli in a Phobic Adult Sample: A Neuroimaging Study
Reprinted from: *J. Clin. Med.* **2019**, *8*, 2139, doi:10.3390/jcm8122139 131

Tanya Guitard, Stéphane Bouchard, Claude Bélanger and Maxine Berthiaume
Exposure to a Standardized Catastrophic Scenario in Virtual Reality or a Personalized Scenario in Imagination for Generalized Anxiety Disorder
Reprinted from: *J. Clin. Med.* **2019**, *8*, 309, doi:10.3390/jcm8030309 143

Jessica Isbely Montana, Marta Matamala-Gomez, Marta Maisto, Petar Aleksandrov Mavrodiev, Cesare Massimo Cavalera, Barbara Diana, Fabrizia Mantovani and Olivia Realdon
The Benefits of emotion Regulation Interventions in Virtual Reality for the Improvement of Wellbeing in Adults and Older Adults: A Systematic Review
Reprinted from: *J. Clin. Med.* **2020**, *9*, 500, doi:10.3390/jcm9020500 159

Nansi López-Valverde, Jorge Muriel Fernández, Antonio López-Valverde, Luis F. Valero Juan, Juan Manuel Ramírez, Javier Flores Fraile, Julio Herrero Payo, Leticia A. Blanco Antona, Bruno Macedo de Sousa and Manuel Bravo
Use of Virtual Reality for the Management of Anxiety and Pain in Dental Treatments: Systematic Review and Meta-Analysis
Reprinted from: *J. Clin. Med.* **2020**, *9*, 1025, doi:10.3390/jcm9041025 181

Nansi López-Valverde, Jorge Muriel Fernández, Antonio López-Valverde, Luis F Valero Juan, Juan Manuel Ramírez, Javier Flores Fraile, Julio Herrero Payo, Leticia A Blanco Antona, Bruno Macedo de Sousa and Manuel Bravo
Retraction: Lopez-Valverde, N.; et al. Use of Virtual Reality for the Management of Anxiety and Pain in Dental Treatments: Systematic Review and Meta-Analysis. *J. Clin. Med.* 2020, *9*, 1025
Reprinted from: *J. Clin. Med.* **2020**, *9*, 2404, doi:10.3390/jcm9082404 199

Monia Cabinio, Federica Rossetto, Sara Isernia, Francesca Lea Saibene, Monica Di Cesare, Francesca Borgnis, Stefania Pazzi, Tommaso Migliazza, Margherita Alberoni, Valeria Blasi and Francesca Baglio
The Use of a Virtual Reality Platform for the Assessment of the Memory Decline and the Hippocampal Neural Injury in Subjects with Mild Cognitive Impairment: The Validity of Smart Aging Serious Game (SASG)
Reprinted from: *J. Clin. Med.* **2020**, *9*, 1355, doi:10.3390/jcm9051355 201

Ngeemasara Thapa, Hye Jin Park, Ja-Gyeong Yang, Haeun Son, Minwoo Jang, Jihyeon Lee, Seung Wan Kang, Kyung Won Park and Hyuntae Park
The Effect of a Virtual Reality-Based Intervention Program on Cognition in Older Adults with Mild Cognitive Impairment: A Randomized Control Trial
Reprinted from: *J. Clin. Med.* **2020**, *9*, 1283, doi:10.3390/jcm9051283 215

Roberta Bevilacqua, Elvira Maranesi, Giovanni Renato Riccardi, Valentina Di Donna, Paolo Pelliccioni, Riccardo Luzi, Fabrizia Lattanzio and Giuseppe Pelliccioni
Non-Immersive Virtual Reality for Rehabilitation of the Older People: A Systematic Review into Efficacy and Effectiveness
Reprinted from: *J. Clin. Med.* **2019**, *8*, 1882, doi:10.3390/jcm811882 227

Jessica Isbely Montana, Cosimo Tuena, Silvia Serino, Pietro Cipresso and Giuseppe Riva
Neurorehabilitation of Spatial Memory Using Virtual Environments: A Systematic Review
Reprinted from: *J. Clin. Med.* **2019**, *8*, 1516, doi:10.3390/jcm8101516 241

Elisa Pedroli, Filippo La Paglia, Pietro Cipresso, Caterina La Cascia, Giuseppe Riva and Daniele La Barbera
A Computational Approach for the Assessment of Executive Functions in Patients with Obsessive–Compulsive Disorder
Reprinted from: *J. Clin. Med.* **2019**, *8*, 1975, doi:10.3390/jcm8111975 . . . . **267**

Cosimo Tuena, Silvia Serino, Léo Dutriaux, Giuseppe Riva and Pascale Piolino
Virtual Enactment Effect on Memory in Young and Aged Populations: A Systematic Review
Reprinted from: *J. Clin. Med.* **2019**, *8*, 620, doi:10.3390/jcm8050620 . . . . **281**

About the Editors

Giuseppe Riva is Full Professor (tenure position) of General Psychology and Communication Psychology at the Catholic University of Milan, Italy and Head Researcher of the the Applied Technology for Neuro-Psychology Laboratory—ATN-P Lab., Istituto Auxologico Italiano, Verbania, Italy. In the ATN-P Lab., he conducted extensive research and published many papers on methods and assessment tools in psychology and the use of virtual reality and the internet in medicine and in training.

Silvia Serino is Marie Skłodowska-Curie Research Fellow at MySpaceLab (University Hospital Lausanne, CHUV). She obtained her PhD in Psychology at the Università Cattolica del Sacro Cuore in Milan (Italy) in 2015 with a thesis investigating the role of spatial processing for the cognitive system. Her main research interest is the study of the interactions between body and space, which are important for action and memory. Toward this aim, she employed different techniques from cognitive psychology, including psychophysics experiments, virtual reality simulations, and physiological recordings in both healthy participants and individuals presenting deficits in spatial and body representations, as a model for investigating how body and spatial representations interact.

She is Editor and reviewer of several international journals in the field of cognitive psychology and cognitive neuroscience. She published more than 120 papers on recognized journals about the complex relationship between space, body, and memory, and in pathological conditions (e.g., neurodegenerative diseases), also exploiting the use of virtual reality as an "embodied tool" for investigating high-level cognitive processes.

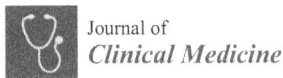

Editorial

Virtual Reality in the Assessment, Understanding and Treatment of Mental Health Disorders

Giuseppe Riva [1,2] and Silvia Serino [1,3,*]

1. Humane Technology Lab, Università Cattolica del Sacro Cuore, 20123 Milan, Italy; giuseppe.riva@unicatt.it
2. Istituto Auxologico Italiano, IRCCS, U.O. di Neurologia e Neuroriabilitazione, Ospedale S. Giuseppe, 28824 Piancavallo, Italy
3. MySpace Lab, Department of Clinical Neuroscience, University Hospital Lausanne (CHUV), 1011 Lausanne, Switzerland
* Correspondence: silvia.serino@unicatt.it

Received: 21 October 2020; Accepted: 22 October 2020; Published: 26 October 2020

Abstract: Computer scientists usually describe virtual reality (VR) as a set of fancy hardware and software technologies. However, psychology and neuroscience are starting to consider VR as the most advanced form of human-computer interaction allowing individuals to act, communicate and become present in a computer-generated environment. In this view, the feeling of "being there" experienced during a VR experience can become a powerful tool for personal change: it offers a dynamic and social world where individuals can live and share a specific experience. For this reason, the use of VR in mental health shows promise: different researches support its clinical efficacy for conditions including anxiety disorders, stress-related disorders, obesity and eating disorders, pain management, addiction and schizophrenia. However, more research is needed to transform the promises of VR in a real clinical tool for mental health. This Special Issue aims to present the most recent advances in the mental health applications of VR, as well as their implications for future patient care.

Keywords: virtual reality; mental health; presence

Computer scientists usually describe virtual reality (VR) as a set of fancy hardware and software technologies [1]: a computer or mobile device (e.g., a smartphone) with a graphics card capable of interactive third-dimensional (3D) visualization, controllers, and a head-mounted display (HMD) embedding one or more trackers. This short description clearly identifies the core technological parts of a VR system [2]: input devices, output devices, and the virtual environment. Input devices comprise all the sensors and trackers that sense the individual's actions (e.g., hand and head movements) allowing the user to interact with the virtual environment. Output devices include all the technologies (e.g., head-mounted displays or CAVEs) that provide continuous computer-generated information to the user. Finally, the virtual environment (VE) is the 3D simulated scenario generated by the computer or the mobile device. VEs are designed to be explored, so users can interact (e.g., moving, pushing, picking, rotating, etc.) with their contents. In multi-user virtual environments (MUVEs) two or more users can share the same simulated scenario and communicate and/or interact inside it. To allow communication and interaction between users, MUVEs use avatars—personalized graphical representations of the individuals—that are directly controlled by their movements in real time. Embodied virtual agents, on the other hand, are graphical representations of the individuals controlled by the computer itself using an artificial intelligence program.

However, psychology and neuroscience are starting to consider VR as the most advanced form of human-computer interaction because it allows individuals to act, communicate and become present in a computer-generated environment [3,4]. In this view, the feeling of "being there" experienced during a VR experience can become a powerful tool for personal change [5,6]: it offers a dynamic and social world where individuals can live and share a specific experience. For this reason, the use of VR in mental health shows promise: different researches support its clinical efficacy for conditions including anxiety disorders, stress-related disorders, obesity and eating disorders, pain management, addiction and schizophrenia [7–9]. However, the use of VR in clinical practice has long been limited by two main factors: the lack of usability and the cost of virtual tools [10,11].

The first generation of VR devices, available between 1990 and 2015, was characterized by a series of significant shortcomings - low display resolution, limited field of view, and uncomfortable designs—producing different side effects to their users. In particular, motion sickness (due to low display quality) and neck pains (due to the weight of the HMD), limited the use of this technology in a clinical setting. Moreover, the first VR systems required expensive HMDs paired with equally expensive high-end computers usually costing 20,000/50,000 USD. Finally, developing and using a VR experience required a significant technical knowledge that was typically unavailable in hospitals and/or clinical centers.

2016 saw the release of the first generation of HMDs targeted at consumers. The Oculus Rift—an HMD developed and manufactured by Oculus VR, a division of Facebook Inc., and sold for 600 USD—marked a new generation of VR devices (see Table 1) that is revolutionizing how VR is used in general. In a few years, the cost of a complete VR device—including input, output, and 3D graphic computation—dropped by tens of thousands of dollars to just a few hundred, the price of the cheapest standalone VR systems [12]. However, more research is needed to transform the promises of VR in a real clinical tool for mental health. This Special Issue aims to present the most recent advances in the mental health applications of VR, as well as their implications for future patient care.

In most cases, VR is used as a "simulative tool" to recreate ecologically valid scenarios reproducing feared/critical situations (i.e., fear of speaking in front of an audience) with a precise control over the stimuli delivery according both to therapeutic strategies and patients' needs [3,4]. In this way, patients can enter simulations of the situations that are extremely dangerous to experience in real-life (i.e., fear of heights), thus extending the boundaries of existing treatments. Moreover, VR permits the repeated delivery of the same scenarios while allowing the anxiety to attenuate, graded in difficulty and customized for each specific patient. VR-based treatments including simulations have been successfully implemented and tested in different clinical trials, especially for treating anxiety disorders [13–17], stress-related disorders [18], phobias [19], and post-traumatic stress disorders [20,21].

In order to further explore the potential of VR in the exposure therapy for anxiety disorders, in the current Special Issue Guitard et al. [22] compared the traditional exposure using imagination through a personalized catastrophic scenario to exposure in VR with a standardized scenario in 28 patients suffering from generalized anxiety disorder (GAD). In both cases, a neutral scenario served as a baseline. Their results indicated that the standardized virtual scenario induced higher anxiety when compared to the neutral one, thus suggesting the possibility of using it for the treatment of patients suffering from GAD.

In the same vein, Peñate et al. [23] tested whether the exposure to virtual phobic stimuli in a group of 32 patients with specific phobias (i.e., small animals) would activate the same brain regions as the exposure to real image stimuli. A specific inspection of the amygdala and insula detected higher activations in response to real images, but those areas have been activated also in response to virtual stimuli. Globally, these findings gave additional support for the use of virtual stimuli in cue-exposure treatments for phobias.

Table 1. Commercially available VR devices.

Mobility Required	PC Based				Mobile Based			Console Based	Standalone		
System	Oculus Rift S	HTC Cosmos/ Vive Pro/ Pro Eye	Valve Index	HP Reverb G2	Samsung Gear VR	Google Cardboard	Google Daydream	PlayStation VR	Xiaomi MI VR	Oculus Quest 2	Lenovo VR Classroom 2
Cost (USD)	399	699/ 1199/ 1599	99	599	99	10–50	69–149	299	199	299	399
Hardware Requirements	High-End PC (>1000 USD)	High-End PC (>1000 USD)	High-End PC (>1000 USD)	High-End PC (>1000 USD)	High-End Samsung Phone (>600 USD)	Middle/Highend Android Phone or iPhone (>299 USD)	High-End Android Phone (>499 USD)	PS4 (299 USD) or PS4 Pro (399 USD)	None (Internal Snapdragon 821 processor)	None (Internal Snapdragon XR2 processor)	None (Internal Snapdrag on 835 processor)
Resolution	2560 × 1440	2880 × 1660	2880 × 1660	2160 × 2160 (per eye)	2560 × 1440	Depends on the phone (minimum 1024 × 768)	Depends on the phone (minimum 1920 × 1080)	1920 × 1080	2560 × 1440	2560 × 1920 (per eye)	2160 × 1920
Refresh Rate	80 Hz	90 Hz	120/144Hz	90 Hz	60 Hz	60 Hz	90 Hz minimum	120 Hz	72 Hz	90 Hz	75 Hz
Field of View	115 degrees	110 degrees	130 degrees	114 degrees	101 degrees	from 70 degrees	96 degrees	100 degrees	90 degrees	100 degrees	110 degrees
Body Tracking	*High*: head tracking (rotation) and volumetric tracking (full room size—15 × 15 ft—movement)	*High*: head tracking (rotation) and volumetric tracking (full room size—15 × 15 ft—movement)	*High*: head tracking (rotation) and volumetric tracking (full room size—15 × 15 ft—movement)	*High*: head tracking (rotation) and volumetric tracking (full room size—15 × 15 ft—movement)	*Medium*: head tracking (rotation)	*Medium*: head tracking (rotation)	*Medium*: head tracking (rotation)	*Medium/High*: head tracking (rotation) and positional tracking (forward/backward)	*Medium*: head tracking (rotation)	*Medium/High*: head tracking (rotation) and volumetric tracking (full room size—15 × 15 ft—movement)	*Medium/High*: head tracking (rotation)
User Interaction with VR	*High* (using controllers)	*Very High* (using controllers and eye tracking)	*High* (using controllers)	*High* (using controllers)	Medium (using gaze, a built-in pad or joystick)	*Low* (using gaze or a button)	*Medium* (using gaze or a joystick)	*High* (using a joystick or controllers)	*Medium* (using gaze, a built-in pad or joystick)	*High* (using controllers or hand tracking)	*Medium* (using gaze, a built-in pad or joystick)
Software Availability	Oculus Store	Steam Store	Steam Store	Steam Store and Windows Mixed Reality Store	Oculus Store	Google Play or IOS Store	Google Play	PlayStation Store	Oculus Store	Oculus Store	Google Play and Lenovo ThinkReality

VR: virtual reality; PC: Personal Computer

Moreover, Montana et al. [24] critically reviewed 11 VR-based trainings for the enhancement of emotion regulation strategies and wellbeing in young and older adults. Included trainings covered different techniques, such as the Mindfulness-Based Stress Reduction protocol, the biofeedback and neurofeedback trainings as methods for the regulation of physiological arousal, and the promotion of outdoor/indoor activities for the enhancement of subjective wellbeing. Globally, the use of VR in this research field is promising since it allows individuals to learn emotion regulation strategies in the context of life-like virtual environments.

Finally, Lopez-Valverde et al. [25] critically reviewed 31 studies and provided additional evidence to the idea that VR can be used as an effective distraction method able reduce pain and anxiety in patients undergoing a variety of dental treatments.

An expanding area of research is the exploitation of VR for delivering cognitive assessment and trainings in neurological conditions, i.e., patients suffering from neurodegenerative diseases or post-stroke individuals. VR has a prominent place among other advanced technologies offering crucial advantages for implementing cognitive trainings [26–30]. Patients can perform cognitive exercises in controlled and secure environments, where it is possible to calibrate the difficulty/intensity of the tasks according to specific patients' needs. Virtual exercises mimic real-world tasks (i.e., ecological validity) and they offer greater chances for transferring learnt abilities to real life [31]. These environments offer also a multisensory stimulation (i.e., vision, touch, motor), with a fruitful rebound on brain plasticity [27]. Several systematic reviews and meta-analyses indicated the efficacy VR for cognitive interventions for individuals with cognitive impairments and Alzheimer's Disease [32,33], for alleviating motor and non-motor symptoms of Parkinson's Disease [34], or for improving spatial neglect (i.e., failure respond to contralateral stimuli) in post-stroke individuals [35].

In this perspective, in this Special Issue, Tuena et al. [36] and Montana et al. [37] focused their efforts in reviewing experimental studies about the use of VR as an instrument for implementing navigational assessment tasks and trainings. Tuena et al. [36] systematically reviewed 31 experimental studies about the so-called "virtual enactment effect", thus providing further support about the "embodied" potential of VR. Indeed, Brooks and colleagues [38] pioneered the idea that the active navigation in virtual environments by means of input tools could be considered as an analogous to the "enactment effect" thanks to the subsequent enhancement of memory performances by motor information. This systematic review shaded light on the key role of the sensorimotor systems for spatial and episodic memory assessment and rehabilitation by emphasizing the crucial role played by VR in future cognitive interventions. Montana and colleagues [37] critically reviewed 16 VR-based trainings for patients with spatial memory disorders (such as, patients with mild cognitive impairment, Alzheimer's disease, traumatic brain injury, multiple sclerosis, stroke, etc.). Although further studies are needed to strengthen the methodological quality of studies in this research area, promising results about the possibility of using VR to deliver training to improve navigation and orientation abilities in several disorders were discussed. In a similar vein, Bevilacqua et al. [39] focused their work on reviewing existing randomized controlled trials in the field of VR-based training for geriatric population, considering only non-immersive systems. The idea is that non-immersive systems have shown to be highly accepted by older people. They critically reviewed 11 trials, thus suggesting that the application of VR has globally a positive impact on the rehabilitation of the most predominant geriatric syndromes.

In the same research domain, Thapa et al. [40] demonstrated the efficacy of an immersive VR-based cognitive training in a sample of 68 individuals with mild cognitive impairment. The proposed VR-based training (three times/week, 100 min each session) included four types of VR game-based contents to improve different cognitive functions (i.e., attention, memory and processing speed). Results indicated that the experimental group exhibited a significant improvement in executive functions, in the gait speed and in the mobility after the training. Finally, Cabinio et al. [41] tested the potential of a novel smart aging serious game (SASG) in discriminating older adults suffering from amnestic mild cognitive impairment from cognitively healthy controls. Results showed similar discriminating abilities for SASG and gold standard tests, and a greater discrimination ability compared to non-specific neuropsychological tests.

As concern the use of VR as "assessment tool", Alcañiz Raya et al. [42] investigated the possibility of discriminating children with autism spectrum disorder (ASD) from typically developed children through body movements' data analysis in a real-simulated imitation task implemented in VR. Their results indicated the feasibility of applying machine learning methods and VR-based ecological tasks to identify body movements' biomarkers that could contribute to improving ASD diagnosis.

In the same vein, Pedroli et al. [43] tested 29 patients with obsessive-compulsive disorder (OCD) and 29 controls with traditional neuropsychological tests and a validated protocol implemented in VR (virtual multiple errands test—VMET) for the assessment of executive functions. They demonstrated the possibility of discriminating OCD patients from controls using scores from three neuropsychological tests and two indices from VMET, opening a novel scenario for future protocols based on VR-based assessment tool and computational techniques.

In the last 40 years, VR has offered innovative solutions also for assessing and treating body representation disturbances in eating and weight-disorders [4,44,45]. One of the most recent trends for treating body representation disturbances in patients suffering from anorexia nervosa (AN) is the exploitation of the so-called VR-based body ownership illusions [46–48]. Advances in technology permits the experimental induction of embodying an entire virtual body thanks to a multisensory stimulation experienced both on own real body and on the fake one in a synchronous way.

In this Special Issue, Porras Garcia et al. [49], Scarpina et al. [50], Provenzano et al. [51] and Matamala-Gomez et al. [52] induced in participants the feeling of being the owner of another fake virtual body and investigated the impact of such illusion in modulating body percept. Porras Garcia et al. [49] introduced some variations to the traditional illusion to further increase its illusory strength; they applied the synchronous multisensory stimulation on the entire participants' body, and they created a real-size virtual body, based on each participants' silhouette. They found that participants showed higher levels of body concerns and body anxiety after owning the larger-size body, than after owning the real-size one. The synchronous visuo-tactile group had higher scores in comparison to the asynchronous one, although the differences did not reach statistical significance. Scarpina et al. [50] employed the traditional virtual body ownership illusion in 15 participants with obesity and in a sample of normal-weight participants. Results indicated that participants with obesity as well as controls successfully experienced the illusion; both groups reported a decrease in the estimation of the abdomen's circumference (congruently with avatar size) after the synchronous condition. Globally, these studies encouraged further research exploiting the use of VR as an "embodied tool" for modulating body representations in clinical populations, specifically in terms of its potential therapeutic use [46].

In addition, Provenzano et al. [51] applied the illusion with some modifications: they individualized the avatar according to participants' bodies and the evaluated the effect of the embodiment strength using both explicit (i.e., the perceptual and emotional aspects of body image distortion) and implicit (i.e., body temperature) measures. They found that the embodiment was stronger after synchronous stimulation for both groups, but it did not reduce body image distortions in patients with AN. They found that the illusion succeeded in eliciting affective reactions: patients with AN experienced more negative emotions after embodying the fattest avatar.

VR-based bodily illusions are useful also for modulating the pain threshold in healthy subjects, with potential therapeutic implications for individuals with chronic pain. Matamala-Gomez et al. [52] aimed at deeper understanding the mechanisms of visual distortion on pain response in 27 healthy participants; in particular, they reproduced the telescoping effect in amputees (i.e., phantom limbs can be perceived as gradually retracting inside the stump). Results indicated that embodying a distorted virtual arm increased an autonomic response (i.e., skin conductance response) to a threatening event (i.e., virtual needle) with respect to embodying a normal control arm, but when participants embodied a reddened-distorted virtual arm, the skin conductance response was comparatively reduced in response to the threat. These findings provided further support to the use of VR for the modulation of pain responses by systematically changing the representation of the telescoped limb, with crucial implications for its use in integrated treatments to reduce chronic pain in clinical population.

Finally, a recent Cochrane review indicated that VR could play a role to provide schizophrenic patients with customized interventions able to increase their compliance by enhancing their cognitive skills [53]. Findings from studies carried out so far are promising, but there is an urgent need of high-quality studies.

In this domain, in this Special Issue, Drori et al. [54] presented and tested a novel VR paradigm to investigate the sense of reality (SoR), i.e., the ability to discriminate between true and false perceptions, that is a central criterion in the assessment of neurological and psychiatric health. They induced hallucination-like visual experiences and tested their effects using both objective and subjective measures of SoR. Results indicated a novel psychophysical link between the sensitivity to alterations of reality and prodromal psychotic symptoms.

In the same perspective, Stern et al. [55] focused their attention on one aspect of the bodily self, namely the sense of agency (i.e., the feeling of controlling our body's actions). Starting from literature suggesting that the sense of agency is impaired in psychosis, with stress influencing this relationship, they found that an increased alteration of the virtual hand was significantly associated with a decrease in subjective ratings of sense of agency and body ownership. Moreover, they found that sense of agency was not related to the trait anxiety neither to induced stress.

In conclusion, while VR applications such as those discussed in the articles above are addressing very specific ways of supporting mental health, we believe that a new era in computing, one that aims directly at improving people's psychological mental health will only be possible when we will able to exploit all the potential of this exciting technology. More, the design goal of achieving VR experiences for assessment and treatment in mental health requires an interdisciplinary approach, integrating knowledge and ideas from disciplines such as computer graphic, neuroscience, social and cognitive psychology, multi-sensory perception, cognition, multimedia development, and healthcare. In order to build VR tools which can effectively improve our approach to mental health, it will be necessary to incorporate and integrate ongoing insights from these fields into next-generation research exploiting all the dimensions of VR. In fact, VR is at the same time a simulative technology, a cognitive technology, and an embodied technology [3]. These features will make VR the perfect tool for experiential assessment and learning with great clinical potential. We hope that this new breed of artifacts will build on the work described in this special issue.

Author Contributions: Conceptualization, writing—review and editing, G.R. and S.S. All authors have read and agreed to the published version of the manuscript.

Funding: This research received no external funding.

Conflicts of Interest: The authors declare no conflict of interest.

References

1. Riva, G. Virtual reality in clinical psychology. *Ref. Modul. Neurosci. Biobehav. Psychol.* **2020**. [CrossRef]
2. Parsons, T.; Gaggioli, A.; Riva, G. Virtual reality for research in social neuroscience. *Brain Sci.* **2017**, *7*, 42. [CrossRef] [PubMed]
3. Riva, G.; Wiederhold, B.K.; Mantovani, F. Neuroscience of virtual reality: From virtual exposure to embodied medicine. *Cyberpsychol. Behav. Soc. Netw.* **2019**, *22*, 82–96. [CrossRef]
4. Riva, G.; Baños, R.M.; Botella, C.; Mantovani, F.; Gaggioli, A. Transforming experience: The potential of augmented reality and virtual reality for enhancing personal and clinical change. *Front. Psychiatry* **2016**, *7*, 164. [CrossRef] [PubMed]
5. Schubring, D.; Kraus, M.; Stolz, C.; Weiler, N.; Keim, D.A.; Schupp, H. Virtual reality potentiates Emotion and task effects of alpha/beta brain oscillations. *Brain Sci.* **2020**, *10*, 537. [CrossRef] [PubMed]
6. Muratore, M.; Tuena, C.; Pedroli, E.; Cipresso, P.; Riva, G. Virtual reality as a possible tool for the assessment of self-awareness. *Front. Behav. Neurosci.* **2019**, *13*, 62. [CrossRef]

7. Riva, G. Virtual reality. In *The Palgrave Encyclopedia of the Possible*; Springer International Publishing: Cham, Switzerland, 2020; pp. 1–10.
8. Valmaggia, L. The use of virtual reality in psychosis research and treatment. *World Psychiatry* **2017**, *16*, 246–247. [CrossRef]
9. Jerdan, S.W.; Grindle, M.; van Woerden, H.C.; Kamel Boulos, M.N. Head-mounted virtual reality and mental health: Critical review of current research. *JMIR Serious Games* **2018**, *6*, e14. [CrossRef]
10. Lindner, P.; Miloff, A.; Hamilton, W.; Reuterskiöld, L.; Andersson, G.; Powers, M.B.; Carlbring, P. Creating state of the art, next-generation Virtual Reality exposure therapies for anxiety disorders using consumer hardware platforms: Design considerations and future directions. *Cogn. Behav. Ther.* **2017**, *46*, 404–420. [CrossRef]
11. Zanier, E.R.; Zoerle, T.; Di Lernia, D.; Riva, G. Virtual reality for traumatic brain injury. *Front. Neurol.* **2018**, *9*, 345. [CrossRef]
12. Realdon, O.; Serino, S.; Savazzi, F.; Rossetto, F.; Cipresso, P.; Parsons, T.D.; Cappellini, G.; Mantovani, F.; Mendozzi, L.; Nemni, R.; et al. An ecological measure to screen executive functioning in MS: The picture interpretation test (PIT) 360°. *Sci. Rep.* **2019**, *9*, 5690. [CrossRef] [PubMed]
13. Carl, E.; Stein, A.T.; Levihn-Coon, A.; Pogue, J.R.; Rothbaum, B.; Emmelkamp, P.; Asmundson, G.J.; Carlbring, P.; Powers, M.B. Virtual reality exposure therapy for anxiety and related disorders: A meta-analysis of randomized controlled trials. *J. Anxiety Disord.* **2019**, *61*, 27–36. [CrossRef]
14. Meyerbröker, K.; Emmelkamp, P.M. Virtual reality exposure therapy in anxiety disorders: A systematic review of process-and-outcome studies. *Depress. Anxiety* **2010**, *27*, 933–944. [CrossRef] [PubMed]
15. Opriş, D.; Pintea, S.; García-Palacios, A.; Botella, C.; Szamosközi, Ş.; David, D. Virtual reality exposure therapy in anxiety disorders: A quantitative meta-analysis. *Depress. Anxiety* **2012**, *29*, 85–93. [CrossRef] [PubMed]
16. Powers, M.B.; Emmelkamp, P.M. Virtual reality exposure therapy for anxiety disorders: A meta-analysis. *J. Anxiety Disord.* **2008**, *22*, 561–569. [CrossRef]
17. Cavalera, C.; Pepe, A.; Zurloni, V.; Diana, B.; Realdon, O. A short version of the state shame and guilt scale (SSGS-8). *TPM Test. Psychom. Methodol. Appl. Psychol.* **2017**, *24*, 99–106.
18. Serino, S.; Triberti, S.; Villani, D.; Cipresso, P.; Gaggioli, A.; Riva, G. Toward a validation of cyber-interventions for stress disorders based on stress inoculation training: A systematic review. *Virtual Real.* **2014**, *18*, 73–87. [CrossRef]
19. Botella, C.; Fernández-Álvarez, J.; Guillén, V.; García-Palacios, A.; Baños, R. Recent progress in virtual reality exposure therapy for phobias: A systematic review. *Curr. Psychiatry Rep.* **2017**, *19*, 42. [CrossRef] [PubMed]
20. Botella, C.; Serrano, B.; Baños, R.M.; Garcia-Palacios, A. Virtual reality exposure-based therapy for the treatment of post-traumatic stress disorder: A review of its efficacy, the adequacy of the treatment protocol, and its acceptability. *Neuropsychiatr. Dis. Treat.* **2015**, *11*, 2533. [CrossRef]
21. Gonçalves, R.; Pedrozo, A.L.; Coutinho, E.S.F.; Figueira, I.; Ventura, P. Efficacy of virtual reality exposure therapy in the treatment of PTSD: A systematic review. *PLoS ONE* **2012**, *7*, e48469. [CrossRef]
22. Guitard, T.; Bouchard, S.; Bélanger, C.; Berthiaume, M. Exposure to a standardized catastrophic scenario in virtual reality or a personalized scenario in imagination for generalized anxiety disorder. *J. Clin. Med.* **2019**, *8*, 309. [CrossRef] [PubMed]
23. Peñate, W.; Rivero, F.; Viña, C.; Herrero, M.; Betancort, M.; De la Fuente, J.; Álvarez-Pérez, Y.; Fumero, A. The Equivalence between virtual and real feared stimuli in a phobic adult sample: A neuroimaging study. *J. Clin. Med.* **2019**, *8*, 2139. [CrossRef] [PubMed]
24. Montana, J.I.; Matamala-Gomez, M.; Maisto, M.; Mavrodiev, P.A.; Cavalera, C.M.; Diana, B.; Mantovani, F.; Realdon, O. The benefits of emotion regulation interventions in virtual Reality for the improvement of wellbeing in adults and older adults: A systematic review. *J. Clin. Med.* **2020**, *9*, 500. [CrossRef]
25. López-Valverde, N.; Muriel Fernández, J.; López-Valverde, A.; Valero Juan, L.F.; Ramírez, J.M.; Flores Fraile, J.; Herrero Payo, J.; Blanco Antona, L.A.; Macedo de Sousa, B.; Bravo, M. Use of virtual reality for the Management of anxiety and pain in dental treatments: Systematic review and meta-analysis. *J. Clin. Med.* **2020**, *9*, 3086. [CrossRef]
26. Bohil, C.J.; Alicea, B.; Biocca, F.A. Virtual reality in neuroscience research and therapy. *Nat. Rev. Neurosci.* **2011**, *12*, 752–762. [CrossRef]
27. Perez-Marcos, D.; Bieler-Aeschlimann, M.; Serino, A. Virtual reality as a vehicle to empower motor-cognitive neurorehabilitation. *Front. Psychol.* **2018**, *9*, 2120. [CrossRef]

28. Repetto, C.; Serino, S.; Macedonia, M.; Riva, G. Virtual reality as an embodied tool to enhance episodic memory in elderly. *Front. Psychol.* **2016**, *7*, 1839. [CrossRef]
29. Riva, G.; Mantovani, F.; Gaggioli, A. Presence and rehabilitation: Toward second-generation virtual reality applications in neuropsychology. *J. Neuroeng. Rehabil.* **2004**, *1*, 9. [CrossRef]
30. Rizzo, A.S.; Kim, G.J. A SWOT analysis of the field of virtual reality rehabilitation and therapy. *Presence Teleoper. Virtual Environ.* **2005**, *14*, 119–146. [CrossRef]
31. Parsons, T.D.; Carlew, A.R.; Magtoto, J.; Stonecipher, K. The potential of function-led virtual environments for ecologically valid measures of executive function in experimental and clinical neuropsychology. *Neuropsychol. Rehabil.* **2017**, *27*, 777–807. [CrossRef] [PubMed]
32. Coyle, H.; Traynor, V.; Solowij, N. Computerized and virtual reality cognitive training for individuals at high risk of cognitive decline: Systematic review of the literature. *Am. J. Geriatr. Psychiatry* **2015**, *23*, 335–359. [CrossRef]
33. García-Betances, R.I.; Arredondo Waldmeyer, M.T.; Fico, G.; Cabrera-Umpiérrez, M.F. A succinct overview of virtual reality technology use in Alzheimer's disease. *Front. Aging Neurosci.* **2015**, *7*, 80.
34. Clay, F.; Howett, D.; FitzGerald, J.; Fletcher, P.; Chan, D.; Price, A. Use of immersive virtual reality in the assessment and treatment of Alzheimer's disease: A systematic review. *J. Alzheimer's Dis.* **2020**, *75*, 1–21.
35. Pedroli, E.; Serino, S.; Cipresso, P.; Pallavicini, F.; Riva, G. Assessment and rehabilitation of neglect using virtual reality: A systematic review. *Front. Behav. Neurosci.* **2015**, *9*, 226. [CrossRef]
36. Tuena, C.; Serino, S.; Dutriaux, L.; Riva, G.; Piolino, P. Virtual enactment effect on memory in young and aged populations: A systematic review. *J. Clin. Med.* **2019**, *8*, 620. [CrossRef]
37. Montana, J.I.; Tuena, C.; Serino, S.; Cipresso, P.; Riva, G. Neurorehabilitation of spatial memory using virtual environments: A systematic review. *J. Clin. Med.* **2019**, *8*, 1516. [CrossRef]
38. Brooks, B.M. The specificity of memory enhancement during interaction with a virtual environment. *Memory* **1999**, *7*, 65–78. [CrossRef]
39. Bevilacqua, R.; Maranesi, E.; Riccardi, G.R.; Di Donna, V.; Pelliccioni, P.; Luzi, R.; Lattanzio, F.; Pelliccioni, G. Non-immersive virtual reality for rehabilitation of the older people: A systematic review into efficacy and effectiveness. *J. Clin. Med.* **2019**, *8*, 1882. [CrossRef] [PubMed]
40. Thapa, N.; Park, H.J.; Yang, J.-G.; Son, H.; Jang, M.; Lee, J.; Kang, S.W.; Park, K.W.; Park, H. The effect of a virtual reality-based intervention program on cognition in older adults with mild cognitive impairment: A randomized control trial. *J. Clin. Med.* **2020**, *9*, 1283. [CrossRef]
41. Cabinio, M.; Rossetto, F.; Isernia, S.; Saibene, F.L.; Di Cesare, M.; Borgnis, F.; Pazzi, S.; Migliazza, T.; Alberoni, M.; Blasi, V. The use of a virtual reality platform for the assessment of the memory decline and the hippocampal neural injury in subjects with mild cognitive impairment: The validity of smart aging serious game (SASG). *J. Clin. Med.* **2020**, *9*, 1355. [CrossRef]
42. Alcañiz Raya, M.; Marín-Morales, J.; Minissi, M.E.; Teruel Garcia, G.; Abad, L.; Chicchi Giglioli, I.A. Machine learning and virtual reality on body movements' behaviors to classify children with autism spectrum disorder. *J. Clin. Med.* **2020**, *9*, 1260. [CrossRef] [PubMed]
43. Pedroli, E.; La Paglia, F.; Cipresso, P.; La Cascia, C.; Riva, G.; La Barbera, D. A computational approach for the assessment of executive functions in patients with obsessive-compulsive disorder. *J. Clin. Med.* **2019**, *8*, 1975. [CrossRef] [PubMed]
44. Riva, G.; Gaudio, S.; Serino, S.; Dakanalis, A.; Ferrer-García, M.; Gutiérrez-Maldonado, J. Virtual reality for the treatment of body image disturbances in eating and weight disorders. In *Body Image, Eating, and Weight*; Springer: Berlin/Heidelberg, Germany, 2018; pp. 333–351.
45. Riva, G.; Gutiérrez-Maldonado, J.; Dakanalis, A.; Ferrer-García, M. Virtual reality in the assessment and treatment of weight-related disorders. In *Virtual Reality for Psychological and Neurocognitive Interventions*; Rizzo, A.S., Bouchard, S., Eds.; Springer: New York, NY, USA, 2019; pp. 163–193.
46. Serino, S.; Dakanalis, A. Bodily illusions and weight-related disorders: Clinical insights from experimental research. *Ann. Phys. Rehabil. Med.* **2017**, *60*, 217–219. [CrossRef] [PubMed]
47. Serino, S.; Pedroli, E.; Keizer, A.; Triberti, S.; Dakanalis, A.; Pallavicini, F.; Chirico, A.; Riva, G. Virtual reality body swapping: A tool for modifying the allocentric memory of the body. *Cyberpsychol. Behav. Soc. Netw.* **2016**, *19*, 127–133. [CrossRef]
48. Keizer, A.; van Elburg, A.; Helms, R.; Dijkerman, H.C. A virtual reality full body illusion improves body image disturbance in anorexia nervosa. *PLoS ONE* **2016**, *11*, e0163921. [CrossRef]

49. Porras Garcia, B.; Ferrer Garcia, M.; Olszewska, A.; Yilmaz, L.; González Ibañez, C.; Gracia Blanes, M.; Gültekin, G.; Serrano Troncoso, E.; Gutiérrez Maldonado, J. Is this my own body? Changing the perceptual and affective body image experience among college students using a new virtual reality embodiment-based technique. *J. Clin. Med.* **2019**, *8*, 925. [CrossRef]
50. Scarpina, F.; Serino, S.; Keizer, A.; Chirico, A.; Scacchi, M.; Castelnuovo, G.; Mauro, A.; Riva, G. The effect of a virtual-reality full-body illusion on body representation in obesity. *J. Clin. Med.* **2019**, *8*, 1330. [CrossRef]
51. Provenzano, L.; Porciello, G.; Ciccarone, S.; Lenggenhager, B.; Tieri, G.; Marucci, M.; Dazzi, F.; Loriedo, C.; Bufalari, I. Characterizing body image distortion and bodily self-plasticity in anorexia nervosa via visuo-tactile stimulation in virtual reality. *J. Clin. Med.* **2020**, *9*, 98. [CrossRef]
52. Matamala-Gomez, M.; Nierula, B.; Donegan, T.; Slater, M.; Sanchez-Vives, M.V. Manipulating the perceived shape and color of a virtual limb can modulate pain responses. *J. Clin. Med.* **2020**, *9*, 291. [CrossRef] [PubMed]
53. Välimäki, M.; Hätönen, H.M.; Lahti, M.E.; Kurki, M.; Hottinen, A.; Metsäranta, K.; Riihimäki, T.; Adams, C.E. Virtual reality for treatment compliance for people with serious mental illness. *Cochrane Database Syst. Rev.* **2014**, *10*. [CrossRef]
54. Drori, G.; Bar-Tal, P.; Stern, Y.; Zvilichovsky, Y.; Salomon, R. UnReal? Investigating the sense of reality and psychotic symptoms with virtual reality. *J. Clin. Med.* **2020**, *9*, 1627. [CrossRef] [PubMed]
55. Stern, Y.; Koren, D.; Moebus, R.; Panishev, G.; Salomon, R. Assessing the relationship between sense of agency, the bodily-self and stress: Four virtual-reality experiments in healthy individuals. *J. Clin. Med.* **2020**, *9*, 2931. [CrossRef] [PubMed]

Publisher's Note: MDPI stays neutral with regard to jurisdictional claims in published maps and institutional affiliations.

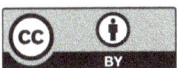

© 2020 by the authors. Licensee MDPI, Basel, Switzerland. This article is an open access article distributed under the terms and conditions of the Creative Commons Attribution (CC BY) license (http://creativecommons.org/licenses/by/4.0/).

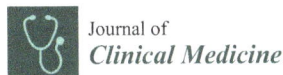

Article

The Effect of a Virtual-Reality Full-Body Illusion on Body Representation in Obesity

Federica Scarpina [1,2,*,†], Silvia Serino [3,*,†], Anouk Keizer [4], Alice Chirico [5], Massimo Scacchi [6,7], Gianluca Castelnuovo [2,5], Alessandro Mauro [1,8] and Giuseppe Riva [3,5]

1. Istituto Auxologico Italiano, IRCCS, U.O. di Neurologia e Neuroriabilitazione, Ospedale S. Giuseppe, 28824 Piancavallo, Italy
2. Istituto Auxologico Italiano, IRCCS, Laboratorio di Psicologia, Ospedale S. Giuseppe, 28824 Piancavallo, Italy
3. Istituto Auxologico Italiano, IRCCS, Laboratorio Sperimentale di Ricerche Tecnologiche Applicate alla Psicologia, 20149 Milano, Italy
4. Experimental Psychology/Helmholtz Institute, Faculty of Social and Behavioural Sciences, Utrecht University, 3584 Utrecht, The Netherlands
5. Psychology Department, Università Cattolica del Sacro Cuore, 20123 Milan, Italy
6. Istituto Auxologico Italiano, IRCCS, U.O. di Medicina Generale, Ospedale S. Giuseppe, 28824 Piancavallo, Italy
7. Department of Clinical Sciences and Community Health, University of Milan, 20122 Milan, Italy
8. "Rita Levi Montalcini" Department of Neuroscience, University of Turin, 10124 Turin, Italy
* Correspondence: federica.scarpina@gmail.com (S.F.); s.serino@auxologico.it (S.S.)
† These authors equally contributed to this work.

Received: 19 July 2019; Accepted: 22 August 2019; Published: 28 August 2019

Abstract: Background. The effective illusory ownership over an artificial body in modulating body representations in healthy and eating disorders population has been repeatedly reported in recent literature. In this study, we extended this research in the field of obesity: specifically, we investigated whether ownership over a virtual body with a skinny abdomen might be successfully experienced by participants affected by obesity. **Methods.** Fifteen participants with obesity and fifteen healthy-weight participants took part at this study in which the VR-Full-Body Illusion was adopted. The strength of illusion was investigated through the traditional Embodiment Questionnaire, while changes in bodily experience were measured through a body size estimation task. **Results.** Participants with obesity as well as healthy-weight participants reported to experience the illusion. About the body size estimation task, both groups reported changes only in the estimation of the abdomen's circumference after the experimental condition, in absence of any another difference. **Discussion.** Participants with obesity reported to experience the illusion over a skinny avatar, but the modulation of the bodily experience seems controversial. Future lines of research exploiting this technique for modulating body representations in obesity, specifically in terms of potential therapeutic use, were discussed.

Keywords: body representation; obesity; health; virtual reality; full body illusion

1. Introduction

The efficacy of the illusory ownership over an artificial body (i.e., body-ownership illusion) as a method for modulating body representations in both healthy such as [1–6] and clinical population (such as individuals suffering of eating disorders [7,8], Complex Regional Pain Syndrome [9] and Disturbed Body Integrity [10,11] has been repeatedly reported in recent literature. Indeed, since from the traditional Rubber Hand Illusion [12], it was speculated if bodily illusions might be adopted in therapeutic settings [13–17] for enhancing positive rehabilitative outcomes. More recently, the research about body ownership illusions moves from the embodiment of a single body part (such as the hand [12] or the foot [10], towards the entire body. For example, in the Virtual Reality-Full Body Illusion (VR-FBI) [2–5] participants experience the illusion of ownership towards a full-body avatar. Traditionally, the avatar is showed with different physical dimensions (i.e., thinner or larger) respect to the participants. Interestingly, when participants experience successfully the illusion, they generally perceive themselves as fatter or thinner than they really are, according to the characteristics of embodied virtual body [2–5]. An example was offered by Normand and colleagues (2011) [18], who induced embodiment over a virtual body with a larger abdomen in a sample of males; immediately after this experience, participants perceived their own body as larger than the real physical dimensions, congruently with the embodied avatars' characteristics. The illusion seemed to work also in the opposite direction: female participants who embodied avatars with skinny bodies tended to perceive their own bodies as slimmer [2–5].

As concerns eating disorders, there are in literature some interesting but preliminary studies investigating the use of body-ownership illusions as a method for exploring the boundaries of bodily self in affected individuals. For example, Eshkevari and colleagues [19] found an increased malleability of the bodily experience for individuals with eating disorders, who rated to experience the Rubber Hand Illusion higher than the healthy controls. Keizer and colleagues [7] applied the VR-FBI in a sample of individuals affected by Anorexia Nervosa, revealing that participants who experience ownership over a different virtual body reported a significant decrease in their body-size distortions too. In the 2016, our group presented a single-case study about a female individual affected by severe obesity, who experienced high level of body dissatisfaction and showed consistent distortions in the estimation of her own body-size parts [20]. We reported that both components (body dissatisfaction and body-size distortions) improved after experiencing the VR-FBI. In our knowledge, this single case study is still the only unique attempt to exploit this illusion in the context of obesity; thus, if body-ownership illusion could successfully modulate body representation in individuals affected by obesity is still an open question.

In the current study, we used a VR-FBI [1,2,20] as a technique for inducing illusory ownership over a virtual body with a skinny abdomen in a sample of individuals affected by obesity, compared to a group of healthy-weight individuals. Thus, in this study, participants saw the slim abdomen of the avatar through VR googles. When the experimenter stroked participants on their abdomen, delivering a tactile stimulation, they saw this stroking on the avatar's abdomen (i.e., the visual input). In line with previous studies [1,2,20], two conditions were administered for all participants: the experimental condition, in which the touch and the vision of the touch were *synchronized*; the temporal coherence between the sensory input onset generally elicits the illusory ownership over the artificial body; and the control condition, in which the two perceived stimuli are *asynchronized*, since there was a temporal delay between the visual and tactile input onset. To measure the potential changes in the perceptual component of body parts representations, we adopted the Body Part Size Estimation Task [1,20]. Participants were asked to estimate their height, and the width and the circumference of three different body parts (shoulders, abdomen, and hips), at three time points: before the VR-FBI, representing the baseline, and after both the two (synchronous and asynchronous) conditions of visuo-tactile stimulation. Moreover, in line with the traditional literature [1–12,20,21], we adopted the Embodiment Questionnaire [1]: this questionnaire, administered after both stimulation conditions, allows to measure the strength of illusion in terms of: (1) *Ownership* over the virtual body; (2) *Self-location*, i.e., being in the same location of the virtual body; and (3) *Sense of agency* over the virtual body.

Considering the previous results about healthy individuals [1–5,18], we might expect that all participants experienced successfully the VR-FBI after the synchronous visuo-tactile stimulation (i.e., the experimental condition), but not after the asynchronous (i.e., control) condition. Moreover, about the Body Part Size Estimation Task [1,20], there would be a decrease in body size estimations compared to the baseline (i.e., before the VR-FBI took place); indeed, when the illusion emerged, healthy-weight individuals should perceive themselves slimmer than real physical dimensions, accordingly with the avatar's dimension. Similarly, if the illusion might be efficiently induced also for individuals affected by obesity, we might expect to find a difference in the estimation of their body parts after the synchronous, but not the asynchronous condition.

2. Methods

The study was conducted in compliance with the Helsinki's Declaration (of 1975, as revised in 2008), was approved by the Ethics Review Board of the Università Cattolica del Sacro Cuore (Catholic University of the Sacred Heart, Milan, Italy). Subjects volunteered to participate; they received verbal explanation of the procedures and gave informed written consent, were free to withdraw at will and were naïve to the rationale of the experiment.

Participants. All participants were female and right-handed. None of them had previously experience with bodily illusions and were naïve to the rationale of this experiment. Fifteen individuals affected by obesity and fifteen female healthy-weight individuals took part in the study (Table 1). Participants affected by obesity were individuals at the first week of a diagnostic hospitalization, before a rehabilitative treatment for losing weight. We adopted the same inclusion criteria of our previous studies [22–24]. All subjects were nonsmokers and free from gastrointestinal, cardiovascular, psychiatric, or metabolic disorders or any concurrent medical condition not related to obesity, according to routinely clinical assessment. In addition, weight and height were measured to the nearest 0.1 kg and 0.1 cm, respectively, using standard methods. BMI was expressed as body mass (kg)/ height (m^2). Obesity was defined for any BMI over 30 kg/m^2. Healthy-weight participants were recruited through convenience and snowball sampling—In particular, students from the Catholic University of Milan were invited during lessons and asked to refer friends. No economical compensation was given. The same above-mentioned inclusion criteria were adopted, except for the BMI that was between 18.5 and 25 kg/m^2.

VR-FBI. In this experiment we used the same protocol of our previous studies [1–20]. During the entire procedure, participants were kindly asked to avoid any movements; this set-up did not track participants' movement and the avatar was not responsive. All participants were invited to stand upright and wear the head-mounted display (Oculus Rift DK2) to experience the VR-FBI. The Oculus Rift DK2D (compatible with the developed application) was connected to a portable computer (HP TRUE VISION with CPU Intel® Core™i7). The virtual room was developed with the software Unity3D (www.unity3d.com), while the avatar was modelled using the software MakeHuman (http://www.makehuman.org/). To experience the illusion, all participants were exposed to two different conditions. During the *synchronous* condition (i.e., the experimental condition), the experimenter provided a visuo-tactile stimulation on participants' abdomen with a brush attached to the motion-tracking device (i.e., Razer Hydra) for 90 s, while a synchronous stimulation was delivered on virtual abdomen (i.e., the virtual touch provided on the abdomen of the virtual body). In the *asynchronous* condition (i.e., the control condition) the experimenter provided the same visuo-tactile stimulation on participants' abdomen for 90 s, but there was a delay in the corresponding virtual touch (i.e., absence of synchronization between tactile and visual stimulation). In particular, in the asynchronous condition the touch on participants' abdomen was actually recorded by pressing a button on the Razer Hydra at the beginning of the movement. This procedure stopped the image seen by the participants as soon as the touch ended, and then it was replayed in VR when the experimenter finished each touch. Also, this stimulation lasted for 90 s.

All participants were exposed to these two conditions in a counterbalanced order in a within subject-design. They were requested to wear the head-mounted display (i.e., Oculus) to visualize in a first-person perspective the virtual body of a female avatar by looking down at the abdomen of virtual body (i.e., the stimulated body part). They saw the body of a young woman (approximately 25 years old) with a thin abdomen (i.e., with a different shape/size in comparison to the actual body of participants) standing upright in a stimulus-free room was used to induce the full body illusion (Figure 1).

The waist circumference of the avatar was 73.95 cm: the waist circumference of the avatar was significantly smaller respect to the mean waist circumference of both the healthy-weight participants [t(14) = 23.021; $p < 0.001$; mean = 100.18; SD = 4.41)] and participants affected by obesity [t(14) = 18.094; $p < 0.001$; mean = 140.18; SD = 14.24)]. Thus, the avatar was perceptively skinner respect to both groups of participants.

Table 1. Means and standard deviation (in brackets) were reported about demographical and clinical information, percentage of misestimation at the baseline for both groups. In bold, when p value was <0.05. Age and Education are reported in years; body parts physical dimensions were reported in cm.

	Participants with Obesity	Healthy Weight Participant	t	p Value	d
Age	32 (6)	29 (8)	0.97	0.33	0.4
Education	14 (3)	16 (1)	1.97	0.058	0.35
BMI	45 (6.69)	22 (1.66).	12.63	**<0.001**	4.71
Body parts physical dimensions					
Height	161.91 (8.15)	164.52 (9.31)	0.81	0.42	0.29
Width					
Shoulders	48.15 (7.8)	39.7 (1.82)	4.079	**<0.001**	1.49
Abdomen	42.57 (7.12)	29.7 (3.81)	6.16	**<0.001**	2.25
Hips	48.44 (6.12)	35.64 (2.6)	7.44	**<0.001**	2.72
Circumference					
Shoulders	121.15 (12.87)	88.7 (6.86)	8.61	**<0.001**	3.14
Abdomen	130.24 (14.73)	83.27 (9.8)	10.27	**<0.001**	3.75
Hips	140.46 (14.23)	100.17 (4.41)	10.46	**<0.001**	3.82
Body Parts Size Estimation Task: percentage of misestimation—Baseline					
Height	3.2 (3.73)	0.74 (4.31)	1.86	0.76	0.61
Width					
Shoulders	−10.8 (21.86)	−2.19 (14.54)	1.71	0.1	0.46
Abdomen	−1.6 (20.92)	0.13 (23.12)	0.22	0.82	0.07
Hips	6.8 (23.66)	10.37 (22.24)	0.62	0.5	0.15
Circumference					
Shoulders	16.2 (27.6)	39.45 (18.94)	2.69	**0.012**	0.98
Abdomen	6.5 (30.61)	24.43 (15.03)	3.96	**<0.001**	0.74
Hips	7.5 (22.07)	26.08 (15.84)	2.64	**0.013**	0.96

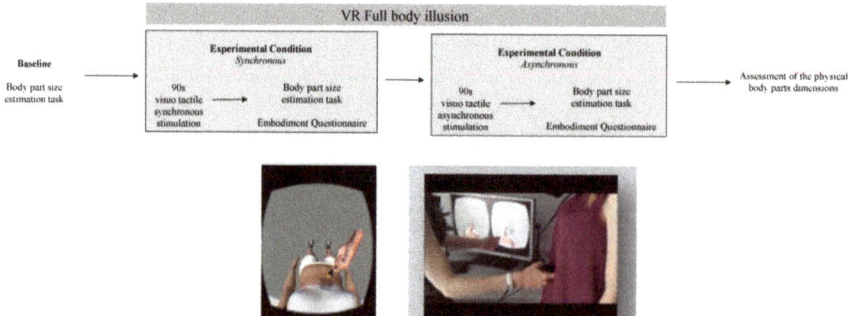

Figure 1. Graphical representation of the VR experimental time-line (upper part) and set-up (below up).

Embodiment Questionnaire. After both the synchronous visuo-tactile stimulation (experimental condition) and the asynchronous visuo-tactile stimulation (control condition), participants were required to fill the Embodiment Questionnaire [1], that it is routinely adopted to assess how participants subjectively experienced the illusion. It consisted of 20 items. Participants rated each statement on a 7-point Likert scale (range from 1 to 7), with higher scores indicating a stronger illusion. The questionnaire allows us to investigate the strength of illusion in terms of: (1) *ownership*, i.e., over the virtual body; (2) *self-location*, i.e., being in the same location of the virtual body; and (3) *sense of agency* over the virtual body. The three components were obtained by calculating the mean scores from the corresponding items.

Body Part Size Estimation Task. Before the illusion (i.e., the baseline) and after both the synchronous visuo-tactile stimulation (experimental condition) and the asynchronous visuo-tactile stimulation (control condition), participants were asked to estimate their own body parts, according to the procedure explained in our previous work [1]. Participants were asked to stand in front of a wall and to estimate the horizontal width of their own shoulders, abdomen, and hips by placing adhesive stickers: the stickers should represent the estimated distance between the left and the right side of the target body part. They were explicitly asked to not look at their body to avoid that they used it as a "reference" for making the estimates. Furthermore, they were asked to estimate the circumference of the above-mentioned three parts of their body by placing a piece of rope in a circle/oval on the floor. Moreover, participants estimated their height using an adhesive marker they placed on the wall. Also, in this case, they were explicitly asked to not use their own body as a reference to estimate their height. At the end of the entire experiment, the experimenter measured the actual width and circumference of the targeted body parts. The order of body parts (height, shoulders, abdomen, hips) and type of estimation (width, circumference) was counterbalanced over participants. For each body part and type of estimation, we calculated the percentage of misestimation according to the formula proposed by Keizer and colleagues [7]:

$$\textit{percentage of misestimation} = [(\textit{estimated size} - \textit{actual size})/\textit{actual size}] \times 100$$

According to the formula, a negative result suggested an underestimation, while a positive result an overestimation.

Data Analyses. Differences in demographical and clinical aspects were examined through an Independent samples t-test. For the embodiment questionnaire a Repeated Measure ANOVA with the within factors of *Condition* (i.e., synchronous vs. asynchronous) and of *Subscale* (i.e., ownership, location and agency) and the between factor of *Group* (participants with obesity vs. healthy weight participants) was conducted.

For the Body Part Size Estimation Task, we first explored any possible difference between the two groups in the estimation of the body parts at the baseline through an independent sample *t*-test. Successively, for each body part, a Repeated Measure ANOVA was run with the within factor of *Condition* (i.e., baseline, synchronous asynchronous) and the between factor of *Group* (participants with obesity vs. healthy weight participants), to verify the effect of VR_FBI on the body estimation. A significant main effect of *Condition*, and specifically between the baseline and the synchronous condition, but not between baseline and asynchronous, would suggest the effect of VR-FBI on the body size estimation; in case of significant interaction *Group*Condition*, the effect of *Condition* would emerge differently between individuals affected by obesity and healthy-weight individuals. In this case, for the two groups independently we performed post-hoc two independent sample t-tests: in the first one, the error in the synchronous condition was compared to the baseline; in the second, the error in the asynchronous condition. A difference was considered significant if the *p* value was below the Bonferroni's corrected threshold of 0.025 (0.05/2).

3. Results

Demographical and clinical aspects. Obese and healthy weight participants did not differ in *Age* and *Education level*, as showed in Table 1. As expected, participants affected by obesity had a significantly higher *BMI* than healthy weight participants. Moreover, for all considered body parts, except for height, individuals affected by obesity had higher physical dimensions than controls.

Embodiment Questionnaire. No main effect of *Group* (participants with obesity M = 3.58; SD = 1.87; healthy-weigh participants M = 3.82; SD = 1.39) emerged [$F(1,28) = 0.25$; $p = 0.62$; $\eta\rho^2 = 0.009$). The main effect of *Subscale* (ownership M = 3.56; SD = 1.48; location M = 4.04; SD = 1.49; agency M = 3.49; SD = 1.85) [$F(2, 56) = 3.13$; $p = 0.051$; $\eta\rho^2 = 0.1$) was marginally significant, but not the main effect of *Condition* (synchronous M = 3.86; SD = 1.53; asynchronous M = 3.54; SD = 1.71) [$F(1, 28) = 1.71$; $p = 0.2$; $\eta\rho^2 = 0.05$). Interestingly, an interaction *Condition*Subscale* [$F(2, 56) = 3.8$; $p = 0.028$; $\eta\rho^2 = 0.12$) emerged. Thus, we performed three paired sample t-tests in which for each subscale (ownership, location and agency) we compared the scores at the two *Conditions* (synchronous vs. asynchronous). A significant difference (Bonferroni corrected p-value 0.05/3 = 0.016) emerged for the *location* subscale [$t(29) = 2.69$; $p = 0.012$], but not for the *ownership* subscale [$t(29) = 1.32$; $p = 0.19$] or for the *agency* subscale [$t(29) = 0.41$; $p = 0.68$] (Figure 2).

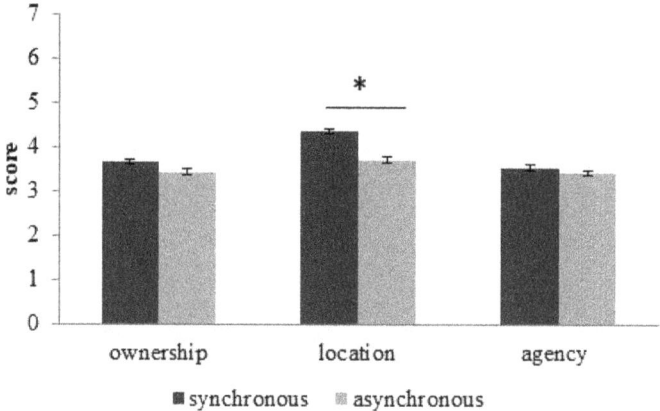

Figure 2. About the Embodiment questionnaire, means of the score and standard error (bars) were showed for each subscale (ownership, location and agency) in the synchronous (dark grey) and asynchronous (light grey) conditions. * indicates a significant difference according to the Bonferroni-corrected *p* value of 0.016.

The interactions *Condition*Group* [$F(1,28) = 0.26$; $p = 0.61$; $\eta\rho^2 = 0.009$) and *Subscale*Group* [$F(2, 56) = 0.14$; $p = 0.86$; $\eta\rho^2 = 0.005$) were not significant. Finally the second level-interaction *Group*Condition*Subscale* was not significant [$F(2,56) = 0.52$; $p = 0.59$; $\eta\rho^2 = 0.018$]. The absence of any difference between groups suggested that both participants with obesity and healthy-weight participants reported similar scores in the Embodiment Questionnaire after the induction of the VR-FBI, but it should be noticed that it is true independently from the condition (experimental/synchronous vs. control/asynchronous). However, all participants reported a stronger illusion in the experimental/synchronous condition with respect to the control/asynchronous condition in terms of self-location: in other words, when in the experimental condition, participants reported a stronger feeling to be in the same spatial location of the avatar with respect to the control condition.

Body Parts Size Estimation Task. As reported in the Table 1, at the baseline, analyses revealed a significant difference between the two groups in the estimation of the circumference of the shoulders, abdomen and hips, but not in the estimation of their width; moreover, no difference emerged in the estimation of the height. Specifically, as suggested by means reported in the Table 1, the healthy-weight participants showed a significant larger percentage of misestimation of the circumference of the three body parts than the participants with obesity.

Focusing on height, a significant main effect of *Group* emerged ($F(1, 26) = 4.67$; $p = 0.04$; $\eta\rho^2 = 0.15$), showing that individuals affected by obesity (M = 3.16; SD = 1.07) had a significant overestimation compared to the controls (M = −0.004; SD = 0.99), in absence of main effect of *Condition* (baseline

M = 1.9; SD = 3.72; synchronous M = 1; SD = 4.91; asynchronous M = 1.6; SD = 4.47) ($F(2, 52) = 1.82$; $p = 0.17$; $\eta\rho^2 = 0.06$) or a significant interaction *Group*Condition* ($F(2,52) = 2.88$; $p = 0.88$; $\eta\rho^2 = 0.41$). Thus, the VR-FBI did not change the height estimation for both groups.

For shoulder width estimation no main effect of *Group* (participants with obesity M = −10.24; SD = 4.32; healthy-weigh participants M = −4.58; SD = 4.67) ($F(1, 24) = 0.78$; $p = 0.38$; $\eta\rho^2 = 0.032$) or *Condition* (baseline M = −5.35; SD = 3.65; synchronous M = −8.52; SD = 3.42; asynchronous M = −8.36; SD = 3.15) ($F(2,48) = 1.38$; $p = 0.26$; $\eta\rho^2 = 0.055$) was found. Instead, a significant interaction *Group*Condition* ($F(2,48) = 3.5$; $p = 0.038$; $\eta\rho^2 = 0.12$) emerged. Post-hoc comparison for participants affected by obesity did not show a difference in the horizontal estimation of the shoulders between the baseline and the synchronous condition ($t(13) = 0.049$; $p = 0.62$), nor between the baseline and the asynchronous condition ($t(13) = 1.13$; $p = 0.27$). Instead, in the controls a significant difference emerged between the baseline and the synchronous condition ($t(12) = 2.58$; $p = 0.024$), but not between the baseline and the asynchronous condition ($t(12) = 2.36$; $p = 0.035$), when we adopted the Bonferroni corrected p value threshold (0.05/2 = 0.025) (Figure 3). Thus, these results show that the illusion affected shoulder width estimation of healthy-weight controls but not of individuals affected by obesity. However, as shown in Figure 3, it should be noticed that controls show a larger error after the synchronous and the asynchronous (even though the difference did not reach the significance) stimulation with respect to the baseline: this result was in contrast with the previous literature [1,2,5,18], in which it was generally reported a reduction of the error after the VR-FBI manipulation.

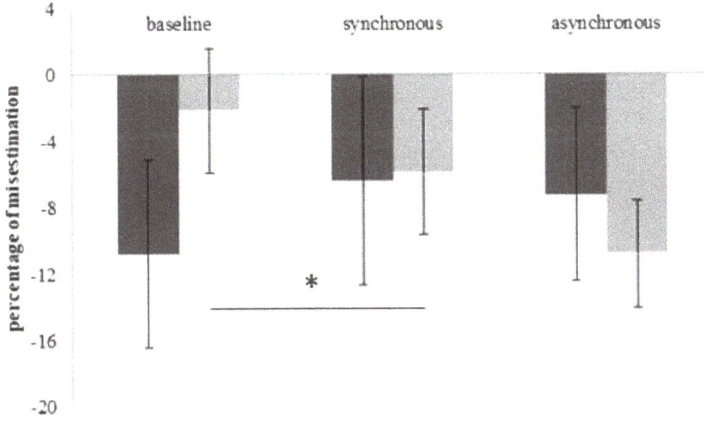

Figure 3. About the horizontal estimation of the shoulders, means of the percentage of misestimation and standard error (bars) were showed for participants affected by obesity (dark grey bars) and healthy-weight participants (light grey) for the three experimental conditions. * indicates a significant difference according to the Bonferroni-corrected p value of 0.025.

For width estimation of the abdomen, no main effect of *Group* (participants with obesity M = −4.49 SD = 5.39; healthy-weigh participants M = −1.29; SD = 5.79) ($F(1, 26) = 0.16$; $p = 0.68$; $\eta\rho^2 = 0.006$) or *Condition* (baseline M = −0.006; SD = 3.77; synchronous M = −4.93; SD = 4.29; asynchronous M = −3.73; SD = 4.53) ($F(2, 52) = 2.12$; $p = 0.13$; $\eta\rho^2 = 0.07$) emerged; moreover no significant interaction *Group*Condition* ($F(2, 52) = 1.21$; $p = 0.3$; $\eta\rho^2 = 0.04$) was found. Thus, the FBI did not change the width estimation of the abdomen for both groups.

For width estimation of the hips, we found a main effect of *Group* ($F(1, 24) = 8.33$; $p = 0.008$; $\eta\rho^2 = 0.25$): participants affected by obesity (M = 15.03; SD = 3.55) overestimated this body part with respect to the controls (M = 0.49; SD = 3.55). However, no main effect of *Condition* (baseline M = −9.47;

SD = 2.91; synchronous M = 4.94; SD = 2.54; asynchronous M = 8.87; SD = 3.02) (F(2, 48) = 2.37; p = 0.1; $\eta\rho^2$ = 0.09) or interaction *Group*Condition* (F(2, 48) = 2.54; p = 0.08; $\eta\rho^2$ = 0.09) emerged. This result suggested that VR-FBI did not change the width estimation of the hips for both groups.

For circumference estimation of shoulders, a significant main effect of *Group* was found (F(1, 28) = 4.86; p = 0.036; $\eta\rho^2$ = 0.14) confirming the previous results; in general, healthy-weight participants (M = 31.98; SD = 5.48) overestimated this body part compared to the participants affected by obesity (M = 14.88; SD = 5.48). Interestingly, a significant main effect of *Condition* emerged (F(2, 56) = 3.17; p = 0.049; $\eta\rho^2$ = 0.10): however, when the post-hoc t-test comparisons adopting the Bonferroni corrected p value threshold (0.05/2 = 0.025) were performed, no significant difference between the baseline (M = 27.81; SD = 4.32) and the synchronous condition (M = 19.91; SD = 4.53) (t(29) = 2.2; p = 0.036) or the baseline and the asynchronous condition (M = 22.58; SD = 4) (t(29) = 1.41; p = 0.16) emerged. Moreover, no significant interaction *Group*Condition* emerged (F(1, 26) = 1.64; p = 0.2; $\eta\rho^2$ = 0.05).

For estimation of the circumference of the abdomen, a significant main effect of *Group* emerged (F(1, 23) = 19.95; p < 0.001; $\eta\rho^2$ = 0.46): in line with the previous results, healthy-weight participants (M = 21.84; SD = 3) reported a significant overestimation of their body size compared to participants with obesity (M = 2.44; SD = 3.13), in absence of any main effect of *Condition* (baseline M = 13.14; SD = 2.91; synchronous M = 11.07; SD = 2.81; asynchronous M = 12.2; SD = 2.14) (F(2, 46) = 0.31; p = 0.73; $\eta\rho^2$ = 0.013) or a significant interaction *Group*Condition* (F(2, 46) = 0.97; p = 0.38; $\eta\rho^2$ = 0.04).

For estimation of the circumference of the hips, no main effect of *Group* (participants with obesity corrected M = 16.73; SD = 4.13; healthy-weight participants corrected M = 6.61; SD = 3.84) (F(1, 26) = 3.21; p = 0.08; $\eta\rho^2$ = 0.11) was found. However, we observed a main effect of *Condition* (F(2, 52) = 3.51; p = 0.037; $\eta\rho^2$ = 0.11): a significant difference between the baseline (M = 15.51; SD = 3.6) and the synchronous condition (M = 8.89; SD = 3.07) (t(28) = 2.6; p = 0.014) was found. Instead, no difference emerged between the baseline and the asynchronous condition (M = 10.6; SD = 2.86) (t(28) = 1.94; p = 0.06) (Figure 4). No significant interaction *Group*Condition* (F(2, 52) = 2.17; p = 0.12; $\eta\rho^2$ = 0.07) was found. Thus, according to these results, for both groups, changes in the estimation of the hips circumference emerged after the synchronous (but not the asynchronous) condition, with respect to the baseline. Specifically, as shown in Figure 4, after the illusion was induced in the synchronous condition, all participants reported a reduction of the error in the estimation of the hips' circumference, in line with our hypothesis.

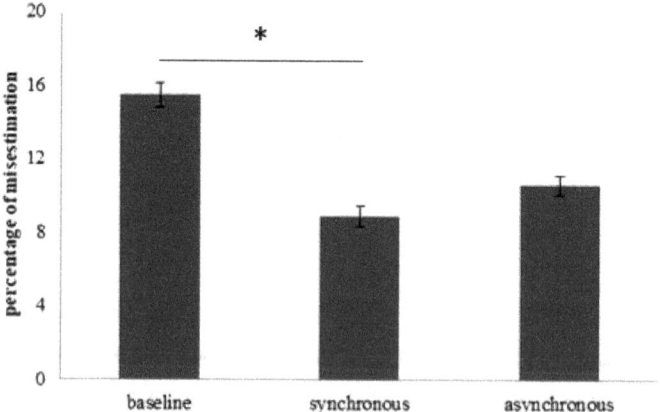

Figure 4. About the circumference estimation of the hips, means of the percentage of misestimation and standard error (bars) were showed for the three experimental condition (baseline, synchronous and asynchronous). * indicates a significant difference according to the Bonferroni-corrected p value of 0.025.

4. Discussion

The aim of the present work was to investigate for the first time in literature the potential changes in body representations induced by the illusionary ownership over a virtual skinny body (i.e., the VR-FBI) in a sample of individuals affected by obesity in comparison with a group of healthy weight individuals. We adopted two measures: the Embodiment Questionnaire [1] to study the strength of the bodily illusion; and the Body Part Size Estimation Task [1] to verify if the illusion might induce a modulation of body representations in our participants.

First, we found that VR-FBI was efficiently induced in individuals with obesity with the same strength of the healthy weight individuals. Indeed, there was no significant difference between the two groups as concerns the scores obtained from the Embodiment Questionnaire [1]. However, for all participants, it should be noted that we found a significant difference in the *self-location* subscale, but not in the *ownership* and *agency* subscales, between the two experimental conditions, suggesting that also in the asynchronous condition (and thus not only the synchronous one) all individuals experience the illusion of ownership. To this regard, it was already reported that a first-person perspective of a realistic virtual body substituting participants' own body might be sufficient to generate an illusory feeling of ownership, with changes in body representations, in absence of any multisensory stimulation [25], as reported also for the Rubber Hand Illusion [26]. Thus, the asynchronous stimulation is not a "*neutral condition*", since it can affect body representations [27]. As concerns the self-location subscale, we did not expect specific differences between the two conditions, since our paradigm did not experimentally manipulate the spatial location. However, higher scores in self-location subscale could drive higher embodiment over the virtual body, as Maselli and Slater [25] emphasized a strict relationship between the sense of ownership and the feeling of self-location towards the virtual body. Moreover, there is an ongoing debate about what subjective components, such as body dissatisfaction [5] or bodily sensory experience [2,28–30]—That were not directly measured by the questionnaire—might enhance or impede to experience the bodily illusion [2,28–31]. Moreover, as recently stated by Tamè and colleagues [28] about the Rubber Hand Illusion, even though individuals report the *feeling* like the fake hand is part of their own body, "*they do not believe that it really is*": this aspect should be taken in account also when individuals are asked to rate their experience of ownership towards an avatar.

The second other main result regarded the possible modulation of body representations, when measured through the Body Part Size Estimation Task [1], due to the bodily illusion. According to the results, an interesting pattern emerged considering the estimation of the circumference of the hips: both healthy weight individuals and individuals affected by obesity shown a reduction of the error after the synchronous, but not the asynchronous, condition, with respect to the baseline. This result seems to suggest that the illusion can efficiently modulate body representations in individuals affected by obesity, specifically in terms of the circumference of the hips, as well as in controls. In other words, affected individuals perceived themselves to have skinner hips after they have embodied a skinny avatar. However, such an effect did not emerge for the other body parts investigated in this study. How might this pattern of results be interpreted? We might observe that the hips represent a very significant and critical body part, not only in obesity but also in healthy weight participants, and specifically in women, in which there is a propensity to accumulate fat on the hips and buttocks (the "feminine gynecoid" type) instead of a more central distribution on the abdomen, that is typically observed in males [32–34]. Thus, it makes sense to believe that from a clinical point of view this body part is quite important and perhaps more sensitive than other body parts, such as the shoulders. Second, it should be noted that during the experimental procedure, participants looked toward the avatar's lower part, that was clearly skinner than the own physical body dimension. Considering that, it should be carefully clarified the psychological meaning of this difference. Indeed, it cannot be excluded that the presence of a skinny avatar would might enhance (and not mitigate) the negative feelings towards the body. In this sense, the therapeutic applicability of bodily illusions in obesity should require future investigation in which also psychological and clinical factors, as well as the outcome of the weight loss program, should be taken in account. For example, it should be investigated if the alteration of body parts size estimation might be related to other psychological factors, such as fear and worries about the success of the treatment as well as the subjective level of perceived social stigma [35,36] since they could be negative consequences on efficacy of rehabilitative intervention, as well as the most recent study about the effect of bodily illusions on social cognition [31]. Indeed, Guardia and colleagues [37] described the single case of an individual affected by obesity who did not update her body image to the "new" physical body dimensions after a massive weight loss; in other words, the patient continued to describe her body as larger as before the treatment [37–39].

Overall, this study provided preliminary evidence that individuals with obesity can experience the VR-FBI, and that the illusion can induce a modulation of body representations only for specific body parts.

However, some caveats should be considered not only in the interpretation of our data but also for future investigation. First, a higher number of participants is mandatory to verify the reproducibility of our results.

When we investigate the application of the bodily illusion in the obesity, we should take in account not only the psychological and emotional components associated to this procedure, but also the cognitive process on which bodily illusions ground, that is the *multisensory integration* [40]. Specifically, the illusion can be efficiently induced only when the two stimuli (in this case, tactile and visual input) are perceived temporally synchronous; in other words, they are perceived as unique temporal event. For humans, multisensory integration is very critical, since it seems to be implicated in several cognitive processes, such as taste perception [41], flavor perception [42–44], but also bodily awareness [45,46] and sense of agency [47]. Focusing on bodily illusions, and specifically the asynchronous stimulation, the recognition of the delay between stimuli might depend on the subjective efficacy of the multisensory integration process, with effect on the induction and the strength of the illusion e.g., [25,27,48,49]. In obesity, the research about alteration of primary [50–52] and multiple sensory inputs [24–56] is still in its infancy. However, it was reported that individuals affected by obesity show an alteration of multisensory process, with possible effects of the ability in recognizing two stimuli (and overall, two events) as concurrent and concomitant [24–56]. Thus, future research needs to fully explore the relationship between the alteration in the experience of bodily illusions and altered multisensory integration.

Focusing on the VR-FBI, two aspects should be taken in account. The first regards the dimension of the avatar. In this work, we adopted an avatar with a skinny body, in line with our previous studies [1,20]. However, it should be verified if different dimensions of avatar (thus, a larger avatar as well as an avatar with bodily dimensions equivalent to the physical one) would affect differently body parts size estimation. In fact, in healthy individuals, while it was reported that a correct feeling of ownership was observed for images of hands with veridical and enlarged dimension respect to the physical one in healthy individuals, but absent in case of reduced dimensions, in the Rubber Hand Illusion [57,58]. Instead, the illusion emerged with both large and small full bodies in VR-FBI [55,59]. We reported that the two groups differed in the estimation of body size at the baseline. Interestingly, the healthy weight participants reported a significant larger error for the circumference of the three body parts of shoulders, abdomen and hips in respect to the participants with obesity. As expected, for all considered body parts, except for the height, individuals affected by obesity had higher physical dimensions than controls; thus, bodily dimensions were dramatically different between groups. However, the distortion of the body parts circumference observed in the healthy weight participants was quite different respect to that of the participants with obesity. As previously mentioned, the physical reduction of body size dimensions is a goal of the rehabilitative program for losing weight, and it is reasonable to think that individuals with obesity might be more aware about their own physical body than healthy weight individuals, who otherwise are generally described to have a negative feeling and high level of concerns about their own body [60]. Moreover, it should be noted the body size distortions are highly present also in healthy population [60]. However, as reviewed by Costantini and Haggard [40], pre-existing body representations play a crucial in body ownership. Indeed, the ownership towards an external object is due not only to the simultaneity of the sensory (visual-tactile) stimulation, but also to the match between the visual image of the body part/whole body adopted in the illusion and its existing subjective cognitive representation, i.e., the perceptual body representation [61] or offline stored knowledge about own body [62]. Nevertheless, when we ask individuals to judge the dimension of body parts, perhaps we are measuring the perceptual dimension together *plus* the feelings, concerns and preoccupation about those body parts [22–63], affecting the judgement itself. The second aspect regards the fact that during this experiment, in line with previous research [2–5], participants did not move as well as avatar was static. However, brain seems to be more responsive to human action than to static images [64], with possible implications on changes in body representations [65,66]. Thus, in the future perspectives, body representations changes might be investigated when embodiment towards an avatar is induced through a visuo-motor integration (the virtual body is seen to move synchronously with the own body), instead of a visuo-tactile integration (as done in the present study), taking advantage of motion sensors technology. Nevertheless, in case of motion, the presence of cybersickness during the VR experiment should be carefully measured, specifically when clinical condition like obesity, in which dizziness and falls are generally experience [67], are tested.

Finally, even though it is out of the scope of this work, we would like to underline some criticisms relative to the two measures (i.e., Body size estimation task and Embodiment Questionnaire) adopted in this study. About the Body parts size estimation task, it should be noticed that height (i.e., a vertical measurement taken from the top of the body to its base), horizontal (from the left of the body to the right) and circumferential (a measurement taken around the body) estimations ground on different neural mechanisms about spatial processing [68]. For example, a task in which we are required to identify the midline of a horizontal line would be solved adopting counting strategies, that instead might not be so useful when we have to estimate where is the center of a circle [69]. This aspect should be taken in account when a task about the estimation of body parts or whole body is chosen as measure of the illusion. Moreover, it should be noted that in the Body Size Estimation Task [1–20], participants are explicitly required to estimate the horizontal distance between the left and right side of each body part placing adhesive stickers on the wall. To avoid that they used their body as a reference for giving a correct body size estimation, we explicitly required participants to do not look at their own body during the task. This task has clear advantages: it's economical and traditionally adopted in clinical settings [70,71]. However, participants are fully aware that they have to focus on their own body to solve the task, and possible overcome side effect of negative attitudes on the judgment might reduce the illusion effect. Adopting more implicit measures in which a lower level of subjective awareness about the judgment [72] is required, should strengthen our results. A similar criticism can be arisen about the Embodiment Questionnaire [1], since it allows us to assess exclusively the subjective (and thus explicit and aware) experience of the illusion.

5. Conclusions

In this manuscript we presented the first investigation on the effect of a VR-FBI [2–5,17,18,20] on body representations in obesity. Indeed, only one single case study about VR-FBI on body representations in obesity [20] was reported in literature. Our results revealed that individuals affected by obesity might efficiently experience the illusory ownership over an entire virtual body, with possible changes on the estimation of the circumference of the hips. Thus, VR-FBI might be a promising tool to be adopted in rehabilitative settings [8,17], also in obesity. However, this work represents the first step in the field: future research should verify if and in which clinical and psychological circumstances as well as experimental conditions the illusion can efficiently modulate body representation in obesity.

Author Contributions: Conceptualization, S.F., S.S. and R.G.; Data curation, C.A., S.M., C.G. and M.A.; Formal analysis, S.F.; Funding acquisition, R.G.; Investigation, S.F., S.S. and C.A.; Methodology, S.F., S.S. and K.A.; Software, C.A.; Supervision, M.A.; Writing—Original draft, S.F. and S.S.; Writing—Review & editing, K.A., S.M., C.G., M.A. and R.G.

Funding: This research was funded by the Italian MIUR (Ministero dell'Università e della Ricerca Italiana) research project "Unlocking the memory of the body: Virtual Reality in Anorexia Nervosa" (Grant no. 201597WTTM).

Acknowledgments: This paper was partially supported by the Italian MIUR (Ministero dell'Università e della Ricerca Italiana) research project "Unlocking the memory of the body: Virtual Reality in Anorexia Nervosa" (Grant no. 201597WTTM).

Conflicts of Interest: The authors declare no conflict of interest.

References

1. Serino, S.; Scarpina, F.; Dakanalis, A.; Keizer, A.; Pedroli, E.; Castelnuovo, G.; Chirico, A.; Catallo, V.; Di Lernia, D.; Riva, G. The Role of Age on Multisensory Bodily Experience: An Experimental Study with a Virtual Reality Full-Body Illusion. *Cyberpsychol. Behav. Soc. Netw.* **2018**, *21*, 304–310. [CrossRef] [PubMed]
2. Petkova, V.I.; Ehrsson, H.H. If I were you: Perceptual illusion of body swapping. *PLoS ONE* **2008**, *3*, e3832. [CrossRef]
3. Slater, M.; Spanlang, B.; Sanchez-Vives, M.V.; Blanke, O. First person experience of body transfer in virtual reality. *PLoS ONE* **2010**, *5*, e10564. [CrossRef] [PubMed]
4. Serino, S.; Pedroli, E.; Keizer, A.; Triberti, S.; Dakanalis, A.; Pallavicini, F.; Chirico, A.; Riva, G. Virtual Reality Body Swapping: A Tool for Modifying the Allocentric Memory of the Body. *Cyberpsychol. Behav. Soc. Netw.* **2016**, *19*, 127–133. [CrossRef] [PubMed]
5. Preston, C.; Ehrsson, H.H. Implicit and explicit changes in body satisfaction evoked by body size illusions: Implications for eating disorder vulnerability in women. *PLoS ONE* **2018**, *13*, e0199426. [CrossRef] [PubMed]
6. Valzogher, C.; Mazzurega, M.; Zampini, M.; Pavani, F. Incongruent multisensory stimuli alter bodily self-consciousness: Evidence from a first-person perspective experience. *Acta Psychol.* **2018**, *191*, 261–270. [CrossRef] [PubMed]
7. Keizer, A.; van Elburg, A.; Helms, R.; Dijkerman, H.C. A Virtual Reality Full Body Illusion Improves Body Image Disturbance in Anorexia Nervosa. *PLoS ONE* **2016**, *11*, e0163921. [CrossRef] [PubMed]
8. Serino, S.; Polli, N.; Riva, G. From avatars to body swapping: The use of virtual reality for assessing and treating body-size distortion in individuals with anorexia. *J. Clin. Psychol.* **2019**, *75*, 313–322. [CrossRef] [PubMed]
9. Jeon, B.; Cho, S.; Lee, J.H. Application of virtual body swapping to patients with complex regional pain syndrome: A pilot study. *Cyberpsychol. Behav. Soc. Netw.* **2014**, *17*, 366–370. [CrossRef]
10. Lengeenhager, B.; Hilti, L.M.; Brugger, P. Disturbed body integrity and the "rubber foot illusion". *Neuropsychology* **2015**, *29*, 205–211. [CrossRef]
11. Kaplan, R.A.; Enticott, P.G.; Hohwy, J.; Castle, D.J.; Rossell, S.L. Is body dysmorphic disorder associated with abnormal bodily self-awareness? A study using the rubber hand illusion. *PLoS ONE* **2014**, *9*, e99981. [CrossRef]
12. Botvinick, M.; Cohen, J. Rubber hands 'feel' touch that eyes see. *Nature* **1998**, *391*, 756. [CrossRef] [PubMed]
13. Moseley, G.L.; Gallace, A.; Spence, C. Bodily illusions in health and disease: Physiological and clinical perspectives and the concept of a cortical 'body matrix'. *Neurosci. Biobehav. Rev.* **2012**, *36*, 34–46. [CrossRef] [PubMed]
14. Gutiérrez-Maldonado, J.; Wiederhold, B.K.; Riva, G. Future Directions: How Virtual Reality Can Further Improve the Assessment and Treatment of Eating Disorders and Obesity. *Cyberpsychol. Behav. Soc. Netw.* **2016**, *19*, 148–153. [CrossRef] [PubMed]
15. Riva, G. Virtual reality in the treatment of eating and weight disorders. *Psychol. Med.* **2017**, *47*, 2567–2568. [CrossRef] [PubMed]
16. Freeman, D.; Reeve, S.; Robinson, A.; Ehlers, A.; Clark, D.; Spanlang, B.; Slater, M. Virtual reality in the assessment, understanding and treatment of mental health disorders. *Psychol. Med.* **2017**, *47*, 2393–2400. [CrossRef] [PubMed]
17. Serino, S.; Dakanalis, A. Bodily illusions and weight-related disorders: Clinical insights from experimental research. *Ann. Phys. Rehabil. Med.* **2017**, *60*, 217–219. [CrossRef]
18. Normand, J.M.; Giannopoulos, E.; Spanlang, B.; Slater, M. Multisensory stimulation can induce an illusion of larger belly size in immersive virtual reality. *PLoS ONE* **2011**, *6*, e16128. [CrossRef] [PubMed]

19. Eshkevari, E.; Rieger, E.; Longo, M.R.; Haggard, P.; Treasure, J. Increased plasticity of the bodily self in eating disorders. *Psychol. Med.* **2012**, *42*, 819–828. [CrossRef]
20. Serino, S.; Scarpina, F.; Keizer, A.; Pedroli, E.; Dakanalis, A.; Castelnuovo, G.; Chirico, A.; Novelli, M.; Gaudio, S.; Riva, G. A Novel Technique for Improving Bodily Experience in a Non-operable Super-Super Obesity Case. *Front. Psychol.* **2016**, *7*, 837. [CrossRef]
21. Tsakiris, M.; Haggard, P. The Rubber Hand Illusion Revisited: Visuotactile Integration and Self-Attribution. *J. Exp. Psychol. Hum. Percept. Perform.* **2005**, *31*, 80–91. [CrossRef] [PubMed]
22. Scarpina, F.; Castelnuovo, G.; Molinari, E. Tactile mental body parts representation in obesity. *Psychiatry Res.* **2014**, *220*, 960–969. [CrossRef] [PubMed]
23. Scarpina, F.; Cau, N.; Cimolin, V.; Galli, M.; Castelnuovo, G.; Priano, L.; Pianta, L.; Corti, S.; Mauro, A.; Capodaglio, P. Body-scaled action in obesity during locomotion: Insights on the nature and extent of body representation disturbances. *J. Psychosom. Res.* **2017**, *102*, 34–40. [CrossRef]
24. Scarpina, F.; Migliorati, D.; Marzullo, P.; Mauro, A.; Scacchi, M.; Costantini, M. Altered multisensory temporal integration in obesity. *Sci. Rep.* **2016**, *6*, 28382. [CrossRef] [PubMed]
25. Maselli, A.; Slater, M. The building blocks of the full body ownership illusion. *Front. Hum. Neurosci.* **2013**, *7*, 83. [CrossRef] [PubMed]
26. Rohde, M.; Luca, M.; Ernst, M.O. The rubber hand illusion: Feeling of ownership and proprioceptive drift Do not go hand in hand. *PLoS ONE* **2011**, *6*, e21659. [CrossRef] [PubMed]
27. Perez-Marcos, D.; Martini, M.; Fuentes, C.T.; Rivas, A.I.B.; Haggard, P.; Sanchez-Vives, M.V. Selective distortion of body image by asynchronous visuotactile stimulation. *Body Image* **2018**, *24*, 55–61. [CrossRef] [PubMed]
28. Tamè, L.; Linkenauger, S.A.; Longo, M.R. Dissociation of feeling and belief in the rubber hand illusion. *PLoS ONE* **2018**, *13*, e0206367. [CrossRef] [PubMed]
29. Blanke, O.; Metzinger, T. Full-body illusions and minimal phenomenal selfhood. *Trends Cognit. Sci.* **2009**, *13*, 7–13. [CrossRef]
30. David, N.; Fiori, F.; Aglioti, S.M. Susceptibility to the rubber hand illusion does not tell the whole body-awareness story. *Cognit. Affect. Behav. Neurosci.* **2014**, *14*, 297–306. [CrossRef]
31. Maister, L.; Slater, M.; Sanchez-Vives, M.V.; Tsakiris, M. Changing bodies changes minds: Owning another body affects social cognition. *Trends Cognit. Sci.* **2015**, *19*, 6–12. [CrossRef] [PubMed]
32. Champe, P.C.; Richard, A. *Harvey Lippincott's Illustrated Reviews: Biochemistry*, 3rd ed.; Lippincott, Williams & Wilkins: Baltimore, ML, USA, 2003.
33. Zavorsky, G.S.; Murias, J.M.; Kim do, J.; Gow, J.; Sylvestre, J.L.; Christou, N.V. Waist-to-hip ratio is associated with pulmonary gas exchange in the morbidly obese. *Chest* **2007**, *131*, 362–367. [CrossRef] [PubMed]
34. Janjic, C. Android-type obesity and gynecoid-type obesity. *Praxis* **1996**, *85*, 1578–1583. [PubMed]
35. Puhl, R.M.; Heuer, C.A. Obesity stigma: Important considerations for public health. *Am. J. Public Health* **2010**, *100*, 1019–1028. [CrossRef] [PubMed]
36. Puhl, R.M.; Suh, Y. Health Consequences of Weight Stigma: Implications for Obesity Prevention and Treatment. *Curr. Obes. Rep.* **2015**, *4*, 182–190. [CrossRef] [PubMed]
37. Guardia, D.; Metral, M.; Pigeyre, M.; Bauwens, I.; Cottencin, O.; Luyat, M. Body distortions after massive weight loss: Lack of updating of the body schema hypothesis. *Eat. Weight Disord.* **2013**, *18*, 333–336. [CrossRef] [PubMed]
38. Dakanalis, A.; Gaudio, S.; Serino, S.; Clerici, M.; Carrá, G.; Riva, G. Body-image distortion in anorexia nervosa. *Nat. Rev. Dis. Primers* **2016**, *2*, 16026. [CrossRef]
39. Riva, G.; Gaggioli, A.; Dakanalis, A. From body dissatisfaction to obesity: How virtual reality may improve obesity prevention and treatment in adolescents. *Stud. Health Technol. Inform.* **2013**, *184*, 356–362.
40. Costantini, M.; Haggard, P. The rubber hand illusion: Sensitivity and reference frame for body ownership. *Conscious. Cognit.* **2007**, *16*, 229–240. [CrossRef]
41. Slocombe, B.G.; Carmichael, D.A.; Simner, J. Cross-modal tactile-taste interactions in food evaluations. *Neuropsychologia* **2016**, *88*, 58–64. [CrossRef]
42. Auvray, M.; Spence, C. The multisensory perception of flavor. *Conscious. Cognit.* **2008**, *17*, 1016–1031. [CrossRef] [PubMed]
43. Wallace, M.T. Multisensory Perception: The Building of Flavor Representations. *Curr. Biol.* **2015**, *25*, R986–R988. [CrossRef] [PubMed]

44. Spence, C. Multisensory flavor perception. *Cell* **2015**, *161*, 24–35. [CrossRef] [PubMed]
45. Salomon, R.; Noel, J.P.; Łukowska, M.; Faivre, N.; Metzinger, T.; Serino, A.; Blanke, O. Unconscious integration of multisensory bodily inputs in the peripersonal space shapes bodily self-consciousness. *Cognition* **2017**, *166*, 174–183. [CrossRef] [PubMed]
46. Tsakiris, M. The multisensory basis of the self: From body to identity to others. *Q. J. Exp. Psychol.* **2017**, *70*, 597–609. [CrossRef] [PubMed]
47. Pyasik, M.; Burin, D.; Pia, L. On the relation between body ownership and sense of agency: A link at the level of sensory-related signals. *Acta Psychol.* **2018**, *185*, 219–228. [CrossRef] [PubMed]
48. Maselli, A.; Kilteni, K.; López-Moliner, J.; Slater, M. The sense of body ownership relaxes temporal constraints for multisensory integration. *Sci. Rep.* **2016**, *6*, 30628. [CrossRef] [PubMed]
49. Kilteni, K.; Maselli, A.; Kording, K.P.; Slater, M. Over my fake body: Body ownership illusions for studying the multisensory basis of own-bodyperception. *Front. Hum. Neurosci.* **2015**, *9*, 141. [CrossRef] [PubMed]
50. Szalay, C.; Aradi, M.; Schwarcz, A.; Orsi, G.; Perlaki, G.; Németh, L.; Hanna, S.; Takács, G.; Szabó, I.; Bajnok, L.; et al. Gustatory perception alterations in obesity: An fMRI study. *Brain Res.* **2012**, *1473*, 131–140. [CrossRef]
51. Stafford, L.D.; Whittle, A. Obese Individuals Have Higher Preference and Sensitivity to Odor of Chocolate. *Chem. Senses* **2015**, *40*, 279–284. [CrossRef]
52. Holinski, F.; Menenakos, C.; Haber, G.; Olze, H.; Ordemann, J. Olfactory and Gustatory Function After Bariatric Surgery. *Obes. Surg.* **2015**, *25*, 2314–2320. [CrossRef] [PubMed]
53. Preston, C.; Ehrsson, H.H. Illusory changes in body size modulate body satisfaction in a way that is related to non-clinical eating disorder psychopathology. *PLoS ONE* **2014**, *9*, e85773. [CrossRef] [PubMed]
54. Holmes, N.P.; Snijders, H.J.; Spence, C. Reaching with alien limbs: Visual exposure to prosthetic hands in a mirror biases proprioception without accompanying illusions of ownership. *Percept. Psychophys.* **2006**, *68*, 685–701. [CrossRef] [PubMed]
55. Piryankova, I.V.; Wong, H.Y.; Linkenauger, S.A.; Stinson, C.; Longo, M.R.; Bülthoff, H.H.; Mohler, B.J. Owning an overweight or underweight body: Distinguishing the physical, experienced and virtual body. *PLoS ONE* **2014**, *9*, e103428. [CrossRef] [PubMed]
56. Wan, X.; Spence, C.; Mu, B.; Zhou, X.; Ho, C. Assessing the benefits of multisensory audiotactile stimulation for overweight individuals. *Exp. Brain Res.* **2014**, *232*, 1085–1093. [CrossRef] [PubMed]
57. Pavani, F.; Zampini, M. The role of hand size in the fake-hand illusion paradigm. *Perception* **2007**, *36*, 1547–1554. [CrossRef] [PubMed]
58. Kilteni, K.; Normand, J.M.; Sanchez-Vives, M.V.; Slater, M. Extending body space in immersive virtual reality: A very long arm illusion. *PLoS ONE* **2012**, *7*, e40867. [CrossRef] [PubMed]
59. Van der Hoort, B.; Guterstam, A.; Ehrsson, H.H. Being Barbie: The size of one's own body determines the perceived size of the world. *PLoS ONE* **2011**, *6*, e20195. [CrossRef]
60. Schwartz, M.B.; Brownell, K.D. Obesity and body image. *Body Image* **2004**, *1*, 43–45. [CrossRef]
61. Longo, M.R.; Azañón, E.; Haggard, P. More than skin deep: Body representation beyond primary somatosensory cortex. *Neuropsychologia* **2010**, *48*, 655–668. [CrossRef]
62. Riva, G. The Neuroscience of Body Memory: From the Self through the Space to the Others. *Cortex* **2018**, *104*, 241–260. [CrossRef] [PubMed]
63. Smeets, M.A.; Klugkist, I.G.; Rooden, S.V.; Anema, H.A.; Postma, A. Mental body distance comparison: A tool for assessing clinical disturbances in visual body image. *Acta Psychol.* **2009**, *132*, 157–165. [CrossRef] [PubMed]
64. Peuskens, H.; Vanrie, J.; Verfaille, K.; Orban, G.A. Specificity of regions processing biological motion. *Eur. J. Neurosci.* **2005**, *21*, 2864–2875. [CrossRef] [PubMed]
65. Vocks, S.; Legenbauer, T.; Rüddel, H.; Troje, N.F. Static and dynamic body image in bulimia nervosa: Mental representation of body dimensionsand biological motion patterns. *Int. J. Eat. Disord.* **2007**, *40*, 59–66. [CrossRef] [PubMed]
66. Cazzato, V.; Siega, S.; Urgesi, C. "What women like": Influence of motion and form on esthetic body perception. *Front. Psychol.* **2012**, *3*, 235. [CrossRef]
67. Corna, S.; Aspesi, V.; Cau, N.; Scarpina, F.; Gattini Valdés, N.; Brugliera, L.; Cimolin, V.; Capodaglio, P. Dizziness and Falls in Obese Inpatients Undergoing Metabolic Rehabilitation. *PLoS ONE* **2017**, *12*, e0169322. [CrossRef]

68. Jewell, G.; McCourt, M.E. Pseudoneglect: A review and meta-analysis of performance factors in line bisection tasks. *Neuropsychologia* **2000**, *38*, 93–110. [CrossRef]
69. Girardi, M.; McIntosh, R.D.; Michel, C.; Vallar, G.; Rossetti, Y. Sensorimotor effects on central space representation: Prism adaptation influences haptic and visual representations in normal subjects. *Neuropsychologia* **2004**, *42*, 1477–1487. [CrossRef]
70. Probst, M.; Vandereycken, W.; Vanderlinden, J.; Van Coppenolle, H. The significance of body size estimation in eating disorders: Its relationship with clinical and psychological variables. *Int. J. Eat. Disord.* **1998**, *24*, 167–174. [CrossRef]
71. Shafran, R.; Fairburn, C.G. A new ecologically valid method to assess body size estimation and body size dissatisfaction. *Int. J. Eat. Disord.* **2002**, *32*, 458–465. [CrossRef]
72. Longo, M.R. Implicit and Explicit Body Representations. *Eur. Psychol.* **2015**, *20*, 6–15. [CrossRef]

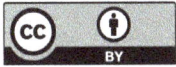

© 2019 by the authors. Licensee MDPI, Basel, Switzerland. This article is an open access article distributed under the terms and conditions of the Creative Commons Attribution (CC BY) license (http://creativecommons.org/licenses/by/4.0/).

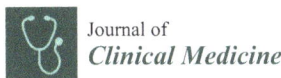

Article

Characterizing Body Image Distortion and Bodily Self-Plasticity in Anorexia Nervosa via Visuo-Tactile Stimulation in Virtual Reality

Luca Provenzano [1,2,†], Giuseppina Porciello [1,2,†,*], Sofia Ciccarone [1,2], Bigna Lenggenhager [3], Gaetano Tieri [2,4], Matteo Marucci [1,2,5], Federico Dazzi [6], Camillo Loriedo [7] and Ilaria Bufalari [2,8,*]

1. Department of Psychology, "Sapienza" University of Rome, 00185 Rome, Italy; luca.provenzano@uniroma1.it (L.P.); sofia.ciccarone@uniroma1.it (S.C.); matteo.marucci@uniroma1.it (M.M.)
2. IRCCS, Santa Lucia Foundation, 00142 Rome, Italy; gaetano.tieri@gmail.com
3. Department of Psychology, University of Zurich, 8050 Zurich, Switzerland; bigna.lenggenhager@gmail.com
4. Virtual Reality Lab, University of Rome Unitelma-Sapienza, 00161 Rome, Italy
5. BrainTrends Ltd., Applied Neuroscience, Gallicano nel Lazio (RM), 00010 Rome, Italy
6. Department of Human Sciences, Lumsa University, 00193 Rome, Italy; federicodazzi@hotmail.com
7. Clinica Psichiatrica, "Sapienza" University of Rome, 00185 Rome, Italy; camillo.loriedo@uniroma1.it
8. Department of Developmental and Social Psychology, "Sapienza" University of Rome, 00185 Rome, Italy
* Correspondence: ilaria.bufalari@uniroma1.it (I.B.); giuseppina.porciello@uniroma1.it (G.P.)
† These authors contributed equally to this work.

Received: 4 December 2019; Accepted: 19 December 2019; Published: 30 December 2019

Abstract: We combined virtual reality and multisensory bodily illusion with the aim to characterize and reduce the perceptual (body overestimation) and the cognitive-emotional (body dissatisfaction) components of body image distortion (BID) in anorexia nervosa (AN). For each participant (20 anorexics, 20 healthy controls) we built personalized avatars that reproduced their own body size, shape, and verisimilar increases and losses of their original weight. Body overestimation and dissatisfaction were measured by asking participants to choose the avatar that best resembled their real and ideal body. Results show higher body dissatisfaction in AN, caused by the desire of a thinner body, and no body-size overestimation. Interpersonal multisensory stimulation (IMS) was then applied on the avatar reproducing participant's perceived body, and on the two avatars which reproduced increases and losses of 15% of it, all presented with a first-person perspective (1PP). Embodiment was stronger after synchronous IMS in both groups, but did not reduce BID in participants with AN. Interestingly, anorexics reported more negative emotions after embodying the fattest avatar, which scaled with symptoms severity. Overall, our findings suggest that the cognitive-emotional, more than the perceptual component of BID is severely altered in AN and that perspective (1PP vs. 3PP) from which a body is evaluated may play a crucial role. Future research and clinical trials might take advantage of virtual reality to reduce the emotional distress related to body dissatisfaction.

Keywords: anorexia nervosa; body image distortion; body dissatisfaction; embodiment; virtual reality; interpersonal multisensory stimulation

1. Introduction

Anorexia nervosa (AN) affects mostly adolescent and young women [1], has the highest mortality rate among all psychiatric disorders [2] and is largely resistant to currently available treatments [3]. A core clinical symptom of AN is body image distortion (BID), which impacts onset, prognosis, and relapse [4]. Body image is a multifaceted construct that comprises body-related perception, expectations, thoughts, feelings, and actions [5,6] which are represented in dedicated neural circuitries [7–10]. In AN, BID affects both perceptual and cognitive-emotional components of the body representation [11], i.e., patients typically overestimate their body size [12] and report higher body dissatisfaction [13] than healthy controls (HC) [14].

The use of new sophisticated and biometrically plausible distortion methods, made possible by immersive virtual reality contexts, has paved the way for precisely measuring body overestimation e.g., [15], whereas the development of interpersonal multisensory stimulation (IMS) paradigms has increased insights into the plasticity of the bodily self [15,16]. In IMS paradigms, participants typically experience a tactile stimulation on their own body synchronously with an observed touch at the corresponding body part on another individual's body [17–19] which leads to the illusory sensation of ownership toward the latter (termed embodiment), as evidenced by subjective, behavioral, and physiological measures [20–24].

IMS paradigms have been extended to virtual avatars observed from a first-person perspective (1PP) [25], even of different sizes [26], which might lead to a change in one's own body perception according to the avatar size [27]. Specifically, in HC identification with a slim virtual body reduces not only the overestimation of the own body size but also increases body satisfaction [28], while identification with an obese avatar induces body dissatisfaction [28].

Embodiment illusions might thus represent a promising tool to reduce BID in AN. Preliminary results in this field suggest that, in AN patients, illusory ownership of a fake hand is enhanced [29] and leads to a reduction in hand-size overestimation [30]. Also, embodying a normal body mass index (BMI) avatar reduces overestimation of shoulders, abdomen, and hips [31]. However, this effect occurs after both synchronous (experimental condition) and asynchronous (control condition) IMS, suggesting that it might not be due to the embodiment per se, but rather to purely visual effects.

Thus, the few existing studies using embodiment illusions in AN patients tentatively suggest that a normalization of BID is possible. Yet, it is still unclear how robust the effect is, to what degree it is linked to embodiment per se and how such illusions affect and interact with the affective-emotional components of body representation, which are central to BID [11,32].

Here, we addressed these issues by: (i) individualizing the avatars for each of our participant' body (unlike previous studies); (ii) assessing the embodiment strength both at the explicit (questionnaires, e.g., [19,33]) and implicit level (body temperature, e.g., [34], but see [35] for a critical account), and (iii) measuring both perceptual and emotional aspects of BID before and after the embodiment of three different sized avatars was induced. We tested young females with AN and low-BMI age-matched HC with no diagnosis of eating disorders.

We expected AN patients to overestimate their body size [12] and to show higher body dissatisfaction than HC [13], as indexed by clinical measures (clinical questionnaires' scores) and by the higher discrepancy between one's own perceived and ideal body [36]. Furthermore, according to Eshkevari and colleagues [29], we expected higher bodily self-plasticity (namely higher embodiment measured both at the implicit and explicit level) in AN patients compared to HC. Importantly, we hypothesized that body dissatisfaction would decrease in AN patients as an effect of embodying a body which corresponds or is thinner than the perceived one [28]. Lastly, we expected that embodying an avatar larger than the perceived one would enhance negative emotions in AN patients more than HC.

2. Materials and Methods

2.1. Participants

A total of 21 female patients diagnosed with AN and 22 age-matched HC were recruited. All AN patients were diagnosed with anorexia nervosa (restricting type) by the Department of Psychiatry and Eating Disorder of the Hospital Policlinico Umberto I, which followed the criteria of Diagnostic and Statistical Manual of Mental Disorder—5 [37]. One AN patient was later excluded because of diagnostic migration, i.e., the diagnosis changed from AN to major depression as primary disorder with a secondary eating disorder component. Two HC were excluded for technical problems. A total of 20 AN patients ((mean ± standard error (SE)) (age = 23.30 ± 7.61, BMI = 15.87 ± 1.12)) and 20 HC (age = 23.85 ± 3.23, BMI = 18.98 ± 1.01) finally participated in the study. For the HC, the presence and/or history of any eating disorder and/or other psychiatric disorders constituted an exclusion criterion, whereas a BMI score in the lower normal range (i.e., between 17 and 21) was an inclusion criterion. The study was approved by the Ethical Committees of Policlinico Umberto I and IRCCS Santa Lucia Foundation and in accordance with the ethical standards of the 2013 Declaration of Helsinki. All the participants read and signed the informed consent.

2.2. Procedure

The experiment consisted of two sessions: a pre-experimental (Section 2.3) and an experimental session (Section 2.4), with about one week break in between, in which the individualized avatars were created.

2.3. Pre-Experimental Session

This session lasted about one hour. Participants filled out a series of questionnaires presented in randomized order on a computer using E-Prime® 2.0 software. The Eating Disorder Inventory—2 (EDI-2) [38], the Body Shape Questionnaire (BSQ) [39], the Body Uneasiness Test (BUT) [40], and the Bulimic Investigatory Test, Edinburgh (BITE) [41] were used to assess the symptoms severity of the eating disorder pathology, whereas the Symptom Checklist-90-R (SCL-90-R) [42] was used to check for the presence of others psychiatric symptoms (see Supplementary Materials for detailed information).

Subsequently, a female experimenter measured circumferences and lengths of selected body parts of each participants and took pictures of participants' body standing up (front, back, and profile view) with a Nikon D40 mounted on a tripod. Participants' pictures and body measures served to create the avatars personalized for each participant.

Avatars Modelling

A 3D modelling software (MakeHumans, open source tool for making 3d characters) was used to recreate the personalized avatar that matched participants' real body in terms of height, shape, and body size and two more avatars that reproduced verisimilar loss of 30% and gain of 50% of the original weight (Figure 1, panel A). Specifically, Adobe Photoshop 7.0 (Adobe Systems Incorporated, San Jose, CA, USA) was used to create highly detailed skin, clothes, and material textures. Subsequently, these three avatars were imported into 3dsMax (Autodesk Inc., Mill Valley, CA), a 3D modelling and animation software, which we used to create a continuum of 28 avatars incrementing in size in steps of 3%, starting from the thinnest (−30%) to the fattest avatar (+50%). One set of 28 standing avatars facing the participants was created for subsequent task, i.e., the Avatar selection task (please see Section 2.4.1) in which participants could choose the avatar that best resembled their own body by observing it from a 3PP. We decided to present a set of avatars going from −30% to +50% of the original body size in order to not end up with unrealistically thin bodies (especially in the case of the AN) and to be able to measure the presence of body overestimation in the range suggested by a recent meta-analysis [12]. Another set of avatars was created lying on a deck chair (Figure 1, panel B) and used for inducing the embodiment (please see Section 2.4.3).

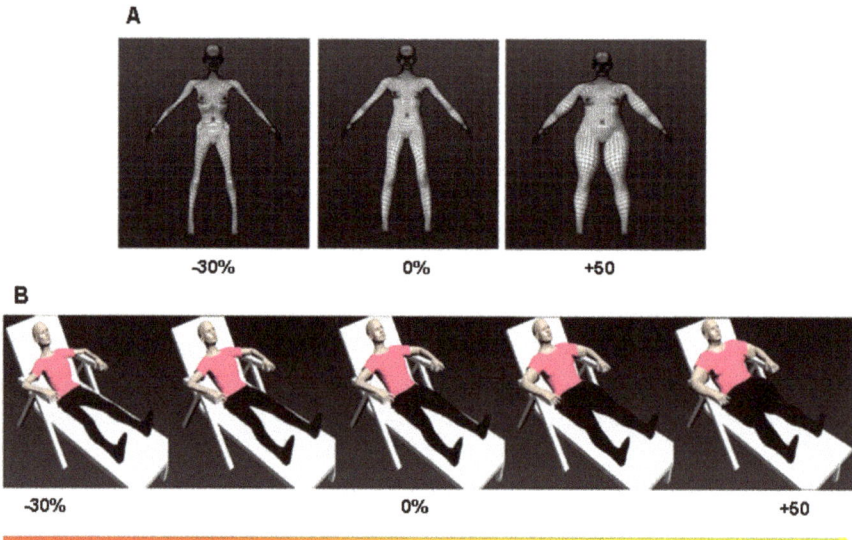

Figure 1. Creation of 3D Stimuli. (**A**) Example of three customized avatars built according to the participant's body measures and pictures: an avatar that reproduced participant's real body (avatar 0%), a thinner avatar (avatar −30%), and fatter avatar (+50%). (**B**) Example of avatars selection extracted from the continuum of avatars lying on a deck chair and increasing in size in steps of 3%, starting from the thinnest (−30%) to the fattest avatar (+50%).

2.4. Experimental Session

This session lasted about two hours (see Figure 2 for an illustration of the procedure). Participants first performed the Avatar selection task (Section 2.4.1). Then they put on clothes that matched the avatar's outfit and lay down on the deck chair to perform the perceived and ideal body tasks (Section 2.4.2). Afterward, participants experienced synchronous and asynchronous IMS (Section 2.4.3) with three different body size avatars (Avatar 0%., i.e., the avatar they chose in the Avatar selection task; Avatar −15% and Avatar +15%, i.e., an avatar 15% thinner and one 15% fatter than the one reproducing their own perceived body) in separate runs, counterbalanced across participants. Within each run participants received synchronous and asynchronous IMS in separate blocks (counterbalanced across participants) with the same avatar size. Immediately after each IMS block, participants performed the perceived body task (first 6 blocks) or the ideal body task (second 6 blocks, or vice versa). Then, we collected explicit and implicit measurements of embodiment (Section 2.4.4) and the emotional response (Section 2.4.5) to the IMS. At the end participants were also asked to rate the avatars in terms of similarity and attractiveness (Section 2.4.6).

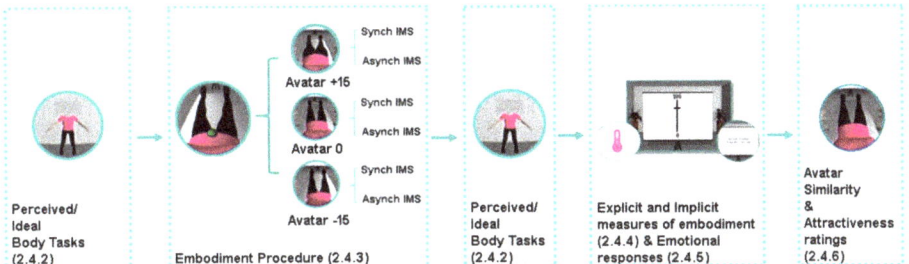

Figure 2. Experimental procedure. After selecting the avatar most similar to their perceived body and the one most resembling their ideal body, participants were enrolled in embodiment blocks in which synchronous and asynchronous interpersonal multisensory stimulation (IMS) were applied to three different bodies (the perceived body, −15% thinner body, +15% fatter body). After each embodiment block participants repeated the perceived and ideal body tasks to measure the effects of the embodiment of different sized avatars on body dissatisfaction. Explicit and implicit measures of the embodiment illusion, as well as the emotional response after being exposed to a/synchronous touching of different sized avatars were recorded after each embodiment block. At the end of the experiment we asked participants to rate from a first-person perspective the three avatars in terms of similarity to their own body and overall attractiveness.

All the experimental tasks were done in a virtual scenario that reproduced the actual experimental room, i.e., a 5 × 8 meters furnished room with a deck chair, identical to the one participant sat on during the experiment, and a 1.5 × 1.5 meters screen where questionnaires were projected.

2.4.1. Avatar Selection Task

Participants were asked to choose the avatar that best fits their own body from a continuum ranging from a body that was 30% thinner to another one that was +50% fatter than the actual body, i.e., the body that was reproduced on the bases of each participant's body size and shape. Participants initially saw the avatar in the middle of this continuum and were specifically instructed to explore all the continuum before choosing the avatar's body that best resembled their own in terms of shape and size. In this task, participants were standing up and the avatars were presented in a specular congruence with respect to their actual body, i.e., from a 3PP, as if they were looking at themselves in a mirror. The selected avatar (0% Avatar), the one 15% fatter (+15% Avatar) and the one 15% thinner (−15% Avatar) than the 0%, were used as virtual body stimuli for the embodiment blocks (Section 2.4.3).

2.4.2. Perceived and Ideal Body Tasks: Body Dissatisfaction

To assess participants' body dissatisfaction immediately before and after the IMS we asked them to choose the avatar which best resembled their real (perceived body task) and ideal (ideal body task) body in terms of size/shape/weight along the −30%–+50% continuum (Figure 3A). Differently from the avatar selection task, however, judgments were performed while participants were laying down on the deck chair and avatars were projected standing up in front of them, i.e., from a 3PP. As these tasks were performed before and immediately after IMS, participants were left lying on the desk chair to avoid disrupting any induced feelings of ownership over the avatar's body.

A Perceived/Ideal Body Task

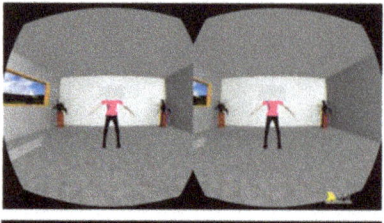

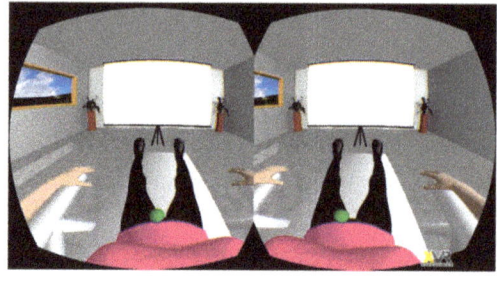

B Embodiment Procedure

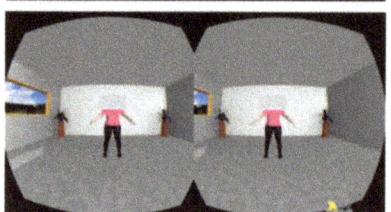

Figure 3. (**A**) Perceived/ideal body task. In separate blocks, participants choose the avatar which was the most similar to their own body (perceived body task) and the avatar which best resembled their ideal body (ideal body task) along a continuous of avatars presented from a third-person perspective (3PP). Each task comprised two trials presented in counterbalanced order: in one trial participants started the selection from the thinnest avatar (upper part of panel A), in the other from the fattest one (lower part of panel A). (**B**) Embodiment procedure. During the embodiment procedure a three minute of a/synchronous visuo-tactile stimulation was delivered. During the embodiment participants observed one of three different avatars from a first-person perspective (1PP). A virtual ball was programmed to touch the avatar on three different spots around the belly button in eight different ways (single touches and stroking movements).

Each task (perceived and ideal body task) comprised two trials, presented in counterbalanced order: in one trial participants started the selection from the thinnest avatar, in the other from the fattest one. Trials' scores were then averaged for the final score. The discrepancy between the size of the ideal and the perceived body, calculated as the absolute difference between the two, was considered an index of participants' body dissatisfaction.

2.4.3. Embodiment Procedure

During the IMS procedure participants saw the body from a 1PP (Figure 3B) through a head-mounted display (Oculus Rift Developers Kit Dk1, Oculus VR, Menlo Park, CA, USA). Thus, the virtual body replaced the participant's body in space. A calibration was performed to assure a proper positioning of the virtual camera and a precise overlap between the touch felt on the abdomen and the one observed on the avatar. Then, three minutes of visuo-tactile IMS were applied to the participant's and the avatar's body. The IMS was performed by a female experimenter, who received through headphones audio cues indicating the time and the location of each touch.

For the experimental condition (Synchronous-IMS), we aimed to reach the maximal multisensory congruence between the real and the virtual body. Thus, in the synchronous condition the observed and felt touch matched in time and location, and we tracked participants' head movements online to adjust visual perspective. However, as the visuo-proprioceptive congruence given by observing an avatar from a 1PP can be enough to induce feelings of ownership over a virtual body [43], we also aimed to reduce the possible occurrence of such illusory effects in the asynchronous control condition. Thus, we tried to boost the discrepancy in the control condition by delivering touches that were asynchronous in both time and location, as previous studies found that this stimulation was effective in maximizing the difference between synchronous and asynchronous conditions (see for example [44,45]) and we locked participant's head tracking during the asynchronous IMS.

During visual-tactile stimulation, the participants were asked not to move their head and look at the belly that was stimulated. Before starting the stimulation, the experimenter made sure that the participant always looked at the virtual abdomen by continuously checking: (i) the orientation of the participants' head (which had to be directed toward their real belly), and (ii) the virtual scenario on the PC monitor (where the virtual abdomen always had to be positioned in the center of the monitor).

2.4.4. Explicit and Implicit Measures of Embodiment

As an explicit measure of embodiment, we used a self-reported questionnaire adapted from previous studies [19,33] assessing the strength of the illusion on three different components: Ownership, i.e., the sense of virtual body being one's own; Agency i.e., the sense of being in control of the virtual body; and Referred Touch, i.e., the feeling of directly being touched by the seen ball (see Supplementary Materials for the complete list of items). As an implicit measure of embodiment, we recorded participants' body temperature, taken through an infrared thermometer (IFR 100, Microlife AG, Widnau, CH, precision: ± 0.2 °C, 32.0–42.2 °C) under participants' right armpit immediately after each block of IMS to compare ratings taken after synchronous vs. asynchronous embodiment blocks. Since we wanted to exclude participants with altered body temperature (due for example to febrile illness) we also took the body temperature before the experimental session started.

2.4.5. Measure of Emotional Response Induced by Embodiment

Valence and intensity of the emotional response induced by being exposed to a/synchronous touching of the three differently sized avatars were assessed by a visual analogue scale (VAS) ranging from "very negative" (0) to "very positive" (100) presented after both synchronous and asynchronous IMS.

2.4.6. Similarity and Attractiveness Ratings of the Avatars

As part of the final debriefing procedure, we checked how the −15%, 0%, and +15% avatars used during the embodiment blocks were actually perceived by the participants. Therefore, we asked participants to verbally rate on 0–100 VAS how much the three avatars resembled their own body (similarity ratings) and how attractive they thought these were (attractiveness ratings). The avatars were presented from a 1PP while participants were still laying down on the deck chair. Thus, ratings were collected while there was a spatial congruence between the actual participant's body and the avatar's body, i.e., while participants observed the three avatars replacing their own body in space.

3. Results

Data were analyzed using STATISTICA version 8.0 (StatSoft, Tulsa, OK, USA). Significance was set at $p < 0.05$. The Duncan test was used for post-hoc comparisons. Bayes Factors were calculated by means the open-source software JASP [46] which allows quantification of evidence in favor of the alternative or null hypothesis.

3.1. Baseline Measures

Descriptive statistics and independent sample *t*-tests were used for group comparisons of the demographical variables, eating disorder pathology and all the other baseline measures (Table 1).

Patients with anorexia nervosa (AN) reported higher symptoms severity scores in all scales (the Eating Disorder Inventory (EDI)—drive for thinness, EDI—body dissatisfaction scales, Body Shape Questionnaire (BSQ), Body Uneasiness Test—Global Severity Score (BUT GSI), but not at the EDI—bulimia, and at the Bulimic Investigatory Test, Edinburgh (BITE)). Patients with AN also had a lower body mass index (BMI) compared to healthy controls (HC). Body dissatisfaction (calculated as perceived minus ideal body) was higher in AN patients than in HC. While both groups were accurate and did not differ on the estimation of their perceived body, AN patients considered a thinner body as ideal compared to HC (see Table 2 for detailed statistics).

Table 1. Means (M) and standard deviations (SD) of demographic and eating disorders variables for the two groups (healthy controls-HC, and anorexics-AN), and results of the *t*-tests.

Demographic and Eating Disorder Variables							
	HC (N = 20)		AN (N = 20)				
	M	SD	M	SD	t	df	p
Age	23.85	3.23	23.30	7.60	0.29	38	0.767
BMI	18.94	0.98	15.86	1.12	9.22	38	0.001
EDI—drive for thinness	2.00	3.54	13.05	7.42	−6.01	38	0.001
EDI—bulimia	0.40	0.99	0.95	2.19	−1.02	38	0.313
EDI—body dissatisfaction	4.00	3.66	13.10	7.15	−5.07	38	0.001
BSQ	64.55	17.13	118.75	32.89	−6.54	38	0.001
BUT GSI	0.93	0.28	2.58	1.01	−7.07	37	0.001
BITE Symptoms	6.10	3.97	11.80	6.41	−3.38	38	0.002
BITE Severity	1.15	1.18	2.80	3.96	−1.79	38	0.082

BMI = Body Mass Index; EDI = Eating Disorder Inventory; BSQ = Body Shape Questionnaire; BUT GSI = Body Uneasiness Test, General Symptom Index subscale, BITE = Bulimic Investigatory Test, Edinburgh.

Table 2. Means (M) and standard deviations (SD) of perceived body, ideal body, and body dissatisfaction (perceived body minus ideal body) tasks measured at the baseline of the two groups (healthy controls-HC, and anorexic patients-AN), and results of the *t*-tests, i.e., *p*-values (p) and Bayesian factors (BF). Values are expressed as a % of the real bodies of the participants (100 is the real body size).

Perceived, Ideal and Body Dissatisfaction Measures								
	HC		AN					
Task	M	SD	M	SD	t	df	p	BF
Perceived Body	101.65	8.02	102.85	14.06	−0.33	38	0.742	0.32
Ideal Body	94.65	1.38	87.10	1.59	2.28	38	0.028	2.26
Body Dissatisfaction	8.45	7.85	19.95	12.97	−3.39	38	0.002	20.90

3.2. Explicit and Implicit Measures of Embodiment

Three separate 2 × 2 × 3 ANOVAs were run for each component (i.e., Ownership, Agency, and Referral of Touch) of the illusion, each with the factors Group, IMS, and Avatar. They revealed a main effect of IMS for the Ownership, Agency, and Referral of Touch (all Fs > 13.34; all ps < 0.001; all ηs2 > 0.259), suggesting a stronger illusion for synchronous as compared to the asynchronous IMS. We also found a main effect of Avatar on Ownership (F (1,38) = 7.85, $p < 0.001$, η2= 0.171)), with participants reporting higher scores for the +15% Avatar ((mean ± SE) (39.38 ±1.89)) compared to the 0% (33.78 ± 2.26) and to the −15% (32.08 ± 2.27) (all ps < 0.001). All the other main and interaction effects were not significant (all Fs< 3.35 all ps > 0.084).

The same 2 × 2 × 3 ANOVA run on the body temperature revealed a main effect of IMS (F (1,38) = 1.80, $p = 0.002$, η2 = 0.221)) showing a lower body temperature after the synchronous stimulation (34.91 ± 0.14) compared to the asynchronous one (35.02 ± 0.13). None of the other main and interaction effects were significant (all Fs < 1.27, all ps > 0.287). Please see Supplementary Materials for additional analyses.

These results suggest that there was no group dependent difference in how avatars were embodied and therefore a comparable level of bodily self-plasticity between AN and HC.

3.3. Body Dissatisfaction after Embodiment

A 2 × 2 × 3 ANOVA with Group (AN, HC) as between-and IMS (synchronous, asynchronous) and Avatar (−15%, 0%, +15%) as within-subjects factors showed no significant main or interaction effects (all Fs < 3.39, all ps > 0.073, all η2 < 0.065). Given that classical null hypothesis testing is not the ideal statistical tool for drawing conclusions about non-significant results [47,48], we also performed a Bayesian ANOVA which allows quantification of evidence in favor of the alternative or null hypothesis. The full model including main effects and the interaction between them provides evidence in favor of the null hypothesis ($BF_{10} = 8.131 \times 10^{-5}$), suggesting that embodiment of avatars of different body sizes did not change body dissatisfaction in AN and HC.

3.4. Emotional Response after Embodiment

The 2 × 2 × 3 ANOVA on the emotional ratings with the factors Group, IMS, and Avatar revealed a main effect of IMS (F (1,38) = 18.01, $p < 0.001$, η2 = 0.321), explained by more positive emotions following synchronous (59.44 ± 3.34) compared to the asynchronous (44.34 ± 2.93) IMS. The Avatar × Group interaction was also significant (F (2,76) = 7.21, $p < 0.001$, η2 = 0.159) (Figure 4) and shows that independently of the IMS, AN patients felt more negative emotions after being exposed to the +15% Avatar (44.71 ± 3.95) compared to the −15% Avatar (53.59 ± 4.50) ($p = 0.017$). The opposite trend was true for the HC who showed significantly more negative emotional response after being exposed to the −15% (50.02 ± 4.49) compared to the +15% (58.60 ± 3.95; $p = 0.020$) and marginally to the 0% Avatar (56.88 ± 3.99; $p = 0.057$). Finally, AN patients experienced more negative emotions to the +15% Avatar (44.71 ± 3.95) than HC (58.60 ± 3.95; $p = 0.040$). No other main or interaction effects were significant (all Fs < 3.73, all ps > 0.061). These results suggest that differently from the HC group, AN patients experienced negative emotions when they observed an avatar replacing their own body in space which reproduced a verisimilar increase in weight of 15%, with respect to the one that reproduced verisimilar decrease of weight of the same magnitude. This happened independently from the type of IMS used to induce the embodiment.

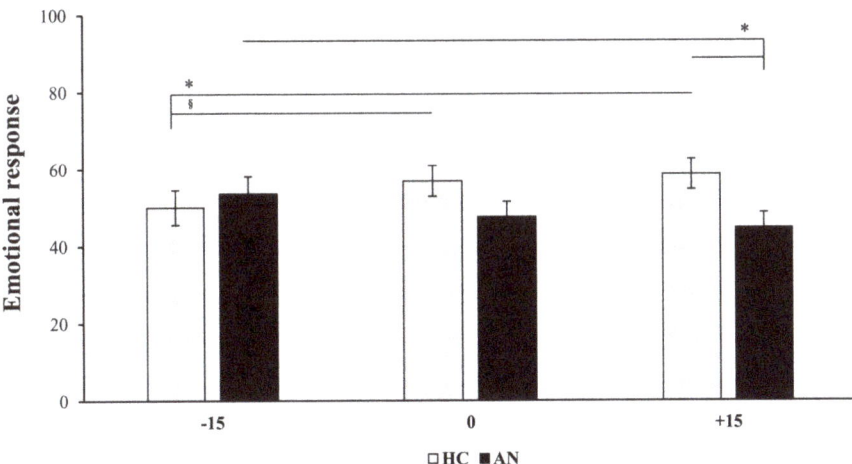

Figure 4. Emotional response after embodiment. Graph showing the effect of the interaction between avatar size (−15%; 0%; +15%) and group (healthy controls—HC; patients with anorexia nervosa—AN) on the emotional scale ranging from 0 (very negative emotions) to 100 (very positive emotions). Error bars represent standard error of mean. * = $p < 0.05$, § = marginally significant ($p = 0.057$).

3.5. Avatars' Similarity and Attractiveness Ratings

The 2 × 3 ANOVA with the factors Group and Avatar performed on the similarity ratings revealed a main effect of the Avatar (F (2,76) = 39.14, $p < 0.001$, η2 = 0.50): participants perceived the 0% (66.82 ± 3.26) and the +15% Avatar (69.37 ± 3.91) as more similar to their real body than the −15% Avatar (33.72 ± 4.52) (all ps < 0.001) (Figure 5, panel A). All the other main and interaction effects were not significant (all Fs < 0.59; all ps > 0.446). These results show that an increase in weight of 15% with respect to one's own perceived body size might pass unobserved in both patients and controls, while a loss of weight of similar magnitude is detected.

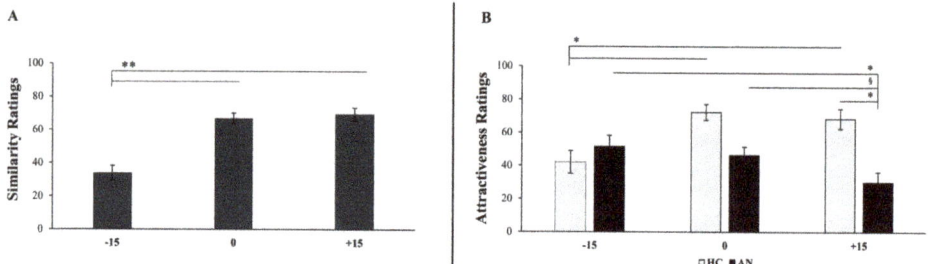

Figure 5. (**A**) Avatars' similarity ratings. Graph showing the main effect of Avatar size (−15%; 0%; +15%) on similarity ratings given during the observation of the avatars from a 1PP. (**B**) Avatars' attractiveness ratings. Graph showing the effect of the interaction between Avatar size (−15%; 0%; +15%) and Group (healthy controls, HC; patients with anorexia nervosa, AN) on attractiveness ratings given during the observation of the avatars from a 1PP. Error bars represent standard error of mean. ** = $p < 0.001$, * = $p < 0.05$, § = marginally significant, i.e., $p = 0.058$.

The same ANOVA performed on the attractiveness ratings revealed a main effect of Group (F (1,38) = 12.07, $p = 0.001$, η2 = 0.241). HC rated the avatars as more attractive than AN (60.87 ± 3.71 vs. 42.63, ± 3.71). The Avatar × Group interaction was also significant (F (2,76) = 9.47, $p < 0.001$, η2 = 0.119) (Figure 5, panel B). AN considered the +15% Avatar as the least attractive ((30.10 ± 5.99) vs. the −15% Avatar (51.45 ± 6.83; $p = 0.016$) and the 0% Avatar (46.35 ± 4.82; $p = 0.058$). HC instead considered the −15% Avatar as the least attractive ((42.00 ± 6.83) vs. the 0% Avatar (72.25 ± 4.82; $p < 0.001$) and +15% Avatar (68.35 ± 5.99; $p = 0.002$)). The main effect of Avatar was not significant (F (2,76) = 2.74, $p = 0.070$). These results show that a loss of 15% of body weight is associated in AN patients to an increase in body attractiveness with respect to the perceived body weight (even though marginally) and to a verisimilar gain of the same magnitude in body weight, while it results in a decrease in body attractiveness with respect to the same categories of virtual bodies in HC participants.

3.6. Correlations between +15% Avatar Emotional Response and Symptoms Severity

Finally, we tested, separately for each group, whether the emotions experienced with the exposure to the +15% Avatar (which was considered highly similar to the self and minimally attractive (Section 3.5)), was associated to self-reported body shape preoccupations, as indexed by the Body Shape Questionnaire (BSQ), and to the presence of abnormal body image concerns and eating behaviors, as indexed by the global severity index of the Body Uneasiness Test (BUT-GSI). We found that in AN patients, there was a significant correlation between the emotions experienced with the +15% Avatar and the strength of the concerns about the body shape (r = 0.62; $p = 0.004$; BF_{10}= 14.05). Also, the correlation between the emotions experienced with the +15% Avatar and the BUT-GIS was significant (r = 0.69; $p = 0.001$; BF_{10} = 37.07). These correlations therefore suggested that the higher the symptoms' severity was, the higher the negative emotional experience with the +15% Avatar (Figure 6, right panels). No significant correlation was found in the HC group (all rs < 0.05; all ps > 0.826; BFs_{10} < 0.283), Figure 6, left panels).

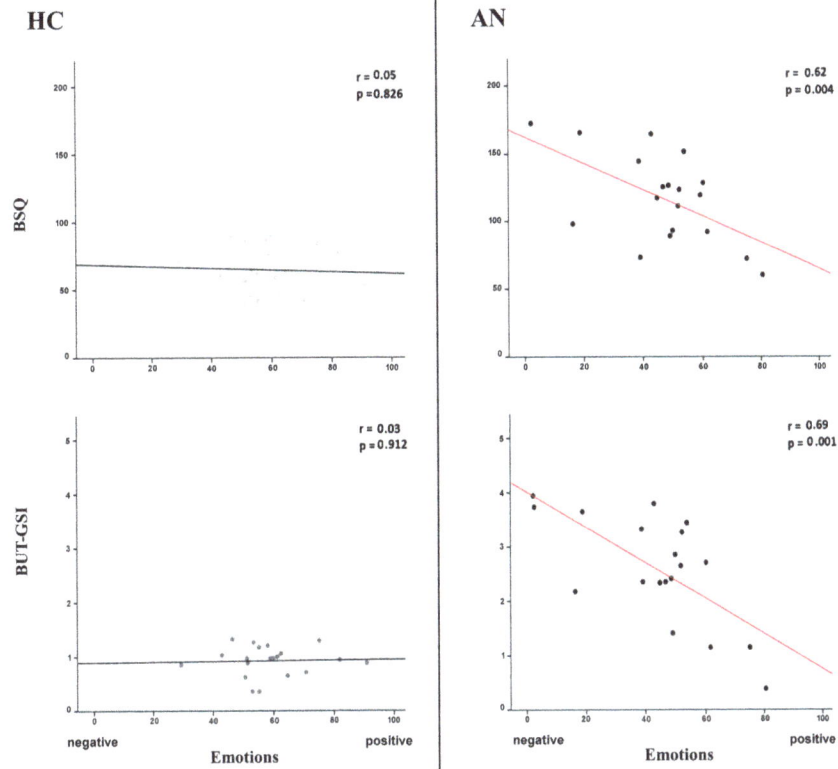

Figure 6. Correlations between +15% Avatar emotional response and symptoms severity. Scatterplots showing correlations between emotional changes after the exposure to the +15% Avatar and severity symptoms scores in the two groups. In the group of patient with anorexia nervosa (AN), the +15% Avatar emotional index correlated significantly with scores at the Body Shape Questionnaire (BSQ) and with the global severity index of the Body Uneasiness Test (BUT-GSI), while correlations were not significant in the healthy control (HC) group.

4. Discussion

We aimed to characterize, and eventually reduce, perceptual and cognitive-emotional components of body image distortion (BID) in AN using virtual bodies and embodiment illusion. To the best of our knowledge, only one study [49] investigated the body image in AN by: (i) using biometric self-avatars and (ii) reproducing the daily life experience of looking at oneself in the mirror. No studies instead coupled the creation of biometric self-avatars with multisensory bodily illusion paradigms.

Our results confirm that AN patients show higher body weight/shape concerns, drive for thinness (self-report questionnaires) and body dissatisfaction (perceptual minus ideal body size) compared to HC. However, body dissatisfaction in AN was not caused by a body overestimation, as suggested by previous literature [12]. Indeed, both AN patients and HC were accurate and did not differ in estimating the size of their real bodies, but AN patients desired a thinner body than HC. Although unexpected, these results are in line with a recent study [49] that adopted a virtual reality (VR) approach similar to the present one. Molbert and colleagues [49] measured body overestimation in AN by using a body scanner to create 3D avatars that faithfully reproduced participants' real body and then manipulated these avatars to reproduce weight gains and losses. Analogously to our findings, results from this study show that AN patients perceived their body similar to the HC but, differently from them, they desired a thinner body. Thus, all together these results support the idea that BID in AN is characterized by distorted attitudes concerning the desired body rather than by perceptual overestimation of the body size. Moreover, in agreement with the results of a recent meta-analysis [14], our findings also support the idea that estimation of one's own body size based on depictive methods (i.e., when participants estimate their body size by selecting a visual representation of their own body, like in this study) is less adapt to capture body size overestimation with respect to metric methods (i.e., when participants estimate their body size using quantifiable spatial estimations). This might be due to different features characterizing body representation that are targeted by these two types of methods. According to the body model proposed by Longo [50], the metric measures use both explicit and implicit knowledge of the body while the depictive measures, rely on explicit knowledge only, therefore they might be less automatic and more controllable.

The main aim of the present study was to investigate whether embodiment of differently sized avatars could reduce BID in AN. Therefore, we coupled virtual reality with a visuo-tactile IMS setup to induce embodiment of differently sized avatars, and measured embodiment strength and changes in perceptual and cognitive-emotional components of BID after embodiment induction. We adopted a controlled IMS procedure that differed from previous studies in several ways [15,28] and had the final aim of maximizing the congruence of virtual and real bodily signals. Thus we adopted both the 1PP and the head tracking during the synchronous IMS condition. This was particularly relevant in case of embodiment of bodies that patients might consider unattractive, as the ones reproducing their own weight and maximally in those reproducing a gain of 15% of this weight.

However, differently from [28], we used both synchronous and asynchronous IMS in order to disentangle the effects of embodiment and of observing the avatars from a 1PP. To this aim, we adopted a particular asynchronous control condition, in which we tried to maximize the incongruence between the virtual and real bodily signals. Indeed, the simple visuo-proprioceptive congruence between the real body and avatar's body given by presenting the avatars from a 1PP might result per-se in illusory feelings of ownership of the observed body. Thus, to reduce the possible occurrence of such illusory effects also in the asynchronous control condition, we applied spatio-temporal asynchronous touches as in [44,45]. Also, we locked the head tracking of the virtual camera (differently from [15]), to reduce the visuo-motor congruency between the self and the virtual body and further disrupt possible illusory embodiment in the control condition (see Section 2.4.3 of the methods for details). Instead of using the same avatar size for all participants [28], we created customized avatars, matching actual weight, height, and body parts' dimensions/shape and induced embodiment with the avatar reproducing participant's perceived body size/shape and avatars reproducing realistic loss and gain in weight of 15% with respect to the perceived weight.

Both explicit (scores at the embodiment questionnaire) and implicit (body temperature data) measures of the embodiment suggest that our synchronous visuo-tactile stimulation was effective in inducing higher embodiment compared to the asynchronous one. Specifically, the answers at the self-report questionnaire show higher ratings after the synchronous compared to the asynchronous visuo-tactile stimulation for all the three components of corporal awareness. Participants were more likely to: (i) feel that the avatar's body was their own one (Ownership), (ii) feel in control of its movements (Agency), and (iii) feel that the perceived touch was caused by the virtual one (Referral of Touch). These illusory sensations were independent of group and no interaction with the avatar size was found. Only for the Ownership component there was a main effect of the avatar size, with higher ratings attributed to the fatter avatars compared to both the 0% and the −15% avatar independently of group and type of IMS. Implicit measures of the embodiment mirror the explicit ones, as we found a change in body temperature between synchronous and asynchronous conditions independently of group and avatar size. However, the interpretation that this change in body temperature might be considered an implicit index of embodiment is currently highly debated in the literature [35] and we believe future studies are needed to clearly attribute the occurrence of such change to any evident factor (please see Supplementary Materials for a more detailed discussion on body temperature changes).

All in all, our measures on embodiment strength converge in showing that plasticity of body representation was similar in AN and HC. This result apparently contradicts previous literature which showed stronger bodily illusion for body parts (i.e., hands) in AN compared to HC participants [30]. It has been shown that bodily illusion negatively correlated with interoceptive abilities [29] and that higher bodily plasticity in AN plausibly results from altered multisensory integration of extero-and interocepetive signals [51]. In line with our results, HC and AN showed similar levels of embodiment of full bodies [31]. A conceivable reason for these contrasting results (rubber hand vs. full body illusion) might reside in the body part where touch is delivered. During the full body illusion touch is delivered to a highly salient and problematic body part for AN, i.e., the area around the abdomen. This may cause unpleasant sensations and negative emotions that in turn may dampen the embodiment in AN patients, making it similar to the level experienced by HC. Even though unpleasantness of the touch was not directly assessed in this study, AN patients anecdotally reported it.

An interesting finding of the present study is the fact that, independently of IMS type, AN patients showed more negative feelings after being exposed to the fatter avatar and that the strength of this effect correlated with clinical symptoms' severity. HC, instead, showed more negative emotional reactions toward the thinner avatar, which were unrelated to body concerns and eating disorder measures. This is even more interesting when considering how much the three differently sized avatars were retrospectively considered physically attractive and similar to the self. Both AN and HC participants rated the perceived and the fatter avatars as most similar to themselves (compared to the −15%). However, AN patients found them to be the least attractive (and the −15% as the maximally attractive), while HC rated them as the most attractive (and the −15% as the minimally attractive). Thus, anorexics reacted negatively to fatter avatars which were considered highly self-resembling and less attractive. These results mirror results from a previous study in HC who embodied obese avatars (BMI of 32.3) observed from 1PP [52]. This experience increased body dissatisfaction and negative emotional reactions, and at a neural level changed activity of anterior cingulate cortex and anterior insula. Such regions are known to mediate negative body-related emotional and affective experiences, such as pain and disgust [53,54]. While these results may shed light on negative emotions experienced by anorexics, it is worth noticing that we did not include obese avatars. The personalized avatars increased by 15% were still below the over-weight range, considering the average BMI (18.98) in HC. We would like to notice that both in the synchronous and in the asynchronous IMS blocks the avatars were presented in the 1PP. As we reported above, simple visuo-proprioceptive congruence (1PP) may induce some illusory feelings of embodiment even during asynchronous visuo-tactile stimulation. Even though we introduced spatio-temporal incongruent touches and motor discrepancy to get illusory sensations in the asynchronous condition as low as possible, it is possible that such sensations were able to trigger an emotional response as in the synchronous condition.

Importantly, contrary to our predictions embodiment of differently sized avatars did not significantly change participants' body dissatisfaction. This result stands in contrast with the results of a previous study by Preston and Ehrsson [28] conducted in HC only, which found that embodiment of a standardized slim body decreased body size perception and increased body satisfaction. Several differences may acknowledge for the discrepant results. Here, we measured body size perception with a task based on a visual representation of the body, i.e., participants had to estimate their body size on a customized avatar presented from a 3PP (body image). Instead, in the study by Preston and Ehrsson [28], perception of hip size was estimated by asking participants to indicate the distance on a ruler which reproduced their hip size in the absence of visual feedback (body schema). Participants were quite accurate in our body size estimation task, while participants in Preston and Ehrsson's study [28] overestimated the size of their hips. In line with the above-mentioned discussion about the effectiveness of metric vs. depictive measures in detecting body size overestimation, these contrasting results suggest that IMS might be able to change body schema more than body image.

Absence of changes in body dissatisfaction might also be explained from a theoretical point of view by considering differences between the egocentric frame of reference [55,56], i.e., body perceived from the 1PP based on its present state constituted by interoceptive and exteroceptive inputs, vs. the allocentric frame of reference, i.e., a somatic representation of the body as a 3PP based on beliefs and attitudes related to the body. According to the Allocentric Lock Theory [57], people with AN are locked in their allocentric representation of the body and are unable to update it through egocentric sensory inputs. Indeed, in our study participants experienced embodiment of avatars of different sizes from an egocentric frame of reference, whereas the estimation of real/ideal body size was performed from an allocentric frame of reference. We can speculate that, even if the embodiment of differently sized avatars could have been successful in affecting the body image as experienced from an egocentric frame of reference, the inability for the AN patients to update their allocentric representation of the body through egocentric sensory inputs might have led to no changes in body dissatisfaction induced by the embodiment.

Related to the point above, our results also let us speculate that observing one's own body from a 1PP (as it usually happens when we look down to our own body) or observing its reproduction from a 3PP (as it usually happens in front of a mirror, in pictures or videos) might bias our perception of its dimension. Indeed, when participants judge 3D reproduction of themselves without spatial or specular congruence with the self-body (as in the perceived body task), they are quite good at estimating their own body size. However, when they observe their own body by looking directly at it (as in similarity ratings task) they are more sensible to detect a loss than an increase in weight. Indeed, results from the similarity ratings show that an increase in weight of 15% with respect to one's own perceived body size might pass unobserved in both patients and controls, while a loss of weight of similar magnitude is detected. This shows an asymmetry in how weight loss and gain might be considered by our perceptual system that seems to be detectable only when the to-be-judged body replaces our own in space. Also, our results suggest that the above-mentioned perceptual asymmetry is probably due to how we affectively experience our own body. Indeed, loss of weight is associated in controls to a decrease in body attractiveness, while in anorexic patients it is associated to an increase in body attractiveness. An increase of 15% in body weight is instead considered as attractive as the perceived body weight, both in patients and controls. If we focus on patients only, our results also suggest that when dealing with the affective component of the body, it does not matter whether one's own body size is observed from a detached third-person perspective (ideal body task) or through directly looking at it (attractiveness ratings). One's own perceived body size seem to be considered less desirable and attractive than a simulated loss of weight of 15%. On the same line, the simulated illusory experience of a gain in one's own body weight is negatively experienced by anorexic patients, but not by controls (results from the emotional response task).

Overall, the present study suggests that the cognitive-emotional component of body image and not the perceptual one is severely altered in AN. Despite the inability to reduce body dissatisfaction in AN patients, our procedure was successful in inducing a strong embodiment of differently sized avatars, as measured at both the explicit and implicit level, and in enhancing negative emotional responses of anorexics to the fattest avatar which scaled with symptoms' severity.

Future research and clinical trials should aim at changing the distorted cognitive-emotional components of body image through the internalization of a normal weight body and the reduction of the emotional distress caused by weight gain, more than at changing the perceptual ones. Additionally, even if one should be cautious in using stimuli of enlarged bodies, virtual reality could be used to gradually expose and habituate AN patients to healthier versions of their bodies and to act as an intermediary step prior to the in vivo body image exposure, as some therapeutic protocols are already showing (see [58] for a review).

Supplementary Materials: The following are available online at http://www.mdpi.com/2077-0383/9/1/98/s1.

Author Contributions: G.P. and I.B. designed research; G.T. and M.M. implemented the virtual reality setup; L.P., S.C., I.B. and G.P. created the experimental stimuli; L.P. and S.C. collected and processed the experimental data; L.P., G.P., S.C., and I.B. analyzed data; F.D. and C.L. verified the diagnosis and provided clinical support to the anorexic patients; I.B. supervised the work. All authors discussed the results and commented on the manuscript. L.P., G.P. and I.B. wrote the manuscript, B.L. critically revised it. All authors have read and agreed to the published version of the manuscript.

Acknowledgments: We thank all participants who took part in this study. Particular thanks go to those with AN who, make research on AN possible. I.B. was funded by the Italian Ministry of Health (GR-2011-02351798). B.L. was supported by the Swiss National Science Foundation (nr. 170511), GP was supported "Progetti per Avvio alla Ricerca 2019", "Sapienza" University of Rome (Prot. Num. AR21916B890A9214) and SC was supported by "Progetti per Avvio alla Ricerca 2019", "Sapienza" University of Rome (Prot. Num. AR11916B88D6817C).

Conflicts of Interest: The authors report no financial or other relationship relevant to the subject of this article.

References

1. Gaudio, S.; Brooks, S.J.; Riva, G. Nonvisual multisensory impairment of body perception in anorexia nervosa: A systematic review of neuropsychological studies. *PLoS ONE* **2014**, *9*, e110087. [CrossRef] [PubMed]
2. Arcelus, J. Mortality Rates in Patients with Anorexia Nervosa and Other Eating Disorders. *Arch. Gen. Psychiatry* **2011**, *68*, 724. [CrossRef] [PubMed]
3. Cornelissen, K.K.; Bester, A.; Cairns, P.; Tovée, M.J.; Cornelissen, P.L. The influence of personal BMI on body size estimations and sensitivity to body size change in anorexia spectrum disorders. *Body Image* **2015**, *13*, 75–85. [CrossRef] [PubMed]
4. Farrell, C.; Lee, M.; Shafran, R. Assessment of body size estimation: A review. *Eur. Eat. Disord. Rev.* **2005**, *13*, 75–88. [CrossRef]
5. Urgesi, C.; Fornasari, L.; Canalaz, F.; Perini, L.; Cremaschi, S.; Faleschini, L.; Thyrion, E.Z.; Zuliani, M.; Balestrieri, M.; Fabbro, F.; et al. Impaired configural body processing in anorexia nervosa: Evidence from the body inversion effect. *Br. J. Psychol.* **2014**, *105*, 486–508. [CrossRef]
6. Cash, T.F. Body image: Past, present, and future. *Body Image* **2004**, *1*, 1–5. [CrossRef]
7. Peelen, M.V.; Downing, P.E. The neural basis of visual body perception. *Nat. Rev. Neurosci.* **2007**, *8*, 636–648. [CrossRef]
8. Gandolfo, M.; Downing, P.E. Causal Evidence for Expression of Perceptual Expectations in Category-Selective Extrastriate Regions. *Curr. Biol.* **2019**, *29*, 1–5. [CrossRef]
9. Moreau, Q.; Pavone, E.F.; Aglioti, S.M.; Candidi, M. Theta synchronization over occipito-temporal cortices during visual perception of body parts. *Eur. J. Neurosci.* **2018**, *48*, 2826–2835. [CrossRef]
10. Moreau, Q.; Parrotta, E.; Era, V.; Martelli, M.; Candidi, M. Role of the occipito-temporal Theta rhythm in hand visual identification. *J. Neurophysiol.* **2019**. [Epub ahead of print]. [CrossRef]
11. Cash, T.F.; Deagle, E.A. The nature and extent of body-image disturbances in anorexia nervosa and bulimia nervosa: A meta-analysis. *Int. J. Eat. Disord.* **1997**, *22*, 107–125. [CrossRef]
12. Gardner, R.M.; Brown, D.L. Body size estimation in anorexia nervosa: A brief review of findings from 2003 through 2013. *Psychiatry Res.* **2014**, *219*, 407–410. [CrossRef] [PubMed]
13. Keel, P.K.; Dorer, D.J.; Franko, D.L.; Jackson, S.C.; Herzog, D.B. Postremission predictors of relapse in women with eating disorders. *Am. J. Psychiatry* **2005**, *162*, 1–6. [CrossRef] [PubMed]
14. Mölbert, S.C.; Klein, L.; Thaler, A.; Mohler, B.J.; Brozzo, C.; Martus, P.; Karnath, H.O.; Zipfel, S.; Giel, K.E. Depictive and metric body size estimation in anorexia nervosa and bulimia nervosa: A systematic review and meta-analysis. *Clin. Psychol. Rev.* **2017**, *57*, 21–31. [CrossRef] [PubMed]
15. Piryankova, I.V.; Wong, H.Y.; Linkenauger, S.A.; Stinson, C.; Longo, M.R.; Bülthoff, H.H.; Mohler, B.J. Owning an overweight or underweight body: Distinguishing the physical, experienced and virtual body. *PLoS ONE* **2014**, *9*, e103428. [CrossRef] [PubMed]
16. Berlucchi, G.; Aglioti, S.M. The body in the brain revisited. *Exp. Brain Res.* **2010**, *200*, 25–35. [CrossRef] [PubMed]
17. Porciello, G.; Bufalari, I.; Minio-Paluello, I.; Di Pace, E.; Aglioti, S.M. The 'Enfacement' illusion: A window on the plasticity of the self. *Cortex* **2018**, *104*, 261–275. [CrossRef]
18. Botvinick, M.; Cohen, J. Rubber hands "feel" touch that eyes see. *Nature* **1998**, *391*, 756. [CrossRef]

19. Lenggenhager, B.; Tadi, T.; Metzinger, T.; Blanke, O. Video ergo sum: Manipulating bodily self-consciousness. *Science* **2007**, *317*, 1096–1099. [CrossRef]
20. Sforza, A.; Bufalari, I.; Haggard, P.; Aglioti, S.M. My face in yours: Visuo-tactile facial stimulation influences sense of identity. *Soc. Neurosci.* **2010**, *5*, 148–162. [CrossRef]
21. Bufalari, I.; Sforza, A.L.; Di Russo, F.; Mannetti, L.; Aglioti, S.M. Malleability of the self: Electrophysiological correlates of the enfacement illusion. *Sci. Rep.* **2019**, *9*, 1–14. [CrossRef] [PubMed]
22. Fusaro, M.; Tieri, G.; Aglioti, S. Influence of cognitive stance and physical perspective on subjective and autonomic reactivity to observed pain and pleasure: An immersive virtual reality study. *Conscious. Cogn.* **2019**, *67*, 86–97. [CrossRef] [PubMed]
23. Porciello, G.; Holmes, B.S.; Liuzza, M.T.; Crostella, F.; Aglioti, S.M.; Bufalari, I. Interpersonal Multisensory Stimulation reduces the overwhelming distracting power of self-gaze. *Sci. Rep.* **2014**, *4*, 6669. [CrossRef] [PubMed]
24. Mino-Paluello, I.; Porciello, G.; Gandolfo, M.; Boukarras, S.; Aglioti, S.M. The Enfacement illusion boosts facial mimicry. *Cortex* **2019**, *123*, 113–123. [CrossRef] [PubMed]
25. Maselli, A.; Slater, M. The building blocks of the full body ownership illusion. *Front. Hum. Neurosci.* **2013**, *7*, 1–15. [CrossRef] [PubMed]
26. Van der Hoort, B.; Guterstam, A.; Ehrsson, H.H. Being barbie: The size of one's own body determines the perceived size of the world. *PLoS ONE* **2011**, *6*, e20195. [CrossRef]
27. Normand, J.M.; Giannopoulos, E.; Spanlang, B.; Slater, M. Multisensory stimulation can induce an illusion of larger belly size in immersive virtual reality. *PLoS ONE* **2011**, *6*, e16128. [CrossRef]
28. Preston, C.; Ehrsson, H.H. Illusory changes in body size modulate body satisfaction in a way that is related to non-clinical eating disorder psychopathology. *PLoS ONE* **2014**, *9*, e85773. [CrossRef]
29. Eshkevari, E.; Rieger, E.; Longo, M.R.; Haggard, P.; Treasure, J. Increased plasticity of the bodily self in eating disorders. *Psychol. Med.* **2012**, *42*, 819–828. [CrossRef]
30. Keizer, A.; Smeets, M.A.M.; Postma, A.; van Elburg, A.; Dijkerman, H.C. Does the experience of ownership over a rubber hand change body size perception in anorexia nervosa patients? *Neuropsychologia* **2014**, *62*, 26–37. [CrossRef]
31. Keizer, A.; Van Elburg, A.; Helms, R.; Dijkerman, H.C. A virtual reality full body illusion improves body image disturbance in anorexia nervosa. *PLoS ONE* **2016**, *11*, e0163921. [CrossRef] [PubMed]
32. Sepúlveda, A.R.; Botella, J.; León, J.A. Body-image disturbance in eating disorders: A meta-analysis. *Psychol. Spain* **2002**, *6*, 83–95.
33. Tieri, G.; Tidoni, E.; Pavone, E.F.; Aglioti, S.M. Body visual discontinuity affects feeling of ownership and skin conductance responses. *Sci. Rep.* **2015**, *5*, 17139. [CrossRef] [PubMed]
34. Tieri, G.; Gioia, A.; Scandola, M.; Pavone, E.F.; Aglioti, S.M. Visual appearance of a virtual upper limb modulates the temperature of the real hand: A thermal imaging study in Immersive Virtual Reality. *Eur. J. Neurosci.* **2017**, *45*, 1141–1151. [CrossRef] [PubMed]
35. De Haan, A.M.; Van Stralen, H.E.; Smit, M.; Keizer, A.; Van der Stigchel, S.; Dijkerman, H.C. No consistent cooling of the real hand in the rubber hand illusion. *Acta Psychol. (Amst.)* **2017**, *179*, 68–77. [CrossRef] [PubMed]
36. Mohr, H.M.; Röder, C.; Zimmermann, J.; Hummel, D.; Negele, A.; Grabhorn, R. Body image distortions in bulimia nervosa: Investigating body size overestimation and body size satisfaction by fMRI. *Neuroimage* **2011**, *56*, 1822–1831. [CrossRef]
37. American Psychiatric Association. *Diagnostic and Statistical Manual of Mental Disorder*, 5th ed.; American Psychiatric Association: Arlington, VA, USA, 2013.
38. Garner, D. *Eating Disorder Inventory-2: Professional Manual*; Psychological Assessment Resources Inc: Odessa, Finland, 1991.
39. Cooper, P.; Taylor, M.; Sc, B.; Cooper, Z.; Fairburn, C.G. The Development and Validation of the Body Shape Questionnaire. *Int. J. Eat. Disord.* **1987**, *6*, 485–494. [CrossRef]
40. Cuzzolaro, M.; Vetrone, G.; Marano, G.; Garfinkel, P.E. The Body Uneasiness Test (BUT): Development and validation of a new body image assessment scale. *Eat. Weight Disord.* **2006**, *11*, 1–13. [CrossRef]
41. Henderson, M.; Freeman, C.P.L. A Self-rating Scale for Bulimia the "BITE". *Br. J. Psychiatry* **1987**, *150*, 18–24. [CrossRef]

42. Derogatis, L.R. *Symptom Checklist-90-R: Administration, Scoring & Procedure Manual for the Revised Version of the SCL-90*; National Computer Systems: Minneapolis, MN, USA, 1994.
43. Slater, M.; Spanlang, B.; Sanchez-Vives, M.V.; Blanke, O. First person experience of body transfer in virtual reality. *PLoS ONE* **2010**, *5*, e10564. [CrossRef]
44. Apps, M.A.J.; Tsakiris, M. The free-energy self: A predictive coding account of self-recognition. *Neurosci. Biobehav. Rev.* **2014**, *44*, 85–97. [CrossRef] [PubMed]
45. Bufalari, I.; Lenggenhager, B.; Porciello, G.; Holmes, B.S.; Aglioti, S.M. Enfacing others but only if they are nice to you. *Front. Behav. Neurosci.* **2014**, *8*, 1–12. [CrossRef] [PubMed]
46. Love, J.; Selker, R.; Marsman, M.; Jamil, T.; Dropmann, D.; Verhagen, J.; Ly, A.; Gronau, Q.F.; Šmíra, M.; Epskamp, S.; et al. JASP: Graphical statistical software for common statistical designs. *J. Stat. Softw.* **2019**, *88*, 1–17. [CrossRef]
47. Dienes, Z. Using Bayes to get the most out of non-significant results. *Front. Psychol.* **2014**, *5*, 1–17. [CrossRef] [PubMed]
48. Dienes, Z. How Bayes factors change scientific practice. *J. Math. Psychol.* **2016**, *72*, 78–89. [CrossRef]
49. Mölbert, S.C.; Thaler, A.; Mohler, B.J.; Streuber, S.; Romero, J.; Black, M.J.; Zipfel, S.; Karnath, H.O.; Giel, K.E. Assessing body image in anorexia nervosa using biometric self-avatars in virtual reality: Attitudinal components rather than visual body size estimation are distorted. *Psychol. Med.* **2017**, *48*, 1–12. [CrossRef]
50. Longo, M.R. *Perceptual and Emotional Embodiment: Foundations of Embodied Cognition Volume 1*; Routledge: London, UK, 2015.
51. Pollatos, O.; Kurz, A.L.; Albrecht, J.; Schreder, T.; Kleemann, A.M.; Schöpf, V.; Kopietz, R.; Wiesmann, M.; Schandry, R. Reduced perception of bodily signals in anorexia nervosa. *Eat. Behav.* **2008**, *9*, 381–388. [CrossRef]
52. Preston, C.; Ehrsson, H.H. Illusory obesity triggers body dissatisfaction responses in the insula and anterior cingulate cortex. *Cereb. Cortex* **2016**, *26*, 4450–4460. [CrossRef]
53. Jabbi, M.; Bastiaansen, J.; Keysers, C. A Common Anterior Insula Representation of Disgust Observation, Experience and Imagination Shows Divergent Functional Connectivity Pathways. *PLoS ONE* **2008**, *3*, e2939. [CrossRef]
54. Wiech, K.; Lin, C.; Brodersen, K.H.; Bingel, U.; Ploner, M.; Tracey, I. Anterior Insula Integrates Information about Salience into Perceptual Decisions about Pain. *J. Neurosci.* **2010**, *30*, 16324–16331. [CrossRef]
55. Galati, G.; Lobel, E.; Vallar, G.; Berthoz, A.; Pizzamiglio, L.; Le Bihan, D. The neural basis of egocentric and allocentric coding of space in humans: A functional magnetic resonance study. *Exp. Brain Res.* **2000**, *133*, 156–164. [CrossRef] [PubMed]
56. Haggard, P.; Longo, M.R.; Aza, E. More than skin deep: Body representation beyond primary somatosensory cortex. *Neuropsychologia* **2010**, *48*, 655–668.
57. Riva, G. Neuroscience and eating disorders: The allocentric lock hypothesis. *Med. Hypotheses* **2012**, *78*, 254–257. [CrossRef] [PubMed]
58. Koskina, A.; Campbell, I.C.; Schmidt, U. Reviews Exposure therapy in eating disorders revisited. *Neurosci. Biobehav. Rev.* **2013**, *37*, 193–208. [CrossRef] [PubMed]

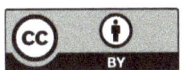

© 2019 by the authors. Licensee MDPI, Basel, Switzerland. This article is an open access article distributed under the terms and conditions of the Creative Commons Attribution (CC BY) license (http://creativecommons.org/licenses/by/4.0/).

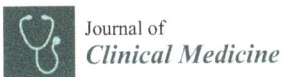

Article

UnReal? Investigating the Sense of Reality and Psychotic Symptoms with Virtual Reality

Gad Drori [1,*], Paz Bar-Tal [1], Yonatan Stern [1,2], Yair Zvilichovsky [1] and Roy Salomon [1]

[1] Gonda Brain Research Center, Bar-Ilan University, Ramat Gan 5290002, Israel; bartalpaz@gmail.com (P.B.-T.); yoniastern@gmail.com (Y.S.); zvilich@gmail.com (Y.Z.); roy.salomon@biu.ac.il (R.S.)
[2] Psychology Department, University of Haifa, Haifa 3498838, Israel
* Correspondence: gadidrori@gmail.com

Received: 15 April 2020; Accepted: 20 May 2020; Published: 28 May 2020

Abstract: Distortions of reality, such as hallucinations, are common symptoms of many psychiatric conditions. Accordingly, sense of reality (SoR), the ability to discriminate between true and false perceptions, is a central criterion in the assessment of neurological and psychiatric health. Despite the critical role of the SoR in daily life, little is known about how this is formed in the mind. Here, we propose a novel theoretical and methodological framework to study the SoR and its relation to psychotic symptoms. In two experiments, we employed a specialized immersive virtual reality (VR) environment allowing for well-controlled manipulations of visual reality. We first tested the impact of manipulating visual reality on objective perceptual thresholds (just noticeable differences). In a second experiment, we tested how these manipulations affected subjective judgments of reality. The results revealed that the objective perceptual thresholds were robust and replicable, demonstrating that SoR is a stable psychometric property that can be measured experimentally. Furthermore, reality alterations reduced subjective reality judgments across all manipulated visual aspects. Finally, reduced sensitivity to changes in visual reality was related to self-reported prodromal psychotic symptoms. These results provide evidence for the relevance of SoR in the assessment of psychosis and other mental disorders in which reality is distorted.

Keywords: sense of reality; virtual reality; hallucinations; psychosis; derealization

1. Introduction

1.1. Sense of Reality

We normally and intuitively trust our sensory representation of the world to closely correspond to what "is really there" [1,2]. We term this correspondence "reality", and differentiate it from other states in which our representations of the world do not match the environment, such as dreaming and hallucinations. Intriguingly, we seem to possess a capacity to judge whether our sensory experience corresponds to the world or not, i.e., a sense of reality (SoR). This capacity is a critical aspect of the human mind, allowing us to guide our actions based on meaningful sensory signals. Abnormal SoR processing may lead to a disparity between experience and reality, resulting in hallucinations (false perceptions), which is a core symptom of psychosis. However, while SoR is an important criterion in the assessment of neurological and psychiatric health [3–5], we know little regarding its underlying cognitive mechanisms.

Previous work has focused on the mechanisms allowing the separation of internally and externally generated information in memory (i.e., source monitoring) (e.g., [6,7]). Source monitoring paradigms typically evaluate the ability to remember the source of a stimuli (e.g., was this word previously seen or imagined?) (e.g., [8]). This research has been based on the proposition that hallucinations are grounded in failures to discriminate the source of the information correctly (i.e., perception vs. imagery or memory). Thus, while the discrimination of imagery, perception, and memory has been studied extensively (e.g., [5,9,10]), the ability to discriminate between real and false perceptions in real time (i.e., perceptual reality monitoring) is poorly understood. This discrimination is essential as distortions of perceptual reality in the form of hallucinations or illusions originating from neurological, psychiatric, pharmacological, medical, or psychological origins are commonplace [11,12]. Despite the importance of this issue, there is scarce knowledge regarding 'how do we decide what is real?', or in other words, 'how do we form a SoR?'

1.2. A Theoretical Framework of SoR

There is growing evidence that perception is an inferential process [13–15]. For instance, "predictive coding" frameworks suggest that perception arises through a process of inferences (*predictions*) about the likely causes of sensory information (i.e., *likelihood*). These *predictions* are based on previous experience, through which higher levels in the hierarchy attempt to predict the signals arising from the lower levels [14,16,17]. When an unusual sensory event (e.g., a pink elephant) violates predictions, a *prediction error* arises and propagates through the hierarchy until it is either "predicted away" at higher levels (e.g., I'm wearing pink glasses) or the generative model is updated (e.g., pink elephants exist) [15,18]. Perception is thus a process of inference based on our experientially acquired model of the world. Therefore, we suggest that SoR can be viewed as a probabilistic inference based on the magnitude of prediction errors expressing the fit between a given sensory signal and our model of the world [19,20]. For a given sensory event, the magnitude of the prediction error is the probability of the perception being "real" in light of one's model of the world. Thus, viewing a "pink elephant" could be taken as a veridical perception, an optical aberration, or a hallucination, based on one's model of the world.

1.3. Failures of SoR as a Conceptual Framework

Hallucinations (i.e., false perceptions) are a perplexing symptom of many psychiatric and neurological disorders. Advances in neuroscience and computational psychiatry relate hallucinations to breakdowns of predictive processes [20–22]. For example, overreliance on predictions, favoring prior expectations over sensory evidence, may lead to hallucinations [21,23,24]. On the other hand, the overweighting of sensory signals and deficient predictive processes, enabling the structuring of experience, may cause a sense of alienation from one's own actions and thoughts, causing passivity symptoms [25–27].

Intriguingly, hallucinations can be experienced with or without insight into their nature as false perceptions. For example, patients with Charles Bonnet syndrome experience complex hallucinations yet typically identify these as hallucinations [28]. Contrarily, psychotic patients often lose the ability to discern between real and hallucinatory percepts, which has been linked to poorer prognosis [29] and reduced cognitive abilities [30,31]. Thus, psychiatric hallucinations and pseudo-hallucinations include a sensory aspect (i.e., unusual or non-veridical perceptual experience) and a metacognitive aspect related to insight (i.e., assessment of the validity of the perceptual experience). Indeed, depersonalization and derealization syndromes found in several psychiatric conditions produce a sense of "unrealness" in the absence of hallucinations, suggesting a deficit in SoR without the aberrant perceptual experience [32,33]. Thus, failures of the sense of reality leading to hallucinations, depersonalization, and derealization may be driven by either abnormal prediction error signaling impacting bottom-up sensory processing, or top-down predictions affecting the subjective experience of "unrealness", or a combination of these two. Critically, psychosis typically presents both abnormal sensory experiences as well as diminished insight regarding the implausibility of these experiences. These various manifestations of psychopathology highlight the need for a better understanding of the different components of SoR.

1.4. Modeling SoR Using Virtual Reality

SoR was previously challenging to test experimentally as visual manipulations of reality were limited to specific instances, such as prism glasses or still image manipulations (e.g., [34,35]). Here, we developed and tested a novel ecological approach to the study of the SoR, using immersive virtual reality (VR). Virtual reality is now widely employed in scientific studies [36,37] and can be used to manipulate variables that could not otherwise be manipulated (e.g., [38,39]). We created a realistic immersive environment (*UnReal*, Figure 1) in which we can manipulate different visual aspects of reality, creating hallucination like visual stimuli. Importantly, the virtual reality environment allows us to parametrically manipulate such aspects, enabling us to alter reality slightly or massively. For example, we can reduce the height of the participants' first person viewpoint on the world (*shrink* condition) or increase it (*grow* condition), inducing experiences of changes of *self*, which occur in hallucinatory states (e.g., *Alice in Wonderland* syndrome [40]). Furthermore, we can also induce minute changes, which are barely noticeable by the participants, thus resembling derealization-like states.

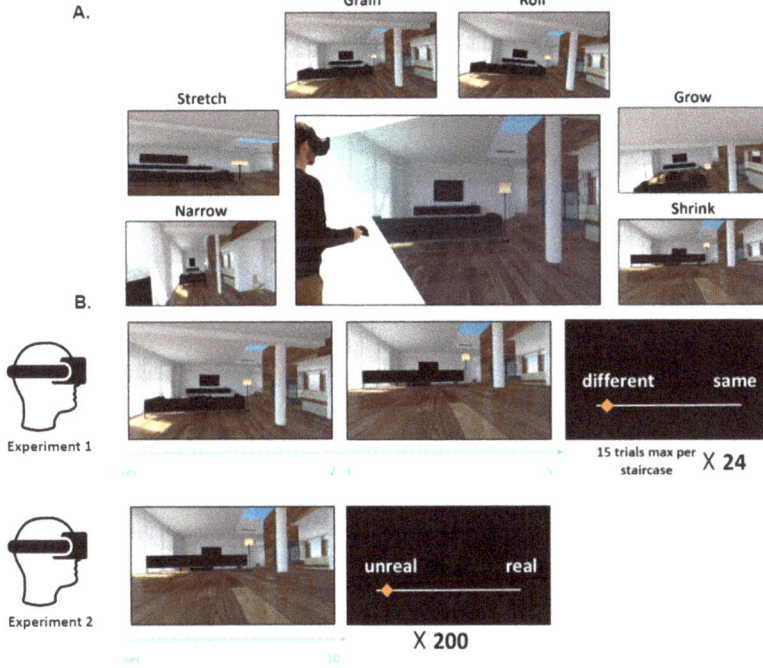

Figure 1. Experimental setup and design. (**A**) Center, illustrative image of the experimental setup and visual scenario. Participants donned a head-mounted display (HMD) and viewed the immersive virtual environment in 360° around them. The images on the sides and bottom represent the six types of alterations of the visual aspects employed, at the highest magnitude of alteration shown, for comparison, on a similar section of the virtual room. (**B**) Trial flow for the experiments. (Top) In Experiment 1, a virtual reality (VR) environment appeared for 2 s, followed by a black screen and then a second VR environment. Subsequently, participants were presented a question screen asking them to report if the two VR environments were identical or not. (Bottom). In Experiment 2, participants viewed a VR environment, which could be altered or unaltered. In each trial, they were required to judge on a continuous scale how 'real' the environment felt to them.

We selected several aspects of reality to be examined in this project, based on the phenomenology of distorted visual reality as found in psychiatric, neurological, medical, and pharmacological states [11,12,41]. These alterations of reality broadly fall into three domains: (1) *Perceptual* changes, in which the visual appearance (e.g., graininess) of the scene is manipulated; (2) laws of *nature*, in which we manipulate the visual aspects of the laws of nature (e.g., stretching of the physical world); and (3) changes of *self*, in which we manipulate the participants' sense of self through conflicts between visual signals and self-related information (e.g., changes in the first person perspective). Alterations of reality in these domains are hallmarks of the phenomenology of hallucinations in psychedelic, neurological, and psychiatric states [42–44].

1.5. The Present Study: Goals and Predictions

We report the results of two experiments investigating SoR and psychotic symptoms using immersive VR. In experiment 1, we tested the objective psychophysical sensitivity of participants to such alterations by measuring the just noticeable differences (JNDs) between altered and unaltered environments and how these are related to self-reported psychosis symptoms. In experiment 2, we tested the impact of these alterations on the subjective experience of participants, by having them make explicit reality judgments. We hypothesized that psychophysical measures of sensory processing (JNDs) would be stable within participants (low within-subject variance), demonstrating that SoR exhibits robust psychometric properties. Furthermore, we examined whether these measures of SoR are correlated to self-reported prodromal psychotic symptoms, especially for manipulations of the self that are known to be linked to schizophrenia spectrum psychosis [25,27,45]. Finally, we hypothesized that alterations of reality would consistently reduce subjective reality judgments, and this decrease will be related to the magnitude of alteration. Thus, by creating hallucination-like sensory experiences in virtual reality, we examined the impact of parametric induction of distortions on objective and subjective measures of SoR.

2. Methods

2.1. Participants

Thirty healthy participants took part in two experiments: Fifteen participated in experiment 1 (10 women, mean age 24.8 years, SD = 4.3 years) and 15 in experiment 2 (6 women, mean age 26.6 years, SD = 3.8 years). All of them were naïve to the purpose of the experiment, had normal or corrected-to-normal vision, and no self-reported psychiatric or neurological history. All participants gave written informed consent and received payment for their participation (40–50 NIS/~$15 US). The study was performed in accordance with the ethical standards of the Declaration of Helsinki, and the ethics committee of the Gonda Multidisciplinary Brain Research Center approved the experimental protocols.

2.2. Hardware

Both experiments were performed on an Intel core i7 processor and 32 GB of RAM computer running in-house software (*UnReal*, built using Unity 2018.3.2). The participants wore a head-mounted display (HMD-HTC Vive) during the experiment. Motion tracking was performed using the HTC VIVE (1.0) system. Subjects responded using the HTC VIVE touch sensitive controller (all VR hardware was manufactured by Valve Corp., Washington, DC, USA).

2.3. Experimental Design

To test the SoR experimentally, we constructed an immersive virtual environment in which we could experimentally manipulate different aspects of reality in a highly controlled fashion (*UnReal*). Here, we used an indoor variant of the *UnReal* environment modeled as an apartment with a high polygon and realistic appearance. The environment contained numerous objects and furniture as well as an animated cat (see Figure 1A for example). The participants were positioned at the center of the room, and observed the environment in 360° from a stationary point. We used a within-subject design in which all participants in each experiment underwent the same experimental protocol.

2.4. Virtual Environment

Unity 2018.3.2 was used to construct an environment that would reflect a normative space. The use of a Polybox's Lounge & Kitchen Pack Asset from Unity Asset Store Environment with real depth and width processing was selected, and additional furniture and accessories were added to make the room realistic. The room's width, length, and height were 13.2, 24.7, and 3.36, respectively, in the Unity unit system. The camera position was ~8.5 from the right wall when the camera was facing the TV, and 11.5 units from the TV itself.

2.5. Alterations of Reality

In order to test the impact of altered reality, we took advantage of the possibilities of VR to induce specific and well-controlled alterations of different aspects of visual reality. Specifically, we manipulated three domains of reality using six aspects (Figure 1A). (1) In the perceptual domain, we manipulated: (a) Graininess of the visual display (*grain*), and (b) the degree of the tilt of the virtual space (*roll*); (2) in the laws of nature domain: (c) Stretching and (d) narrowing of the width dimension of the virtual space (*stretch* and *narrow*); and (3) in the self domain: (e) Elevating and (f) lowering the participants' first person perspective (*grow* and *shrink*). As mentioned above, these specific alterations were selected based on the phenomenology of distorted visual reality as found in psychiatric, neurological, medical, and pharmacological states and their applicability within immersive virtual reality (see Supplementary Material and Figure S1 for technical details of the implementation of the alterations).

2.6. Experiment 1: Psychophysics of Virtually Altered Reality

2.6.1. Experimental Procedure

To assess SoR, in each trial, participants were successively immersed in two virtual environments (2-s duration each), with a black screen displayed (1-s duration) between them (Figure 1B). Critically, the two environments were identical except that one of the environments included an alteration in one of the aspects of reality mentioned above, whereas the other environment was unaltered. Participants then judged whether the environments were 'different' or 'same' in a classic psychophysics two-alternative forced choice (2AFC) paradigm. We employed a 1-up/ 2-down staircase procedure [46] to derive the JND for each of the aspects of reality. After each response, the alteration level either increased (if the participant judged environments as identical) or decreased (if the participant judged environments as different), by 40% of the current alteration. There were 6 such staircase procedures (one for each condition), which appeared four times each, thus totaling in 24 randomly intermingled staircases each containing only one type of alteration.

Preceding the experimental task, participants were instructed regarding the use of the VR system, the response controllers, as well as the course of the experiment. Then, they performed a training session in which they were acclimated to the VR environment, the experimental task, and response controllers, which lasted until they reported acclimation to the task (26 trials max). To avoid VR motion sickness effects [47], they were instructed to report any discomfort and could stop the experiment at any stage.

2.6.2. Questionnaires

Following task completion, participants completed two self-report questionnaires. The *Cardiff Anomalous Perceptions Scale* (CAPS) and the *Prodromal Questionnaire Brief Version* (PQ-B). The CAPS is a 32-item validated and reliable questionnaire of perceptual anomalies, with subscales of distress, intrusiveness, and frequency of anomalous perceptual experiences [48,49]. The PQ-B primarily serves as an initial screener questionnaire for prodromal or early psychotic symptoms. The PQ-B examines the existence of thoughts and experiences that describe cardinal symptoms of psychosis, such as suspicion, grandiosity, disorganized communication, unconventional thinking, disruptions in perception, difficulties in social functioning, and difficulties in academic or occupational functioning [50,51].

2.7. Experiment 2: Subjective Assessment of Virtually Altered Reality

Experimental Procedure

Experiment 2 examined the effects of altered reality on participants' subjective phenomenological experience of reality. In each trial, participants were placed in the center of the virtual environment and instructed to explore it in 360° degrees while standing in one spot. To ensure exploration, they were instructed to search for a target object (a teddy bear). Each trial lasted 10 s or until participants found the object, after which the room disappeared, and the response screen appeared. Participants provided a subjective rating of how 'real' or 'unreal' the environment felt on a continuous scale of 0–100 (Figure 1B). Each participant performed 200 trials. Sixty trials displayed the environment without alteration, while 140 trials included an alteration of reality in one of the aspects manipulated in experiment 1. Importantly, in each trial, only a single aspect of reality was manipulated. For each aspect of reality, there were four magnitudes of alteration (Supplementary Material Figure S1), which were identical across participants and whose values were based on a pilot study. Each magnitude for each aspect occurred five times, and the order was pseudo-randomized.

Similar to experiment 1, participants were first instructed regarding the use of the VR system, the response controller, and exposed to the environment and equipment until they felt comfortable. Then, they performed a training block of 15 trials, which were excluded from analysis, which included 3 trials with a large change in reality, 2 with mid-level magnitudes of alterations, and 10 with no alterations to practice responses.

2.8. Data Analysis

2.8.1. Experiment 1

Data was processed using in-house Matlab scripts [52]. Statistical analyses were done using JASP 0.11 [53]. To calculate JNDs, for each participant, we averaged the last five trials of each staircase to compute the mean parameter values that the staircase converged on. For each aspect of alteration, these JND values were used to calculate the variance and mean of the JNDs per condition, across the staircase procedures. Conditions with negative numerical scales (e.g., shrink, narrow) were converted to absolute values so that all JNDs represented the absolute distance from zero (i.e., from the unaltered condition). It should be noted that comparison across aspect ratings in both experiments was meaningful only for pairs of aspects that shared a similar scale. Therefore, *grow* and *shrink* JNDs were compared using a paired t-test and null effects were assessed using the Bayesian paired t-test, while the remaining aspects could not be directly compared. The within-subject variance of the JNDs in each aspect was calculated across the four staircases. The rate of convergence for each aspect was calculated by averaging the number of steps it took in each staircase until convergence. Pearson's r was used to test for correlations between JNDs across the different aspects. Spearman's Rho was used to test for correlations between JNDs and the CAPS and PQ-B questionnaires.

2.8.2. Experiment 2

The subjective ratings of reality in experiment 2 were averaged across participants for each magnitude of manipulation and each aspect separately. These mean values were then used for observing the change in reality ratings across ascending levels of reality manipulations in a repeated measures ANOVA (where normality was violated, a non-parametric Friedman test was performed and Greenhouse–Geisser corrections were applied when required). Pearson's r was used to test for correlations between subjective ratings of reality across aspects. Where possible, we compared subjective judgments using a paired t-test on the difference between the *real* and first level of alteration (which corresponded to the largest reduction in subjective judgements).

3. Results

3.1. Experiment 1

The average JNDs and their within-subject variance can be seen in Table 1 (see Table S3 for full descriptive statistics).

Table 1. Descriptive statistics for experiment 1.

	JND					
	Narrow	Stretch	Shrink	Grow	Roll	Grain
Mean	0.09	0.12	0.04	0.05	2.57	0.01
Std. Deviation	0.06	0.06	0.03	0.03	2.37	0.05
Minimum	0.04	0.07	0.01	0.01	0.31	0.03
Maximum	0.24	0.29	0.12	0.12	9.5	0.19
	Within-Subject Variability					
	Narrow	Stretch	Shrink	Grow	Roll	Grain
Mean	0.003	0.004	0.001	8.0e-4	0.93	0.002
Std. Deviation	0.003	0.009	0.002	0.002	1.05	0.003
Minimum	0	0	0	0	0.003	0
Maximum	0.008	0.04	0.007	0.006	3.92	0.01
	Convergence Rate					
	Narrow	Stretch	Shrink	Grow	Roll	Grain
Mean	5.99	8.73	7.03	6.57	5.74	6.76
Std. Deviation	1.47	0.91	1.6	1.98	2.23	1.76
Minimum	3	7	4	3	1	4
Maximum	9	10	9.5	9.75	10	10

Overall, participants showed very stable JNDs with little within-subject variability. For example, the average JND for *narrow* was ($M = 0.09$) and the average within-subject variability was ($SD^2 = 0.003$). In *stretch*, the average JND was ($M = 0.12$) and the average within-subject variance was ($SD^2 = 0.004$). The exception to this low variance was *roll*, which showed larger variance: ($M = 2.57$, $SD^2 = 0.93$). Thus, the average variability of the JNDs for all but one condition was approximately ~2.5% of the mean JND (8.2% including *roll*). This demonstrates the visual sensitivity to changes across different aspects of reality alteration and their relative consistency within participants. The *roll* condition showed greater within-subject (and between-subject) variability. We suspect this may have occurred due to some participants' compensating for the visual manipulation of *roll* by tilting their heads in the opposite direction. In addition to the consistency of the JNDs themselves, the number of trial steps needed for the staircase procedure to converge was also similar across aspects. Convergence rates ranged from 5.7 to 8.7 (trial steps) across conditions. For instance, the average *grow* and *grain* convergence rates were ($M = 6.5$, $SD = 1.98$; $M = 6.7$, $SD = 1.76$), respectively. The average convergence rate across all aspects was ($M = 6.8$, $SD = 1.05$), indicating that our staircase procedure was effective at uncovering perceptual thresholds across conditions (see Figure 2A,B. for examples of convergence rates for *grow* and *grain* and Table 1 for all conditions). Combined, the measure of within-subject variability along with the consistent convergence rate of the staircase procedures implies that perceptual thresholds of SoR exhibit stable psychometric properties that can be measured experimentally.

Examining the correlations between JNDs across the different aspects (see the correlation matrix in Figure 2D and the example correlation in Figure 2E), they exhibited high, positive, and significant correlations ranging from 0.22 to 0.95 ($M = 0.61$, $SD = 0.25$). Thus, participants with high sensitivity in one aspect were also likely to be sensitive in another aspect and vice versa. An outlier to this pattern was the *grain* aspect, which showed low levels of correlations with all other aspects ($M = 0.31$, $SD = 0.05$). Next, directly comparing JNDs for the *grow* and *shrink* aspects, which share a common parameter scale (see Figure 2C), a paired t-test revealed no significant difference between the two ($M_{Grow} = 0.05$, $SD_{Grow} = 0.03$; $M_{Shrink} = 0.04$, $SD_{Shrink} = 0.03$, $t(14) = -0.66$, $p = 0.51$, Cohen's $d = -0.17$). Bayesian analysis provided moderate evidence ($BF_{10} = 0.31$) for there being no difference in the perceptual sensitivity for vertical changes in both directions.

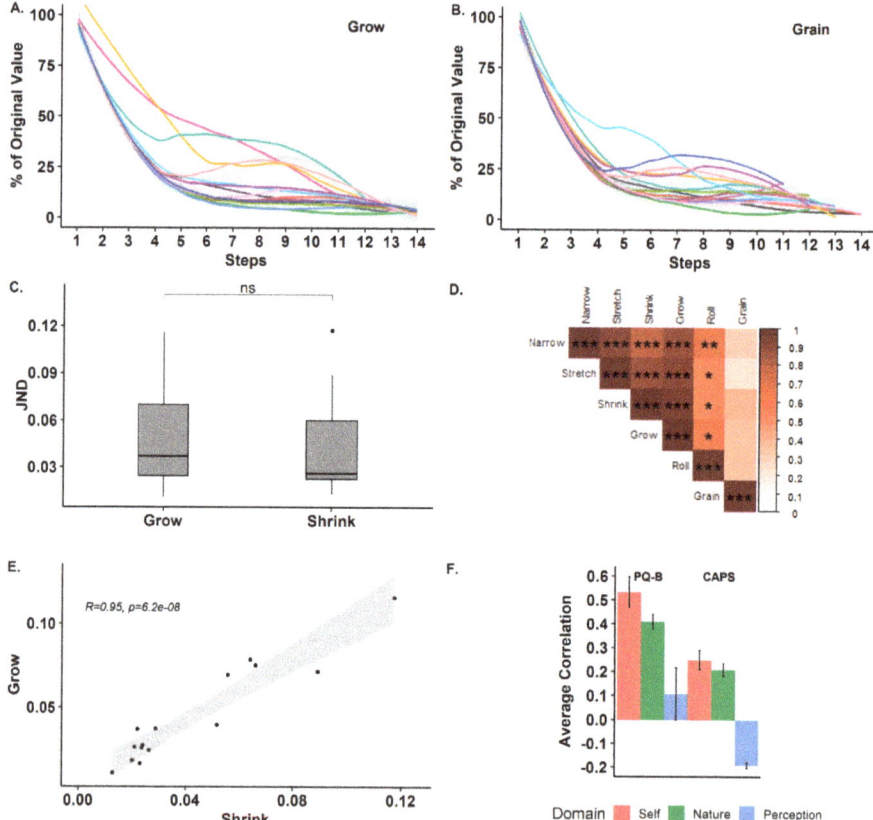

Figure 2. Perceptual thresholds for reality alterations. (**A**,**B**). Convergence rates of the staircase procedure in aspects *grow* and *grain*, respectively. Y-axis shows the magnitude of the reality alteration and the x-axis denotes the number of iterations. Note individual participants (colored lines) converged towards a stable perceptual threshold. (**C**) A comparison between JNDs of *grow* and *shrink* aspects that shared a common scale. (**D**) Pearson correlation matrix between JNDs across all aspects. Note high, positive, and significant correlations were found between all aspects' JNDs, with the exception of *grain*. (**E**) Example of correlation between participants' *grow* and *shrink* JNDs. (**F**). Averaged correlations of The *Cardiff Anomalous Perceptions Scale* (CAPS) and the *Prodromal Questionnaire Brief Version* (PQ-B) scores with JNDs shown by aspect domains (i.e., self, nature, perception).

Clinical questionnaires (CAPS and PQ-B) showed low overall scores ($M_{CAPS} = 3$, $SD_{CAPS} = 4.24$, $M_{PQ-B} = 2.8$, $SD_{PQ-B} = 3.78$) as expected in a non-clinical cohort (see Table S2 for detailed CAPS and PQ-B scores with subscales) [48,50]. Importantly, however, an analysis of the correlations between CAPS and PQ-B, with perceptual sensitivity to alterations, found that JNDs in the *grow* condition were significantly correlated with the PQ-B general score (*Spearman's Rho* = 0.61, $p = 0.015$), indicating that participants showing higher levels of psychotic symptoms also had reduced discrimination between 'real' and 'unreal' perceptions of *self*. Furthermore, the *grow* condition showed a high positive but non-significant (Spearman's Rho = 0.45, $p = 0.09$) correlation with the CAPS general score, indicating that reduced sensitivity to changes in the first person perspective (1PP) is related to abnormal perceptual experiences (see Table S1 for the full correlation matrix with subscales).

3.2. Experiment 2 (Subjective Reality Rating)

The analysis of subjective reality ratings revealed several findings. First, for the unaltered condition (*real*), the mean reality ratings were the highest ($M = 77.21$, $SD = 12.32$), demonstrating the validity of our experimental paradigm. Second, increasing magnitudes of alteration reduced the subjective reality ratings significantly for all aspects. For example, in the *grow* aspect, ratings dropped from ($M = 75$, $SD = 13.99$) in the unaltered condition to ($M = 9.57$, $SD = 8.47$) in the largest alteration magnitude, with a repeated measures ANOVA revealing a significant difference in ratings across alteration magnitudes ($F_{Grow}(2.39,14) = 79.32$, $p_{Grow} < 0.001$, $\eta^2_{Grow} = 0.77$). All other aspects showed similar patterns: ($\chi^2_{Shrink}(4) = 54.15$, $p_{Shrink} < 0.001$, $\eta^2_{Shrink} = 0.8$; $\chi^2_{Grain}(4) = 40.05$, $p_{Grain} < 0.001$, $\eta^2_{Grain} = 0.8$; $\chi^2_{Roll}(4) = 20.32$, $p_{Roll} < 0.001$, $\eta^2_{Roll} = 0.22$; $F_{Stretch}(4,14) = 91.91$, $p_{Stretch} < 0.001$, $\eta^2_{Stretch} = 0.78$; $F_{Narrow}(2.63,14) = 136.15$, $p_{Narrow} < 0.001$ $\eta^2_{Narrow} = 0.84$). Figure 3A–F show the average change in the ratings of subjective reality in all aspects for all levels of alteration. The *roll* condition showed a more linear reduction of reality judgments across the selected magnitudes. We note, however, that in the current design, the manipulations in different aspects are on different scales (based on a pilot experiment) and thus comparisons between different aspects are not possible, apart from the *grow* and *shrink* conditions. We thus compared the mean reduction in subjective ratings in *grow* and *shrink* between the *real* and first alteration magnitude (as this included the largest decrease in ratings across all conditions). Interestingly, in contrast with the similarity of their JNDs, a paired t-test indicated that the initial drop in reality ratings was significantly larger for the *grow* condition ($M_{Grow} = 32.12$, $SD_{Grow} = 23.19$) than for the *shrink* condition, ($M_{Shrink} = 21.18$, $SD_{Shrink} = 20.81$, $t(14) = -2.26$, $p = 0.04$, Cohen's $d = -0.58$, Figure 3I). Indicating that while objective perceptual sensitivity was similar, identical modulations of 1PP in the *grow* and *shrink* conditions had a differential impact on subjective reality judgments (see Table 2 and Table S4 for full descriptive statistics of the subjective ratings of reality across aspects and levels).

Third, the correlations in the reality ratings between different aspects of alteration were high, positive, and significant. Correlations between aspects ranged from 0.42 to 0.93 ($M = 0.72$, $SD = 0.17$, Figure 3G), indicating that participants' subjective judgments were similar across the different aspects. That is, participants judging the environment to be unrealistic in one aspect were also likely to do so in another aspect.

Finally, despite the fact that experiments 1 and 2 were conducted in different cohorts, we were curious regarding the relation between the objective sensitivity to alterations of reality (JNDs) and the effects of these alterations on subjective judgments. To this end, we superimposed the average JND for each aspect onto their respective average subjective ratings plot. Interestingly, for most aspects, the average JNDs (i.e., the perceptual sensitivity to a change in this aspect of reality) was found between *real* and the first magnitude of reality alteration (red diamonds in Figure 3A–F). The *roll* condition was an exception to this, with the JND found between the first and second alteration magnitudes (Figure 3C). Thus, in several aspects, the mean perceptual threshold corresponded to the point in which subjective judgments were massively reduced (e.g., *stretch*, Figure 3D). However, other aspects showed a more graded reduction of subjective reality judgments taking place at magnitudes larger than the liminal perceptual level (e.g., *narrow*, Figure 3A).

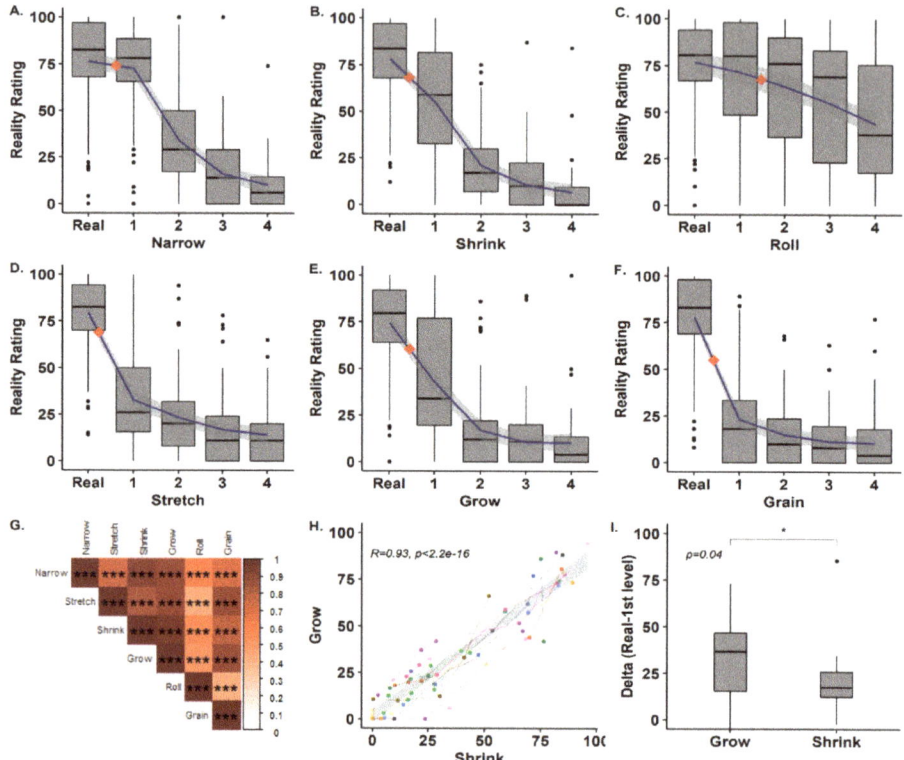

Figure 3. Subjective judgments of reality. (**A–F**) Changes in subjective reality affected the ratings of Sense of Reality (SoR) in a relatively consistent manner. Reality ratings for unaltered environments were highest while ratings for altered environments were reduced, suggesting a consistent tuning curve for SoR. (**G**) Subjective ratings for all aspects showed high, positive, and significant correlations. (**H**) Example of the correlation between participants' subjective rating of *grow* and *shrink*. (**I**) Significant difference between the drop in subjective ratings for *grow* and *shrink*, indicating an asymmetrical response for inducing changes in the first person perspective (1PP).

Table 2. Descriptive statistics for experiment 2.

	Subjective Ratings											
Alteration	Narrow		Stretch		Shrink		Grow		Roll		Grain	
Magnitude	Mean	SD	Mean	SD	Mean	SD	Mean	SD	Mean	SD	Mean	SD
Real	76.84	10.42	79.42	14.34	76.26	15.85	75	13.99	76.96	12.95	78.78	12.51
1	72.59	12.68	32.88	14.46	55.08	19.4	42.88	18.35	71.41	17.7	22.99	16.72
2	33.89	16.27	23.2	13.8	20.96	10.98	16.93	13.2	63.68	25.19	14.95	13.24
3	17.92	11.54	16.67	12.5	14.31	11.67	13.68	12.4	55.2	28.97	11.65	10.61
4	9.63	8.59	14.09	9.015	5.76	7.92	9.57	8.47	43.79	24.82	10.47	12.02

4. Discussion

SoR is a fundamental and ubiquitous criterion in assessing mental health, but it has been difficult to assess experimentally. This is mainly due to the lack of experimental paradigms allowing for well-controlled manipulations of reality. Employing immersive VR and a novel methodological framework, we demonstrated that both objective and subjective measures of SoR can

4.1. The Psychophysics of SoR

In the first experiment, we examined the objective perceptual sensitivity (JNDs) to different aspects of altered reality. Our results revealed several interesting findings. First, objective perceptual thresholds for detecting alterations of reality (JND) were highly consistent within subjects, with within-subject variability in most aspects on an order of (~2.5%) of the mean JND magnitude. In addition, convergence rates were also similar across aspects. These findings suggest that JNDs for the alterations of reality are a robust and replicable psychometric measure. Furthermore, the high and significant correlations between all aspects, apart from *grain*, suggest that the perceptual thresholds across the conditions may rely on similar cognitive processes. Contrarily, JNDs in the *grain* condition were not significantly correlated with JNDs in the other conditions, suggesting that it may have been achieved in a different manner. Importantly, the PQ-B questionnaire responses, probing prodromal symptoms, were highly correlated with perceptual thresholds in the *self* domain (Figure 2F). This indicates that participants with higher ratings of psychosis-like experiences also showed lower sensitivity to changes in manipulation of the first person perspective. This finding is especially interesting given the well-established link between altered self-related processing and psychosis [25,27,45,54]. Similarly, JNDs in the *self* domain were also positively, but non-significantly, correlated with the CAPS questionnaire scores, providing converging evidence for the relationship between perceptual thresholds for reality alterations and clinical symptoms. These correlations, found in healthy participants with low levels of symptoms, are likely to be accentuated in clinical populations, and provide preliminary evidence for the viability of SoR as a diagnostic criterion.

4.2. Subjective Modulation of SoR

The second experiment measured the impact of alterations of reality on subjective judgments of reality. As predicted, we found that when the virtual environment was unaltered, most participants reported higher levels of reality judgments ($M = 77.21$, $SD = 12.32$). Furthermore, increasing magnitudes of reality alterations reduced the subjective judgments of reality (Figure 3A–F). However, as can be seen in Figure 3A–F, there were several outlier participants, which gave extremely low ratings during the *real* condition. It seems that these participants did not accept the basic premise of the task (e.g., accepting the baseline unaltered VR environment as realistic). We note that our results are robust and significant despite this; however, future experiments may benefit from prescreening for such participants.

The different aspects of reality modulated showed different rates of decrease as a function of the alteration magnitude. We note, however, that the current experiment does not allow direct comparisons between the different aspects as they use different scales (e.g., angle for the *roll* condition and percentage of height for *grow*). However, *grow* and *shrink* used the same measure and scaling factor, allowing a direct comparison between them. As predicted, when the participants' 1PP was elevated (*grow*) this reduced reality judgments significantly more than a similar magnitude of 1PP reduction (*shrink*, Figure 3I). This finding is compatible with a predictive coding framework, and specifically the notion that alterations for which we have more experience will have a smaller impact on SoR. Given that we have more experience with the reduction of our 1PP (through sitting and laying down); this had less impact on SoR compared with the *grow* condition for which we have less experience. Indeed, 1PP is considered a fundamental component of the sense of self [43]. Changes in the bodily-self have been found in both neurological (e.g., [55]) and psychiatric [27,56] conditions in which hallucinations are prevalent. Furthermore, experimentally induced changes in the sense of self impact perceptual awareness and self-consciousness [57–59].

Comparing the mean JNDs from the first experiment with the subjective judgments from experiment 2 revealed that for some aspects, the JND marked the point of the greatest reduction in subjective reality (i.e., *stretch*, *grow*, and *grain*). Thus, the perceptual threshold coincided with the subjective experience of reality, as one may expect. However, in other aspects, the largest reduction occurred at larger alteration magnitudes than the JND (i.e., *shrink*, *roll*, and *narrow*). This suggests that subjective judgments are not completely dependent on the objective threshold in certain aspects of reality. We therefore propose that JNDs can be used as standardized units to allow comparisons of SoR across the different aspects. Future experiments will capitalize upon this finding by employing participants' JNDs to normalize the levels of alterations across conditions. In turn, this will allow comparison of the impact of different alterations of reality, allowing the modeling of one's implicit model of expectations of the world. For example, this method would allow us to compute how a change in the self (e.g., 1PP modulation—*grow*) compares to an alteration in a more perceptual aspect (e.g., *grain*), as they will share a common scale.

The broader implications of this study may potentially go beyond providing a novel approach for investigating mechanisms of SoR. The current paradigm (*UnReal*) may allow both laboratory and online gathering of large data sets in diverse cohorts, enabling a starting point for a mechanistic model of SoR. The availability of a reliable mechanistic model of SoR and its clinical and behavioral correlates is bound to provide researchers and clinicians with a new set of conceptual as well as practical tools to address research questions in a large variety of neuropsychiatric and neurological disorders involving hallucinatory or dissociative symptoms. In turn, this may lead to useful measures to further support clinical diagnoses and enable clinicians to develop and employ more accurately targeted treatments, such as new neurocognitive markers for the early detection of psychosis. Finally, our paradigm may allow for the development of novel VR-based therapeutic interventions that enhance and restore SoR in clinical populations with deficits of SoR, similar to approaches in other neurological and psychiatric conditions [60–62].

4.3. Limitations

The current experiments were aimed to test our novel approach to the study of SoR and its relation to psychosis. A central limitation here is that the objective and subjective measurements of SoR were conducted in separate cohorts, thus direct within-subject comparisons were not possible. Future studies will employ both tasks within the same cohort. Furthermore, the PQ-B and CAPS questionnaires were used only in the first experiment, thus the relationship between subjective judgments and clinical symptoms of psychosis and hallucinations is yet to be assessed. Finally, both studies had low numbers of participants and thus suffered from low statistical power, which in turn limited our ability to examine individual differences, such as the effects of age and gender. Further, higher powered studies including clinical populations are needed to validate and extend these findings regarding SoR and psychosis.

4.4. Summary

The present study investigated the SoR and its relation to psychotic symptoms. By inducing hallucination-like visual experiences and testing objective and subjective measures of SoR, we found a novel psychophysical link between sensitivity to alterations of reality and prodromal psychotic symptoms. These results provide evidence for the utility of this ecological and immersive VR methodology for the scientific study of SoR and a novel tool for psychiatric clinical assessment. Future studies may employ the *UnReal* paradigm to build computational models as well as investigate the neural substrates of SoR in healthy and clinical populations. As SoR is a central benchmark in determining psychiatric and neurological wellbeing, it is critical that we acquire a fuller understanding of how SoR is constructed by the brain and mind, allowing us to provide better diagnostic and therapeutic tools.

Supplementary Materials: The following are available online at http://www.mdpi.com/2077-0383/9/6/1627/s1, Figure S1: Visual display of alterations, Table S1: Correlation matrix of JNDs and clinical questionnaires, Table S2: Descriptive statistics of Questionnaire Responses. Table S3. Descriptive statistics of JNDs across aspects, Table S4. Descriptive statistics of Subjective ratings across aspects.

Author Contributions: Conceptualization, R.S.; methodology, R.S., G.D. and P.B.-T.; software, Y.Z.; formal analysis, G.D. and R.S.; investigation, G.D., P.B.-T. and R.S.; resources, R.S.; data curation, G.D., P.B.-T. and R.S.; writing—original draft preparation, G.D., Y.S., P.B.-T. and R.S.; writing—review and editing, G.D., Y.S., P.B.-T. and R.S.; visualization, G.D., P.B.-T. and R.S.; project administration, G.D.; funding acquisition, R.S.; All authors have read and agreed to the published version of the manuscript.

Funding: This research and the APC were funded by a donation from the Charles Roven Foundation to Roy Salomon.

Conflicts of Interest: The authors declare no conflict of interest.

References

1. Metzinger, T. How does the brain encode epistemic reliability? Perceptual presence, phenomenal transparency, and counterfactual richness. *Cogn. Neurosci.* **2014**, *5*, 122–124. [CrossRef] [PubMed]
2. Ratcliffe, M. *Feelings of Being: Phenomenology, Psychiatry and the Sense of Reality*; Oxford University Press: Oxford, UK, 2008; ISBN 0-19-920646-5.
3. APA. *DSM 5*; American Psychiatric Association: Arlington, VA, USA, 2013.
4. Barnes, J.; Boubert, L.; Harris, J.; Lee, A.; David, A.S. Reality monitoring and visual hallucinations in Parkinson's disease. *Neuropsychologia* **2003**, *41*, 565–574. [CrossRef]
5. Bentall, R.P.; Baker, G.A.; Havers, S. Reality monitoring and psychotic hallucinations. *Br. J. Clin. Psychol.* **1991**, *30*, 213–222. [CrossRef] [PubMed]
6. Johnson, M.K. Reality monitoring: An experimental phenomenological approach. *J. Exp. Psychol. Gen.* **1988**, *117*, 390. [CrossRef]
7. Johnson, M.K.; Hashtroudi, S.; Lindsay, D.S. Source monitoring. *Psychol. Bull.* **1993**, *114*, 3. [CrossRef]
8. Raye, C.L.; Johnson, M.K. Reality monitoring vs. discriminating between external sources of memories. *Bull. Psychon. Soc.* **1980**, *15*, 405–408. [CrossRef]
9. Garrison, J.R.; Bond, R.; Gibbard, E.; Johnson, M.K.; Simons, J.S. Monitoring what is real: The effects of modality and action on accuracy and type of reality monitoring error. *Cortex* **2017**, *87*, 108–117. [CrossRef]
10. Simons, J.S.; Garrison, J.R.; Johnson, M.K. Brain Mechanisms of Reality Monitoring. *Trends Cogn. Sci.* **2017**, *21*, 462–473. [CrossRef]
11. Ohayon, M.M. Prevalence of hallucinations and their pathological associations in the general population. *Psychiatry Res.* **2000**, *97*, 153–164. [CrossRef]
12. Blanke, O.; Pozeg, P.; Hara, M.; Heydrich, L.; Serino, A.; Yamamoto, A.; Higuchi, T.; Salomon, R.; Seeck, M.; Landis, T.; et al. Neurological and robot-controlled induction of an apparition. *Curr. Biol.* **2014**, *24*, 2681–2686. [CrossRef]
13. Rao, R.P.N.; Ballard, D.H. Predictive coding in the visual cortex: A functional interpretation of some extra-classical receptive-field effects. *Nat. Neurosci.* **1999**, *2*, 79. [CrossRef] [PubMed]
14. Clark, A. Whatever next? Predictive brains, situated agents, and the future of cognitive science. *Behav. Brain Sci.* **2013**, *36*, 181–204. [CrossRef] [PubMed]
15. Friston, K. The free-energy principle: A rough guide to the brain? *Trends Cogn. Sci. (Regul. Ed.)* **2009**, *13*, 293–301. [CrossRef] [PubMed]
16. de Lange, F.P.; Heilbron, M.; Kok, P. How do expectations shape perception? *Trends Cogn. Sci.* **2018**, *22*, 764–779. [CrossRef] [PubMed]
17. Friston, K.J.; Stephan, K.E. Free-energy and the brain. *Synthese* **2007**, *159*, 417–458. [CrossRef]
18. Wiese, W.; Metzinger, T.K. *Vanilla PP for Philosophers: A Primer on Predictive Processing*; Philosophy and Predictive Processing; MIND Group: Frankfurt am Main, Germany, 2017; ISBN 978-3-95857-302-4.
19. Lau, H. Consciousness, Metacognition, & Perceptual Reality Monitoring. *PsyArXiv* **2019**. [CrossRef]
20. Fletcher, P.C.; Frith, C.D. Perceiving is believing: A Bayesian approach to explaining the positive symptoms of schizophrenia. *Nat. Rev. Neurosci.* **2008**, *10*, 48–58. [CrossRef]
21. Corlett, P.R.; Horga, G.; Fletcher, P.C.; Alderson-Day, B.; Schmack, K.; Powers, A.R. Hallucinations and Strong Priors. *Trends Cogn. Sci.* **2019**, *23*, 114–127. [CrossRef]
22. Sterzer, P.; Adams, R.A.; Fletcher, P.; Frith, C.; Lawrie, S.M.; Muckli, L.; Petrovic, P.; Uhlhaas, P.; Voss, M.; Corlett, P.R. The Predictive Coding Account of Psychosis. *Biol. Psychiatry* **2018**, *84*, 634–643. [CrossRef]
23. Powers, A.R.; Mathys, C.; Corlett, P.R. Pavlovian conditioning–induced hallucinations result from overweighting of perceptual priors. *Science* **2017**, *357*, 596–600. [CrossRef]

24. Griffin, J.D.; Fletcher, P.C. Predictive Processing, Source Monitoring, and Psychosis. *Annu. Rev. Clin. Psychol.* **2017**, *13*, 265–289. [CrossRef]
25. Frith, C.; Done, D. Experiences of alien control in schizophrenia reflect a disorder in the central monitoring of action. *Psychol. Med.* **2009**, *19*, 359–363. [CrossRef] [PubMed]
26. Ford, J.M.; Palzes, V.A.; Roach, B.J.; Mathalon, D.H. Did I do that? Abnormal predictive processes in schizophrenia when button pressing to deliver a tone. *Schizophr. Bull.* **2014**, *40*, 804–812. [CrossRef] [PubMed]
27. Salomon, R.; Progin, P.; Griffa, A.; Rognini, G.; Do, K.Q.; Conus, P.; Marchesotti, S.; Bernasconi, F.; Hagmann, P.; Serino, A. Sensorimotor Induction of Auditory Misattribution in Early Psychosis. *Schizophr. Bull.* **2020**. [CrossRef] [PubMed]
28. Teunisse, R.J.; Zitman, F.G.; Cruysberg, J.R.M.; Hoefnagels, W.H.L.; Verbeek, A.L.M. Visual hallucinations in psychologically normal people: Charles Bonnet's syndrome. *Lancet* **1996**, *347*, 794–797. [CrossRef]
29. Perivoliotis, D.; Grant, P.M.; Peters, E.R.; Ison, R.; Kuipers, E.; Beck, A.T. Cognitive insight predicts favorable outcome in cognitive behavioral therapy for psychosis. *Psychosis* **2010**, *2*, 23–33. [CrossRef]
30. Gerretsen, P.; Menon, M.; Mamo, D.C.; Fervaha, G.; Remington, G.; Pollock, B.G.; Graff-Guerrero, A. Impaired insight into illness and cognitive insight in schizophrenia spectrum disorders: Resting state functional connectivity. *Schizophr. Res.* **2014**, *160*, 43–50. [CrossRef]
31. Nair, A.; Palmer, E.C.; Aleman, A.; David, A.S. Relationship between cognition, clinical and cognitive insight in psychotic disorders: A review and meta-analysis. *Schizophr. Res.* **2014**, *152*, 191–200. [CrossRef]
32. Baker, D.; Hunter, E.; Lawrence, E.; Medford, N.; Patel, M.; Senior, C.; Sierra, M.; Lambert, M.V.; Phillips, M.L.; David, A.S. Depersonalisation disorder: Clinical features of 204 cases. *Br. J. Psychiatry* **2003**, *182*, 428–433. [CrossRef]
33. Sass, L.; Pienkos, E.; Nelson, B.; Medford, N. Anomalous self-experience in depersonalization and schizophrenia: A comparative investigation. *Conscious. Cogn.* **2013**, *22*, 430–441. [CrossRef]
34. Harris, C.S. Adaptation to displaced vision: Visual, motor, or proprioceptive change? *Science* **1963**, *140*, 812–813. [CrossRef]
35. Mudrik, L.; Breska, A.; Lamy, D.; Deouell, L.Y. Integration without awareness. *Psychol. Sci.* **2011**, *22*, 764. [CrossRef]
36. Bohil, C.J.; Alicea, B.; Biocca, F.A. Virtual reality in neuroscience research and therapy. *Nat. Rev. Neurosci.* **2011**, *12*, 752–762. [CrossRef]
37. Sanchez-Vives, M.V.; Slater, M. From presence to consciousness through virtual reality. *Nat. Rev. Neurosci.* **2005**, *6*, 332–339. [CrossRef] [PubMed]
38. Krugwasser, A.R.; Harel, E.V.; Salomon, R. The boundaries of the self: The sense of agency across different sensorimotor aspects. *J. Vis.* **2019**, *19*, 14. [CrossRef] [PubMed]
39. Salomon, R.; Fernandez, N.; van Elk, M.; Vachicouras, N.; Sabatier, F.; Tychinskaya, A.; Llobera, J.; Blanke, O. Changing motor perception by sensorimotor conflicts and body ownership. *Sci. Rep.* **2016**, *6*, 25847. [CrossRef] [PubMed]
40. Blom, J.D. Alice in Wonderland syndrome. *Neurol. Clin. Pract.* **2016**, *6*, 259–270. [CrossRef]
41. Bentall, R. The Illusion of Reality: A Review and Integration of Psychological Research on Hallucinations. *Psychol. Bull.* **1990**, *107*, 82–95. [CrossRef]
42. Preller, K.H.; Vollenweider, F.X. Phenomenology, Structure, and Dynamic of Psychedelic States. In *Behavioral Neurobiology of Psychedelic Drugs*; Halberstadt, A.L., Vollenweider, F.X., Nichols, D.E., Eds.; Current Topics in Behavioral Neurosciences; Springer: Berlin/Heidelberg, Germany, 2018; pp. 221–256. ISBN 978-3-662-55880-5.
43. Blanke, O.; Metzinger, T. Full-body illusions and minimal phenomenal selfhood. *Trends Cogn. Sci.* **2009**, *13*, 7–13. [CrossRef] [PubMed]
44. Dudley, R.; Aynsworth, C.; Mosimann, U.; Taylor, J.-P.; Smailes, D.; Collerton, D.; McCarthy-Jones, S.; Urwyler, P. A comparison of visual hallucinations across disorders. *Psychiatry Res* **2019**, *272*, 86–92. [CrossRef]
45. Parnas, J. Self and schizophrenia: A phenomenological perspective. *Self Neurosci. Psychiatry* **2003**, *1*, 217–241.
46. Levitt, H. Transformed up-down methods in psychoacoustics. *J. Acoust. Soc. Am.* **1971**, *49*, 467–477. [CrossRef]
47. Hettinger, L.J.; Riccio, G.E. Visually induced motion sickness in virtual environments. *Presence: Teleoperators Virtual Environ.* **1992**, *1*, 306–310. [CrossRef]

48. Bell, V.; Halligan, P.W.; Ellis, H.D. The Cardiff Anomalous Perceptions Scale (CAPS): A new validated measure of anomalous perceptual experience. *Schizophr. Bull.* **2005**, *32*, 366–377. [CrossRef] [PubMed]
49. Bell, V.; Halligan, P.W.; Pugh, K.; Freeman, D. Correlates of perceptual distortions in clinical and non-clinical populations using the Cardiff Anomalous Perceptions Scale (CAPS): Associations with anxiety and depression and a re-validation using a representative population sample. *Psychiatry Res.* **2011**, *189*, 451–457. [CrossRef] [PubMed]
50. Loewy, R.L.; Pearson, R.; Vinogradov, S.; Bearden, C.E.; Cannon, T.D. Psychosis risk screening with the Prodromal Questionnaire—Brief version (PQ-B). *Schizophr. Res.* **2011**, *129*, 42–46. [CrossRef]
51. Kline, E.; Wilson, C.; Ereshefsky, S.; Tsuji, T.; Schiffman, J.; Pitts, S.; Reeves, G. Convergent and discriminant validity of attenuated psychosis screening tools. *Schizophr. Res.* **2012**, *134*, 49–53. [CrossRef]
52. MATLAB. *MATLAB 9.6.0.(R2019a)*; The MathWorks Inc.: Natick, MA, USA, 2019.
53. JASP Team. *JASP (Version 0.11.1) [Computer Software]*; Department of Psychological Methods: Amsterdam, The Netherlands, 2019.
54. Nelson, B.; Thompson, A.; Yung, A.R. Basic Self-Disturbance Predicts Psychosis Onset in the Ultra High Risk for Psychosis "Prodromal" Population. *Schizophr. Bull.* **2012**, *38*, 1277–1287. [CrossRef]
55. Blanke, O.; Mohr, C. Out-of-body experience, heautoscopy, and autoscopic hallucination of neurological origin: Implications for neurocognitive mechanisms of corporeal awareness and self-consciousness. *Brain Res. Rev.* **2005**, *50*, 184–199. [CrossRef]
56. Nelson, B.; Fornito, A.; Harrison, B.J.; Yücel, M.; Sass, L.A.; Yung, A.R.; Thompson, A.; Wood, S.J.; Pantelis, C.; McGorry, P.D. A disturbed sense of self in the psychosis prodrome: Linking phenomenology and neurobiology. *Neurosci. Biobehav. Rev.* **2009**, *33*, 807–817. [CrossRef]
57. Faivre, N.; Vuillaume, L.; Bernasconi, F.; Salomon, R.; Blanke, O.; Cleeremans, A. Sensorimotor conflicts alter metacognitive and action monitoring. *Cortex* **2020**, *124*, 224–234. [CrossRef]
58. Salomon, R.; Noel, J.-P.; Łukowska, M.; Faivre, N.; Metzinger, T.; Serino, A.; Blanke, O. Unconscious integration of multisensory bodily inputs in the peripersonal space shapes bodily self-consciousness. *Cognition* **2017**, *166*, 174–183. [CrossRef] [PubMed]
59. Park, H.-D.; Bernasconi, F.; Bello-Ruiz, J.; Pfeiffer, C.; Salomon, R.; Blanke, O. Transient modulations of neural responses to heartbeats covary with bodily self-consciousness. *J. Neurosci.* **2016**, *36*, 8453–8460. [CrossRef] [PubMed]
60. Perruchoud, D.; Pisotta, I.; Carda, S.; Murray, M.M.; Ionta, S. Biomimetic rehabilitation engineering: The importance of somatosensory feedback for brain–machine interfaces. *J. Neural Eng.* **2016**, *13*, 041001. [CrossRef] [PubMed]
61. Lubianiker, N.; Goldway, N.; Fruchtman-Steinbok, T.; Paret, C.; Keynan, J.N.; Singer, N.; Cohen, A.; Kadosh, K.C.; Linden, D.E.; Hendler, T. Process-based framework for precise neuromodulation. *Nat. Hum. Behav.* **2019**, *3*, 436–445. [CrossRef] [PubMed]
62. Freeman, D.; Reeve, S.; Robinson, A.; Ehlers, A.; Clark, D.; Spanlang, B.; Slater, M. Virtual reality in the assessment, understanding, and treatment of mental health disorders. *Psychol. Med.* **2017**, *47*, 2393–2400. [CrossRef]

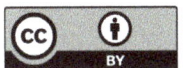

© 2020 by the authors. Licensee MDPI, Basel, Switzerland. This article is an open access article distributed under the terms and conditions of the Creative Commons Attribution (CC BY) license (http://creativecommons.org/licenses/by/4.0/).

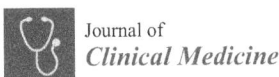

Article

Machine Learning and Virtual Reality on Body Movements' Behaviors to Classify Children with Autism Spectrum Disorder

Mariano Alcañiz Raya [1], Javier Marín-Morales [1], Maria Eleonora Minissi [1], Gonzalo Teruel Garcia [1], Luis Abad [2] and Irene Alice Chicchi Giglioli [1,*]

[1] Instituto de Investigación e Innovación en Bioingeniería (i3B), Universitat Politècnica de Valencia, 46022 Valencia, Spain; malcaniz@i3b.upv.es (M.A.R.); jamarmo@i3b.upv.es (J.M.-M.); meminiss@upvnet.upv.es (M.E.M.); gonzaloteruelg@gmail.com (G.T.G.)

[2] Red Cenit, Centros de Desarrollo Cognitivo, 46020 Valencia, Spain; lam@redcenit.com

* Correspondence: alicechicchi@i3b.upv.es

Received: 26 March 2020; Accepted: 23 April 2020; Published: 26 April 2020

Abstract: Autism spectrum disorder (ASD) is mostly diagnosed according to behavioral symptoms in sensory, social, and motor domains. Improper motor functioning, during diagnosis, involves the qualitative evaluation of stereotyped and repetitive behaviors, while quantitative methods that classify body movements' frequencies of children with ASD are less addressed. Recent advances in neuroscience, technology, and data analysis techniques are improving the quantitative and ecological validity methods to measure specific functioning in ASD children. On one side, cutting-edge technologies, such as cameras, sensors, and virtual reality can accurately detect and classify behavioral biomarkers, as body movements in real-life simulations. On the other, machine-learning techniques are showing the potential for identifying and classifying patients' subgroups. Starting from these premises, three real-simulated imitation tasks have been implemented in a virtual reality system whose aim is to investigate if machine-learning methods on movement features and frequency could be useful in discriminating ASD children from children with typical neurodevelopment. In this experiment, 24 children with ASD and 25 children with typical neurodevelopment participated in a multimodal virtual reality experience, and changes in their body movements were tracked by a depth sensor camera during the presentation of visual, auditive, and olfactive stimuli. The main results showed that ASD children presented larger body movements than TD children, and that head, trunk, and feet represent the maximum classification with an accuracy of 82.98%. Regarding stimuli, visual condition showed the highest accuracy (89.36%), followed by the visual-auditive stimuli (74.47%), and visual-auditive-olfactory stimuli (70.21%). Finally, the head showed the most consistent performance along with the stimuli, from 80.85% in visual to 89.36% in visual-auditive-olfactory condition. The findings showed the feasibility of applying machine learning and virtual reality to identify body movements' biomarkers that could contribute to improving ASD diagnosis.

Keywords: autism spectrum disorder; body movements; repetitive behaviors; virtual reality; machine learning

1. Introduction

1.1. Autism Spectrum Disorder and Repetitive Behaviors

Autism spectrum disorder (ASD) is a neurodevelopmental disorder mainly based on impairments in social communication and interactions' abilities and on the presence of restricted, repetitive patterns of behavior, interests, or activities [1]. It affects 1 in 160 children [2] and its symptomatology tends to appear from two to four years old, although in some cases it is possible to detect in six months old toddlers [3,4]. ASD studies primarily examine the weaknesses in social interaction abilities', and less on the stereotyped and repetitive motor behaviors that also affect educational, social, and daily life [1,5].

Repetitive behaviors (RBs) are defined as heterogeneous observable motor stereotyped or repetitive sequences characterized by rigidity, invariance, inappropriateness, and being purposeless [6,7]. RBs can occur currently with small changes of the routine or in presence of new and unknowns stimuli to reduce subjective arousal and to cope with unfamiliar events, to maintain homeostasis [8–10].

Furthermore, RBs can be classified into two groups: common behaviors and complex behaviors [11]. Common behaviors are for example nail-biting, thumb sucking, and hair twirling and they tend to be also frequent in typical development population (TD), particularly situations that might cause stress or anxiety [12]. On the other hand, complex behaviors include more complex stereotypies, such as flapping hands, fingers wiggling, head spinning and banging, stamping the feet, and high levels of head movement and body rocking. Although complex RBs are possible to find in TDs, complex head spinning and banging, arm flapping, finger wiggling, and body rocking are mostly related to ASD; indeed, ASD individuals tend to exhibit RBs more frequently and severely than age-matched TD controls [13–15].

Several studies have demonstrated the high presence of RBs behaviors in ASD, ranging from 60% to 100% of cases [13–15]. The relevance of this study lies in understanding if movement features and frequency can be used as a diagnostic biomarker to classify children with and without ASD.

1.2. Traditional Assessment in ASD: Advantages and Limitations

Traditional ASD assessment and diagnosis involve qualitative and quantitative measures, such as semi-structured behavioral task observations (Autism Diagnostic Observation Schedule, ADOS) [16] and structured interview (Autism Diagnostic Interview-Revised, ADI-R) [17].

ADOS consists of several structured and semi-structured tasks on communication, use of imagination, social interaction, play, and restrictive and repetitive behavior analysis. The examiner introduces to the child one task at a time, observing whether ASD symptoms are manifested [16]. ADI-R is a semi-structured interview for family caregivers, who answer to questions related to communication, social interaction, and restricted, repetitive, and stereotyped behaviors [17] (see Materials and Methods for a detailed description of both ADOS and ADI-R). Since in ADOS examiner has to judge a child's performance giving scoring and rating, evaluation relies on the examiner's expertise and subjectivity; likewise, in ADI-R ASD diagnosis is based on caregivers' reports rather than on objective evaluation. Although these measures have been always considered as the gold standard for ASD assessment [18], they present some limitations [19,20].

Regarding ADOS and ADI-R, limitations are related to the absence of both objective assessment methods and the ecological validity of the setting. Examiners need to be trained and prepared to avoid inappropriate task presentation and administration, which might cause symptoms over- or under-interpretation, providing misleading outcomes [21,22]. Moreover, traditional assessment methods might not tap and conceal compensatory capabilities that have been already developed by the child [23], and social desirability [24] might affect responses veracity to tests. Because of social desirability bias, individuals might respond to tasks or questions in a manner conceived as favorable by others [25]. Likewise, in semi-structured interviews, such as ADI-R, family caregivers might report differently certain child's behaviors according to their interpretation and will [26].

Furthermore, traditional ASD assessment takes place in settings that lack ecological validity (i.e., laboratory) [27–29], and results do not mirror performance in real life [30,31]. Indeed, in ASD assessment at a laboratory, children might have learned how to behave according to specific rules and scripts [32]. Concerning RB traditional assessment limitations, direct observation consists of watching individual behavioral sequences, and several weaknesses affect measure reliability, such as difficulties in observing high-speed RBs, analyzing two concomitant RBs, detecting RB sequence beginning, ending, and environmental antecedents [18]. Paper-and-pencil rating scales report RBs frequency and intensity from caregivers' general observations and impressions, yielding objective methodological issues related to self-report measures, that, as well as in ADI-R, are not accurate and do not properly tap individual RBs characteristics [33,34]. Finally, video-based RB assessment is an off-line RB coding procedure made by experts. Although a video-based procedure is more reliable than direct observation methods and paper-and-pencil procedures, it is laborious, and it takes a long time [33]; moreover, the examiner's coding ability depends on individual levels of training and expertise [21].

To overcome the lack of ecological validity, and to avoid the use of subjective observational diagnostic methods in ASD, there is a need to automatically quantify and assess RBs, that could be fulfilled using technology [35,36]. Indeed, item-independent methods can grant accurate estimation of RB incidence and co-occurrence [9,35,36], and new technologies, such as virtual reality, can provide more ecological validity and controlled methodologies.

1.3. Implicit Methods: Biomarkers as Supports for ASD Assessment

Recent advances in social cognitive neuroscience (SCN) shed light on how humans analyze and report beliefs, feelings, and behaviors [37]. SCN is a research area that studies biological processes and related cognition-based elements [38], and it is showing that social interactions rely on implicit psychophysiological processes uncontrolled by conscious awareness [39].

Implicit measures tend to assess automatic biological processes outside conscious awareness [38] that ensue from the interaction with environmental external stimuli and their internal processing. Such biomarkers are a valid alternative to explicit measures, which cannot tap implied brain processes on their own [40]. Thus, to overcome explicit measure weaknesses in the ASD diagnosis, more recent research has included biomarkers along with traditional assessment techniques [41,42].

To date, the available utmost biomarkers to study unconscious processes are the electrodermal activity (EDA) [43,44], the functional magnetic resonance imaging (fMRI) [45], the functional near-infrared spectroscopy (fNIRS) [46], the electroencephalography (EEG) [47], the eye tracking [48], and the heart rate variability (HRT) [49]. In ASD assessment, fMRI research showed that ASD is related to hyperactivity in neural activation and alterations in the cingulate posterior cortex and portions of the insula [50]; whereas EEG research suggested that in social context ASD individuals exhibit greater activity in the left hemisphere [51]. Furthermore, recently developed technological tools, such as cameras and/or sensors, allowed the detection and classification of behavioral biomarkers, as body movements [52].

Initial studies on RBs with such devices showed that more automatic and objective assessment is possible, achieving the recognition of RBs [19,33,36,53–58]. For instance, to disentangle RBs from other movements in ASD, three wireless accelerometers placed on six ASD children's wrists and chest in two different settings were able to accurately identify respectively in lab and classroom 86% and 89.5% of spontaneous hand flapping and body rocking cases [33].

Also, RGB color camera equipped with depth sensor and microphones array for simulated-hand flapping discernment was used in a laboratory setting; the application of the dynamic time warping (DTW) algorithm on-camera recorded data showed that it can recognize and isolate all simulated hand flapping instances, leading to claim that RBs detection is possible even involving sensors that not have necessarily to be worn [19].

1.4. Repetitive Behaviors Recognition in ASD

To overcome issues related to traditional RB assessment [18,19], a new research area about movement analysis based on video recordings and automatic tagging has emerged [19,33,36,53–58].

The first attempt has been developing systems that involve video recordings and accelerometers placed on the subject's body to register movements and to transmit data via wireless [35,36,54,59–61].

These measures have yielded promising results in RB classification, although some studies have involved typical population and not ASD individuals [61], and to our knowledge, no studies have assessed RBs involving quantitative methods and have compared them between ASD and other clinical populations. However, accelerometer and video-based methods are expensive in terms of time and effort, and ASD children might feel as uncomfortable wearing accelerometers. For this reason, this work involved an RGB-D camera for real-time analysis. RGB-D camera is a video recording device able to augment the conventional image with depth information, related to how much the recorded moving body is far from the sensor.

Owing to deep learning and big data techniques [62–64], algorithms have been developed that can estimate real-time subjects' posture and categorize automatically their movements. Over the last decades, great progress has been made in posture estimation and modern technologies, allowing classifying postures regardless of the worn clothes and the considered point of view [65–69]. Furthermore, machine-learning methods (ML) are improving the predictive value of motor behavioral biomarkers' measures in ASD, enhancing the development of objective measures in the diagnostic standpoint [70,71]. For example, Crippa et al. (2015) developed a ML to discriminate preschool children with ASD from children with typical development using a simple upper-limb reach-to-drop task. The resulting model showed an accuracy rate of 96.7%, suggesting that ML can be a useful method of classification and discrimination in the diagnosis process [70].

1.5. Use of Virtual Reality in ASD

Virtual reality (VR) is a three-dimensional computer-generated environment that allows users to experience simulated and unreal worlds. VR provides ecological validity to experienced situations and consequent users' reactions, becoming promising in psychological assessment, training, and treatment [72,73].

Over the last two decades, the VR market has deeply grown because of the broad amount of enterprise birth and consequent wide offer of virtual devices. Overall, head-mounted displays (HMDs) are the most important, affordable, and available in the VR market [74]. However, a different VR device has been suggested as more suitable to our target (ASD children): the CAVE-Automatic Virtual Environment (CAVE™) that is a semi-immersive room where 3 to 6 rear-projected surfaces are installed [74–78].

As a semi-immersive system, CAVE™ overcomes users' risk to experience cyber-sickness that is the possible user's discomfort because of sensory-motor incongruence and cognitive dissonance in the virtual world [79]. Furthermore, specifically to ASD children, CAVE system can overcome the significant restrictions of HMDs that, on one hand, are not suitable for small heads, and on the other, can affect and worsen their sensory and cognitive difficulties [80,81]. Previous studies on feasibility, safety of use, and learning skills of CAVE environments in children with ASD have showed no significant negative effect differences between ASD and TD children and improvements in various skills (e.g., pedestrian crossing) [82].

Regardless of the involved technology and the brand, VR systems share three main features: immersion, interaction, and sense of being present in the environment [83–88]. Immersion refers to system capability to isolate the user from reality [86,88]. Interaction allows users to interact with virtual objects in real-time through control sticks or gloves, providing engagement, motivation, and fun [84,89]. Sense of presence is a consequence of immersion and real-time interaction, and it is defined as the psychological feeling related to the sensation of being physically in the virtual environment, even though the awareness of not being there [88,90–94]. Finally, another feature to consider, less addressed in studies and especially in ASD population, concerns the perception and interaction with virtual agents. Virtual agents have been mainly used in social trainings and interventions showing positive results on skills in ASD children [82]. These positive results suggest that virtual agents are perceived not as cartoons or passive objects to watch, but actively as an intentional being that wants to communicate with the child and with mutually directed behaviors. To our knowledge, one study examined the perception of ASD children in the interaction with a virtual agent for performing a task (pick up flowers) [95]. The quantitative data (accuracy and reaction times) showed that ASD children could complete the task and the qualitative data showed that most of the ASD children perceived the virtual agent as an intentional being with mutually directed behavioral intentions, able to engage and motivate the ASD peer.

There is a great involvement of VR in psychological ASD treatment and it taps all important field macro-areas, such as clinical psychology, neuropsychology, and cognitive and motor rehabilitation [75,85,96–105]. Specifically, treatment studies, applying VR to ASD, mainly referred to social competence [101,102,104], emotional recognition [103], and anxiety and phobias [105] showing initial positive effects of this technique. Regarding ASD VR assessment, it has been less addressed and mainly focused on social communication and interaction symptoms. For example, it has been observed that during a virtual interview about personal life, ASD children looked less to social avatars than their TD control peers, identifying correctly 76% of ASD cases [102]. Also, ASD children made atypical social judgments on the kindness of faces photographs in a virtual environment compared to TD controls [103]. Despite VR potential in ASD assessment has already been strengthened [75], to our knowledge, no one has investigated whether it is possible to disentangle ASD in a VR experience using RBs movement analysis.

Starting from these premises, the main aim of this study is to discriminate ASD children from children with typically developing through body movements' data analysis in a multimodal VR experience, characterized by three stimuli: visual, auditory, and olfactory. Applying ML methods to the dataset, we explored: (a) If through movement data it is possible to discriminate between the two populations; (b) which body parameters better discriminate between the two populations; and (c) which virtual stimuli condition better discriminate body parameters between the two populations.

2. Materials and Methods

2.1. Participants

This study included a sample of 49 children between the ages of 4 and 7 years; 24 children with a diagnosis of ASD (age: 5.13 ± 1.35; male = 21, female = 3) and 25 with a typical development (TD) (age: 4.86 ± 0.91; male = 16, female = 9).

The ASD group sample was provided by the Development Neurocognitive Centre, Red Cenit, Valencia, Spain. TD and ASD participants presented an individual assessment report that included the ADOS-2 and ADI-R tests [16,17,21]. TD group was recruited by a management company through mailings to families.

To participate in the study, family caregivers received written information about the study and were required to give their written consent. Ethical Committee of the Polytechnic University of Valencia approved the study. The study procedure was in accordance with the ethical standards of the institutional and national research committee and with the 1964 Helsinki declaration and its later amendments or comparable ethical standards.

2.2. Psychological Assessment

The following test and scales have been administered to participants and their family caregivers.

2.2.1. Autism Diagnostic Observation Schedule (ADOS-2)

The Autism Diagnostic Observation Schedule (ADOS) [16,21] is a semi-structured set of observation tasks that measure autism symptoms in social relatedness, communication, play, and repetitive behaviors. A standardized severity score within these domains can be calculated to compare autism symptoms across the different modules, which differ in age and linguistic level. From the trained psychologist observation of these behaviors, the items are scored between 0 to 3 (from no evidence of abnormality related to autism to definitive evidence) and from the sum of scores are obtained two specific indexes (social affectation and restricted and repetitive behavior) and an ASD's global total index. The ADOS-2 presents excellent test-retest reliability (0.87 for the social affectation index, 0.64 for the repetitive behavior index, and 0.88 for the total global index). In the study, the assessment was performed using module 1.

2.2.2. Autism Diagnostic Interview-Revised (ADI-R)

The ADI-R [17] is a semi-structured interview for family caregivers, designed to provide the developmental history framework for a lifetime to detect the presence of ASD for individuals from early childhood to adult life. It consists of 111 questions with three separate domains: communication, social interaction and restricted, repetitive and stereotyped behaviors. The answers are scored on a 0–3 Likert scale, from the absence of the behavior to a clear presentation of the determined behavior. ADI-R presents a high test-retest reliability ranging from 0.93 to 0.97.

2.3. The Multimodal Virtual Environment (VE) and the Imitation Tasks

The multimodal VE consisted of a simulated city street intersection and was divided into three experimental stimuli conditions: visual (V), visual-auditory (VA), and visual-auditory-olfactory (VAO) (Figure 1a).

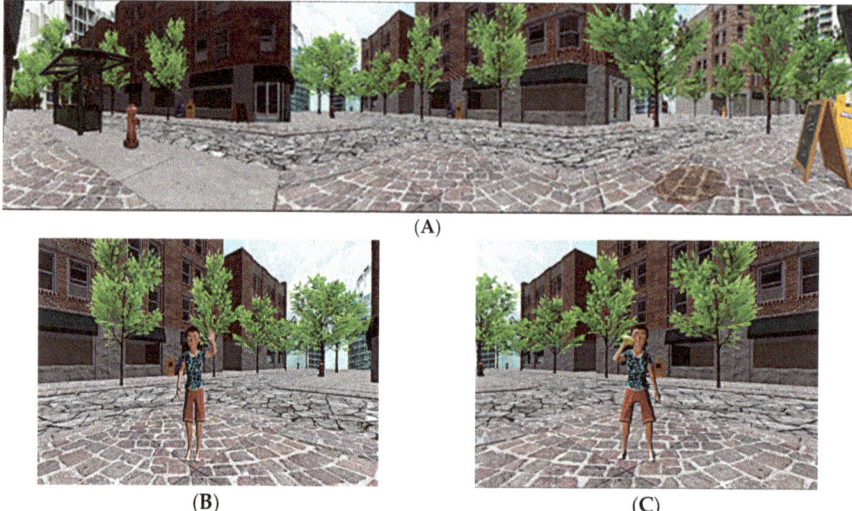

Figure 1. The virtual environment. (**A**) City street intersection; (**B**) visual (V) condition, boy's avatar saying hello; (**C**) visual-auditory-olfactory (VAO) condition, boy's avatar eating a muffin.

First, in the V condition, a boy's avatar appeared from the left side of the surface CAVE™, walking to the middle of the virtual environment, where he stopped and waved to say hello to the participant three times, just before to leave the virtual scene disappearing from behind (Figure 1b).

Next, a girl's avatar appeared in the center of the surface CAVE™, walking to the right of the virtual scene, where she also stopped and repeated the three waves to say hello to the participant, just before leaving the virtual scene disappearing from behind. This sequence was identically repeated three times.

Consecutively, in the second VA stimuli condition, the same avatars appeared in the same first order from the same directions, and they danced over an animated disco song for 10 s three times.

Finally, in the last condition (VAO), the same avatars from the two previous conditions, in the same order and from the same directions, bit a buttered muffin, accompanied with an artificial butter odor (Figure 1c). In the three stimuli conditions, participants were asked to imitate the actions performed by the avatars. Specifically, in the first virtual condition, they should wave three times, dance three times in the second virtual condition, and they should imitate the action of biting a muffing three times.

The selection of the stimuli and the gradual exposition to the three stimuli conditions depended on the hyper-and-hypo sensitivities to sensory stimuli of the ASD population. More in detail, with respect to visual and auditive stimuli (e.g., bright lights or noisy sounds), ASD population presented a hypersensitivity [106,107]; conversely, they present hypo-sensitiveness to olfactive stimuli [108,109]. Sensory hyper-and-hypo sensitivities consequently can affect the information processing in ASD and it has been suggested it may cause RBs [110,111].

The Institute for Research and Innovation in Bioengineering (i3B) of the Polytechnic University of Valencia (UPV) developed the 3D modeling. The environment was projected inside a three surfaces Cave Assisted Virtual Environment (CAVE™) with dimensions of 4 × 4 × 3 mt. It was equipped with three ceiling ultra-short lens projectors, which can project a 100° image from just 55 cm and a Logitech Speaker Z906 500W 5.1 THX sound system (Logitech, Canton of Vaud, Switzerland) (Figure 2).

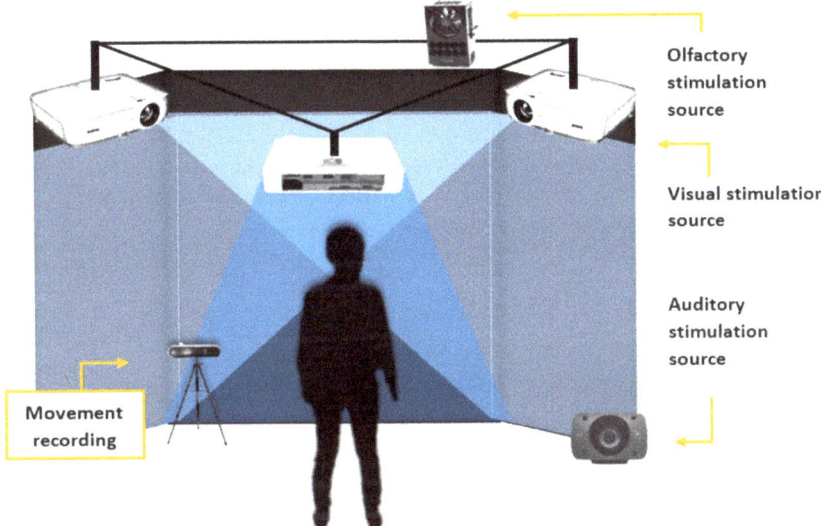

Figure 2. Experimental setting.

2.4. The Olfactory System

Olorama Technology™ (www.olorama.com) a wireless freshener delivered the olfactory stimuli. It can encompass until 12 scents arranged in 12 pre-charged channels, which can be selected and triggered by employing a UDP packet. The device includes a programmable fan time system that controls the duration and intensity of the scent delivery. In the VAO condition, we used a butter scent to evocate the real muffin smell. The scent valve was opened all the time during the last stimuli condition (VAO).

2.5. Experimental Procedure

First, the family caregivers of participants were informed about the general objectives of the research, and, before the experimental session, the setting was also shown and explained to them.

Second, the participant was accompanied in the CAVE™, by the researcher, and by his or her family caregiver according to the child's needs. The participant was placed in the middle of the virtual room, standing in front of the central surface at 1.5 m. The presentation order of VR stimuli conditions for all participants was: visual, visual-auditory, and visual-auditory-olfactory. Before each stimuli VR condition, a two-minute baseline was recorded, and subsequently, the stimuli VR experience condition was presented. The presentation order was maintained the same for all participants to avoid and prevent sensory overload and stress that they could experience.

The total duration of the experiment was of 14 min, and each stimulus condition lasted 2 min and 40 s. Movement recording was turned on during the virtual experience. The researcher monitored the child state during the entire experiment.

2.6. Behavioural Motor Assessment and Data Processing

In the experiment design, it was proposed to use an efficient method to estimate the pose in real-time using an RGB-D camera. The participant's experiment was recorded using an Intel® RealSense™ camera D435 (FRAMOS, Munich, Germany) and Intel RealSense SDK 2.0 (Intel RealSense Technology, Santa Clara, CA, USA) with the cross-platform support. This camera has a depth sensor that uses stereo vision to calculate it. It works like a USB and is equipped with a pair of depth sensors, an RGB sensor, an infrared project a great global image obturator (91.2° × 65.5° × 100.6°).

The detection of the body joints in each frame of the recording was calculated using the deep learning algorithm OpenPose [112], which includes the 2D position related to the video and a confidence level for each joint identification between 0 and 1. The skeleton (Figure 3) includes 25 joints that can be divided into different parts of the body: head (0 nose, 15/16 eyes and 17/18 ears), trunk (1 neck and 8 mid hip), arms (2/5 shoulders, 3/6 elbows and 4/7 wrists), legs (9/12 hips, 10/13 knees, 11/14 ankles), and feet (19/22 big toes, 20/23 small toes and 21/24 heels). After detecting the skeleton, the 3D position of each joint during the experiment was obtained using the depth information of the camera. A computer with an Nvidia GTX1060 graphics card with the NVIDIA Pascal architecture capable of executing neural networks very efficiently in a compact size was used.

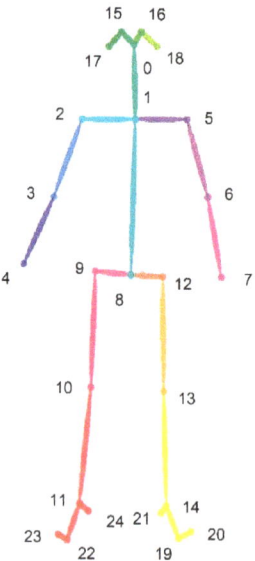

Figure 3. Joint virtual disposition.

After extracting the 3D position of the body's joints from all the experiments, the data recording was segmented for each stimulus condition, excluding the samples of the joints that have a confidence below 0.5. The displacement of the joints was computed using the Euclidean distance between consecutive frames. Finally, the level of movement of a joint during a stimulus was characterized by computing the mean of all displacement.

2.7. Statistical Analysis

First, to characterize behavior differences between ASD and TD children on each stimuli condition, we analyzed the movement frequency of each joint. Since data followed a non-normal distribution (Shapiro-Wilk test: $p < 0.05$), Wilcoxon signed-rank tests were applied.

Second, we applied a set of machine learning models to analyze if the frequency of the movement could discriminate between ASD and TD children. The body was divided into five parts: head (joints 15, 16, 17, and 18), trunk (joints 1 and 8), arms (joints 2, 3, 4, 5, 6, and 7), legs (9, 10, 11, 12, 13, and 14), and feet (19, 20, 21, 22, 23, and 24). The machine learning analysis based on 24 features-based dataset included the five body parts, one related to the whole body, the three stimuli conditions (V, VA, VAO) and one related to the entire experiment. Because of a large number of features, a reduction strategy was adopted to decrease the dimensions in each dataset. Principal component analysis method (PCA) was applied to select features that explain 95% of the variability of the dataset. Finally, a supervised machine-learning model was developed using the PCA features in each dataset.

To implement the models, support vector machine (SVM)-based pattern recognition with a leave-one-subject-out (LOSO) cross-validation procedure has been applied [113]. Within the LOSO scheme, the training set was normalized by subtracting the median value and dividing by the median absolute deviation over each dimension. In each iteration, the validation set consisted of one specific subject and it was normalized using the median and deviation of the training set. We used a C-SVM optimized using a Gaussian Kernel function, changing the parameters of cost and gamma using a vector with seven parameters logarithmically spaced between 0.1 and 1000. Also, a SVM recursive feature elimination (SVM-RFE) procedure was included in a wrapper approach. RFE was performed on the training set of each fold and we computed the median rank for each feature among all folds. In particular, a nonlinear SVM-RFE was implemented, which includes a correlation bias reduction strategy in the feature elimination procedure [114]. To analyze the performance of the models, a set of metrics were considered: accuracy, i.e., percentage of subjects who correctly recognized, true positive rate, i.e., percentage of actual ASD subjects recognized as ASD, true negative rate, i.e., percentage of actual control subjects recognized as controls, and Cohen's kappa, which describes the performance of the model from 0 to 1, 0 being a random class assignation and 1 a perfect classification. The model was optimized to achieve best Cohen's kappa. The algorithms were implemented using Matlab© R2016a and LIBSVM toolbox [115].

3. Results

3.1. Analysis of Total Movement

Figure 4 shows the body joints' significant differences obtained applying Wilcoxon signed-rank. In V stimuli condition, 4 joints of the legs, 2 of the head and 1 of the trunk presented higher movements in ASD population than TD children. In VA stimuli condition, 1 joint of the legs and 2 of the head also presented higher movements in ASD population than TD children. Also in VAO stimuli condition, 3 joints of the head presented the same tendency. Conversely, 1 joint of the head (16) presented lower movement in ASD population in the visual condition baseline (BL_V) and in visual-auditive-olfactive condition baseline (BL_VAO).

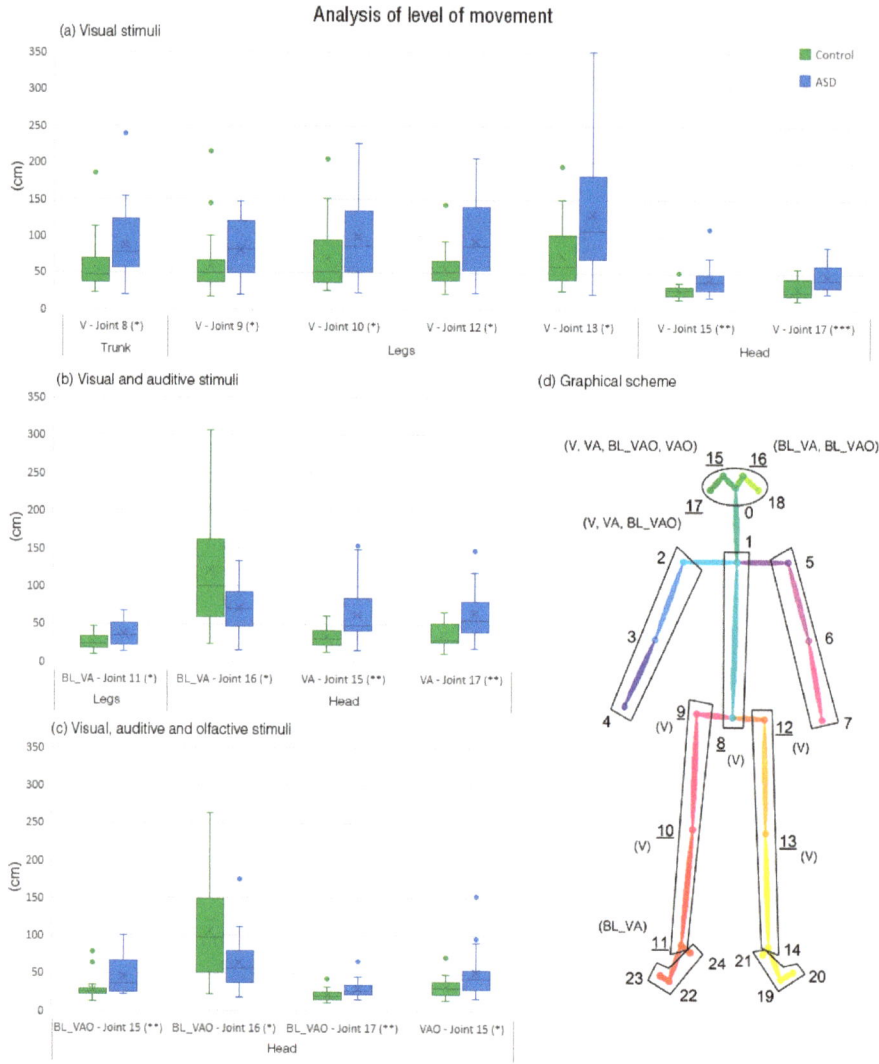

Figure 4. Analysis of the level of movement of joints that presents statistical differences: (**a**) Boxplot of joints in visual stimuli; (**b**) boxplot of joints in visual and auditory stimuli; (**c**) boxplot of joints in visual, auditory, and olfactory stimuli; (**d**) scheme of the joints including the stimuli where differences are found. Note. * $p < 0.05$. ** $p < 0.01$. *** $p < 0.001$.

3.2. ASD Classification Performance

Tables 1 and 2 show the performance of the computed machine learning models, considering the combination of a set of joints and virtual stimuli conditions. Regarding body parameters, the models including the head and trunk joints presented an accuracy of 82.98% and unbalanced confusion matrices. Conversely, the model that uses the feet joints present the same accuracy (82.98%) and a balanced confusion matrix. In addition, the models including arms and legs movements achieved a lower accuracy than the other body joints (74.47% and 72.4% respectively). Finally, the model including all joints and virtual stimuli conditions showed the lowest accuracy (70.21%) and the lower true positives (45.45%).

Table 1. Overview of the accuracy of each model considering the stimuli and set of joints.

		Stimuli			
		V	VA	VAO	All
Set of Joints	Head	80.85%	82.98%	89.36%	82.98%
	Trunk	70.21%	72.34%	76.60%	82.98%
	Arms	87.23%	78.72%	65.96%	74.47%
	Legs	61.70%	63.83%	74.47%	72.34%
	Feet	78.72%	78.72%	65.96%	82.98%
	All	89.36%	74.47%	70.21%	70.21%

Table 2. Detailed level of autism spectrum disorder (ASD) recognition of each model including accuracy, true positive rate (TPR), true negative rate (TNR), Cohen's Kappa and PCA featured selected.

Stimuli	Set of Joints	Accuracy	TPR	TNR	Kappa	PCA Features Selected
All	All	70.21%	45.45%	92.00%	0.39	1/20
V	All	89.36%	100.00%	80.00%	0.79	1/14
VA	All	74.47%	59.09%	88.00%	0.48	2/12
VAO	All	70.21%	63.64%	76.00%	0.40	3/12
All	Head	82.98%	100.00%	68.00%	0.67	1/11
All	Trunk	82.98%	63.64%	100.00%	0.65	2/8
All	Arms	74.47%	90.91%	60.00%	0.50	1/15
All	Legs	72.34%	68.18%	76.00%	0.44	3/8
All	Feet	82.98%	81.82%	84.00%	0.66	2/13
V	Head	80.85%	68.18%	92.00%	0.61	1/6
V	Trunk	70.21%	81.82%	60.00%	0.41	1/3
V	Arms	87.23%	72.73%	100.00%	0.74	1/8
V	Legs	61.70%	45.45%	76.00%	0.22	1/5
V	Feet	78.72%	54.55%	100.00%	0.56	2/6
VA	Head	82.98%	63.64%	100.00%	0.65	3/6
VA	Trunk	72.34%	72.73%	72.00%	0.45	1/3
VA	Arms	78.72%	95.45%	64.00%	0.58	1/8
VA	Legs	63.83%	45.45%	80.00%	0.26	1/4
VA	Feet	78.72%	72.73%	84.00%	0.57	2/6
VAO	Head	89.36%	77.27%	100.00%	0.78	2/6
VAO	Trunk	76.60%	68.18%	84.00%	0.53	2/3
VAO	Arms	65.96%	50.00%	80.00%	0.30	2/7
VAO	Legs	74.47%	68.18%	80.00%	0.48	1/5
VAO	Feet	65.96%	45.45%	84.00%	0.30	2/7

Regarding the influence of the virtual stimuli conditions, the V presented the highest accuracy in the study (89.36%), showing that it is the most relevant stimuli of the experiment. In the VA stimuli, the accuracy decrease to 74.47%, and in VAO to 70.21%. Furthermore, the head joints showed the most consistent performance along with the stimuli, from 80.85% in V to 89.36% in VAO, suggesting that it is the most important part of the body to discriminate ASD population. The trunk joints present also a consistent accuracy, from 70.21% in V to 76.60% in VAO, but the discriminate performance is considerably lower than using the head. All the models used three features or less after applying the automatic feature selection procedure.

4. Discussion

ASD is diagnosed according to qualitative clinician judgments, based on symptoms, through semi-structured observations and interviews (ADOS; ADI-R). Given the qualitative nature of the traditional tools, researchers have focused on improving methods of diagnosis and assessment, pointing out the predictive value of behavioral biomarkers, as more objective and quantitative measures. This study aimed, first, to compare tracked body movements data during a multimodal VR stimulation between ASD and TD children. Second, it was verified which body areas might be relevant for the discrimination between the two populations. Third, the study investigated which virtual stimuli condition better discriminate body areas between the two populations. To reach these aims, we applied a machine learning procedure [70] to body movements' analysis of a multimodal VR experience, composed of three stimuli conditions: visual, visual-auditive, and visual-auditive-olfactory.

The study included a preliminary analysis of the frequency distribution of body movements to investigate the differences between groups and a broad set of supervised ML models combining body parameters and stimuli conditions to evaluate the discriminability between ASD and TD children using movement. Results can be discussed on four points: (1) The significant differences between the two groups on body movements; (2) machine learning methods on body movements and features used; (3) the influence of stimuli conditions; and (4) limitations and future studies.

4.1. Body Movement Parameters' Differences between Groups

The first aim was to identify differences in terms of body movements between children with ASD and TD children. Figure 4 showed significant differences in15 body joints and 13 of them have showed that ASD children present more body movements than TD children. In particular, 4 legs' joints, 2 head's joints and 1 trunk's joint in V condition, 1 legs' joints and 2 head's joints in VA condition, and 4 head's joints in VAO condition showed higher movements, suggesting that ASD children have performed more head and legs' movements than TD children during the imitation tasks. Previous studies that showed that head tilting, legs flapping, as well as bilateral repetitive movements involving legs walking represent two or more movements features related to ASD children confirm the presence of larger body movements' in ASD than in TD children [8,10]. However, only one joint in the head showed higher movement in TD children than ASD children during the baselines of VA and VAO. This result is partially in opposition to the scientific literature but as mentioned in the introduction, common and complex body movements are also present in TD children. To improve the quantitative methods to discriminate ASD from TD children using body movements' frequencies, we applied machine-learning techniques developing 24 models, combining body joint parts and virtual stimuli conditions. In the next section, we deeply discuss the results.

4.2. Machine Learning Methods on Body Movements and Features Used

Concerning the recognition using different parts of the body, the best classification accuracy reached 82.98% for the head parameter by using only one feature selection method, and the same accuracy was achieved for body and foot parameters by using two features' selection method, independently by the specific stimuli condition. Interesting results have also resulted from the model including arms and legs that achieved a classification accuracy of 74.47% and 72.34%, respectively. The results are consistent with the scientific literature that has identified head spinning and banging, body rocking, and stamping the feet, three of the main stereotypies and repetitive movements are related to ASD [8]. Furthermore, these results showed that ML could provide an effective solution to best describe body movements' differences of participant groups' classification during imitation tasks, while the traditional statistical methods (e.g., mean age comparisons) could fail to deal with such complex tasks. To our knowledge, only two previous studies have investigated the predictive value to discriminate between children with and without ASD using an imitation task [70,71]. Both studies focused on the analysis of arm and hand movements during a simple reach-to-drop imitation task, reaching a maximum classification accuracy of 96.7% and 93.8%, respectively. Our study focused on a more complex real-simulated imitation task, composed of three imitation subtasks, waving, dancing, and eating and tracking all body movements.

Thus, the present findings show the feasibility and applicability of a ML method for correctly classifying preschool children with ASD based on real-simulated imitation tasks. In the standard diagnosis of toddlers it is particularly difficult to evaluate repetitive and stereotyped behaviors. The application of technologies, such as cameras and sensors, might have potential clinical applications to support diagnosis providing accurate quantitative methods along with the qualitative traditional methods. Finally, the use of cameras and sensors are more convenient, less expensive, and less invasive technologies than fMRI and EEG to implement in clinical settings.

4.3. The Influence of Stimuli Conditions

Regarding the virtual stimuli conditions, head showed to be the core body movement in the groups' classification during the three stimuli conditions, achieving the best classifications' accuracy of 89.36% in VAO condition, 82.98% in VA condition, and 80.85% in V condition. These results suggest that the greater the sensory stimulation, the greater the stereotypies and repetitive movements, allowing to discriminate children with ASD from TD children. The different classification accuracy among the three stimuli conditions is consistent with previous studies on the sensory sensitivity overload of ASD patients to multimodality stimuli [116–119]. Specifically, ASD patients have shown lower-functioning abilities to filter process and integrate simultaneous information compared to TD subjects [116]. For example, during multiple auditory tones, tasks matched with single visual-flash stimulus ASD patients perceived more flashes than those are presented [117]. Furthermore, EEG studies on ASD patients showed that the amplitude is higher and the latency in the response is delayed than TD subjects [118,119]. Other multimodal sensory stimulations achieved a good accuracy classification between the two groups, resulting in stereotypes and repetitive movements of the trunk (VAO: 76.60%), legs (VAO: 74.47%), arms and feet (VA: 78.72%). Finally, arms and feet movements showed a high accuracy of 87.23 and 78.72 respectively in the classification between groups during the unimodal visual condition.

In general, V condition including all the body achieved the best accuracy (89.36%), including a 100% true positive rate and using only 1 feature of PCA, in contrast to VA (74.47%) and VAO (70.21%). These results, on one hand, highlight that real-simulated imitation activities that can occur in daily life, such as waving (V), dancing (VA), and eating (VAO) allow evaluating body movements discriminating ASD and TD children. Previous studies on discriminating ASD and TD children using imitation tasks have used simple reach-to-grasp and drop arm movement tasks [70] or a hand movement task to target in laboratory settings [71] and our study aimed to investigate whole-body movements in more complex real-simulated scenarios and tasks.

On the other hand, the predominance of the visual influence can depend on the fact that V stimuli was the first condition and could have generated a wow-effect in the subjects. Finally, the model that includes all the data achieved an accuracy of 70.21% with a 45.45% of true positive rate, showing that the feature selection procedures have a critical role to achieve good performance in biomarkers development. This result could suggest that the implemented virtual tasks could fail in detecting RB behaviors.

4.4. Limitations and Future Studies

Despite the promising results, some methodological limitations of the present exploratory study should be reported. The main limitation is the limited sample sizes of participants for each group. Future studies on larger sample sizes could allow validating the ML method, providing also the possibility to test the model. As ASD is a heterogeneous condition, the possibility of training the model with larger groups of ASD and children with typical neurodevelopment would be useful to improve the generalization of the model to a wide condition range of ASD. Also, other comparisons studies, including other neurodevelopment disorders with movement impairments, as the attention deficit hyperactivity disorder, could be valuable by ML for understanding if these groups present similar body movements that are distinct for the different neurodevelopment conditions (e.g., intellectual disability [120]. Indeed, taking also into account different neurodevelopment conditions could improve the specificity of the classifiers for ASD rather than for neurodevelopment disorders in general.

Furthermore, the experimental groups were not matched on measures related to the intelligence quotient performance, cognitive abilities, and motor comorbidities (e.g., dyspraxia), limiting the confidence that the experimental differences observed in the experiment were due to a diagnosis of ASD, and not to differences in other cognitive or non-cognitive factors. Future studies will consider matching these factors in order to improve the reliability and validity of the model results.

Finally, regarding the stimuli conditions, the order of presentation (V-VA-VAO) was not counterbalanced because of the hyper-sensitiveness of ASD children to multiple stimuli [105–108]. Future studies including counterbalanced conditions following high and low children functioning are needed.

5. Conclusions

The present study represents, to our knowledge, the first attempt to discriminate ASD children from children with typical neurodevelopment using body movements parameters of an imitation VR task and machine learning. The significant predictive values of our classification approach might be valuable to support ASD diagnosis, as well as the use of more objective methods and ecological tasks VR-aided along with traditional assessment.

Author Contributions: All authors have contributed to the manuscript as described below: M.A.R. and L.A. designed the study, and M.A.R., L.A., and I.A.C.G. supervised the whole study. Movements' data processing was conducted by J.M.-M. as well as the statistical analyses. The manuscript was originally written by I.A.C.G., M.E.M., G.T.G., and J.M.-M. and the final manuscript was revised by M.A.R. and I.A.C.G. All authors assisted in the revision process. All authors have read and agreed to the published version of the manuscript.

Funding: This work was supported by the Spanish Ministry of Economy, Industry, and Competitiveness funded project "Immersive virtual environment for the evaluation and training of children with autism spectrum disorder: T Room" (IDI-20170912) and by the Generalitat Valenciana funded project REBRAND (PROMETEO/2019/105). Furthermore, this work was co-founded by the European Union through the Operational Program of the European Regional development Fund (ERDF) of the Valencian Community 2014–2020 (IDIFEDER/2018/029).

Acknowledgments: We thank Zayda Ferrer Lluch for the development of virtual reality environments.

Conflicts of Interest: The authors declare no conflict of interest.

References

1. American Psychiatric Association. *Diagnostic and Statistical Manual of Mental Disorders (DSM-5®)*; American Psychiatric Pub: Washington, DC, USA, 2013.
2. World Health Organization. Available online: https://www.who.int/news-room/fact-sheets/detail/autism-spectrum-disorders (accessed on 20 November 2019).
3. Anagnostou, E.; Zwaigenbaum, L.; Szatmari, P.; Fombonne, E.; Fernandez, B.A.; Woodbury-Smith, M.; Buchanan, J.A. Autism spectrum disorder: Advances in evidence-based practice. *Cmaj* **2014**, *186*, 509–519. [CrossRef] [PubMed]
4. Lord, C.; Risi, S.; DiLavore, P.S.; Shulman, C.; Thurm, A.; Pickles, A. Autism from 2 to 9 years of age. *Arch. Gen. Psychiatry* **2006**, *63*, 694–701. [CrossRef] [PubMed]
5. Schmidt, L.; Kirchner, J.; Strunz, S.; Broźus, J.; Ritter, K.; Roepke, S.; Dziobek, I. Psychosocial functioning and life satisfaction in adults with autism spectrum disorder without intellectual impairment. *J. Clin. Psychol.* **2015**, *71*, 1259–1268. [CrossRef]
6. Turner, M. Annotation: Repetitive behaviour in autism: A review of psychological research. *J. Child Psychol. Psychiatry Allied Discip.* **1999**, *40*, 839–849. [CrossRef]
7. Lewis, M.H.; Bodfish, J.W. Repetitive behavior disorders in autism. *Ment. Retard. Dev. Disabil. Res. Rev.* **1998**, *4*, 80–89. [CrossRef]
8. Ghanizadeh, A. Clinical approach to motor stereotypies in autistic children. *Iran. J. Pediatr.* **2010**, *20*, 149.
9. Mahone, E.M.; Bridges, D.; Prahme, C.; Singer, H.S. Repetitive arm and hand movements (complex motor stereotypies) in children. *J. Pediatr.* **2004**, *145*, 391–395. [CrossRef] [PubMed]

10. MacDonald, R.; Green, G.; Mansfield, R.; Geckeler, A.; Gardenier, N.; Anderson, J.; Sanchez, J. Stereotypy in young children with autism and typically developing children. *Res. Dev. Disabil.* **2007**, *28*, 266–277. [CrossRef] [PubMed]
11. Singer, H.S. Motor stereotypies. *Semin. Pediatr. Neurol.* **2009**, *16*, 77–81. [CrossRef]
12. Lidstone, J.; Uljarević, M.; Sullivan, J.; Rodgers, J.; McConachie, H.; Freeston, M.; Leekam, S. Relations among restricted and repetitive behaviors, anxiety and sensory features in children with autism spectrum disorders. *Res. Autism Spectr. Disord.* **2014**, *8*, 82–92. [CrossRef]
13. Bodfish, J.W.; Symons, F.J.; Parker, D.E.; Lewis, M.H. Varieties of repetitive behavior in autism: Comparisons to mental retardation. *J. Autism Dev. Disord.* **2000**, *30*, 237–243. [CrossRef] [PubMed]
14. Campbell, M.; Locascio, J.J.; Choroco, M.C.; Spencer, E.K.; Malone, R.P.; Kafantaris, V.; Overall, J.E. Stereotypies and tardive dyskinesia: Abnormal movements in autistic children. *Psychopharmacol. Bull.* **1990**, *26*, 260–266. [PubMed]
15. Goldman, S.; Wang, C.; Salgado, M.W.; Greene, P.E.; Kim, M.; Rapin, I. Motor stereotypies in children with autism and other developmental disorders. *Dev. Med. Child Neurol.* **2009**, *51*, 30–38. [CrossRef] [PubMed]
16. Lord, C.; Rutter, M.; DiLavore, P.C.; Risi, S.A. *Diagnostic Observation Schedule-WPS (ADOS-WPS)*; Western Psychological Services: Los Angeles, CA, USA, 1999.
17. Lord, C.; Rutter, M.; Le Couteur, A. Autism Diagnostic Interview-Revised: A revised version of a diagnostic interview for caregivers of individuals with possible pervasive developmental disorders. *J. Autism Dev. Disord.* **1994**, *24*, 659–685. [CrossRef]
18. Goldstein, S.; Naglieri, J.A.; Ozonoff, S. *Assessment of Autism Spectrum Disorder*; The Guilford Press: New York, NY, USA, 2009.
19. Gonçalves, N.; Rodrigues, J.L.; Costa, S.; Soares, F. Preliminary study on determining stereotypical motor movements. In Proceedings of the 2012 Annual International Conference of the IEEE Engineering in Medicine and Biology Society, San Diego, CA, USA, 28 August–1 September 2012; pp. 1598–1601.
20. Volkmar, F.R.; State, M.; Klin, A. Autism and autism spectrum disorders: Diagnostic issues for the coming decade. *J. Child Psychol. Psychiatry* **2009**, *50*, 108–115. [CrossRef]
21. Lord, C.; Rutter, M.; DiLavore, P.C.; Risi, S. *Autism Diagnostic Observation Schedule*; Western Psychological Services: Los Angeles, CA, USA, 2001.
22. Reaven, J.A.; Hepburn, S.L.; Ross, R.G. Use of the ADOS and ADI-R in children with psychosis: Importance of clinical judgment. *Clin. Child Psychol. Psychiatry* **2008**, *13*, 81–94. [CrossRef]
23. Torres, E.B.; Brincker, M.; Isenhower, R.W., III; Yanovich, P.; Stigler, K.A.; Nurnberger, J.I., Jr.; José, J.V. Autism: The micro-movement perspective. *Front. Integr. Neurosci.* **2013**, *7*, 32. [CrossRef]
24. Paulhus, D.L. Measurement and Control of Response Bias. In *Measures of Social Psychological Attitudes, Volume 1. Measures of Personality and Social Psychological Attitudes*; Robinson, J.P., Shaver, P.R., Wrightsman, L.S., Eds.; Academic Press: San Diego, CA, USA, 1991; pp. 17–59.
25. Edwards, A.L. *The Social Desirability Variable in Personality Assessment and Research*; Dryden Press: Dryden, ON, Canada, 1957.
26. Möricke, E.; Buitelaar, J.K.; Rommelse, N.N. Do we need multiple informants when assessing autistic traits? The degree of report bias on offspring, self, and spouse ratings. *J. Autism Dev. Disord.* **2016**, *46*, 164–175. [CrossRef]
27. Chaytor, N.; Schmitter-Edgecombe, M.; Burr, R. Improving the ecological validity of executive functioning assessment. *Arch. Clin. Neuropsychol.* **2006**, *21*, 217–227. [CrossRef]
28. Franzen, M.D.; Wilhelm, K.L. Conceptual Foundations of Ecological Validity in Neuropsychological Assessment. In *Ecological Validity of Neuropsychological Testing*; Sbordone, R.J., Long, C.J., Eds.; Gr Press/St Lucie Press Inc.: Delray Beach, FL, USA, 1996; pp. 91–112.
29. Brunswick, E. Symposium of the probability approach in psychology: Representative design and probabilistic theory in a functional psychology. *Psychol. Rev.* **1955**, *62*, 193–217. [CrossRef]
30. Gillberg, C.; Rasmussen, P. Brief report: Four case histories and a literature review of Williams syndrome and autistic behavior. *J. Autism Dev. Disord.* **1994**, *24*, 381–393. [CrossRef] [PubMed]
31. Parsons, S. Authenticity in Virtual Reality for assessment and intervention in autism: A conceptual review. *Educ. Res. Rev.* **2016**, *19*, 138–157. [CrossRef]
32. Francis, K. Autism interventions: A critical update. *Dev. Med. Child Neurol.* **2005**, *47*, 493–499. [CrossRef] [PubMed]

33. Albinali, F.; Goodwin, M.S.; Intille, S.S. Recognizing stereotypical motor movements in the laboratory and classroom: A case study with children on the autism spectrum. In Proceedings of the 11th International Conference on Ubiquitous Computing, Orlando, FL, USA, 30 September–3 October 2009; ACM: New York, NY, USA, 2009; pp. 71–80. [CrossRef]
34. Pyles, D.A.; Riordan, M.M.; Bailey, J.S. The stereotypy analysis: An instrument for examining environmental variables associated with differential rates of stereotypic behavior. *Res. Dev. Disabil.* **1997**, *18*, 11–38. [CrossRef]
35. Min, C.H.; Tewfik, A.H. Novel pattern detection in children with autism spectrum disorder using iterative subspace identification. In Proceedings of the 2010 IEEE International Conference on Acoustics, Speech and Signal Processing, Dallas, TX, USA, 14–19 March 2010; pp. 2266–2269.
36. Min, C.H.; Tewfik, A.H. Automatic characterization and detection of behavioral patterns using linear predictive coding of accelerometer sensor data. In Proceedings of the 2010 Annual International Conference of the IEEE Engineering in Medicine and Biology, Buenos Aires, Argentina, 31 August–4 September 2010; pp. 220–223.
37. Nosek, B.A.; Hawkins, C.B.; Frazier, R.S. Implicit social cognition: From measures to mechanisms. *Trends Cogn. Sci.* **2011**, *15*, 152–159. [CrossRef] [PubMed]
38. Lieberman, M.D. Social cognitive neuroscience. In *Handbook of Social Psychology*; Fiske, S.T., Gilbert, D.T., Lindzey, G., Eds.; John Wiley & Sons Inc.: Hoboken, NJ, USA, 2010; pp. 143–193.
39. Forscher, P.S.; Lai, C.K.; Axt, J.R.; Ebersole, C.R.; Herman, M.; Devine, P.G.; Nosek, B.A. A meta-analysis of procedures to change implicit measures. *J. Pers. Soc. Psychol.* **2019**, *117*, 522–559. [CrossRef]
40. LeDoux, J.E.; Pine, D.S. Using neuroscience to help understand fear and anxiety: A two-system framework. *Am. J. Psychiatry* **2016**, *173*, 1083–1093. [CrossRef] [PubMed]
41. Fenning, R.M.; Baker, J.K.; Baucom, B.R.; Erath, S.A.; Howland, M.A.; Moffitt, J. Electrodermal variability and symptom severity in children with autism spectrum disorder. *J. Autism Dev. Disord.* **2017**, *47*, 1062–1072. [CrossRef]
42. Walsh, P.; Elsabbagh, M.; Bolton, P.; Singh, I. In search of biomarkers for autism: Scientific, social and ethical challenges. *Nat. Rev. Neurosci.* **2011**, *12*, 603. [CrossRef]
43. Nikula, R. Psychological correlates of nonspecific skin conductance responses. *Psychophysiology* **1991**, *28*, 86–90. [CrossRef]
44. Alcañiz Raya, M.; Chicchi Giglioli, I.A.; Marín-Morales, J.; Higuera-Trujillo, J.L.; Olmos, E.; Minissi, M.E.; Abad, L. Application of Supervised Machine Learning for Behavioral Biomarkers of Autism Spectrum Disorder Based on Electrodermal Activity and Virtual Reality. *Front. Hum. Neurosci.* **2020**, *14*, 90. [CrossRef] [PubMed]
45. Cunningham, W.A.; Raye, C.L.; Johnson, M.K. Implicit and explicit evaluation: fMRI correlates of valence, emotional intensity, and control in the processing of attitudes. *J. Cogn. Neurosci.* **2004**, *16*, 1717–1729. [CrossRef] [PubMed]
46. Kopton, I.M.; Kenning, P. Near-infrared spectroscopy (NIRS) as a new tool for neuroeconomic research. *Front. Hum. Neurosci.* **2014**, *8*, 549. [CrossRef] [PubMed]
47. Knyazev, G.G.; Slobodskaya, H.R.; Wilson, G.D. Personality and Brain Oscillations in the Developmental Perspective. In *Advances in Psychology Research*; Shohov, S.P., Ed.; Nova Science Publishers: Hauppauge, NY, USA, 2004; Volume 29, pp. 3–34.
48. Gwizdka, J. Characterizing relevance with eye-tracking measures. In Proceedings of the 5th Information Interaction in Context Symposium, Regensburg, Germany, 26–29 August 2014; pp. 58–67.
49. Nickel, P.; Nachreiner, F. Sensitivity and diagnosticity of the 0.1-Hz component of heart rate variability as an indicator of mental workload. *Hum. Factors* **2003**, *45*, 575–590. [CrossRef] [PubMed]
50. Di Martino, A.; Yan, C.G.; Li, Q.; Denio, E.; Castellanos, F.X.; Alaerts, K.; Deen, B. The autism brain imaging data exchange: Towards a large-scale evaluation of the intrinsic brain architecture in autism. *Mol. Psychiatry* **2014**, *19*, 659. [CrossRef] [PubMed]
51. Van Hecke, A.V.; Lebow, J.; Bal, E.; Lamb, D.; Harden, E.; Kramer, A.; Porges, S.W. Electroencephalogram and heart rate regulation to familiar and unfamiliar people in children with autism spectrum disorders. *Child Dev.* **2009**, *80*, 1118–1133. [CrossRef]
52. Alcañiz, M.L.; Olmos-raya, E.; Abad, L. Uso de entornos virtuales para trastornos del neurodesarrollo: Una revisión del estado del arte y agenda futura. *Medicina (Buenos Aires)* **2019**, *79*, 77–81.

53. Amiri, A.; Peltier, N.; Goldberg, C.; Sun, Y.; Nathan, A.; Hiremath, S.; Mankodiya, K. WearSense: Detecting autism stereotypic behaviors through smartwatches. *Healthcare* **2017**, *5*, 11. [CrossRef]
54. Coronato, A.; De Pietro, G.; Paragliola, G. A situation-aware system for the detection of motion disorders of patients with autism spectrum disorders. *Expert Syst. Appl.* **2014**, *41*, 7868–7877. [CrossRef]
55. Goodwin, M.S.; Intille, S.S.; Velicer, W.F.; Groden, J. Sensor-enabled detection of stereotypical motor movements in persons with autism spectrum disorder. In Proceedings of the 7th International Conference on Interaction Design and Children, Chicago, IL, USA, 11–13 June 2008; pp. 109–112.
56. Goodwin, M.S.; Intille, S.S.; Albinali, F.; Velicer, W.F. Automated detection of stereotypical motor movements. *J. Autism Dev. Disord.* **2011**, *41*, 770–782. [CrossRef]
57. Paragliola, G.; Coronato, A. Intelligent monitoring of stereotyped motion disorders in case of children with autism. In Proceedings of the 2013 9th International Conference on Intelligent Environments, Athens, Greece, 16–17 July 2013; pp. 258–261.
58. Rodrigues, J.L.; Gonçalves, N.; Costa, S.; Soares, F. Stereotyped movement recognition in children with ASD. *Sens. Actuators A Phys.* **2013**, *202*, 162–169. [CrossRef]
59. Madsen, M.; El Kaliouby, R.; Goodwin, M.; Picard, R. Technology for just-in-time in-situ learning of facial affect for persons diagnosed with an autism spectrum disorder. In Proceedings of the 10th International ACM SIGACCESS Conference on Computers and Accessibility, Halifax, NS, Canada, 13–15 October 2008; pp. 19–26.
60. Min, C.H.; Tewfik, A.H.; Kim, Y.; Menard, R. Optimal sensor location for body sensor network to detect self-stimulatory behaviors of children with autism spectrum disorder. In Proceedings of the 2009 Annual International Conference of the IEEE Engineering in Medicine and Biology Society, Minneapolis, MN, USA, 2–6 September 2009; pp. 3489–3492.
61. Westeyn, T.; Vadas, K.; Bian, X.; Starner, T.; Abowd, G.D. Recognizing mimicked autistic self-stimulatory behaviors using hmms. In Proceedings of the Ninth IEEE International Symposium on Wearable Computers (ISWC'05), Osaka, Japan, 11–14 October 2005; pp. 164–167.
62. Simonyan, K.; Zisserman, A. Very deep convolutional networks for large-scale image recognition. *arXiv* **2014**, arXiv:1409.1556.
63. Andriluka, M.; Pishchulin, L.; Gehler, P.; Schiele, B. 2D human pose estimation: New benchmark and state of the art analysis. In Proceedings of the IEEE Conference on Computer Vision and Pattern Recognition, Columbus, OH, USA, 23–28 June 2014; pp. 3686–3693.
64. Lin, T.Y.; Maire, M.; Belongie, S.; Hays, J.; Perona, P.; Ramanan, D.; Zitnick, C.L. Microsoft coco: Common objects in context. In Proceedings of the European Conference on Computer Vision, Zurich, Switzerland, 6–12 September 2014; Springer: Cham, Switzerland, 2014; pp. 740–755.
65. Carreira, J.; Agrawal, P.; Fragkiadaki, K.; Malik, J. Human pose estimation with iterative error feedback. In Proceedings of the IEEE Conference on Computer Vision and Pattern Recognition, Las Vegas, NV, USA, 27–30 June 2016; pp. 4733–4742.
66. Iqbal, U.; Garbade, M.; Gall, J. Pose for action-action for pose. In Proceedings of the 2017 12th IEEE International Conference on Automatic Face & Gesture Recognition (FG 2017), Washington, DC, USA, 30 May–3 June 2017; pp. 438–445.
67. Pfister, T.; Charles, J.; Zisserman, A. Flowing convnets for human pose estimation in videos. In Proceedings of the IEEE International Conference on Computer Vision, Santiago, Chile, 7–13 December 2015; pp. 1913–1921.
68. Toshev, A.; Szegedy, C. Deeppose: Human pose estimation via deep neural networks. In Proceedings of the IEEE Conference on Computer Vision and Pattern Recognition, Columbus, OH, USA, 23–28 June 2014; pp. 1653–1660.
69. Wei, S.E.; Ramakrishna, V.; Kanade, T.; Sheikh, Y. Convolutional pose machines. In Proceedings of the IEEE Conference on Computer Vision and Pattern Recognition, Las Vegas, NV, USA, 27–30 June 2016; pp. 4724–4732.
70. Crippa, A.; Salvatore, C.; Perego, P.; Forti, S.; Nobile, M.; Molteni, M.; Castiglioni, I. Use of machine learning to identify children with autism and their motor abnormalities. *J. Autism Dev. Disord.* **2015**, *45*, 2146–2156. [CrossRef]
71. Wedyan, M.; Al-Jumaily, A.; Crippa, A. Using machine learning to perform early diagnosis of autism spectrum disorder based on simple upper limb movements. *Int. J. Hybrid Intell. Syst.* **2019**, *15*, 195–206. [CrossRef]

72. Burdea, G.C.; Coiffet, P. *Virtual Reality Technology*; John Wiley & Sons: Hoboken, NJ, USA, 2003.
73. Fuchs, H.; Bishop, G. *Research Directions in Virtual Environments*; University of North Carolina at Chapel Hill: Chapel Hill, NC, USA, 1992.
74. Parsons, S.; Mitchell, P.; Leonard, A. The use and understanding of virtual environments by adolescents with autistic spectrum disorders. *J. Autism Dev. Disord.* **2004**, *34*, 449–466. [CrossRef]
75. Parsons, T.D.; Rizzo, A.A.; Rogers, S.; York, P. Virtual reality in paediatric rehabilitation: A review. *Dev. Neurorehabil.* **2009**, *12*, 224–238. [CrossRef] [PubMed]
76. Parsons, T.D. Neuropsychological assessment using virtual environments: Enhanced assessment technology for improved ecological validity. In *Advanced Computational Intelligence Paradigms in Healthcare 6. Virtual Reality in Psychotherapy, Rehabilitation, and Assessment*; Springer: Heidelberg/Berlin, Germany, 2011; pp. 271–289.
77. Bowman, D.A.; Gabbard, J.L.; Hix, D. A survey of usability evaluation in virtual environments: Classification and comparison of methods. *Presence Teleoperators Virtual Environ.* **2002**, *11*, 404–424. [CrossRef]
78. Pastorelli, E.; Herrmann, H. A small-scale, low-budget semi-immersive virtual environment for scientific visualization and research. *Procedia Comput. Sci.* **2013**, *25*, 14–22. [CrossRef]
79. Cobb, S.V.; Nichols, S.; Ramsey, A.; Wilson, J.R. Virtual reality-induced symptoms and effects (VRISE). *Presence Teleoperators Virtual Environ.* **1999**, *8*, 169–186. [CrossRef]
80. Guazzaroni, G. (Ed.) *Virtual and Augmented Reality in Mental Health Treatment*; IGI Global: Hershey, PA, USA, 2018.
81. Wallace, S.; Parsons, S.; Westbury, A.; White, K.; White, K.; Bailey, A. Sense of presence and atypical social judgments in immersive virtual environments: Responses of adolescents with Autism Spectrum Disorders. *Autism* **2010**, *14*, 199–213. [CrossRef]
82. Lorenzo, G.; Lledó, A.; Arráez-Vera, G.; Lorenzo-Lledó, A. The application of immersive virtual reality for students with ASD: A review between 1990–2017. *Educ. Inf. Technol.* **2019**, *24*, 127–151. [CrossRef]
83. Bailenson, J.N.; Yee, N.; Merget, D.; Schroeder, R. The effect of behavioral realism and form realism of real-time avatar faces on verbal disclosure, nonverbal disclosure, emotion recognition, and copresence in dyadic interaction. *Presence* **2006**, *15*, 359–372. [CrossRef]
84. Biocca, F.; Harms, C.; Gregg, J. The networked minds measure of social presence: Pilot test of the factor structure and concurrent validity. In Proceedings of the 4th Annual International Workshop on Presence, Philadelphia, PA, USA, 21–23 May 2001; pp. 1–9.
85. Cipresso, P.; Chicchi Giglioli, I.A.; Alcañiz Raya, M.; Riva, G. The past, present, and future of virtual and augmented reality research: A network and cluster analysis of the literature. *Front. Psychol.* **2018**, *9*, 2086. [CrossRef] [PubMed]
86. Cummings, J.J.; Bailenson, J.N. How immersive is enough? A meta-analysis of the effect of immersive technology on user presence. *Media Psychol.* **2016**, *19*, 272–309. [CrossRef]
87. Skalski, P.; Tamborini, R. The role of social presence in interactive agent-based persuasion. *Media Psychol.* **2007**, *10*, 385–413. [CrossRef]
88. Slater, M. Place illusion and plausibility can lead to realistic behaviour in immersive virtual environments. *Philos. Trans. R. Soc. B Biol. Sci.* **2009**, *364*, 3549–3557. [CrossRef]
89. Sundar, S.S.; Xu, Q.; Bellur, S. Designing interactivity in media interfaces: A communications perspective. In Proceedings of the SIGCHI Conference on Human Factors in Computing Systems, Atlanta, GA, USA, 10–15 April 2010; ACM: New York, NY, USA, 2010; pp. 2247–2256.
90. Baños, R.M.; Botella, C.; Garcia-Palacios, A.; Villa, H.; Perpiñá, C.; Alcaniz, M. Presence and reality judgment in virtual environments: A unitary construct? *Cyber Psychol. Behav.* **2000**, *3*, 327–335. [CrossRef]
91. Baños, R.; Botella, C.; Garcia-Palacios, A.; Villa, H.; Perpiñá, C.; Gallardo, M. Psychological variables and reality judgment in virtual environments: The roles of absorption and dissociation. *Cyber Psychol. Behav.* **2009**, *2*, 143–148. [CrossRef]
92. Bente, G.; Rüggenberg, S.; Krämer, N.C.; Eschenburg, F. Avatar-mediated networking: Increasing social presence and interpersonal trust in net-based collaborations. *Hum. Commun. Res.* **2008**, *34*, 287–318. [CrossRef]
93. Heeter, C. Being there: The subjective experience of presence. *Presence Teleoperators Virtual Environ.* **1992**, *1*, 262–271. [CrossRef]
94. Sanchez-Vives, M.V.; Slater, M. From presence to consciousness through virtual reality. *Nat. Rev. Neurosci.* **2005**, *6*, 332. [CrossRef] [PubMed]

95. Alcorn, A.; Pain, H.; Rajendran, G.; Smith, T.; Lemon, O.; Porayska-Pomsta, K.; Bernardini, S. Social communication between virtual characters and children with autism. In Proceedings of the International Conference on Artificial Intelligence in Education, Auckland, New Zealand, 28 June–1 July 2011; Springer: Berlin, Heidelberg, 2011; pp. 7–14.
96. Mohr, D.C.; Burns, M.N.; Schueller, S.M.; Clarke, G.; Klinkman, M. Behavioral intervention technologies: Evidence review and recommendations for future research in mental health. *Gen. Hosp. Psychiatry* **2013**, *35*, 332–338. [CrossRef] [PubMed]
97. Negut, A.; Matu, S.A.; Sava, F.A.; David, D. Virtual reality measures in neuropsychological assessment: A meta-analytic review. *Clin. Neuropsychol.* **2016**, *30*, 165–184. [CrossRef]
98. Riva, G. Virtual reality in psychotherapy. *Cyber Psychol. Behav.* **2005**, *8*, 220–230. [CrossRef] [PubMed]
99. Valmaggia, L.R.; Latif, L.; Kempton, M.J.; Rus-Calafell, M. Virtual reality in the psychological treatment for mental health problems: An systematic review of recent evidence. *Psychiatry Res.* **2016**, *236*, 189–195. [CrossRef] [PubMed]
100. Mesa-Gresa, P.; Gil-Gómez, H.; Lozano-Quilis, J.A.; Gil-Gómez, J.A. Effectiveness of virtual reality for children and adolescents with autism spectrum disorder: An evidence-based systematic review. *Sensors* **2018**, *18*, 2486. [CrossRef] [PubMed]
101. Cheng, Y.; Ye, J. Exploring the social competence of students with autism spectrum conditions in a collaborative virtual learning environment—The pilot study. *Comput. Educ.* **2010**, *54*, 1068–1077. [CrossRef]
102. Jarrold, W.; Mundy, P.; Gwaltney, M.; Bailenson, J.; Hatt, N.; McIntyre, N.; Swain, L. Social attention in a virtual public speaking task in higher functioning children with autism. *Autism Res.* **2013**, *6*, 393–410. [CrossRef]
103. d'Arc, B.F.; Ramus, F.; Lefebvre, A.; Brottier, D.; Zalla, T.; Moukawane, S.; Leboyer, M. Atypical social judgment and sensitivity to perceptual cues in autism spectrum disorders. *J. Autism Dev. Disord.* **2016**, *46*, 1574–1581. [CrossRef]
104. Hopkins, I.M.; Gower, M.W.; Perez, T.A.; Smith, D.S.; Amthor, F.R.; Wimsatt, F.C.; Biasini, F.J. Avatar assistant: Improving social skills in students with an ASD through a computer-based intervention. *J. Autism Dev. Disord.* **2011**, *41*, 1543–1555. [CrossRef]
105. Maskey, M.; Lowry, J.; Rodgers, J.; McConachie, H.; Parr, J.R. Reducing specific phobia/fear in young people with autism spectrum disorders (ASDs) through a virtual reality environment intervention. *PLoS ONE* **2014**, *9*, e100374. [CrossRef]
106. Baron-Cohen, S.; Ashwin, E.; Ashwin, C.; Tavassoli, T.; Chakrabarti, B. Talent in autism: Hyper-systemizing, hyper-attention to detail and sensory hypersensitivity. *Philos. Trans. R. Soc. B Biol. Sci.* **2009**, *364*, 1377–1383. [CrossRef] [PubMed]
107. Tomchek, S.D.; Huebner, R.A.; Dunn, W. Patterns of sensory processing in children with an autism spectrum disorder. *Res. Autism Spectr. Disord.* **2014**, *8*, 1214–1224. [CrossRef]
108. Ashwin, C.; Chapman, E.; Howells, J.; Rhydderch, D.; Walker, I.; Baron-Cohen, S. Enhanced olfactory sensitivity in autism spectrum conditions. *Mol. Autism* **2014**, *5*, 53. [CrossRef] [PubMed]
109. Dudova, I.; Vodicka, J.; Havlovicova, M.; Sedlacek, Z.; Urbanek, T.; Hrdlicka, M. Odor detection threshold, but not odor identification, is impaired in children with autism. *Eur. Child Adolesc. Psychiatry* **2011**, *20*, 333–340. [CrossRef] [PubMed]
110. Boyd, B.A.; Baranek, G.T.; Sideris, J.; Poe, M.D.; Watson, L.R.; Patten, E.; Miller, H. Sensory features and repetitive behaviors in children with autism and developmental delays. *Autism Res.* **2010**, *3*, 78–87. [CrossRef] [PubMed]
111. Gabriels, R.L.; Agnew, J.A.; Miller, L.J.; Gralla, J.; Pan, Z.; Goldson, E.; Hooks, E. Is there a relationship between restricted, repetitive, stereotyped behaviors and interests and abnormal sensory response in children with autism spectrum disorders? *Res. Autism Spectr. Disord.* **2008**, *2*, 660–670. [CrossRef]
112. Cao, Z.; Hidalgo, G.; Simon, T.; Wei, S.E.; Sheikh, Y. OpenPose: Realtime multi-person 2D pose estimation using Part Affinity Fields. *arXiv* **2018**, arXiv:1812.08008. [CrossRef]
113. Schöllkopf, B.; Smola, A.J.; Williamson, R.C.; Bartlett, P.L. New support vector algorithms. *Neural Comput.* **2000**, *12*, 1207–1245. [CrossRef]
114. Yan, K.; Zhang, D. Feature selection and analysis on correlated gas sensor data with recursive feature elimination. *Sens. Actuators B Chem.* **2015**, *212*, 353–363. [CrossRef]

115. Chang, C.-C.; Lin, C.-J. Libsvm: A Library for Support Vector Machines. *ACM Trans. Intell. Syst. Technol.* **2011**, *2*, 1–27. [CrossRef]
116. O'Neill, M.; Jones, R.S. Sensory-perceptual abnormalities in autism: A case for more research? *J. Autism Dev. Disord.* **1997**, *27*, 283–293. [CrossRef] [PubMed]
117. Foss-Feig, J.H.; Kwakye, L.D.; Cascio, C.J.; Burnette, C.P.; Kadivar, H.; Stone, W.L.; Wallace, M.T. An extended multisensory temporal binding window in autism spectrum disorders. *Exp. Brain Res.* **2010**, *203*, 381–389. [CrossRef] [PubMed]
118. Courchesne, E.; Lincoln, A.J.; Kilman, B.A.; Galambos, R. Event-related brain potential correlates of the processing of novel visual and auditory information in autism. *J. Autism Dev. Disord.* **1985**, *15*, 55–76. [CrossRef] [PubMed]
119. Russo, N.; Foxe, J.J.; Brandwein, A.B.; Altschuler, T.; Gomes, H.; Molholm, S. Multisensory processing in children with autism: High-density electrical mapping of auditory–somatosensory integration. *Autism Res.* **2010**, *3*, 253–267. [CrossRef] [PubMed]
120. Ament, K.; Mejia, A.; Buhlman, R.; Erklin, S.; Caffo, B.; Mostofsky, S.; Wodka, E. Evidence for specificity of motor impairments in catching and balance in children with autism. *J. Autism Dev. Disord.* **2015**, *45*, 742–751. [CrossRef]

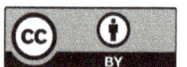

© 2020 by the authors. Licensee MDPI, Basel, Switzerland. This article is an open access article distributed under the terms and conditions of the Creative Commons Attribution (CC BY) license (http://creativecommons.org/licenses/by/4.0/).

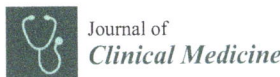

Article

Manipulating the Perceived Shape and Color of a Virtual Limb Can Modulate Pain Responses

Marta Matamala-Gomez [1,2,3,*], Birgit Nierula [1,2,4], Tony Donegan [1], Mel Slater [2] and Maria V. Sanchez-Vives [1,2,5,6]

1. Institut d'Investigacions Biomèdiques August Pi i Sunyer (IDIBAPS), 08036 Barcelona, Spain; bnierula@gmail.com (B.N.); tonydonegan@gmail.com (T.D.); msanche3@clinic.cat (M.V.S.-V.)
2. Event-Lab, Department of Clinical Psychology and Psychobiology, Universitat de Barcelona, 08035 Barcelona, Spain; melslater@gmail.com
3. Dipartamento di Scienze Umane per la Formazione 'Ricardo Massa', Università degli studi Milano-Bicocca, 20126 Milan, Italy
4. Max Planck Institute for Human Cognitive and Brain Sciences, 04103 Leipzig, Germany
5. Departament de Cognició, Desenvolupament i Psicologia de l'Educació, Facultat de Psicologia, Universitat de Barcelona, 08035 Barcelona, Spain
6. Institució Catalana de Recerca i Estudis Avançats (ICREA), 08010 Barcelona, Spain
* Correspondence: marta.matamala10@gmail.com; Tel.: +34-932-275-400 (ext. 4301)

Received: 5 December 2019; Accepted: 18 January 2020; Published: 21 January 2020

Abstract: Changes in body representation may affect pain perception. The effect of a distorted body image, such as the telescoping effect in amputee patients, on pain perception, is unclear. This study aimed to investigate whether distorting an embodied virtual arm in virtual reality (simulating the telescoping effect in amputees) modulated pain perception and anticipatory responses to pain in healthy participants. Twenty-seven right-handed participants were immersed in virtual reality and the virtual arm was shown with three different levels of distortion with a virtual threatening stimulus either approaching or contacting the virtual hand. We evaluated pain/discomfort ratings, ownership, and skin conductance responses (SCRs) after each condition. Viewing a distorted virtual arm enhances the SCR to a threatening event with respect to viewing a normal control arm, but when viewing a reddened-distorted virtual arm, SCR was comparatively reduced in response to the threat. There was a positive relationship between the level of ownership over the distorted and reddened-distorted virtual arms with the level of pain/discomfort, but not in the normal control arm. Contact with the threatening stimulus significantly enhances SCR and pain/discomfort, while reduced SCR and pain/discomfort were seen in the simulated-contact condition. These results provide further evidence of a bi-directional link between body image and pain perception.

Keywords: virtual reality; pain perception; telescoped effect; amputee patients

1. Introduction

Immersive virtual reality (VR) technology has been repeatedly demonstrated to be an effective tool for modulating pain threshold perception in healthy subjects [1,2], and pain ratings in patients with chronic pain [3,4]. This is because multisensory signals, which can be integrated and manipulated in VR environments, influence our perception of pain, in part because nociceptive stimuli activate a wide network of cortical and subcortical areas in the brain, commonly known as the "pain matrix," that are also implicated in the processing of sensory information [5].

Using VR, one can feel immersed (feeling inside of and being able to interact with the virtual world), and present (the subjective illusion of "being there," when placed in the immersed virtual environment despite the knowledge that you are not there) [6] in a multisensory environment that is under the full control of the experimenter [7]. Furthermore, it is possible to induce, through VR, the illusion of owning a virtual body; this refers to the subjective illusion that a body or body part is one's own, which again is facilitated by multisensory feedback such as synchronous visual and tactile stimulation, when the virtual and the real bodies are co-located at the same position [8]. The sense of ownership over a virtual body, or "embodiment," is highly flexible regarding the visual aspect of the body, and it is possible to embody bodies that are quite different from those in real life [9,10]. The virtual body can therefore be designed with the morphological characteristics that the experimenter determines [11]. This allows the exploration of how the visual aspect of the body modulates pain perception. For example, Martini et al. [2] investigated the influence of skin color on pain perception when participants were embodied in a virtual body. They found that participants experienced pain threshold reduction when the virtual arm was represented in red compared to a "normal" or blue color. In addition, another study by the same group showed that virtual arm transparency decreases the pain threshold [12]. It is also possible to alter pain perception and anticipatory responses to pain in healthy subjects by modulating the morphological characteristics of the limb, such as showing a subject's limb becoming smaller or bigger [13]. Moreover, we can reduce pain perception in a patient with chronic pain whose painful limb feels bigger than it really is by reducing the apparent size of their painful limb [14]. This top-down modulation of pain through modification of visual input reveals the potential of VR illusions as a treatment for pain. Additionally, instead of virtual body illusions, other studies have used VR to provide immersive virtual environments as a distractive pain strategy [15,16].

Even though VR is a potential tool for modulating the pain threshold through virtual body illusions in healthy subjects [1,2,12,17–20], this cannot be extrapolated to how these strategies are going to work in chronic pain patients. Indeed, there are some conflicting results about how bodily illusions can reduce chronic pain in clinical populations [21,22]. In this regard, a study conducted with thirteen amputee patients showed that, while phantom pain was reduced after four weeks of mirror therapy training in five amputee patients, eight amputee patients who reported telescopic distortion of the phantom limb (telescopic distortion refers to the feeling that the proximal portion of the amputated limb is missing or has shrunk with the more distal portion floating near, attached to, or 'within' the stump [23,24]), reported a gradual increase in phantom pain perception after the same mirror therapy training [22]. This difference may be due to the different cortical representations of the limb, a phenomenon seen not only in amputees but also in patients with complex regional pain syndrome and other chronic pain conditions [25–29]. The altered representation of the painful part of the body in the brain seems to play a key role in the development and maintenance of chronic pain, and therapies that attempt to reverse these changes have been partially successful, especially in amputee patients [30]. However, few studies have investigated how distorting a representation of a body part affects the sensation of pain. The present study aims to ascertain whether the illusion of ownership over a telescopically distorted virtual arm can modulate pain perception. To study pain, without delivering painful stimuli and avoiding the problems associated with sensitization/adaptation to repeated painful stimuli, we have used a paradigm of anticipatory responses to pain. Since the responses to a threatening stimulus start before skin contact [13], we investigated both the responses to pain when a threatening stimulus touched the virtual hand of the participant and the anticipatory responses to pain as a threatening stimulus approached the virtual hand. In order to deliver an unpleasant sensation to the participants, we used a vibration stimulus attached to the palm associated and triggered by a virtual needle as a threatening stimulus. For this, the skin conductance responses (SCRs), corresponding to the activation of the autonomic nervous system [31], of healthy subjects were recorded while they were embodied in a virtual body in several conditions in which the virtual arm, which was co-located with their real arm, had a normal or a distorted representation. Moreover, as was done in previous investigations [2,32], we wanted to investigate the effects of the redness of a colored telescopically distorted virtual arm on pain both when a threatening stimulus touched the virtual hand of the participant, and the anticipatory response to pain as a threatening stimulus approached the virtual hand.

The current study is a proof-of-concept study that may help us understand the mechanisms of visual distortion of body image, such as the telescoping effect in amputees (the distal part of the phantom limb perceived as shrinking within the stump), and its effect on pain responses.

2. Methods

2.1. Participants

Thirty right-handed, healthy subjects above 18 years of age participated in this study. Three subjects were excluded from further analysis due to an extremely high z-score (>± 2.5) in the SCR data, which led to a final sample size of 27 right-handed subjects (8 males and 19 females; mean age ± SD = 24.7 ± 1.1; mean Edinburgh scale ± SD = 68.7 ± 1.1). The following conditions were considered as inclusion criteria for participation in the study: normal or normal-when-corrected vision, the absence of neurological disorders, no history of chronic pain or other conditions interfering with pain sensitivity, no presence of epilepsy, no medication in use that changed attention to pain or general perception for 24 h before the experiment, and no pregnant women. The experiment was carried out in the installations of the Eventlab for Neuroscience and Technology Laboratory at the University of Barcelona/IDIBAPS. All participants gave written informed consent and received monetary compensation for their participation (12 €). The study was approved by the local ethics committee (Comité Ético de Investigación Clínica de la Corporación Sanitaria Hospital Clínic de Barcelona, HCB/2017/1068) and was carried out according to the Declaration of Helsinki [33].

2.2. Study Design

In order to investigate whether observation of a telescopically distorted representation of the arm alters pain responses and anticipatory responses to pain in healthy subjects, participants completed one experimental session of 20 min. This study was a 3 × 2 within-subject experimental design. The experimental setup is shown in Figure 1A. In this study, there were two main factors. The first factor was Virtual Arm, with three different representations of the virtual arm: (1) the virtual arm represented in a normal position (Control); (2) the virtual arm represented in a distorted position, namely, a shortened virtual forearm shrinking within the arm (telescoped virtual arm) (Distorted); and (3) the virtual arm represented in a distorted position (telescoped virtual arm) and was red (Reddened-Distorted) (see Figure 1B). In all cases, the virtual arm was co-located with the real arm. The telescoped virtual arm representation was created following the graphical representation illustrating telescoping from the 5th edition of *Practical Management of Pain* [34]. In order to explore how these different representations of the virtual arm alter anticipatory responses to pain and pain responses itself, the second factor was *Threatening Stimulus Contact*, with two different types of threatening stimulus: (1) a tactile stimulus that contacted the skin (Real Contact); and (2) a stimulus that approached but did not touch the skin (Simulated Contact). For this, we used a vibrator attached to the palm of the hand of the participants to deliver visuo-tactile stimulations when the threatening stimulus (a virtual needle) contacted the palm of the virtual hand (see Figure 1C). Note that this is a tactile but non-nociceptive stimulus. The three virtual arm representations were combined with the two visually threatening stimulus contacts, resulting in six different conditions, each of which was presented three times. The order of the conditions was randomized among the subjects. Hence, each participant completed a total of 18 virtual arm and threatening stimulus exposures. After each exposure, participants had to indicate their level of sensory intensity (pain intensity) and affective magnitude (unpleasantness/discomfort), assessed using a visual analogue scale (VAS) [35] through a single request: "On a scale from 0 to 100, indicate the level of pain intensity/discomfort that you felt, please." Further, after each exposure, participants had to indicate their level of ownership over the virtual arm [12]. Each stimulus exposure lasted 53 s (Figure 1D). After completing the virtual reality experiment, participants had to complete a questionnaire to evaluate their overall virtual reality experience [36]. In order to measure the electrodermal response when the threatening stimulus eventually touched the skin, and the anticipatory physiological response to an incoming threatening stimulus, the SCR was recorded following exposure to the threatening stimulus [13,37], which in the real contact condition touched the virtual hand and in the simulated contact condition simply approached the virtual hand without contacting it.

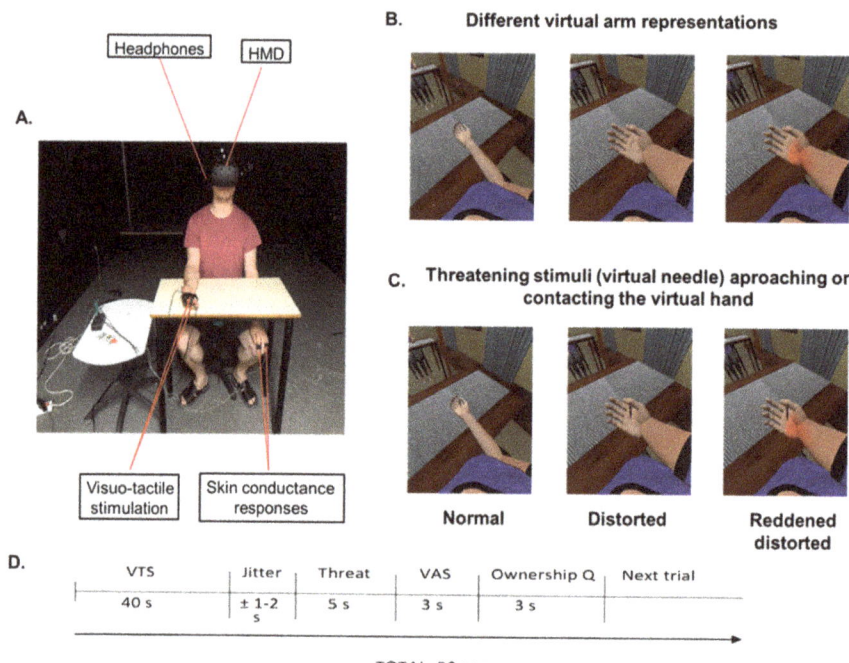

Figure 1. Experimental set-up and virtual arm and threatening stimulus conditions. (**A**) Participants wore a head-mounted display (HMD) that immersed them in a virtual environment. This allowed them to feel embodied in a virtual body, which they saw from a first-person perspective and which was co-located with their real body. Using headphones, participants heard the task instruction, "Pay attention to the right arm placed on the table, please," before each visuo-tactile stimulus phase, which lasted 45 s. During the visuo-tactile stimulation, which was used to induce ownership over the virtual arm, virtual balls tapped the virtual fingers while participants felt, simultaneously, a tactile stimulation (vibration) on their real fingers. To record skin conductance responses after each threatening stimulus, two electrodes were attached to the index and ring fingers of the participants' left hands. (**B**) Different virtual arm representations (virtual arm factor): normal representation, distorted representation (telescoped virtual arm), and reddened-distorted representation of the virtual arm. The distorted representation of the virtual forearm was shrinking within the virtual arm, as occurs with the telescoping effect in amputee patients. However, from a participant's first-person perspective it seems bigger than the normal representation. (**C**) Threatening stimulus (virtual needle) in all three levels of the virtual arm factor. (**D**) Timeline of one experimental trial. Each experimental trial lasted around 53 s and was divided into four parts: First, participants were immersed in an immersive virtual reality (VR) environment in which the virtual arm could either be distorted, reddened and distorted, or in a normal position. To induce ownership over the virtual arm, they received 45 s of synchronous visuo-tactile stimulation. Second, after a jitter of 1–2 s, the threatening event appeared (a virtual needle) for 5 s. Immediately after the threatening event, the VAS appeared on the screen of the HMD. Finally, after the VAS was taken, a question related to ownership over the virtual arm appeared. VTS, visuo-tactile stimulation VAS, visual analogue scale; Ownership Q, ownership questionnaire.

2.3. Apparatus

2.3.1. Head-Mounted Display

We used a head-mounted display (HMD) (Rift Development Kit 2, Oculus, Menlo Park, CA, USA) with a resolution of 960 × 1080 pixels per eye and a nominal horizontal field of view of 100° displayed at 75 Hz to show the virtual environment, which was programmed in Unity 4.5.3 (Unity Technologies, San Francisco, CA, USA). The virtual body was configured to match the gender of the participants (female or male) and was taken from the Rocketbox library (Rocketbox Studios GmbH, Hannover, Germany). The virtual environment was the same during all conditions. Headphones were used in order to allow the participants to follow the task instructions during the experimental sessions (Figure 1A).

2.3.2. Visuo-Tactile Stimulation

To increase the illusion of ownership over the virtual body, we used visuo-tactile stimulation. For this, we delivered tactile stimulation to the participants by using vibrators attached to the middle and index fingers, and to the palm of the right hand, that were controlled by Unity through an Arduino MEGA microcontroller board (Figure 1A). Each vibration had a duration of 1.0 s.

2.3.3. Skin Conductance Responses

To record skin conductance, we attached two electrodes to the index and the ring fingers of the left hands of the participants (Figure 1A). The SCR was recorded at a sampling rate of 256 Hz, using a portable biosignal acquisition device (g.MOBIlab+, g.tec), while the recording and storage of the data was handled by a Simulink model in Matlab 2012b (The MathWorks, Inc., Natick, MA, USA).

2.4. Procedures

2.4.1. Position of the Participants

Participants were seated on a chair with their right arm resting on the table and their left arm hidden under the table, resting on the left leg to ensure that participants only paid attention to their right arm during the experimental session. The right arm of the subject was placed within their field of view. The two vibrators attached to the dorsal distal phalanges of the right index and middle fingers were used in order to deliver visuo-tactile stimulations to induce the ownership illusion over the virtual arm. The other vibrator attached to the palm of the hand was used to deliver visuo-tactile stimulations when the threatening stimulus (the virtual needle) contacted the palm of the virtual hand. Through the HMD, participants were immersed in a virtual reality scenario in which they saw a virtual body from a first-person perspective co-located with their own real body [38]. They heard the task instructions through headphones throughout the experimental session, and their skin conductance was recorded with the two electrodes attached to their left index and ring fingers.

2.4.2. Virtual Reality Scenario

Once participants donned the HMD, the room lights were turned off to allow the participants to be fully immersed in the virtual environment. At the beginning of the experimental session, participants were instructed to look around the virtual room, to describe what they saw, and to look down at their virtual body in order to habituate to the virtual scenario and the virtual body. The right virtual arm was always placed in the field of view of the participants with the palm of the hand facing up to the celling. Once the habituation phase was over, participants were asked to focus their attention on the right virtual arm. During the entire session and before the presentation of each condition, participants listened to the following verbal instruction through the headphones: "Pay attention to the right arm that is located on the table, please." In order to induce the illusory ownership over the virtual body in each different representation of the virtual arm, each representation of the virtual arm included

40 s of visuo-tactile stimulation where participants saw a virtual ball tapping in random order their virtual right index and middle finger whilst feeling a spatiotemporal synchronous vibration on their real right index and middle finger, respectively [39]. During the experimental session, participants were exposed to six conditions in which three representations of the arm were combined with two types of stimulus contact.

2.4.3. Pain Ratings and Ownership Measures

Pain ratings and measures of the degree of ownership over the virtual arm were taken for each of the six conditions to measure the effect of visual distortion on the sensory and anticipatory aspects of pain processing. Once each virtual trial was over, the screen of the HMD turned black and a VAS appeared with a voice instruction asking the participants to judge how strong the pain feels in order to assess the intensity of pain and how discomforting the threatening stimulus was perceived, on a scale ranging from 0 (not discomfort at all/minimum pain intensity) to 100 (worst discomfort/strongest pain intensity imaginable) [13]. Participants' ratings were promptly annotated by the experimenter. After the VAS, a question related to ownership over the virtual arm in each representation appeared in the screen of the HMD, with a voice instruction asking the participant to judge their level of ownership over the virtual arm from −3 (totally disagree) to 3 (totally agree), with the following sentence: "I felt that the virtual arm was my arm" [36]. After the virtual reality exposure, the HMD and the headphones were removed and participants had to fill in a questionnaire concerning the overall virtual reality experience.

2.5. SCR Data Preprocessing

The peak-to-base response amplitude of skin conductance was used as an index of SCR [40–42]. For the assessment of SCRs, the difference between the maximum value detected in a 6 s post-stimulus time window and the baseline (3 s pre-stimulus) was computed, which is comparable with other studies in which a time frame of 1–5 s after stimulus onset was chosen [43–45]. Finally, we obtained the normalized maximum change of the SCR after each stimulus (virtual needle real contact/virtual needle simulated contact). The sample rate to extract SCR data was set to 256 Hz. The data were stored under Matlab and could be opened in the Matlab command windows with g.BSanalyze (gtec). Final SCR data were obtained by using a Matlab graphical user interface (GUI) for feature extraction of the skin conductance signal *(featextractiongui)* in Matlab2012b (The MathWorks, Inc. Natick, MA, USA). Event markers identifying each stimulus type were programmed to automatically register SCR when the stimulus—the virtual needle—contacted (real contact) or approached (simulated contact) the palm of the virtual hand.

2.6. Virtual Reality Experience Questionnaire

Once participants completed the whole VR exposure, they had to fill in a questionnaire related to their VR experience, answering the following statements from −3 (totally disagree) to +3 (totally agree) [36]:

Q1. During the experiment there were moments in which I felt that the virtual balls were touching my real fingers.
Q2. Although the virtual body did not seem to be physically my body, I felt that it could be my own body.
Q3. When I saw the virtual arm distorted, I felt that my own arm was distorted as well.
Q4. During each different representation of the virtual arm, I felt that if I moved my real arm the virtual arm would start moving too.
Q5. During the whole experimental session, I was able to focus my attention to the right arm.

2.7. Data Handling

All statistical tests were performed in Stata 13 (StataCorp LP, College Station, TX, USA). This was a mixed-effects design, with fixed-effects virtual arm (normal, distorted, reddened-distorted) and threat contact (real contact, simulated contact), and random effects over the individual subjects. We analyzed differences in pain ratings and in SCR across conditions with a multilevel mixed-effects linear regression test (the "mixed" function in Stata). Furthermore, in order to observe differences between virtual arm conditions, we ran a pairwise comparison with the Scheffe test for multiple comparisons. Moreover, in order to observe a possible relationship between ownership and pain ratings assessed with the VAS throughout the experiment, we used Spearman's correlation test. In order to observe differences in ownership scores across conditions, we used multilevel mixed-effect ordered logistic regression test (the "meologit" function in Stata). Finally, in order to conduct mediation analyses, we used a seemingly unrelated regression test (the "sureg" function in Stata).

3. Results

3.1. Changes in Shape and Color of the Virtual Arm Modulate SCR after Threatening Stimulus Exposure

Our results show that changes in shape and color of the virtual arm modulated SCR after a threatening stimulus exposure. In this case, the SCR was taken as a proxy of pain responses, as has been established in previous work by Romano and Maravita [13]. Specifically, we observed a higher SCR when the virtual arm was distorted (telescoped virtual arm) compared with the normal virtual arm ($z = -2.93$, $p = 0.003$); we did not find a significant relationship between the shape changes of the virtual arm and SCR, but did find a significant relationship between color changes and SCR. The results show that the red color in the reddened-distorted virtual arm increase anticipatory pain responses, showing a significant difference between normal ($z = -2.93$, $p = 0.014$) and distorted ($z = -4.79$, $p < 0.0001$) virtual arm conditions. Furthermore, in relation to the dependency of the SCR on the threatening stimulus contact, our results showed a significant decrease in SCR when the threatening stimulus approached but did not contact the virtual hand (simulated contact), compared to the real contact condition ($z = -3.08$, $p = 0.002$) (Figure 2). Interestingly, the proportions between SCR in normal virtual arm, those of distorted and reddened-distorted arms, were the same both for the real contact and the simulated contact; however, the absolute values were smaller in the simulated contact. Table 1 summarizes SCR values and p-values for all of the experimental conditions.

Table 1. Values in terms of means, standard error (SE), and p-values indicating mean differences between the different experimental conditions.

Experimental Variable	Virtual Arm			Threat Contact	
	Normal Virtual Arm (1)	Distorted Virtual Arm (2)	Reddened-Distorted Virtual Arm (3)	Real Contact (1)	Simulated Contact (2)
Mean	8.13	10.43	4.49	9.27	6.17
SE	13.20	12.63	9.25	13.60	10.09
p-value	0.014	<0.001			<0.001
Conditions	3 vs. 1	3 vs. 2			2 vs. 1

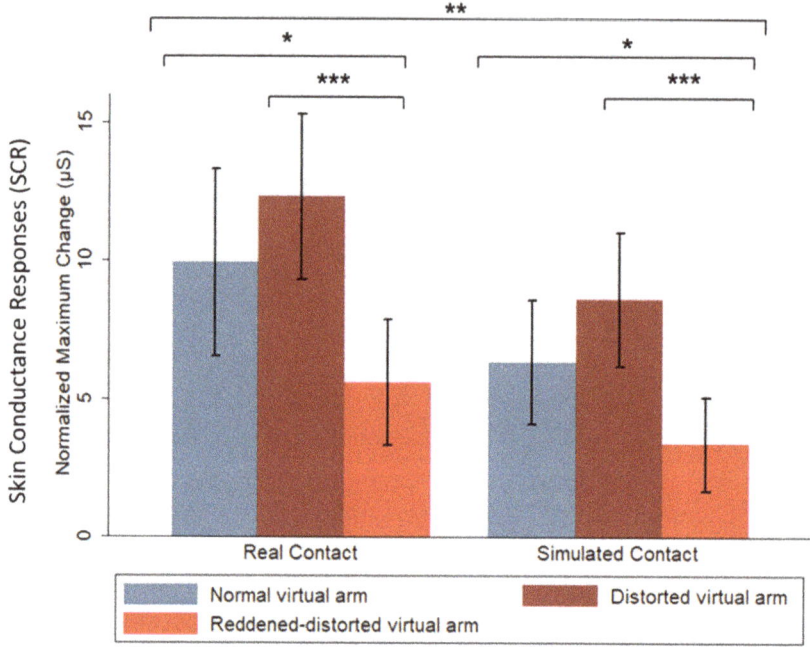

Figure 2. Skin conductance response (SCR) increased when the virtual needle contacted (real contact) the virtual hand in all three virtual arm conditions, while the reddened-distorted virtual arm showed a comparatively decreased SCR in both real and simulated contact of the threatening stimulus. Difference in SCR after the threatening stimulus contacted (real contact) or approached (simulated contact) the virtual hand in all three virtual arm conditions. Bars show mean change in SCR and error bars indicate 95% confidence interval. * $p < 0.05$, ** $p < 0.01$, *** $p < 0.001$.

3.2. Distortion of the Virtual Arm Increase Pain Ratings (VAS) after Threatening Stimulus Exposure

The data obtained in our study show a positive relationship between the level of ownership over the distorted ($r_s = 0.226$, $p < 0.01$) and reddened-distorted ($r_s = 0.225$, $p < 0.01$) virtual arms with the level of pain/discomfort assessed using the VAS. Nevertheless, this positive relationship was not found after the normal virtual arm exposure ($r_s = 0023$, $p = 0.767$) (Figure 3A–C). Thus, in the distorted virtual arm conditions, we found that the higher the level of ownership of the distorted and reddened-distorted virtual arm, the higher the pain/discomfort perception. Furthermore, in agreement with the above results in which we observed a significant difference when the threatening stimulus contacted or approached the virtual arm, again our results show a significant difference in pain/discomfort perception when the threatening stimulus contacted or approached the virtual arm. In particular, we found lower VAS scores when the threatening stimulus approached the virtual hand, but not when it contacted the virtual hand (multilevel effects mixed effects $z = -7.00$, $p < 0.001$).

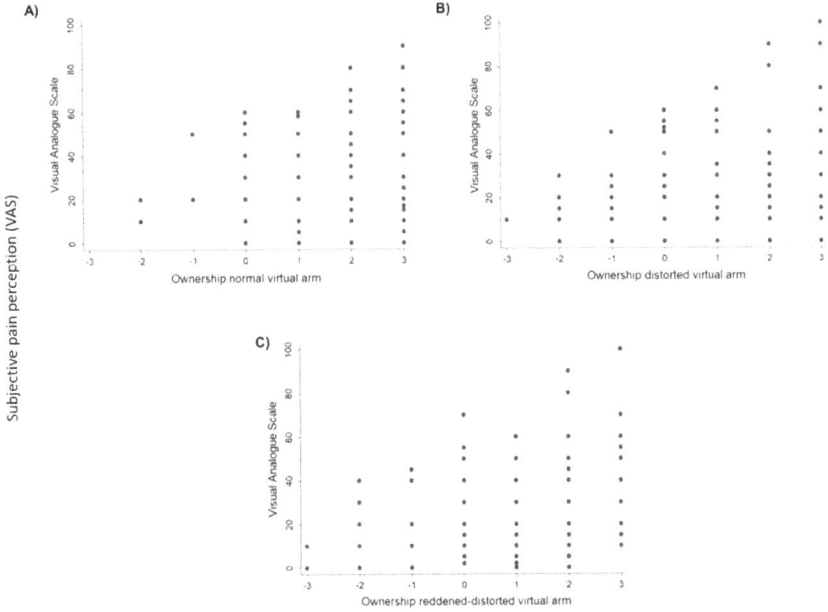

Figure 3. Pain ratings increase with the distortion of the embodied virtual arm. The relationship between pain ratings and ownership levels under the (**A**) normal virtual arm condition (no relationship); (**B**) the distorted virtual arm condition; and (**C**) the reddened-distorted virtual arm condition.

3.3. Dependency of Ownership on Shape and Color Changes of the Virtual Arm after Threatening Stimulus Exposure

The reported levels of ownership show a statistically significant difference between the different representations of the virtual arm, ownership being higher with the normal representation of the virtual arm. Indeed, we found a statistically significant difference in ownership between the normal representation of the virtual arm and both the distorted ($z = -9.16$, $p < 0.001$) and reddened-distorted virtual arm ($z = -8.92$, $p < 0.001$). In addition, contact of the threatening stimulus with the virtual hand significantly increased the level of ownership in all three virtual arm representations compared with simulated contact of the threatening stimulus ($z = -2.30$, $p = 0.021$) (Figure 4A). Table 2 summarizes ownership values and p-values for all of the experimental conditions.

Table 2. Scoring values in terms of mean, standard error (SE) and p-values for all the different experimental conditions.

Experimental Variable	Virtual Arm			Threat Contact	
	Normal Virtual Arm (1)	Distorted Virtual Arm (2)	Reddened-Distorted Virtual Arm (3)	Real Contact (1)	Simulated Contact (2)
Mean	1.89	1.03	1.05	1.42	1.38
SE	1.13	1.49	1.50	1.23	1.49
p-value		<0.001	<0.001		0.021
Condition		2 vs. 1	3 vs. 1		2 vs. 1

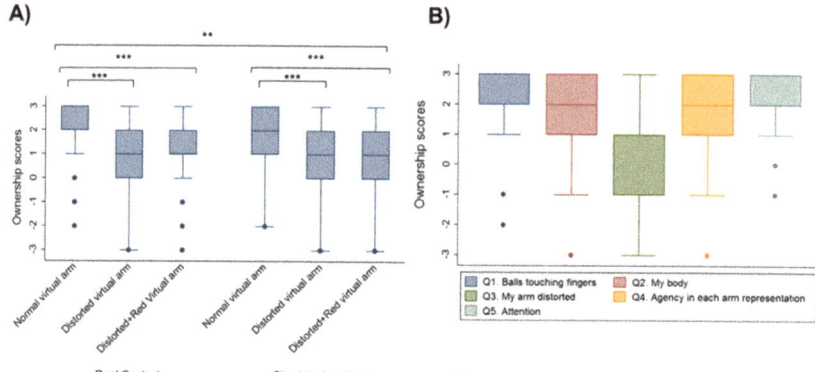

Figure 4. Ownership levels increase with the normal representation of the virtual arm. (**A**) Ownership question ratings after each virtual reality condition exposure show higher ownership scores in the normal virtual arm representation compared with the distorted and reddened-distorted conditions, in both real and simulated contact of the threatening stimulus. (**B**) Questionnaire ratings after the whole virtual reality exposure show that although participants reported high levels of agency and ownership of the virtual body, ownership scores decreased with the distorted virtual arm representation. Boxplots show medians (horizontal lines), interquartile ranges (IQR; boxes), data outside 1.5 × IQR (whiskers), and outliers (o). ** $p < 0.01$, *** $p < 0.001$.

From the results obtained in the final VR questionnaire that participants had to fill in after the VR experience, we found that participants reported high levels of ownership (Q1, Q2) and agency (Q4) of the virtual body and virtual arm. However, we also observed low scores in ownership levels with the distorted virtual arm representation (Q3). Finally, in Q5, which was related to the level of attention towards the virtual arm, participants reported high attention levels of the virtual arm throughout the whole VR exposure (Figure 4B).

We found that ownership (ownership scoring collected during the experimental sessions) mediates differences in SCR, but not subjective pain ratings (VAS), between the different virtual arm conditions. Specifically, we found a significant relationship between the independent factor virtual arm and the mediation variable ownership ($z = -5.39$, $p < 0.001$). Further, we also found a significant relationship between the SCR (dependent variable) and ownership ($z = -2.91$, $p = 0.004$), and between the SCR and the virtual arm factor ($z = -3.34$, $p = 0.001$). We calculated the mediation effect (ME) by the following calculation: ME = regression coefficient between SCR and ownership ($r_s = -1.13$) × regression coefficient between SCR and virtual arm ($r_s = -0.42$). The ME of ownership in SCR between the different virtual arm conditions is 0.472. Although we did not find a relationship between the subjective pain ratings (VAS), as a second dependent variable, and the virtual arm factor ($z = 0.90$, $p = 0.367$), we found a significant relationship between VAS and ownership ($z = 5.31$, $p < 0.001$). Nevertheless, no mediation effects of ownership can be reported in subjective pain responses ratings (VAS) between different virtual arm conditions.

4. Discussion

Through immersive virtual reality, we can induce the sense of owning a virtual arm by using a congruent multisensory correlation between the real and the virtual arm [8,46]. It is known that changes in the color and shape of a virtual arm (that is co-located with the real one) modulate pain threshold in healthy subjects (see [47] for a review). Furthermore, there is some evidence demonstrating that a distorted representation in the brain of the painful part of the body is associated with increased pain perception in chronic pain patients [48,49]. Along these lines, some studies have investigated the role of the representation of the painful part of the body in the brain, such as the telescopic effect in amputees, on pain perception [25,50]. The study by Makin and colleagues [25] highlighted the importance of the preserved representation of the amputated limb in the area of the brain where the former hand was represented [51] as a key factor involved in chronic phantom pain. In their study, the authors suggested that this preserved representation could activate phantom chronic pain through top-down (central to peripheral nervous system) mechanisms. In line with this study, Bultitude and Rafal [26] suggested that the pain in patients with complex regional pain syndrome is a consequence of a distorted representation of the affected limb in the brain. Furthermore, some patients with chronic pain report that the mental representation of their affected body part is somehow distorted in size or posture, or even absent entirely [27–29], which may be associated with a distorted cortical representation of the limb. While early investigations found that visual feedback techniques such as mirror therapy or virtual reality could reduce pain perception in amputee patients [30,52,53], it has also been shown that mirror therapy can exacerbate pain in those amputees that experience the telescopic effect [22].

Here, we conducted a proof-of-concept study in healthy subjects in order to better understand the mechanisms of pain/discomfort in amputee patients that suffer from the telescoping effect. Although the mechanisms for acute and chronic pain are different [54], and amputees and healthy individuals are likely to have significantly different cortical representation of their body [55], this study can contribute to the understanding of the effects of visual distortion of the body on pain. We observed that multisensory integration interventions using VR could be used to manipulate the shape and color of the virtual body representation in order to modulate pain perception and anticipatory responses to pain in healthy subjects. We conclude that autonomic responses (SCR) that act as proxies of pain responses are enhanced when there is a virtual threat (virtual needle) that approaches or eventually touches a virtual arm that feels a part of one's own body. This paradigm can be used in order to explore how changes in the morphological or functional characteristics of the represented virtual body can modulate pain responses while avoiding the problems derived from repetitive painful stimulation, such as sensitization and adaptation. Although existing studies have demonstrated that visual illusions in which arm size is increased or decreased can affect pain perception in both healthy and clinical populations [4,13,56], this is the first study to investigate how being embodied in a virtual body with a distorted virtual arm (simulating the telescopic effect in amputees), affects subjective (pain scores in VAS) and the related physiological responses (SCR) to a threatening event in healthy subjects.

First, regarding the virtual arm factor, we found that being embodied in a distorted virtual arm enhances SCR and pain/discomfort ratings to the threatening event compared with the normal virtual arm condition; these results are in line with later investigations [13] in which the authors found higher SCR while observing a visually magnified hand. Moreover, other studies also found that visual enlargement of the hand being viewed enhanced analgesia by increasing heat-pain thresholds, compared with the visual reduction of the viewed hand [57]. However, the opposite effect was found in clinical populations with chronic pain, in which the visual enlargement of the affected hand increased pain perception compared with the visual reduction of the affected hand [14]. Furthermore, in the former study [57], they also found that visual enlargement of the viewed hand enhanced analgesia by increasing heat-pain thresholds, while visual reduction of the viewed hand reduced analgesia. However, the opposite effect was found in clinical populations with chronic pain, in which the visual enlargement of the affected hand increased pain perception compared with visual reduction of the affected hand [14]. Furthermore, in another study, a negative body image associated with an injured-appearing hand (induced using the rubber hand illusion paradigm) reduced the pain threshold in healthy subjects, but no such increase was seen with a visually distorted (stretched) rubber hand [58]. One possible explanation for the difference is that the distorted rubber hand was not exactly co-located with the real hand of the participant, diminishing the sense of ownership of the rubber hand, as surmised by Nierula and co-authors [17].

In a previous study, Romano and Maravita [13] found that visual distortion of the hand by giving a visual minifying hand feedback increased SCR in healthy subjects, whilst a magnified visual feedback of the hand decreased SCR, which suggests that the visual size increase enhances the cognitive, anticipatory component of pain processing. In our study we also found that SCR was lower in the reddened-distorted virtual arm condition compared with normal and distorted virtual arm conditions. In line with the study from Romano and Maravita [13], we speculate that in our study the red color in the reddened-distorted virtual arm enhanced the cognitive, anticipatory component of pain processing and decreased the SCR to the subsequent threatening stimulus. In fact, it is known that by observing a reddened embodied virtual arm, we can reduce the pain threshold in healthy subjects [2]. Hence, as participants were observing the reddened virtual arm 45 s before the threatening stimulus appeared (visuo-tactile stimulation phase) at the beginning of each condition, we can speculate that the red color caused an anticipatory pain response, resulting in a reduction in SCR following the threatening stimulus being in contact or simulated contact with the virtual arm. This effect could be induced via several mechanisms: on one hand, anticipatory responses to pain could induce the activation of endogenous descending analgesic neural pathways [59], involving subcortical reticular structures that target the dorsal horns of the spinal cord grey matter, reducing afferent noxious signals. This interpretation could be explained by the principle of diffuse noxious inhibitory control, by which a noxious stimulus decreases the response (or increases the threshold) to a subsequent painful stimulus (see [60] for a review). On the other hand, the expectation of the incoming painful stimulus can induce a pre-activation of early somatosensory regions with a subsequently decreased response when the signal from the noxious stimulus arrives at the cortex [61]. Moreover, it is also known that the more certainty regarding a painful stimulus that modulates the expectancy about pain perception, the more the recruitment of attentional resources to the ascending nociceptive input [62]. Hence, one may hypothesize that changes in shape and color of an embodied virtual arm may modulate both physiological and subjective measures of pain responses.

Secondly, in our study we found a generally increased SCR and subjective measure of pain perception when the threatening stimulus touched the virtual hand, and a generally reduced SCR when the threatening stimulus approached but did not touch the virtual hand in all three virtual arm conditions. Our findings differ from those shown in the study by Romano and Maravita [13], in which they observed a reduced SCR with real contact noxious stimuli while observing a magnified hand was associated with increased anticipatory SCR when the noxious stimuli approached the skin without touching it. However, they also observed a general increase in SCR for both real and simulated contact while observing a shrunken vision of the hand. In our study we did not observe such differences in SCR between the different virtual arm conditions. One explanation for this could be the synchronous visuo-tactile stimulation that participants received in their real hand once the threatening stimulus touched the virtual hand. It is well known that through synchronous visuo-tactile stimulation we may induce a sense of ownership over a fake limb, as in the "rubber hand illusion" study [63], over a whole fake body [64] and over a virtual arm [8]. Therefore, we postulate that the fact of receiving tactile stimulation (vibration) at the same place of the real hand, at the same time that the threatening stimulus touched the embodied virtual hand, enhanced the feeling of the virtual needle hurting the virtual arm, thereby enhancing pain perception. Finally, participants experienced higher levels of ownership with the normal virtual arm condition either when the virtual needle touched or approached the virtual arm. Nevertheless, participants reported higher levels of ownership after the normal virtual arm representation in the real contact of the threatening event condition. Once again, this could be explained by the synchronous visuo-tactile stimulation that is induced when the virtual needle touches the virtual hand, which may enhance the sense of ownership over the virtual body [8]. Then, one may postulate that the observed results in the subjective pain responses and physiological responses to the threatening event may be related to the lower ownership responses towards the distorted (telescoped) virtual arm condition.

Finally, mediation effects of ownership ratings in SCR are open to several interpretations. First, this effect confirms that being embodied in a virtual body by providing a virtual body illusion can modulate physiological responses, as has been demonstrated previously [65–67]. Further, modulation of the morphological characteristics of the virtual body modulates physiological responses [68].

Our results show that changing the morphological characteristics of an embodied virtual body while being in a painful or threatening situation may modulate the physiological responses associated with pain, and these can be mediated by the feeling of ownership of the virtual body. While the use of embodiment to change body representations for pain relief has been already discussed (see [47] for a review), no mediation effects of ownership were found for the subjective pain measure (VAS ratings). One explanation of this may be because of the lower ownership ratings, compared to the normal virtual arm representation, obtained in the distorted and in the reddened-distorted virtual arm conditions. Although participants knew that the distorted virtual arm was not their real arm, it still influenced physiological responses of the participants, as has been demonstrated in previous studies [2,18,69]. Hence, even though participants felt less ownership in the distorted virtual arm conditions, physiological responses to pain were still modulated, highlighting the powerful effect of virtual embodiment in modulating body representations and their consequent impact on the modulation of physiological responses of pain responses.

5. Limitations

The present study shows a limitation regarding an unbalance in the participants' genders. It is known that females and males perceive pain differently [70], so although in this study no experimental pain was induced, the threatening event and the distortion of the virtual arm could activate both pain and anticipatory pain responses.

6. Conclusions

The present study investigated the influence of telescoping effects on the perception of pain by inducing such limb distortions in healthy people through VR. Our findings are in line with other studies in which the authors demonstrated that healthy subjects could experience the telescoped effect and the associated telescoping sensations (pain/discomfort) normally experienced by amputee patients through full virtual body illusions. Further, the results of this study demonstrate that the link between body image and pain responses is bi-directional, showing a top-down effect of body image on pain. This bi-directional link has also been reported in other studies [22,25,50,71,72]. Furthermore, our results reinforce the importance of tackling body image distortions when trying to reduce pain responses in chronic pain patients, especially in amputee patients with a telescopic limb sensation, suggesting that VR could be a powerful tool for modulating pain responses by changing the representation of the telescoped limb.

Author Contributions: Conceptualization, M.M.-G., B.N. and M.V.S.-V.; methodology, M.M.-G. and B.N.; software, M.S.; validation, M.V.S.-V.; formal analysis, M.M.-G. and M.S.; investigation, M.M.-G.; resources, M.V.S.-V. and M.S.; data curation, M.M.-G.; writing—original draft preparation, M.M.-G. and T.D.; writing—review and editing, T.D., M.V.S.-V. and M.S.; visualization, M.V.S.-V. and M.S.; supervision, M.V.S.-V.; project administration, T.D.; funding acquisition, M.V.S.-V. and M.S. All authors have read and agreed to the published version of the manuscript.

Funding: The present work was funded by the Agency for Management of University and Research Grants (AGAUR), project number 2017-SGR-01296.

Acknowledgments: We thank Ramón Olivera from the Event-Lab for the virtual reality scenarios, and for technical support.

Conflicts of Interest: The authors declare no conflict of interest.

References

1. Martini, M.; Perez-Marcos, D.; Sanchez-Vives, M.V. Modulation of pain threshold by virtual body ownership. *Eur. J. Pain* **2014**, *18*, 1040–1048. [CrossRef]
2. Martini, M.; Perez-Marcos, D.; Sanchez-Vives, M.V. What Color is My Arm? Changes in Skin Color of an Embodied Virtual Arm Modulates Pain Threshold. *Front. Hum. Neurosci.* **2013**, *7*, 438. [CrossRef]

3. Llobera, J.; González-Franco, M.; Perez-Marcos, D.; Valls-Solé, J.; Slater, M.; Sanchez-Vives, M.V. Virtual reality for assessment of patients suffering chronic pain: A case study. *Exp. Brain Res.* **2013**, *225*, 105–117. [CrossRef] [PubMed]
4. Senkowski, D.; Heinz, A. Chronic pain and distorted body image: Implications for multisensory feedback interventions. *Neurosci. Biobehav. Rev.* **2016**, *69*, 252–259. [CrossRef]
5. Mouraux, A.; Diukova, A.; Lee, M.C.; Wise, R.G.; Iannetti, G.D. A multisensory investigation of the functional significance of the "pain matrix". *Neuroimage* **2011**, *54*, 2237–2249. [CrossRef]
6. Slater, M. Place Illusion and Plausibility Can Lead to Realistic Behaviour in Immersive Virtual Environments. *Philos. Trans. R. Soc.* **2009**, *364*, 3549–3557. [CrossRef] [PubMed]
7. Sanchez-Vives, M.V.; Slater, M. From presence to consciousness through virtual reality. *Nat. Rev. Neurosci.* **2005**, *6*, 332–339. [CrossRef]
8. Slater, M.; Perez-Marcos, D.; Ehrsson, H.H.; Sanchez-Vives, M.V. Towards a digital body: The virtual arm illusion. *Front. Hum. Neurosci.* **2008**, *2*, 6. [CrossRef] [PubMed]
9. Maister, L.; Slater, M.; Sanchez-Vives, M.V.; Tsakiris, M. Changing bodies changes minds: Owning another body affects social cognition. *Trends Cogn. Sci.* **2015**, *19*, 6–12. [CrossRef]
10. Peck, T.C.; Seinfeld, S.; Aglioti, S.M.; Slater, M. Putting yourself in the skin of a black avatar reduces implicit racial bias. *Conscious. Cogn.* **2013**, *22*, 779–787. [CrossRef]
11. Banakou, D.; Groten, R.; Slater, M. Illusory ownership of a virtual child body causes overestimation of object sizes and implicit attitude changes. *Proc. Natl. Acad. Sci. USA* **2013**, *110*, 12846–12851. [CrossRef]
12. Martini, M.; Kilteni, K.; Maselli, A.; Sanchez-Vives, M.V. The body fades away: Investigating the effects of transparency of an embodied virtual body on pain threshold and body ownership. *Sci. Rep.* **2015**, *5*, 13948. [CrossRef]
13. Romano, D.; Maravita, A. The visual size of one's own hand modulates pain anticipation and perception. *Neuropsychologia* **2014**, *57*, 93–100. [CrossRef]
14. Moseley, G.; Parsons, T.; Spence, C. Visual distortion of a limb modulates the pain and swelling evoked by movement. *Curr. Biol.* **2008**, *18*, R1047–R1048. [CrossRef]
15. Hoffman, H.G.; Patterson, D.R.; Carrougher, G.J.; Sharar, S.R. Effectiveness of virtual reality-based pain control with multiple treatments. *Clin. J. Pain* **2001**, *17*, 229–235. [CrossRef] [PubMed]
16. Hoffman, H.G.; Richards, T.L.; Coda, B.; Bills, A.R.; Blough, D.; Richards, A.L.; Sharar, S.R. Modulation of thermal pain-related brain activity with virtual reality: Evidence from fMRI. *Neuroreport* **2004**, *15*, 1245–1248. [CrossRef]
17. Nierula, B.; Martini, M.; Matamala-Gomez, M.; Slater, M.; Sanchez-Vives, M.V. Seeing an Embodied Virtual Hand is Analgesic Contingent on Colocation. *J. Pain* **2017**, *18*, 645–655. [CrossRef]
18. Romano, D.; Llobera, J.; Blanke, O. Size and viewpoint of an embodied virtual body impact the processing of painful stimuli. *J. Pain* **2015**, *17*, 350–358. [CrossRef]
19. Pozeg, P.; Palluel, E.; Ronchi, R.; Solcà, M.; Al-Khodairy, A.W.; Jordan, X.; Kassouha, A.; Blanke, O. Virtual reality improves embodiment and neuropathic pain caused by spinal cord injury. *Neurology* **2017**, *89*, 1894–1903. [CrossRef]
20. Solcà, M.; Ronchi, R.; Bello-Ruiz, J.; Schmidlin, T.; Herbelin, B.; Luthi, F.; Konzelmann, M.; Beaulieu, J.Y.; Delaquaize, F.; Schnider, A.; et al. Heartbeat-enhanced immersive virtual reality to treat complex regional pain syndrome. *Neurology* **2018**, *91*, e479–e489. [CrossRef]
21. Boesch, E.; Bellan, V.; Moseley, G.; Stanton, T. The effect of bodily illusions on clinical pain: A systematic review and meta-analysis. *Pain* **2016**, *157*, 516–529. [CrossRef]
22. Foell, J.; Bekrater-Bodmann, R.; Diers, M.; Flor, H. Mirror therapy for phantom limb pain: Brain changes and the role of body representation. *Eur. J. Pain* **2014**, *18*, 729–739. [CrossRef]
23. Giummarra, M.J.; Gibson, S.J.; Georgiou-Karistianis, N.; Bradshaw, J.L. Central mechanisms in phantom limb perception: The past, present and future. *Brain Res. Rev.* **2007**, *54*, 219–232. [CrossRef]
24. Flor, H.; Nikolajsen, L.; Staehelin Jensen, T. Phantom limb pain: A case of maladaptive CNS plasticity? *Nat. Rev. Neurosci.* **2006**, *7*, 873–881. [CrossRef]
25. Makin, T.R.; Scholz, J.; Filippini, N.; Henderson Slater, D.; Tracey, I.; Johansen-Berg, H. Phantom pain is associated with preserved structure and function in the former hand area. *Nat. Commun.* **2013**, *4*, 1570. [CrossRef]

26. Bultitude, J.H.; Rafal, R.D. Derangement of body representation in complex regional pain syndrome: Report of a case treated with mirror and prisms. *Exp. Brain Res.* **2010**, *204*, 409–418. [CrossRef]
27. Lewis, J.; Kersten, P.; McPherson, K. Wherever is my arm? Impaired upper limb position accuracy in complex regional pain syndrome. *Pain* **2010**, *149*, 463–469. [CrossRef]
28. Melzack, R. Phantom limbs and the concept of a neuromatrix. *Trends Neurosci.* **1990**, *13*, 88–92. [CrossRef]
29. Wand, B.M.; Parkitny, L.; O'Connell, N.E.; Luomajoki, H.; McAuley, J.H.; Thacker, M.; Moseley, G.L. Cortical changes in chronic low back pain: Current state of the art and implications for clinical practice. *Man. Ther.* **2011**, *16*, 15–20. [CrossRef]
30. Ramachandran, V.S.; Altschuler, E.L. The use of visual feedback, in particular mirror visual feedback, in restoring brain function. *Brain* **2009**, *132*, 1693–1710. [CrossRef]
31. Armel, K.C.; Ramachandran, V.S. Projecting sensations to external objects: Evidence from skin conductance response. *Proc. R. Soc. B Biol. Sci.* **2003**, *270*, 1499–1506. [CrossRef]
32. Moseley, G.L.; Arntz, A. The context of a noxious stimulus affects the pain it evokes. *Pain* **2007**, *133*, 64–71. [CrossRef]
33. World Medical Association World Medical Association Declaration of Helsinki: Ethical principles for medical research involving human subjects. *J. Am. Med. Assoc.* **2013**, *310*, 2191–2194. [CrossRef] [PubMed]
34. Nikolajsen, L.; Springer, J.S.; Haroutiunian, S. Phantom Limb Pain. In *Practical Management of Pain*; Elsevier Inc.: Amsterdam, The Netherlands, 2014; Chapter 26; pp. 369–377.e3. ISBN 9780323083409.
35. Price, D.D.; McGrath, P.A.; Rafii, A.; Buckingham, B. The validation of visual analogue scales as ratio scale measures for chronic and experimental pain. *Pain* **1983**, *17*, 45–56. [CrossRef]
36. Kilteni, K.; Groten, R.; Slater, M. The Sense of Embodiment in Virtual Reality. *Presence Teleoperators Virtual* **2012**, *21*, 373–387. [CrossRef]
37. Cheng, Y.; Lin, C.P.; Liu, H.L.; Hsu, Y.Y.; Lim, K.E.; Hung, D.; Decety, J. Expertise Modulates the Perception of Pain in Others. *Curr. Biol.* **2007**, *17*, 1708–1713. [CrossRef]
38. Kilteni, K.; Normand, J.-M.; Sanchez-Vives, M.V.; Slater, M. Extending body space in immersive virtual reality: A very long arm illusion. *PLoS ONE* **2012**, *7*, e40867. [CrossRef]
39. Slater, M.; Perez-Marcos, D.; Ehrsson, H.H.; Sanchez-Vives, M.V. Inducing illusory ownership of a virtual body. *Front. Neurosci.* **2009**, *3*, 214–220. [CrossRef]
40. Breimhorst, M.; Sandrock, S.; Fechir, M.; Hausenblas, N.; Geber, C.; Birklein, F. Do intensity ratings and skin conductance responses reliably discriminate between different stimulus intensities in experimentally induced pain? *J. Pain* **2011**, *12*, 61–70. [CrossRef]
41. Lykken, D.T.; Venables, P.H. Direct measurement of skin conductance: A proposal for standardization. *Psychophysiology* **1971**, *8*, 656–672. [CrossRef]
42. Rhudy, J.L.; Bartley, E.J.; Williams, A.E. Habituation, sensitization, and emotional valence modulation of pain responses. *Pain* **2010**, *148*, 320–327. [CrossRef] [PubMed]
43. Lopes-Machado, E.Z.; De Souza Crippa, J.A.; Hallak, J.E.C.; Guimarães, F.S.; Zuardi, A.W. Electrodermically nonresponsive schizophrenia patients make more errors in the stroop color word test, indicating selective attention deficit. *Schizophr. Bull.* **2002**, *28*, 459–466. [CrossRef] [PubMed]
44. Turpin, G.; Schaefer, F.; Boucsein, W. Effects of stimulus intensity, risetime, and duration on autonomic and behavioral responding: Implications for the differentiation of orienting, startle, and defense responses. *Psychophysiology* **1999**, *36*, 453–463. [CrossRef]
45. Veit, R.; Lotze, M.; Sewing, S.; Missenhardt, H.; Gaber, T.; Birbaumer, N. Aberrant social and cerebral responding in a competitive reaction time paradigm in criminal psychopaths. *Neuroimage* **2010**, *49*, 3365–3372. [CrossRef]
46. Sanchez-Vives, M.V.; Spanlang, B.; Frisoli, A.; Bergamasco, M.; Slater, M. Virtual hand illusion induced by visuomotor correlations. *PLoS ONE* **2010**, *5*, e10381. [CrossRef]
47. Matamala-Gomez, M.; Donegan, T.; Bottiroli, S.; Sandrini, G.; Sanchez-Vives, M.V.; Tassorelli, C. Immersive virtual reality and virtual embodiment for pain relief. *Front. Hum. Neurosci.* **2019**, *13*, 279. [CrossRef]
48. Moseley, G.L.; Flor, H. Targeting Cortical Representations in the Treatment of Chronic Pain. *Neurorehabil. Neural Repair* **2012**, *26*, 646–652. [CrossRef]
49. Lotze, M.; Moseley, G.L. Role of Distorted Body Image in Pain. *Curr. Rheumatol. Reports Curr. Med. Gr. LLC ISSN* **2007**, *9*, 488–496. [CrossRef]

50. Makin, T.R.; Scholz, J.; Henderson Slater, D.; Johansen-Berg, H.; Tracey, I. Reassessing cortical reorganization in the primary sensorimotor cortex following arm amputation. *Brain* **2015**, *138*, 2140–2146. [CrossRef]
51. Schott, G.D. Penfield's homunculus: A note on cerebral cartography. *J. Neurol. Neurosurg. Psychiatry* **1993**, *56*, 329–333. [CrossRef]
52. Tung, M.L.; Murphy, I.C.; Griffin, S.C.; Alphonso, A.L.; Hussey-Anderson, L.; Hughes, K.E.; Weeks, S.R.; Merritt, V.; Yetto, J.M.; Pasquina, P.F.; et al. Observation of limb movements reduces phantom limb pain in bilateral amputees. *Ann. Clin. Transl. Neurol.* **2014**, *1*, 633–638. [CrossRef] [PubMed]
53. Mercier, C.; Sirigu, A. Training With Virtual Visual Feedback to Alleviate Phantom Limb Pain. *Neurorehabil. Neural Repair* **2009**, *23*, 587–594. [CrossRef]
54. Khelemsky, Y. Acute and chronic pain management. In *Anesthesiology and Otolaryngology*; Springer: Berlin/Heidelberg, Germany, 2013; Volume 9781461441, pp. 373–391. ISBN 9781461441847.
55. Palermo, L.; Di Vita, A.; Piccardi, L.; Traballesi, M.; Guariglia, C. Bottom-up and top-down processes in body representation: A study of brain-damaged and amputee patients. *Neuropsychology* **2014**, *28*, 772–781. [CrossRef] [PubMed]
56. Moseley, G.L. I can't find it! Distorted body image and tactile dysfunction in patients with chronic back pain. *Pain* **2008**, *140*, 167–171. [CrossRef] [PubMed]
57. Mancini, F.; Longo, M.R.; Kammers, M.P.M.; Haggard, P. Visual distortion of body size modulates pain perception. *Psychol. Sci.* **2011**, *22*, 325–330. [CrossRef] [PubMed]
58. Osumi, M.; Imai, R.; Ueta, K.; Nobusako, S.; Morioka, S. Negative body image associated with changes in the visual body appearance increases pain perception. *PLoS ONE* **2014**, *9*, e107376. [CrossRef] [PubMed]
59. Fields, H.L.; Basbaum, A.I.; Heinricher, M.M. Central nervous system mechanisms of pain modulation. In *Wall and Melzack's Textbook of Pain*; Saunders: Philadelphia, PA, USA, 2006; pp. 125–142. ISBN 978-0-443-07287-1.
60. Pud, D.; Granovsky, Y.; Yarnitsky, D. The methodology of experimentally induced diffuse noxious inhibitory control (DNIC)-like effect in humans. *Pain* **2009**, *144*, 16–19. [CrossRef]
61. Porro, C.A.; Baraldi, P.; Pagnoni, G.; Serafini, M.; Facchin, P.; Maieron, M.; Nichelli, P. Does anticipation of pain affect cortical nociceptive systems? *J. Neurosci.* **2002**, *22*, 3206–3214. [CrossRef]
62. Brown, C.A.; Jones, A.K. A role for midcingulate cortex in the interruptive effects of pain anticipation on attention. *Clin. Neurophysiol.* **2008**, *119*, 2370–2379. [CrossRef]
63. Botvinick, M.; Cohen, J. Rubber hands' feel 'touch that eyes see. *Nature* **1998**, *391*, 756. [CrossRef]
64. Ehrsson, H.; Petkova, V. If I were you: Perceptual illusion of body swapping. *PLoS ONE* **2008**, *3*, e3832.
65. González-Franco, M.; Peck, T.C.; Rodríguez-Fornells, A.; Slater, M. A threat to a virtual hand elicits motor cortex activation. *Exp. Brain Res.* **2014**, *232*, 875–887. [CrossRef] [PubMed]
66. Kilteni, K.; Grau-Sánchez, J.; Veciana De Las Heras, M.; Rodriguez-Fornells, A.; Slater, M. Decreased corticospinal excitability after the illusion of missing part of the arm. *Front. Hum. Neurosci.* **2016**, *10*, 3423. [CrossRef]
67. Nierula, B.; Spanlang, B.; Martini, M.; Borrell, M.; Nikulin, V.V.; Sanchez-Vives, M.V. Agency and responsibility over virtual movements controlled through different paradigms of brain–computer interface. *J. Physiol.* **2019**. [CrossRef]
68. Bergström, I.; Kilteni, K.; Slater, M. First-Person Perspective Virtual Body Posture Influences Stress: A Virtual Reality Body Ownership Study. *PLoS ONE* **2016**, *11*, e0148060. [CrossRef]
69. Romano, D.; Pfeiffer, C.; Maravita, A.; Blanke, O. Illusory self-identification with an avatar reduces arousal responses to painful stimuli. *Behav. Brain Res.* **2014**, *261*, 275–281. [CrossRef]
70. Fillingim, R.B. Sex, gender, and pain: Women and men really are different. *Curr. Rev. Pain* **2000**, *4*, 24–30. [CrossRef]
71. Schmalzl, L. "Pulling telescoped phantoms out of the stump": Manipulating the perceived position of phantom limbs using a full-body illusion. *Front. Hum. Neurosci.* **2011**, *5*, 5. [CrossRef]
72. Thøgersen, M.; Hansen, J.; Arendt-Nielsen, L.; Flor, H.; Petrini, L. Removing own-limb visual input using mixed reality (MR) produces a "telescoping" illusion in healthy individuals. *Behav. Brain Res.* **2018**, *347*, 263–271. [CrossRef]

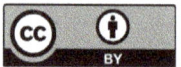

© 2020 by the authors. Licensee MDPI, Basel, Switzerland. This article is an open access article distributed under the terms and conditions of the Creative Commons Attribution (CC BY) license (http://creativecommons.org/licenses/by/4.0/).

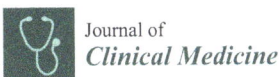

Article

Is This My Own Body? Changing the Perceptual and Affective Body Image Experience among College Students Using a New Virtual Reality Embodiment-Based Technique

Bruno Porras Garcia [1], Marta Ferrer Garcia [1], Agata Olszewska [1], Lena Yilmaz [1], Cristina González Ibañez [1], Mireia Gracia Blanes [1], Gamze Gültekin [1], Eduardo Serrano Troncoso [2,3] and José Gutiérrez Maldonado [1,*]

1. Department of Clinical Psychology and Psychobiology, University of Barcelona, Passeig de la Vall d'Hebron, 171, 08035 Barcelona, Spain
2. Child and Adolescent Psychiatry and Psychology Department, Hospital Sant Joan de Déu of Barcelona; Passeig de Sant Joan de Déu, 2, 08950 Esplugues de Llobregat, Barcelona, Spain
3. Children and Adolescent Mental Health Research Group, Institut de Recerca Sant Joan de Déu, Passeig de Sant Joan de Déu, 2, 08950 Esplugues de Llobregat, Barcelona, Spain
* Correspondence: jgutierrezm@ub.edu

Received: 23 May 2019; Accepted: 25 June 2019; Published: 27 June 2019

Abstract: Body image disturbances (BIDs) have been widely studied using virtual reality (VR) devices that induce a full body illusion (FBI) and allow manipulation of the individual's perceptual and affective experiences of the body. This study aimed to assess whether the induction of the FBI over a virtual body would produce changes in body-related anxiety and BIDs using a new whole-body visuo-tactile stimulation procedure. Fifty non-clinical participants were randomly assigned to synchronous or asynchronous visuo-tactile groups. During the pre-assessment, all participants filled in BIDs and body-anxiety questionnaires. Then, they were embodied into two virtual bodies (VBs): firstly, with their real measurements, and secondly, with a larger-size body. Body image disturbances, body anxiety, fear of gaining weight, and FBI levels were assessed after exposure to each avatar. All participants in both conditions showed higher levels of BIDs and body anxiety after owning the larger-size VB than after owning the real-size VB ($p < 0.05$). The synchronous visuo-tactile group had higher scores, although the differences did not reach statistical significance. This study provides evidence of the usefulness of this new embodiment-based technique to induce changes in BIDs or body anxiety in a non-clinical sample, being suitable for use in future body image interventions.

Keywords: virtual reality; body image disturbances; body anxiety; fear of gaining weight; full body illusion

---

1. Introduction

Body image has been described as a multi-dimensional construct reflecting the mental representation a person has of their physical appearance [1], including perceptual, cognitive, attitudinal, and affective components [2,3]. Likewise, body image disturbances (BIDs) involve dysfunctional cognitions, attitudes, and emotions related to the way in which an individual experiences their own body shape or weight. Body image distortion (the perceptual component) and body image dissatisfaction (the affective component) are the most commonly studied and assessed BIDs [4,5]. Body image distortion refers to the difficulty of precisely estimating one's own body size, whereas body image dissatisfaction refers to the degree a person likes or dislikes their own body [6]. Body image disturbances have also been related to avoidance behaviors and negative checking strategies [7].

Other studies have suggested that body image may be a state rather than a trait and may, therefore, be modifiable, depending on the situation or emotional variables [6,8]. One emotional variable directly related to BID is fear of gaining weight and the resulting state body anxiety. Similarly, an excessive concern with having a thinner body is related to high anxiety levels, and that, consequently, affects BID [9].

Body image disturbances have a high prevalence among eating disorder patients, as well as in non-clinical populations. Regarding body dissatisfaction, previous studies found that 44% of women and 17% of men in European adult samples would like to lose weight [10]. In Spanish college students, 84.2% of young women were not satisfied with their physical appearance and that 70% of women and 52.8% of men desired to reduce their weight [11]. In relation to perceptual body image distortion, previous studies found that both eating disorder (ED) patients and healthy individuals overestimated their BMI by more than two points [12].

Virtual reality (VR) has been successfully used in the assessment and treatment of BID [13]. This technology allows researchers to create real-size 3D simulations of participants' bodies with their specific physical characteristics and place them in VR immersive environments that reproduce real-life situations related to their body image concerns [13,14]. Recent studies have progressed to assessing the effect of inducing the ownership illusion of a virtual body on the experience of one's own body (e.g., [15–18]). To do so, the avatar must elicit feelings of ownership and the participants must recognize themselves in the virtual avatar [17].

To induce these illusory feelings of ownership, it is necessary to synchronize the stimulation of the real body and the false body using different sensory modalities (e.g., visual, tactile, motor, and vestibular) [18]. Visuo-tactile synchronization is one of the most widely studied and best-known methods of eliciting this full body illusion (FBI) and is based on the paradigm of the rubber hand illusion (RHI) [19]. In this paradigm, the participant was first seated in front of a rubber hand which was positioned in the place of their real hidden hand. Next, the participant's non-visible hand was touched as they saw the fake rubber hand being touched synchronously, thus eliciting an illusion of ownership over the fake rubber hand. According to Botvinick and Cohen [19], asynchronous tactile and visual stimulation would significantly reduce this illusion.

Immersive VR devices have been widely used to investigate several important aspects related to FBI, such as the type of multisensory stimulation applied to produce it (e.g., visuo-tactile versus visuomotor stimulation) [20], or the sort of visual perspective from which the virtual body is observed (first versus third person perspective) [16]. Regarding the type of multisensory stimulation, there is no definite agreement in the literature at present about the best method to elicit the illusion. Several authors suggested that this illusion can be elicited using a synchronous visuo-tactile stimulation, in which the participant observes the virtual body or some specific virtual body parts being touched while also feeling touches on their own real body [15,18,21–23]. Other studies have also elicited the FBI by performing synchronous visuomotor stimulation [20,24,25]. Therefore, the results suggest that both visuomotor and visuo-tactile synchronous stimulation can induce the FBI [20], and that the illusion can be strengthened by combining vision, touch, motor control, and proprioception inputs in the same interventions [26].

Regarding the role of visual perspective, participants can either look at themselves in a first-person perspective (1PP) or in a mirror perspective, by observing their virtual bodies in a mirror. While some studies suggest that 1PP is necessary for eliciting FBI [21,25,27], others have also induced it by using a mirror view [16] or third person perspective [28]. Therefore, not only first-person visual perspectives can play an important role in creating the FBI [16].

A considerable number of studies have investigated the role of the FBI in attempts to modify body image disturbances (for extensive recent reviews, see Gutiérrez–Maldonado et al., 13,14), by changing the perceptual experiences of the size and shape of certain body parts [16]. For instance, the FBI was elicited in participants within a virtual avatar with enlarged arms [29]. Similarly, in another study participants felt an enlarged virtual abdomen as their own [22]. In a non-clinical sample, the FBI was elicited in a virtual avatar whose body mass index had been previously modified to have an enlarged or a thinner body [17].

Preston and Ehrsson [15] elicited the FBI in individuals who were exposed to a virtual mannequin body that was manipulated to be slimmer or wider than the individual's real body. In addition, they achieved significant reductions in individuals' perceived body size and increases in body satisfaction levels when participants owned a slim mannequin body. Similarly, Serino et al. [18,30] showed how non-clinical participants [18] and a single case patient with anorexia nervosa (AN) [30], reported significant reductions in the ratio between estimated and actual measurements of body parts after they were embodied into a VR avatar with a skinny abdomen. In a study with a clinical sample, Keizer et al. [23] found that owning a skinny virtual body significantly reduced the perceived body size in AN patients as well as in healthy participants. Additionally, this change in perceived body size was preserved two hours later, especially among the healthy participants. Finally, two previous studies with healthy samples found that owning a larger-size virtual body can produce changes in body representations [22] and can also elicit higher body anxiety levels [31]. Therefore, the use of FBI in VR environments may be a suitable method for manipulating the perceptual and emotional experiences of the body image.

In order to extend our knowledge of the usefulness of VR techniques to modify body image disturbances and body-related anxiety, this study presents a novel VR embodiment-based technique. Among the novelties of the current study are: the use of a visuo-tactile stimulation procedure over the whole body, in both 1PP and mirror view; the reproduction of a real-size virtual body, based on each participant's frontal silhouette, resulting in accurate representations of their actual body; and a realistic simulation of their weight gain through different body parts (e.g., stomach, hips, waist, etc.) based on their real silhouette.

The main aim of the study was to assess whether the induction of the FBI of a virtual body produced changes in body-related anxiety and body image disturbances of non-clinical participants. Participants owned two different virtual bodies (VBs): one with the same body size as their own and another with a larger body size. In addition, participants were randomly assigned to the synchronous or asynchronous visuo-tactile condition.

Based on previous studies (e.g., [22,31]), we expected: first, that owning a larger-size VB would elicit higher body anxiety and body image disturbances than owning the real-size VB in both synch/asynch groups (and that the synchronous group would have higher scores); second, that the visuo-tactile synchronous group would show higher FBI levels in the real-size and larger-size VBs than the asynchronous group.

2. Materials and Methods

2.1. Participants

This study was approved by the ethical committee of the University of Barcelona. The sample was composed of 50 undergraduate students at the University of Barcelona, recruited through campus flyers and advertisements in social network groups. Forty women and 10 men (M_{age} = 21.8, SD = 2.55, M_{BMI} = 22.5, SD = 2.51) participated in the study. Exclusion criteria were self-reported diagnosis of a current ED, a BMI under 17 (moderate thinness) or over 30 (obesity) according to the World Health Organization [32] or a current self-reported severe mental disorder diagnosis (e.g., schizophrenia or bipolar disorder). Each participant was given an identification code in order to guarantee the confidentiality of the data.

2.2. Measures

2.2.1. Assessment of Body Image Disturbances and Body Anxiety

Figural Drawing Scale for Body Image Assessment (BIAS-BD) [12]: This questionnaire allows the use of physical anthropometric dimensions of adult women and men by providing a series of human silhouettes. This questionnaire has two versions (A and B) in which silhouettes are randomized differently to avoid order effect bias. Participants selected, among a set of human silhouettes, the one that was perceived as their body size (perceived silhouette) and the one that was desired to have (desired body size). Then, according to their BMI, the real silhouette was also selected. Body dissatisfaction (BIAS-O) was assessed by calculating the discrepancy between the perceived and desired body sizes. Body distortion (BIAS-X) was assessed by calculating the discrepancy between the perceived and real body sizes. This questionnaire presents good psychometric properties, with a good reliability test-retest ($r = 0.86$) and a good concurrent validity ($r = 0.76$) [12].

Physical Appearance State and Trait Anxiety Scale (PASTAS) [33]: This body anxiety questionnaire comprises two separate self-report scales which measure weight-related and non-weight-related anxiety. In this study, we used the weight scale (W). This questionnaire presents good internal reliability, with a Cronbach's alpha that ranges from 0.82 to 0.92, good test–retest ($r = 0.87$) and good convergent validity indices for the W scale ($r = 0.74$ EDI-BD, $r = 0.62$ EDI-DT) [34].

Visual Analog Scale (VAS)-FGW: This scale ranging from 0 (zero) to 100 (complete) assesses the fear of weight gain that the individual is feeling at a specific moment. The following question was posed to the participants: "On a scale from 0 to 100, rate how afraid you are of gaining weight right now".

2.2.2. Assessment of the Full-Body Illusion (FBI)

VAS-FBI: This visual analog scale ranging from 0 (zero) to 100 (complete) assesses the level of FBI of the virtual body that the individual is feeling at a specific moment. The following question was posed to the participants: "On a scale from 0 to 100, indicate to what extent you felt that the virtual body was your own body". In case a participant asked about the meaning of the previous question, it was clarified that the expression "feeling the virtual body as your own body" referred to whether they had the sense of being the owner of the virtual body.

2.3. Hardware and Software Features

Participants were exposed to an immersive virtual scenario using a head-mounted display (HMD) HTC-VIVE connected to a computer with enough graphic and processor power to move VR environments. Two programs were used to develop the virtual simulations: Blender 2.78 to create the virtual avatars (a man and a woman), and Unity 3D 5.5 to integrate all the elements within a virtual environment, which consisted of an unfurnished room with a large mirror placed in front of the participant's avatar, 1.5 meters away. It was not visible at the beginning of the experiment (first-person perspective) and was activated only during the mirror view condition. In the back part of the room there was a small door, slightly open, which was placed there to avoid any feeling of being trapped inside.

Both male and female avatars wore a standard black t-shirt with black jeans and black trainers, as well as a swimming cap to reduce the idiosyncratic influence of hairstyle.

2.4. Procedure

Pre-assessment: Once they signed the informed consent form, all participants completed a test battery which included the BIAS-BD and PASTAS trait and state questionnaires. All participants were weighed and measured after completing the two questionnaires in order to avoid the possibility that anxiety might affect the questionnaire responses. The BMI was calculated using the classical formula (BMI = weight (kg)/height (m)^2).

Creating the real-size virtual avatar (whole body photograph): The first step in creating the virtual avatar with the real measurements of the participants was to take a frontal view photograph of the whole body of the participant. A high-definition (HD) Logitech camera was used. All participants had to remain still in a marked position, two meters away from the camera, with their arms slightly raised and their legs slightly separated. Once the participant's photo was taken and processed in our program, the experimenters manually overlapped the photo and the virtual body by adapting the height and different body measures of the virtual avatar (e.g., arms, legs, hip, waist, chest, shoulder, etc.)

to the silhouette of the participant. The resulting virtual avatar, which represented the participant's frontal body measurements, will be referred to from now on as the "real-size virtual body". Finally, all participants were located within the avatar's body during the exposure to an immersive VR environment.

Visuo-tactile stimulation procedure: To enhance the illusion of owning the virtual body, an adaptation of the visuo-tactile stimulation procedure used by Keizer et al. [23] was conducted. While the Keizer et al. [23] procedure consisted of applying a tactile stimulation only to the abdomen for 90 seconds, in our study we also induced tactile stimulation over other specific body parts (the upper and lower limbs). Therefore, a series of continuous touches were applied to specific body parts, with a total duration of a minute and a half (15" each for left and right arm, 30" to the abdomen, and 15" each for left and right leg). The experimenter used one of the HTC-VIVE controllers to deliver the touches, while the participants looked at themselves (first-person perspective) while in their virtual bodies. Additionally, after the first-person perspective procedure (1PP), a mirror appeared on the wall in front of the avatar; the participants were asked to look at their avatars reflected in the mirror, while the same visuo-tactile procedure was repeated (mirror view). The complete duration of the visuo-tactile stimulation procedure was three minutes.

The control group asynchronous condition followed the procedure just described (1PP and mirror view) but the experimenter delivered the continuous touches, with a two-second delay, so that the visual feedback was inconsistent between what participants saw and what they really felt. For example, when they were feeling the touch to their forearm, they saw their avatar being touched on the shoulders.

In sum, both groups (synch/asynch) initially answered the test battery in the pre-assessment, then all participants were exposed to two virtual bodies: the first with the same body size as the participant and the second one larger than the participant (see Figure 1). In each body size condition, a visuo-tactile stimulation procedure was applied, using first a 1PP and second using a mirror view. Then, once they had finished the visuo-tactile stimulation procedure, participants answered the VAS-FBI and VAS-FGQ questions orally. Finally, after the last of each body size exposures, they left the VR environment and answered the BIAS-BD and PASTAS questionnaires.

PRE-ASSESSMENT	REAL-SIZE VB	LARGER-SIZE VB
Whole body photography	VAS- Full Body Illusion	VAS- Full Body Illusion
PASTAS Body anxiety State	VAS- Fear of gaining weight	VAS- Fear of gaining weight
BIAS_X (body image distortion)	PASTAS Body anxiety State	PASTAS Body anxiety State
BIAS_O (body image dissatisfaction)	BIAS_X (body image distortion)	BIAS_X (body image distortion)
Weight and height measurement	BIAS_O (body image dissatisfaction)	BIAS_O (body image dissatisfaction)

VITUAL REALITY VISUO-TACTILE STIMULATION PROCEDURE

2 GROUPS

VT ASYNCHRONOUS

VT SYNCHRONOUS

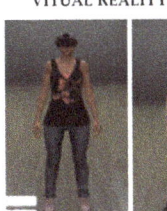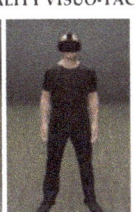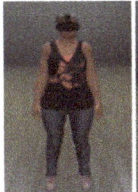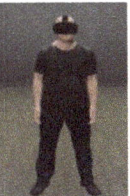

Figure 1. Experimental design scheme. Between-subjects group condition (synchronous versus asynchronous), within-subjects assessment condition (pre-assessment, real-size and larger-size virtual bodies), and dependent variables reported. VT = visuo-tactile, VB = virtual body, VAS = visual analog scales.

2.5. Statistical Analysis

The outcome of the intervention was analyzed with the statistical software IBM SPSS Statistics v.23. Mixed between (group)–within (assessment condition) analyses of variance (ANOVA) were conducted. The assumptions were partially met, since there was homogeneity of variances ($p > 0.05$) as assessed by the Levene's test. The assumption of sphericity was not completely met ($p < 0.05$) for some variables

(VAS_Fear of weight gain), therefore, it was decided to use the Green–House–Geisser corrected test for sphericity instead of this variable. Data were not normally distributed in all the variables assessed by the Kolmogorov–Smirnov test. However, it was decided to run the test regardless, as ANOVA is considered a robust test even in the case of a deviation from normality [35]. Finally, few outliers were detected in both BIDs measures, as assessed by inspection of a boxplot. Statistical analyses were conducted with and without the outliers, and since the results did not significantly differ, it was decided to include them in the analyses.

3. Results

3.1. Descriptive Results

A two-way mixed ANOVA was conducted. Means and standard deviations of all dependent variables were specified for each experimental condition at the different assessment times (Table 1).

Table 1. Descriptive outcomes, means, and standard deviations stated in the visuo-tactile group condition (asynchronous group versus synchronous group) at the different assessment conditions.

	Pre-Assessment		Real-Size VB		Larger-Size VB	
	Asyn-Group $n = 24$ M (SD)	Syn-Group $n = 26$ M (SD)	Asyn-Group $n = 24$ M (SD)	Syn-Group $n = 26$ M (SD)	Asyn-Group $n = 24$ M (SD)	Syn-Group $n = 26$ M (SD)
PASTAS	5.00 (5.87)	5.92 (5.31)	4.96 (5.46)	6.23 (5.77)	5.71 (6.07)	9.15 (6.89)
BIAS_X	9.58 (16,68)	13.65 (16.40)	9.17 (12.22)	12.50 (15.25)	18.54 (18.56)	19.62 (18.92)
BIAS_O	8.75 (18.72)	14.40 (21.81)	7.29 (14.06)	10.60 (19.22)	16.67 (18.57)	18.40 (22.39)
VAS-FBI	-	-	48.33 (20.44)	65.46 (19.15)	42.71 (28.97)	55.58 (23.07)
VAS-FGW	-	-	23.33 (26.77)	33.00 (29.34)	29.79 (29.39)	48.77 (29.48)

Note: Body Image Disturbances (Body Image Distortion-BIAS_X, Body Image Dissatisfaction- BIAS_O), Body Anxiety (PASTAS), fear of gaining weight (VAS-FWG), and full-body illusion (VAS-FBI). VB = Virtual body, Async = Asynchronous, Sync = Synchronous group conditions.

According to the descriptive results, in the pre-assessment, there were no statistically significant group differences ($p > 0.05$) in any of the body anxiety or BID measures. Therefore, it was decided to continue the statistical analyses.

3.2. Statistical Analyses

As shown in Table 2, there were no statistically significant interactions between group and assessment conditions ($p > 0.05$) on body dissatisfaction (BIAS_O), body distortion (BIAS_X), fear of gaining weight (VAS-FGW), and full body illusion (VAS-FBI). However, there was a significant interaction between group and assessment conditions in body anxiety (PASTAS) $F (2, 96) = 3.297$, $p = 0.041$, partial $\eta^2 = 0.064$.

Regarding body anxiety (PASTAS), three additional between-subjects ANOVAs were conducted separately in each assessment condition to follow up the simple effects of group on assessment time. Mean differences (MD) ± standard error (SE) are specified. Body anxiety scores did not differ significantly between the two groups ($p > 0.05$) in the pre-assessment and the real-size virtual body conditions (see Figure 2a). With the larger size virtual body, even though differences between the groups did not reach statistically significance $F (1, 48) = 3.492$, $p = 0.07$, partial $\eta^2 = 0.068$, with a medium effect size according to Cohen [36]; body anxiety scores were higher in the synchronous than in the asynchronous group condition (MD = 3.446 ± SE = 1.84).

Table 2. Mixed between–within subject analysis of variance comparing groups (Group 1-Asynchronous group versus Group 2-Synchronous group) with the different assessment conditions.

	Time x Group			Time of Assessment		
	F	p	η²	F	p	η²
PASTAS	3.297	0.041 *	0.064	8.554	0.001 *	0.151
BIAS_X	0.347	0.707	0.007	11.798	0.001 *	0.197
BIAS_O	0.410	0.665	0.009	8.177	0.001 *	0.148
VAS-FBI	0.312	0.579	0.006	4.130	0.048 *	0.079
VAS-FGW	3.855	0.055	0.074	21.968	0.001 *	0.314

Note: Green–House–Geisser corrected test for sphericity used. * Significant p-values < 0.05.

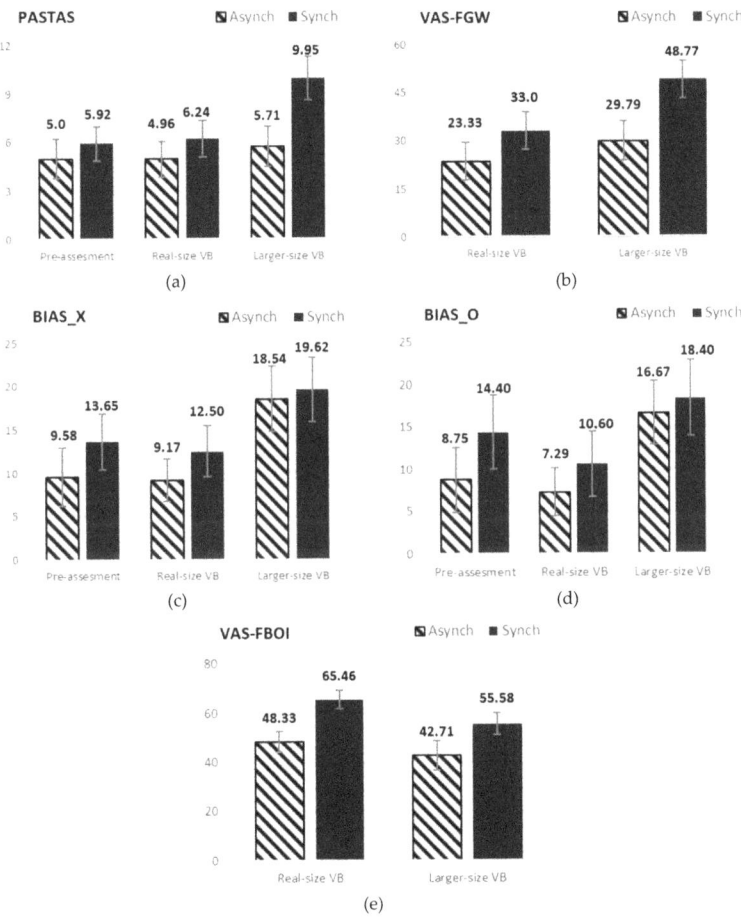

Figure 2. (**a**) Body anxiety mean scores, (**b**) fear of weight gain mean scores, (**c**) body image distortion mean scores, (**d**) body image dissatisfaction mean scores, (**e**) full-body ownership illusion mean scores. Means of the asynchronous and synchronous groups in the three assessment conditions (pre-assessment, real-size virtual body, larger-size virtual body). Error bars represent standard errors. Body image disturbances (Body Image Distortion-BIAS_X, Body Image Dissatisfaction-BIAS_O), Body anxiety (PASTAS), fear of gaining weight (VAS-FWG), and full-body ownership illusion (VAS-FBI). VB = Virtual body.

The main effect of assessment condition (see Table 2) showed that there were statistically significant differences ($p < 0.05$) in body anxiety (PASTAS), body image disturbances (BIAS_X or BIAS_O), fear of weight gain (VAS-FWG), and full body ownership illusion (VAS-FBI) measures.

To analyze the outcomes in more detail, multiple post-hoc tests (pairwise comparisons) were conducted. Mean differences (MD) ± standard error (SE) were specified. As can be seen in Table 3, all the measures were significantly higher in the larger-size VB condition than in both the real-size VB and the pre-assessment (for illustrations see Figure 2a–d). However, the VAS-FBI scores decreased compared with the real-size VB.

Table 3. Post-hoc analyses (pairwise comparison) at the different assessment times (pre-assessment, real-size virtual body and larger-size virtual body).

	Assessment Time Conditions					
	Pre-Assessment versus Real-Size VB		Larger-Size VB versus Real-Size VB		Larger-Size VB versus Pre-Assessment	
	MD	SE	MD	SE	MD	SE
PASTAS	0.133	0.491	1.837 *	0.517	1.970 *	0.584
BIAS_X	0.785	1.717	8.245 *	1.957	7.460 *	1.938
BIAS_O	2.629	1.915	8.588 *	2.133	5.958	2.448
VAS-FBI			−7.755 *	3.816		
VAS-FGW			11.114 *	2.371		

Note: MD = Mean differences, SE = Standard Error. * Significant p-values < 0.05. VB = Virtual body.

Finally, there was a statistically significant main effect of group on the VAS-FBI $F(1, 48) = 7940$, $p = 0.007$, partial $\eta^2 = 0.142$. Regardless of the assessment condition, the synchronous group showed higher levels of FBI than the asynchronous group (see Figure 2e).

4. Discussion

This study aimed to assess whether a visuo-tactile embodiment-based procedure could elicit changes in the body anxiety and body image disturbance responses of healthy participants when owning two different-size virtual bodies. In addition, two different visuo-tactile group conditions were compared (synchronous versus asynchronous visuo-tactile stimulation).

As expected, all participants, regardless of group, showed higher levels of body image disturbances (BIDs) and body anxiety after owning the larger-size virtual body (VB) than after owning with the real-size VB, and the scores were higher in the synchronous visuo-tactile group. Our results support previous findings suggesting that body image is a state rather than a trait, and can, thus, be modified by internal and external stimuli [6], such as owning a larger-size VB. Jakatdar, Cash, and Engle [37] suggested that malleability of the body image is more frequent in ED patients but also occurs in healthy participants, as our data show. Our results contrast with those of previous studies which did not report significant differences on body size estimating tasks before and after owning a larger mannequin/virtual body [15,17]. The differences in the results may be explained by differences in the methodological procedures used. For instance, even though in all the studies there was a larger-size/overweight virtual body condition, in our study, participants previously owned a real-size virtual body that represented their own silhouette, while in two previous studies [15,17], thin/underweight virtual bodies or mannequins were used instead.

In addition, the appearance of the virtual body, i.e., the body shape, may also explain the differences between the present study and previous studies. The appearance of the virtual body may play an important role not only in the eliciting of the illusory feelings of ownership [38,39], but also in eliciting emotional responses in healthy participants [15]. In our study a weight gain proportionally spread over the whole body (e.g., the belly, thighs, waist, arms) was reproduced, resulting in a more realistic increase of weight across the body, and consequently evoking higher anxiety and body image disturbance levels in participants when owning the larger virtual body than when owning the real-size virtual body. In contrast, other studies may have not found similar results because the weight gain was represented less proportionally, for example, by increasing only the stomach size of the mannequin [15]. Additionally, the increase in the weight of our avatar was previously based on the real-size virtual body with the participant's silhouette, allowing a more accurate and natural weight increase in the larger-size virtual body.

Regarding body anxiety levels, our results are in line with those of a previous study by our group [31], in which healthy college students undergoing a synchronous visuomotor procedure reported higher levels of body anxiety and fear of weight gain after owning a larger-size VB than after owning their real-size VB. However, the current study has attempted to overcome some of the limitations reported there, such as the small sample size, the lack of an asynchronous visuomotor procedure, and the lack of a baseline pre-assessment time condition. Furthermore, BID and body anxiety levels did not differ significantly after owning a virtual avatar with participants' real measurements (real-size VB) compared with the pre-assessment. This suggests that, regardless of the type of visuo-tactile stimulation, all participants delivered, perceived, and felt the real-size VB as their own body, even without being aware of it.

According to the differences between the synchronous and asynchronous visuo-tactile groups, there were not statistically significant group differences in BID and body anxiety measures. Interesting non-significant tendencies were found in body anxiety measures. Participants who underwent a synchronous visuo-tactile procedure reported higher body anxiety and fear of gaining weight levels than those in the asynchronous condition, at the larger size VB. One possible explanation for these tendencies, is that some of the body parts that were (in)congruently stimulated (e.g., the stomach or the thighs) are usually reported as body areas of higher concern [40] or weight-related body areas [33]. Previous studies have reported that individuals with ED [40,41] show an attentional preference towards these self-reported unattractive body areas. Therefore, it might be expected that a synchronous visuo-tactile stimulation over those salient body areas with a significant weight gain might elicit a higher more unpleasant anxious response that was not observed at equal levels in the asynchronous group. Consequently, our results suggest that the specific influence of the FBI induced by a synchronous visuo-tactile stimulation over specific body parts may differentially affect body anxiety and BID measures after owning a larger-size VB. Regarding BID measures, our results are in line with previous studies in which inducing a synchronous or asynchronous visuo-tactile stimulation did not affect body distortion levels after owning a skinny virtual body [18], or an underweight or overweight virtual body [17].

Regarding the FBI levels, the synchronous visuo-tactile group showed significantly greater FBI levels in both the real-size VB and larger-size VB than the asynchronous group. Our results are in line with previous studies that compared synchronous versus asynchronous visuo-tactile stimulation procedures for eliciting FBI by owning either a slim virtual body or mannequin body (e.g., [15,16,21,23]) or an overweight virtual body [15,17,22]. However, some important differences between our study and previous research should be noted, such as, for example, the type of visual perspective displayed. In the present study, a combination of both 1PP and a mirror view perspective were used successively in order to strengthen the FBI, in comparison to previous studies that have used only a first-person perspective to elicit the FBI (e.g., [15,21,23]).

Another important difference is the sort of tactile stimulation delivered. A visuo-tactile stimulation procedure over the whole body (abdomen, upper and lower extremities) was delivered in this study, in contrast to previous studies in which the only stimulated body parts were the abdomen or the belly [18,23], or the upper and lower limbs [17]. Additionally, the body posture was also different from the study conducted by Piryankova et al. [17], in which the participants were seated while the upper and lower virtual limbs were touched. In our study, all participants were in a standing position, in which the realism of the virtual avatar is less likely to be affected.

The current study presents some limitations that should be addressed in future research. Body mass index (BMI) was not controlled. Although we excluded participants with obesity (BMI > 30) or who were moderate-to-severely underweight (BMI < 17), previous literature suggested that overweight, compared to healthy weight, individuals present higher body dissatisfaction levels [42]. Another important limitation is that no screening questionnaire or clinical structured interview was used to properly assess the presence of an ED diagnosis or other mental disorders. It should be noted that even though our participants were allocated randomly, the synchronous visuo-tactile group reported slightly higher BID levels than the asynchronous group at the pre-assessment time condition. However, as the group differences did not reach significance, it was decided to continue the statistical analyses. As regards the length of the experiment, participants generally spent one hour in the laboratory. We realize that it may cause fatigue, especially because participants were asked to stand still while the experimenter was running the tactile-stimulation procedure for each body size condition. Following the previous argument, and so as not to lengthen the experiment further, it was decided not to include other body-size conditions such as a slimmer virtual body, as the studies by Preston et al. [15] or Piryankova et al. [17] had done.

These results may have different implications in clinical practice. In the near future, it would be interesting to apply FBI and VR embodiment-based techniques to treat the fear of gaining weight and body anxiety in ED patients, and specifically in anorexia nervosa (AN) patients. One possibility would be to develop an exposure therapy to one's own body, in which an AN patient could own an avatar with their own body silhouette and their BMI would increase gradually, according to a pre-established hierarchy. Additionally, our results support those of previous studies suggesting that VR embodiment-based techniques may be a useful tool for interventions that aim to modify or improve BID levels among healthy participants, or in clinical ED patients (e.g., [23]).

Another interesting approach would be to use VR embodiment-based procedures not only to treat BID, but also to assess it. Following a similar procedure to paper-based figural drawing scale questionnaires (e.g., BIAS-BD, [12]) or human-based 3D computer scales [43,44], participants or ED patients could own a virtual avatar and modify different body parts (or the whole body of the avatar) according to their perceived or desired body size. Additionally, using a VR assessment procedure would also allow the generation of more ecologically valid experimental settings that represent daily life situations: for instance, looking at one's own body in a mirror.

5. Conclusions

This study provides new evidence of the usefulness of VR embodiment-based techniques to induce changes in body image disturbances or body anxiety in a non-clinical sample of college students. Specifically, our findings provide new information about how the influence of the FBI, induced by a synchronous visuo-tactile stimulation, may not only strengthen the FBI when participants own their real-size VB, but may also elicit higher BID and body anxiety levels after owning a larger-size VB, with body anxiety measures being particularly affected by a congruent visuo-tactile stimulation. In addition, a new VR visuo-tactile stimulation procedure over the whole body, which combines first-person perspective and mirror view, is presented and discussed. Finally, this study presents a novel procedure for adapting our virtual avatar bodies based on the real-size frontal silhouettes of our participants, allowing the recreation of a realistic real-size virtual avatar, but even more importantly, the simulation of a more realistic weight gain in our virtual bodies.

The use of VR embodiment-based techniques opens up new possibilities in body image research, some of which are presented and briefly discussed in this article. However, considering the high prevalence of BID among ED patients [12] and among non-clinical populations [10,11], future interventions should continue to focus on understanding and improving the disturbed representations that so many individuals have of their body appearance.

Author Contributions: Conceptualization, B.P.G., M.F.G., A.O., L.Y., C.G.I., M.G.B., G.G., and J.G.M.; methodology, B.P.G.; validation, B.P.G., C.G.I., and M.G.B.; formal analysis, B.P.G.; investigation, B.P.G., M.F.G., C.G.I., M.G.B.; resources, M.F.G., J.G.M.; data curation, B.P.G.; writing—original draft preparation, B.P.G. A.O., L.Y., and G.G. writing—review and editing, B.P.G., M.F.G., E.S.T., J.G.M.; visualization, B.P.G., M.F.G., A.O., L.Y., G.G.; supervision, M.F.G., E.S.T., and J.G.M.; project administration, J.G.M.; funding acquisition, J.G.M.

Funding: This study was funded by the Spanish Ministry of Economy and Competitiveness (MINECO/FEDER/UE/ Project PSI2015-70389-R: Development of reality-based exposure techniques for improving anorexia nervosa treatment) and by the AGAUR, Generalitat de Catalunya, 2017SGR1693.

Conflicts of Interest: The authors declare no conflict of interest. The funders had no role in the design of the study; in the collection, analyses, or interpretation of data; in the writing of the manuscript, or in the decision to publish the results.

References

1. Cash, T.F. Cognitive-behavioural perspectives on body image. In *Body Image: A Handbook of Theory, Research, and Clinical Practice*; Cash, T.F., Pruzinsky, T., Eds.; Guilford Press: New York, NY, USA, 2002; pp. 38–46.
2. Cash, T.F. Cognitive-Behavioral Perspectives on Body Image. In *Body Image: A Handbook of Science, Practice, and Prevention*; Cash, T.F., Smolak, L., Eds.; Guilford Press: New York, NY, USA, 2012; pp. 39–47.
3. Gaudio, S.; Quattrocchi, C.C. Neural basis of a multidimensional model of body image distortion in anorexia nervosa. *Neurosci. Biobehav. Rev.* **2012**, *36*, 1839–1847. [CrossRef] [PubMed]
4. Cash, T.F.; Deagle, E.A. The nature and extent of body-image disturbances in anorexia nervosa and bulimia nervosa: A meta-analysis. *Int. J. Eat. Disord.* **1997**, *22*, 107–126. [CrossRef]
5. Hagman, J.; Gardner, R.M.; Brown, D.L.; Gralla, J.; Fier, J.M.; Frank, G.K.W. Body size overestimation and its association with body mass index, body dissatisfaction, and drive for thinness in anorexia nervosa. *Eat. Weight Disord.* **2015**, *20*, 449–455. [CrossRef] [PubMed]
6. Ferrer-García, M.; Gutiérrez-Maldonado, J. The use of virtual reality in the study, assessment, and treatment of body image in eating disorders and nonclinical samples: A review of the literature. *Body Image* **2012**, *9*, 1–11. [CrossRef] [PubMed]
7. Legenbauer, T.; Thiemann, P.; Vocks, S. Body image disturbance in children and adolescents with eating disorders: Current evidence and future directions. *Z. Kinder. Jugendpsychiatr. Psychother.* **2014**, *42*, 51–59. [CrossRef] [PubMed]
8. Espeset, E.M.S.; Gulliksen, K.S.; Nordbø, R.H.S.; Skårderud, F.; Holte, A. The link between negative emotions and eating disorder behaviour in patients with anorexia nervosa. *Eur. Eat. Disord. Rev.* **2012**, *20*, 451–460. [CrossRef]
9. Maganto Mateo, C.; Cruz Saez, S. La insatisfacción corporal como variable explicativa de los trastornos alimenticios. *Rev. Psicol.* **2002**, *10*, 197–223.
10. Bellisle, F.; Monneuse, M.O.; Steptoe, A.; Wardle, J. Weight concerns and eating patterns: A survey of university students in Europe. *Int. J. Obes. Relat. Metab. Disord.* **1995**, *19*, 723–730.
11. Lameiras Fernández, M.; Calado Otero, M.; Rodríguez Castro, Y.; Fernández Prieto, M. Hábitos alimentarios e imagen corporal en estudiantes universitarios sin trastornos alimentarios. *Rev. Int. Psicol. Clín. Salud* **2003**, *3*, 23–33.
12. Gardner, R.M.; Jappe, L.M.; Gardner, L. Development and validation of a new figural drawing scale for body-image assessment: The BIAS-BD. *J. Clin. Psychol.* **2009**, *65*, 113–122. [CrossRef]
13. Gutiérrez-Maldonado, J.; Wiederhold, B.K.; Riva, G. Future Directions: How Virtual Reality Can Further Improve the Assessment and Treatment of Eating Disorders and Obesity. *Cyberpsychol. Behav. Soc. Netw.* **2016**, *19*, 148–153. [CrossRef] [PubMed]
14. Gutiérrez-Maldonado, J.; Ferrer-García, M.; Dakanalis, A.; Riva, G. Virtual Reality: Applications to Eating Disorders. In *The Oxford Handbook of Eating Disorders*, 2nd ed.; Agras, W.S., Robinson, A.H., Eds.; Oxford University Press: Oxford, UK, 2018; Volume 19, pp. 148–153.
15. Preston, C.; Ehrsson, H.H. Illusory changes in body size modulate body satisfaction in a way that is related to non-clinical eating disorder psychopathology. *PLoS ONE* **2014**, *9*, e85773. [CrossRef] [PubMed]
16. Preston, C.; Kuper-Smith, B.J.; Henrik Ehrsson, H. Owning the body in the mirror: The effect of visual perspective and mirror view on the full-body illusion. *Sci. Rep.* **2015**, *5*, 18345. [CrossRef]

17. Piryankova, I.V.; Wong, H.Y.; Linkenauger, S.A.; Stinson, C.; Longo, M.R.; Bülthoff, H.H.; Mohler, B.J. Owning an overweight or underweight body: Distinguishing the physical, experienced and virtual body. *PLoS ONE* **2014**, *9*, e103428. [CrossRef] [PubMed]
18. Serino, S.; Pedroli, E.; Keizer, A.; Triberti, S.; Dakanalis, A.; Pallavicini, F.; Chirico, A.; Riva, G. Virtual Reality Body Swapping: A Tool for Modifying the Allocentric Memory of the Body. *Cyberpsychol. Behav. Soc. Netw.* **2016**, *19*, 127–133. [CrossRef] [PubMed]
19. Botvinick, M.; Cohen, J. Rubber hands "feel" touch that eyes see. *Nature* **1998**, *391*, 756. [CrossRef] [PubMed]
20. Kokkinara, E.; Slater, M. Measuring the effects through time of the influence of visuomotor and visuotactile synchronous stimulation on a virtual body ownership illusion. *Perception* **2014**, *43*, 43–58. [CrossRef]
21. Petkova, V.I.; Ehrsson, H.H. If I were you: Perceptual illusion of body swapping. *PLoS ONE* **2008**, *3*, e3832. [CrossRef]
22. Normand, J.M.; Giannopoulos, E.; Spanlang, B.; Slater, M. Multisensory stimulation can induce an illusion of larger belly size in immersive virtual reality. *PLoS ONE* **2011**, *6*, e16128. [CrossRef]
23. Keizer, A.; van Elburg, A.; Helms, R.; Dijkerman, H.C. A virtual reality full body illusion improves body image disturbance in anorexia nervosa. *PLoS ONE* **2016**, *11*, e0163921. [CrossRef]
24. Gonzalez-Franco, M.; Perez-Marcos, D.; Spanlang, B.; Slater, M. The contribution of real-time mirror reflections of motor actions on virtual body ownership in an immersive virtual environment. In Proceedings of the IEEE Virtual Reality Conference (VR), Waltham, MA, USA, 20–24 March 2010. [CrossRef]
25. Slater, M.; Spanlang, B.; Sanchez-Vives, M.V.; Blanke, O. First person experience of body transfer in virtual reality. *PLoS ONE* **2010**, *5*, e10564. [CrossRef] [PubMed]
26. Ehrsson, H.H. The Concept of Body Ownership and Its Relation to Multisensory Integration. In *The New Handbook of Multisensory Processes*; Stein, B.E., Ed.; MIT Press: Cambridge, MA, USA, 2012; pp. 775–792.
27. Petkova, V.I.; Khoshnevis, M.; Ehrsson, H.H. The perspective matters! Multisensory integration in ego-centric reference frames determines full-body ownership. *Front. Psychol.* **2011**, *2*, 35. [CrossRef] [PubMed]
28. Preston, C.; Newport, R. How long is your arm? Using multisensory illusions to modify body image from the third person perspective. *Perception* **2012**, *41*, 247–249. [CrossRef] [PubMed]
29. Kilteni, K.; Normand, J.M.; Sanchez-Vives, M.V.; Slater, M. Extending body space in immersive virtual reality: A very long arm illusion. *PLoS ONE* **2012**, *7*, e40867. [CrossRef]
30. Serino, S.; Polli, N.; Riva, G. From avatars to body swapping: The use of virtual reality for assessing and treating body-size distortion in individuals with anorexia. *J. Clin. Psychol.* **2018**, *75*, 313–322. [CrossRef]
31. Ferrer-Garcia, M.; Porras-Garcia, B.; Gonzalez-Ibanez, C.; Gracia-Blanes, M.; Vilalta-Abella, F.; Pla-Sanjuanelo, J.; Gutierrez-Maldonado, J.; Achotegui-Loizate, J.; Riva, G.; Dakanalis, K.; et al. Does owning a "fatter" virtual body increase body anxiety in college students? *Annu. Rev. Cyber Ther. Telemed.* **2017**, *15*, 147–153.
32. World Health Organization. *ICD-10 International Statistical Classification of Diseases and Related Health Problems: Tenth Revision*, 2nd ed.; World Health Organization: Geneva, Switzerland, 2004; Volume 3, ISBN 9241546492.
33. Reed, D.L.; Thompson, J.K.; Brannick, M.T.; Sacco, W.P. Development and validation of the physical appearance state and trait anxiety scale (PASTAS). *J. Anxiety Disord.* **1991**, *5*, 323–332. [CrossRef]
34. Garner, D. *Eating Disorder Inventory-3: Professional Manual*; Psychological Assessment Resources: Lutz, FL, USA, 2004.
35. Schmider, E.; Ziegler, M.; Danay, E.; Beyer, L.; Bühner, M. Is it really robust? Reinvestigating the robustness of ANOVA against violations of the normal distribution assumption. *Methodol. Eur. J. Res. Methods Behav. Soc. Sci.* **2010**, *6*, 147–151. [CrossRef]
36. Cohen, J. *Statistical Power Analysis for the Behavioral Sciences*, 2nd ed.; Lawrence Erlbaum Associates: Hillsdale, NJ, USA, 1988.
37. Jakatdar, T.; Cash, T.; Engle, E. Body-image thought processes: The development and initial validation of the Assessment of Body-Image Cognitive Distortions. *Body Image* **2006**, *3*, 325–333. [CrossRef]
38. Maselli, A.; Slater, M. The building blocks of the full body ownership illusion. *Front. Hum. Neurosci.* **2013**, *7*, 83. [CrossRef]
39. Tsakiris, M.; Carpenter, L.; James, D.; Fotopoulou, A. Hands only illusion: Multisensory integration elicits sense of ownership for body parts but not for non-corporeal objects. *Exp. Brain Res.* **2010**, *204*, 343–352. [CrossRef] [PubMed]
40. Jansen, A.; Nederkoorn, C.; Mulkens, S. Selective visual attention for ugly and beautiful body parts in eating disorders. *Behav. Res. Ther.* **2005**, *43*, 183–196. [CrossRef]

41. Tuschen-Caffier, B.; Bender, C.; Caffier, D.; Klenner, K.; Braks, K.; Svaldi, J. Selective visual attention during mirror exposure in anorexia and bulimia nervosa. *PLoS ONE* **2015**, *10*, e0145886. [CrossRef] [PubMed]
42. Weinberger, N.A.; Kersting, A.; Riedel-Heller, S.G.; Luck-Sikorski, C. Body Dissatisfaction in Individuals with Obesity Compared to Normal-Weight Individuals: A Systematic Review and Meta-Analysis. *Obes. Facts* **2017**, *9*, 424–441. [CrossRef] [PubMed]
43. Cornelissen, K.; Bester, A.; Cairns, P.; Tovée, M.; Cornelissen, P. The influence of personal BMI on body size estimations and sensitivity to body size change in anorexia spectrum disorders. *Body Image* **2015**, *13*, 75–85. [CrossRef] [PubMed]
44. Cornelissen, K.; McCarty, K.; Cornelissen, P.; Tovée, M. Body size estimation in women with anorexia nervosa and healthy controls using 3D avatars. *Sci. Rep.* **2017**, *7*, 15773. [CrossRef] [PubMed]

© 2019 by the authors. Licensee MDPI, Basel, Switzerland. This article is an open access article distributed under the terms and conditions of the Creative Commons Attribution (CC BY) license (http://creativecommons.org/licenses/by/4.0/).

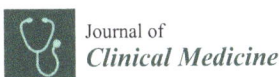

Article

Assessing the Relationship between Sense of Agency, the Bodily-Self and Stress: Four Virtual-Reality Experiments in Healthy Individuals

Yonatan Stern [1,2,*], Danny Koren [1], Renana Moebus [2], Gabriella Panishev [2] and Roy Salomon [2]

1. Psychology Department, University of Haifa, Haifa 3498838, Israel; dkoren@psy.haifa.ac.il
2. Gonda Brain Research Center, Bar-Ilan University, Ramat Gan 5290002, Israel; moebusrenana@gmail.com (R.M.); gabyp97@gmail.com (G.P.); roy.salomon@biu.ac.il (R.S.)
* Correspondence: yoniastern@gmail.com

Received: 3 August 2020; Accepted: 8 September 2020; Published: 11 September 2020

Abstract: The bodily-self, our experience of being a body, arises from the interaction of several processes. For example, embodied Sense of Agency (SoA), the feeling of controlling our body's actions, is a fundamental facet of the bodily-self. SoA is disturbed in psychosis, with stress promoting its inception. However, there is little knowledge regarding the relationship between SoA, stress, and other facets of the bodily-self. In four experiments manipulating embodied SoA using a virtual hand (VH), we examined (1) How is embodied SoA related to other facets of the bodily-self?; and (2) How is SoA impacted by stress? We found that increased alteration of the VH significantly decreased subjective ratings of SoA and body ownership (Exp. 1), supporting the close relation between SoA and body ownership. Interoceptive accuracy and SoA were positively correlated (Exp. 3), connecting awareness to one's actions and cardiac signals. Contrary to our expectations, SoA was not related to trait anxiety (Exp. 3), nor did induced stress impair SoA (Exp. 4). Finally, we found a negative correlation between self-reported prodromal symptoms and SoA. These results strongly support the connection between SoA and the bodily-self. Whereas, SoA was not impaired by stress, and weakly related to psychotic symptoms.

Keywords: sense of agency; metacognition; virtual reality; psychosis; stress; bodily-self

1. Introduction

1.1. Sense of Agency and the Bodily-Self

Experiencing one's self as a physical entity grounded in a body is termed the 'bodily-self' or 'minimal self', emphasizing the fundamental nature of this stratum of selfhood [1–4]. The bodily-self encompasses two related capacities: body ownership and sense of agency (SoA), which are typically seamlessly interwoven into our experience to such a degree that we are typically not explicitly aware of them, rather they are pre-reflective [5,6]. Body ownership, the identification with one's body, relies on the integration of multisensory signals constructing a coherent representation of the self in the present moment. For example, synchronous visual–tactile stimulation can create an illusory sense of body ownership over a rubber hand or a virtual body [7–9]. SoA, the feeling of being in control of one's actions, also relies on multisensory integration but incorporates internal neural efferent signals originating in the agent's volition [10–12].

SoA primarily relies on the comparison of the predicted consequences of our actions (i.e., forwards models) with the actual afferent sensory outcomes via a comparator mechanism (but see other approaches such as Cue Integration, e.g., [13–15] and Postdictive accounts of SoA, e.g., [16,17]). If the predicted and actual outcome of the action match, then SoA arises, whereas if they are incongruent, the outcome will likely be attributed to an external cause [18–20]. For example, while reading this article on a computer screen, when you scroll the mouse with your finger to continue reading, and the screen scrolls, an SoA arises for these actions and outcomes. Importantly, two forms of SoA can be discerned in this example [21,22]. The first, embodied SoA, focuses on the immediate, often pre-reflective, connection between the intention to perform the action and the action itself (i.e., moving your finger) [23]. This form of SoA is inherently tied to the body of the agent that performs the action. The second, non-embodied SoA, focuses on the link between the action performed by the agent (i.e., moving your finger) and the intended outcome (i.e., screen scrolling). This SoA is related to a more general sense of causation, linking an action to its predicted outcome that is often detached spatially and temporally from the agent's body and action. Historically, there has been no clear distinction between these two forms of agency, which are often conflated in the literature [11,24–29]. However, we argue that embodied SoA, with its close affinity to the bodily-self, introduces unique characteristics. The importance of this distinction is intuitively demonstrated by the hypothetical reaction to the failure of each form of agency. Imagine the profound shock and fear you would experience if you intended to move your finger, and it did not move (i.e., embodied SoA). Whereas, if you scrolled your mouse and the screen failed to scroll (i.e., non-embodied SoA), you would likely dismiss it as a problem with your laptop. In line with this distinction, the exclusive focus of the current paper is embodied SoA.

In the literature, various experimental paradigms have been used to examine SoA, yet these diverging paradigms probe different aspects of agency that are often conflated (see [22] for an extensive discussion). Thus, some paradigms (e.g., [30,31]) use an additional actor within the experimental setting, and probe agentic authorship by asking participants whether they or the other actor performed the presented action. While other paradigms have examined the role of active as opposed to passive actions on SoA (e.g., [26,28,32–34]), examining how the agent's volition and the availability of neural efferent signals shape agency. In line with the theoretical suggestion that agency arises primarily from the congruence of predicted and actual sensory outcomes of action ([35–37]), and in line with a well-established line of research examining the effects of sensorimotor congruence on agency (e.g., [28,34,38–41]), the focus of the current paper is on examining how embodied agency is affected by the introduction of conflicts between actions and their visual consequences

1.2. Embodied SoA and Its Metacognition: Exteroceptive and Interoceptive Contributions

In line with our theoretical definition of embodied SoA that focuses on intention and motor actions, experimental operationalizations of embodied SoA use naturalistic representations of the body and focus on the motor action itself. Despite its theoretical and philosophical importance, experimentally examining embodied SoA has been somewhat limited, requiring creativity and ingenuity, such as using mirror set-ups and video systems [31,34], to create realistic distortions of self-generated movements. Recent advances in virtual reality (VR) technology allow for easier, more complex, and better-controlled manipulations of the bodily-self [9,42,43] and embodied SoA [28,44–48]. Such research has enabled significant advances in understanding the cognitive and neural processes by which sensory and motor signals shape the self [1,49,50]. In addition to the integration of exteroceptive signals, research has highlighted the importance of cardiac signals in the formation of the bodily-self. The neural processing of cardiac signals is modified by experimental changes in body ownership [51,52]. Moreover, cardiac signals can be used to induce body ownership over virtual hands [53] and bodies [54]. Within the realm of SoA, cardiac signals have been related to the subjective awareness of motor actions and errors [55,56]. Given the role of cardiac signals in body ownership and actions, we posited that awareness of one's cardiac activity might be linked to awareness of one's actions and embodied SoA.

Within judgments of SoA, we can distinguish between first-order and second-order processes [46,57,58]. First-order processes are related to the initial judgment of agency and include sensitivity—the ability to detect sensorimotor conflicts, and criteria—the decision threshold for asserting agency. Whereas, second-order processes concern the assessment of one's initial judgment and include measures of confidence and metacognition. Importantly, metacognition is a bridge between immediate judgments of agency and reflective awareness and self-knowledge of one's agency [5,57]. Both processes are central in delineating the self and are impaired in psychiatric populations such as psychosis [20,57,58]. Recently, we found that sensitivity and criteria of embodied SoA were both highly correlated across distortions in both the temporal and spatial domains introduced on a virtual hand presentation of self-generated movements [46]. These findings suggest an integrated mechanism of first-order processes that extends beyond specific domains and supports the processing of self-generated actions [4,10].

To briefly summarize, embodied SoA is a fundamental process contributing to our experience of the bodily-self. Accordingly, we hypothesize that SoA will be closely related to other facets of the bodily-self, such as body ownership and interoceptive processing. Furthermore, we expect that SoA and its metacognition will be correlated across domains, pointing to central processing and awareness of embodied actions.

1.3. Open Questions: The Effect of Stress

It is well documented that adverse situations such as stress and anxiety are a contributing factor to a wide range of psychopathological conditions entailing breakdowns of the self. Following trauma, people often experience dissociative states such as depersonalization that entail a deep sense of detachment from themselves, their body, and experiences [59–62]. Likewise, it is widely acknowledged that stress has a prominent role in the inception of psychosis [63–65]. Large-scale epidemiological studies have found that adverse life-events and extreme stress during childhood increase the odds of later psychotic experiences by 2–8 times [66,67]. Psychosis is characterized by disturbance of the minimal self, affecting the basic, pre-reflexive manner in which we experience ourselves, our body, and surroundings [3]. Accordingly, psychosis and disturbance of the bodily-self are closely linked to impaired SoA [68,69]. Across the psychosis continuum, impairments related to SoA are prominent both in the early prodromal phase [70,71] and in chronic schizophrenia patients [20,47]. Despite compelling evidence linking stress to psychosis and impairments of SoA, there is a paucity of experimental research examining how stress affects SoA. Experimentally understanding the effects of stress on SoA may allow us to uncover the underlying mechanisms and better understand the etiological factors affecting impaired SoA.

1.4. The Present Study: Goals and Predictions

The goal of the current study was to investigate two central questions using a VR paradigm of embodied SoA [46]. First, what is the relationship between embodied SoA and other facets of the bodily-self? Second, how is embodied SoA impacted by stress? These two questions were examined in a series of four experiments. Specifically, the following predictions were derived: (1) We hypothesized that increased sensorimotor conflict would significantly decrease subjective ratings of SoA and body ownership (Exp. 1). (2) We hypothesized that SoA processing (sensitivity, criterion and metacognition) would be correlated across different domains of sensorimotor conflict, suggesting a generalized mechanism for embodied SoA (Exp. 2). (3) In line with the role of cardiac signals in the formation of the bodily-self and motor awareness, we expected that interoceptive accuracy and embodied SoA would be positively correlated (Exp. 3). Concerning our second question, given the role of stress in the etiology of disturbances of the self, we expected that stress would be related to impaired SoA. Specifically, (4) we predicted that self-reported trait anxiety, in line with its close relation to stress [72], would be correlated with impaired SoA (Exp. 3). (5) Furthermore, we expected that experimentally manipulated psychosocial stress would affect SoA (Exp. 4). (6) Finally, in line with impairments of SoA in clinical populations with psychosis, we expected to find a correlation between a high presence of self-reported Attenuated Psychotic Symptoms (APS) in healthy individuals and impaired SoA (Exp. 2–4).

2. Participants

Participants in the study were 70 undergraduate students at Bar-Ilan University (37 women) aged 20–48 years (mean 25.4) All participants were right-handed, with normal or corrected-to-normal vision, and self-reported no history of neurological or psychiatric disease. They gave their informed consent to participate in the experiment and in return, were paid or given course credit. The study was approved by the Internal Review Board of Bar-Ilan University and was carried out in accordance with the relevant guidelines and regulations. Participants were excluded from the analysis if they did not have a sufficient number of trials (less than 80%), or failed to comply with instructions (see Supplemental Material Section A for details of participants excluded from each experiment).

3. Procedure

3.1. Experiment 1

In experiment 1 we examined whether increased magnitude of the sensorimotor conflict decreases subjective ratings of SoA and body ownership in order to validate that our experimental paradigm indeed assesses embodied SoA. Fourteen participants performed a VR-based paradigm of recognition of self-generated movements [46]. The technical set-up of the paradigm is described in detail in Krugwasser et al. (2019). In brief, participants' right hand was placed 18 cm below a Leap Motion controller (Leap Motion Inc., San Francisco, CA, USA) and their hand was hidden from them via a barrier. A realistic Virtual Hand (VH) that mimicked the real hand's position and movement was presented on a screen placed in front of the participant, positioned approximately 30 cm from the participant and at the same angle that the real hand was placed behind the barrier (see Figure 1A for set-up). In each trial, participants were presented with a fixation cross (1.5 s) followed by a presentation of the VH (2 s), during which they were instructed to fold only their index finger, while the rest of their hand remained static. A sensorimotor conflict was introduced in some trials by presenting the VH's finger's movement with one of four magnitudes of temporal delay (i.e., 0/100/200/300 ms) between the actual movement and the presentation of the VH's movement. After the presentation of the VH, participants rated their subjective SoA (i.e., "I felt as if the movement presented was my own?"; questions were presented in Hebrew) and body ownership (i.e., "I felt as if the hand presented was my own") on a Likert scale ranging from −3 (i.e., "completely disagree") to 3 (i.e., "completely agree") that were adapted from similar studies [26,28,73,74]. The order of the questions was counterbalanced across participants to avoid confusion. Thirty trials of each magnitude were presented, resulting in a total of 120 trials. A practice block consisting of 15 trials was performed with the experimenter present in order to ensure compliance with task demands at the start of the experiment and was not included in analyses. Trials were not analyzed if a camera malfunction occurred, as reported in the camera logs, if the participant did not respond to one of the questions, or if the reaction time exceeded four seconds.

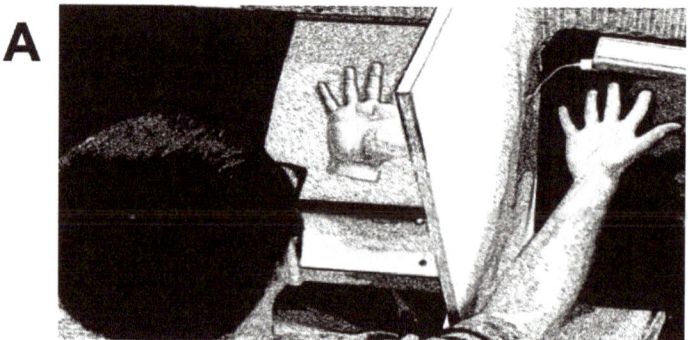

Figure 1. *Cont.*

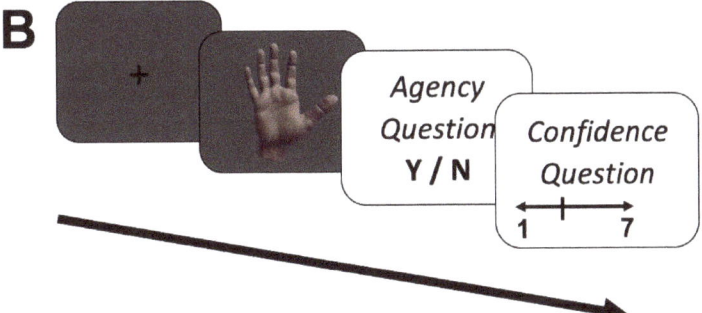

Figure 1. Experimental set-up and trial flow for the experiment. (**A**) Experimental set-up. The participant's hand is hidden from his view by the barrier, and the camera mounted above his hand records movement and presents it on the screen in front of him as a VH. (**B**) Trial flow. In each trial, a fixation cross was followed by a VH that moved with/without an alteration. Following the VH's presentation, in experiments 2–4, participants judged "same"/"not same" in response to the question "Was the movement of the VH identical to my movement?" (i.e., agency question) and rated their confidence in their response to the question, "How confident are you?" (i.e., confidence question) on a scale ranging from 1 (i.e., "not at all") to 7 (i.e., "completely"). In experiment 1, participants rated their subjective experience of SoA (i.e., "I felt as if the movement presented was my own?") and body ownership (i.e., "I felt as if the hand presented was my own?") on a Likert scale ranging from −3 (i.e., "completely disagree") to 3 (i.e., "completely agree"). Please note that across all experiments, the agency question included no explicit mention of the word 'agency'.

3.2. Experiment 2

In experiment 2 we examined whether SoA performance across different sensorimotor domains is correlated, supporting a domain-general mechanism for embodied SoA. Nineteen participants performed the VH paradigm, with three key differences from experiment 1. First, in some trials, the VH was presented with an alteration either in the temporal or spatial domain and in other trials without an alteration. Importantly, alteration in both domains was not presented together in any of the trials. In the temporal domain, as in experiment 1, one of four magnitudes of delay (i.e., 0/100/200/300 ms) between the actual movement and the VH's was inserted. In the spatial domain, an angular deviation of the VH's movement was introduced, with four magnitudes of angular deviation (0°, 6°, 10°, 14°) inserted in the presentation of the bending movement of the index finger. Thus, during a 6° deviation trial the movement of the VH's index finger would diverge in a lateral trajectory (i.e., towards the thumb) from the real index finger's movement by 6°. The finger's motion kinematics were modeled to ensure a natural-looking motion (see [46] for full details). Second, after the presentation of the VH, participants judged whether the VH's movement was identical to their actual movement using a two-alternative forced-choice question (2 AFC), "Was the movement of the VH identical to my movement?" (i.e., agency question), and rated their confidence in their response (i.e., confidence question; see Figure 1B for trial flow). We used this phrasing for the agency question as it probes the psychophysical aspect of SoA (i.e., the sensorimotor correspondence), and is in line with previous studies that have involved altered feedback of self-generated movements [46,75–77], although other approaches using 3 AFC have also been employed (e.g., [24]). Third, participants performed in each domain, 40 trials of the zero (i.e., no alteration) and first magnitude, and 20 trials of the final two magnitudes. Thus, a total of 240 trials in random order were presented.

From this task, we calculated four measures pertaining to SoA and its metacognition. First, we calculated SoA as the proportion of trials in each magnitude of alteration in each domain that participants responded that the VH's movement was identical to their movement. Second, we assessed confidence in SoA by averaging the confidence ratings of the trials with correct SoA (i.e., participants responded that the movement was identical when no alteration was present, or that it was different when an alteration was present). This was extracted for each magnitude of the alteration in each domain. Third, to allow for comparison of performance between domains, a signal detection framework was used to calculate sensitivity and criteria for each domain across the different magnitudes of alteration. Sensitivity reflects the capacity to accurately recognize trials in which the VH's movement was identical to the real hand and trials that it was altered. Criterion reflects the individual's decision boundary in order to judge that the VH movement was identical [78]. Finally, we calculated metacognitive confidence. In contrast to the measure of confidence described above, metacognitive confidence examines whether trials that were correct were rated with higher confidence than trials that were incorrect. This was calculated as the within-participant Goodman–Kruskal gamma correlation [79] between ratings of confidence and correctness of answers, capturing the degree to which confidence was linked to performance [80]. To ensure a sufficient number of observations, metacognitive confidence was calculated across the different magnitudes in each domain, yielding a single value per domain.

Following the completion of the task, participants completed the Prodromal Questionnaire Brief version (PQ-B) [81], as a self-report measure of APS that constitutes mild psychotic symptoms that have been experienced in the past month. We examined the number of items endorsed.

3.3. Experiment 3

In experiment 3 we examined the relation between SoA, interoception and self-reported anxiety. 23 participants performed the VH task identical to the task performed in experiment 2, except for two differences. First, in this experiment, only a temporal delay was administered. Second, 80 trials of each magnitude were administered in random order, resulting in a total of 320 trials. Following the VH task, participants performed a heartbeat tracking task. During the task, they were presented with a fixation cross for three time periods (25, 35, 45 s), in random order. They were instructed to press a button each time they perceived a heartbeat. During this period, the heart rate was recorded. Interoceptive accuracy was calculated as: $\frac{1}{3} \times \sum 1 - \frac{|recorded\ heartbeats - counted\ heartbeats|}{recorded\ heartbeats}$ [82–85]. Accordingly, interoceptive accuracy values range from one, signifying perfect accuracy, to zero. Following the completion of the VH and heartbeat tracking task, they completed both the PQ-B, as in experiment 2, and the State-Trait Anxiety Inventory (STAI) [86]. The ratings of the STAI items were averaged, resulting in a score ranging from 0, reflecting low anxiety, to 4, reflecting high anxiety.

3.4. Experiment 4

In experiment 4 we examined the effects of experimentally induced stress on SoA. Fourteen participants performed a VH task similar to that in experiment 2 except for two differences. First, the VH task was split into two blocks, a 'neutral' block succeeded by a 'stress' block. Second, only the temporal domain was administered. For each magnitude of delay in each of the two blocks, 30 trials were presented, resulting in a total of 240 trials displayed in random order.

To experimentally induce stress, we used an adaptation of well-accepted stress manipulations such as the Trier Social Stress Test [87] and the Montreal Imaging Stress Task [88] that use peer-evaluation and assessment of performance as stressors. Specifically, at the start of the neutral block following the actual practice session with the experimenter, participants were informed that they would now perform a 'practice' block alone that is aimed at acclimating them to the task and that their performance will not be monitored. Following the 'practice' (i.e., neutral) block, the experimenter re-entered the room and briefed the participants that they will now perform the task as a test, and their performance will be monitored. To increase psychosocial stress associated with performing the task as a test, participants were briefed about a fictitious concept of 'physical intelligence', described in such a manner that it is a positive concept related to their self-esteem, and informed that the VH task is a measure of 'physical intelligence'. They were informed that their performance in the current block will be compared to other participants', and that high performers would be recruited for future studies that include high monetary reimbursement (see Supplemental Material Section B for description provided to participants). To further exacerbate social stress, a camera was set up opposite their face and they were informed that their facial expressions would be analyzed during this block, (in effect the camera did not record). Finally, participants were informed that their heart rate would be recorded during this block.

To assess the physiological reaction to the stress induction, during both blocks, heart rate was recorded from three electrodes placed on participants' torso and connected to a G-Nautilus EEG system (250 Hz sampling rate) [89], and heart rate variability (HRV) was calculated. Briefly stated, HRV is a measure of the variability in the duration of succeeding R-peaks and is a robust biomarker of the body's response to stressors [90–92]. Under stress, HRV is typically decreased, whereas during relaxation HRV is relatively high. Physiological stress reactivity was calculated by subtracting the HRV of the neutral block from the stress block. Importantly, negative values of this difference indicated increased stress during the stress block.

Following the completion of both blocks, participants completed a post-experiment interview with the experimenter in which they rated their subjective feeling of stress in the neutral and stress blocks on a Likert scale ranging from 1 (i.e., "not at all") to 5 (i.e., "completely"). Subjective experience of stress was calculated by subtracting the neutral block's score from the stress block's score. In addition, the credibility of the stress induction was assessed in the interview. Finally, participants completed the PQ-B questionnaire.

Importantly, because this task will also be administered to clinical populations such as individuals at 'clinical high-risk' to develop psychosis in the future, we chose a stress manipulation that did not include negative feedback and could be successfully applied to them. Previous findings highlight that this population perceives even mildly stressful situations (i.e., solving simple mathematical problems with feedback introduced as a 'neutral' block) as extremely stressful [93], essentially equating them with the 'stress' block. Furthermore, based on our previous experience with clinical high-risk individuals in experimental settings in which participants were given negative feedback, we sought a mild stress manipulation that would ensure that they would complete the experiment and not leave due to the feedback.

4. Data Analysis

Data were processed using in-house Matlab scripts [94]. Statistical analyses were performed using JASP 0.9 [95]. To assess the effects of different magnitudes of alteration, domains, and blocks on subjective ratings of SoA and body ownership (Exp. 1), as well as SoA accuracy and confidence (Exp. 2–4), a within-subject repeated-measures ANOVA was used. In cases where the assumption of sphericity was violated, we performed Greenhouse–Geisser corrections. Post-hoc comparisons were Bonferroni corrected. To examine the correlations between variables, Pearson correlations were calculated. Finally, Bayesian statistics were used to assess evidence of null results [96,97].

5. Results

5.1. Experiment 1

To examine the effects of magnitude of alteration on subjective ratings of SoA and body ownership, two one-way repeated-measures ANOVAs with the factor magnitude (0/1/2/3) were performed. For SoA we found a significant main effect of magnitude ($F_{3,39} = 6.72$, $p = 0.01$, $\eta^2_p = 0.34$; see Figure 2A), such that as magnitude of alteration increased ratings of SoA decreased. For body ownership we also found a significant main effect ($F_{3,39} = 7.71$, $p = 0.006$, $\eta^2_p = 0.37$; see Figure 2B) similar to that of SoA. Thus, increased alteration of the VH's movement decreased the subjective experience of both SoA and body ownership. To assess if SoA and body ownership were indeed experienced by the participants in the no alteration condition (i.e., M0), we performed a one-sample t-test examining whether M0 ratings significantly differed from the baseline rating of zero. Both SoA ($t_{13} = 4.13$, $p = 0.001$ Cohen's $d = 1.1$) and body ownership ($t_{13} = 4.13$, $p = 0.001$, Cohen's $d = 1.1$) were significantly greater than baseline, further strengthening the ecological validity of the VH paradigm. Finally, to compare the effect of alteration magnitude on SoA as opposed to body ownership, a 2 × 4 repeated-measures ANOVA with the factors magnitude (0/1/2/3) and embodiment aspect (SoA/body ownership) was performed. As expected, the effect of magnitude was significant ($F_{3,39} = 8.03$, $p = 0.006$, $\eta^2_p = 0.38$); however, neither embodiment aspect ($F_{1,13} = 1.29$, $p = 0.28$), nor its interaction with magnitude ($F_{3,13} = 1.36$, $p = 0.27$) were significant. To assess this null finding, we examined the contribution of the embodiment aspect and its interaction with magnitude via the Bayes factor of inclusion ($BF_{Inclusion}$). Briefly stated, $BF_{Inclusion}$ is a measure of the evidence supporting the inclusion of a given factor, by comparing the effect of including or stripping a given factor from a group of models with an equivalent number of parameters [98]. This analysis yielded inconclusive evidence for the inclusion of the embodiment aspect ($BF_{Inclusion} = 2.7$), and moderately supported not including the interaction ($BF_{Inclusion} = 0.11$). To further elucidate the relation between SoA and body ownership, for each participant we examined the correlation between the two ratings on each question. For all participants, the correlation was positive and significant (all p's < 0.005) and the mean correlation across participants was 0.65 (SD = 0.25), with a range of 0.26 to 0.98. Thus, these two facets of the bodily-self are strongly entwined, and both were strongly affected by magnitude of alteration.

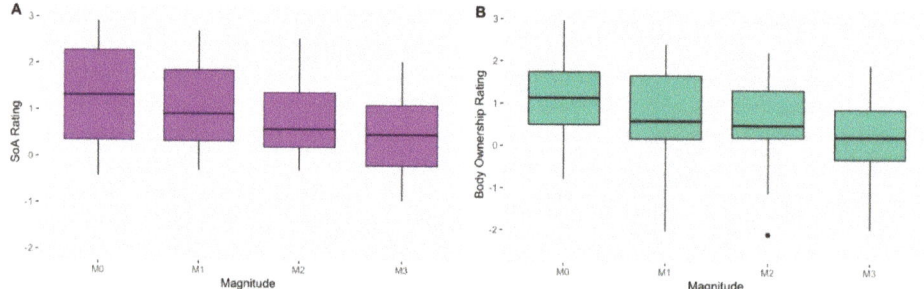

Figure 2. Subjective ratings of SoA (i.e., "I felt as if the movement presented was my own?"; Panel (**A**)) and body ownership (i.e., "I felt as if the hand presented was my own?"; Panel (**B**)) in experiment 1. X-axis is the magnitude of temporal alteration; Y-axis is the subjective rating that ranged from −3 (i.e., "completely disagree") to 3 (i.e., "completely agree").

5.2. Experiment 2

To examine the effects of domain and magnitude of alteration on SoA, a 2 × 4 repeated-measures ANOVA with the factor domain (temporal/spatial) and magnitude (0/1/2/3) was used. A significant main effect of domain was found ($F_{1,54} = 8.87$, $p = 0.008$, $\eta^2_p = 0.33$; see Figure 3A), such that in the temporal domain participants tended to judge VH movements to be identical to their own more than in the spatial domain. Importantly due to the distribution of trials across the magnitude of alteration, this main effect reflects participants' increased tendency to mistake altered trials in the temporal domain. In light of this main effect of domain, in order to examine the effect of magnitude on SoA, we performed a one-way repeated-measures ANOVA with the factor magnitude (0/1/2/3) for each domain separately. In the temporal domain we found a significant main effect of magnitude ($F_{3,54} = 57.44$, $p < 0.001$, $\eta^2_p = 0.76$; see Table S1 in the Supplemental Material for summary statistics and pairwise comparisons), as well as in the spatial domain ($F_{3,54} = 78.35$, $p < 0.001$, $\eta^2_p = 0.81$). As expected, in both domains, as the magnitude of alteration increased, VH movements were correctly judged as not identical to the participants' actual movements. Finally, there was a significant interaction between magnitude and domain ($F_{3,54} = 6.41$, $p < 0.001$, $\eta^2_p = 0.26$). As can be seen in Figure 3A, the differences between domains were most prominent in magnitude one and two, with participants showing a greater tendency to misattribute movements in the temporal domain in these magnitudes.

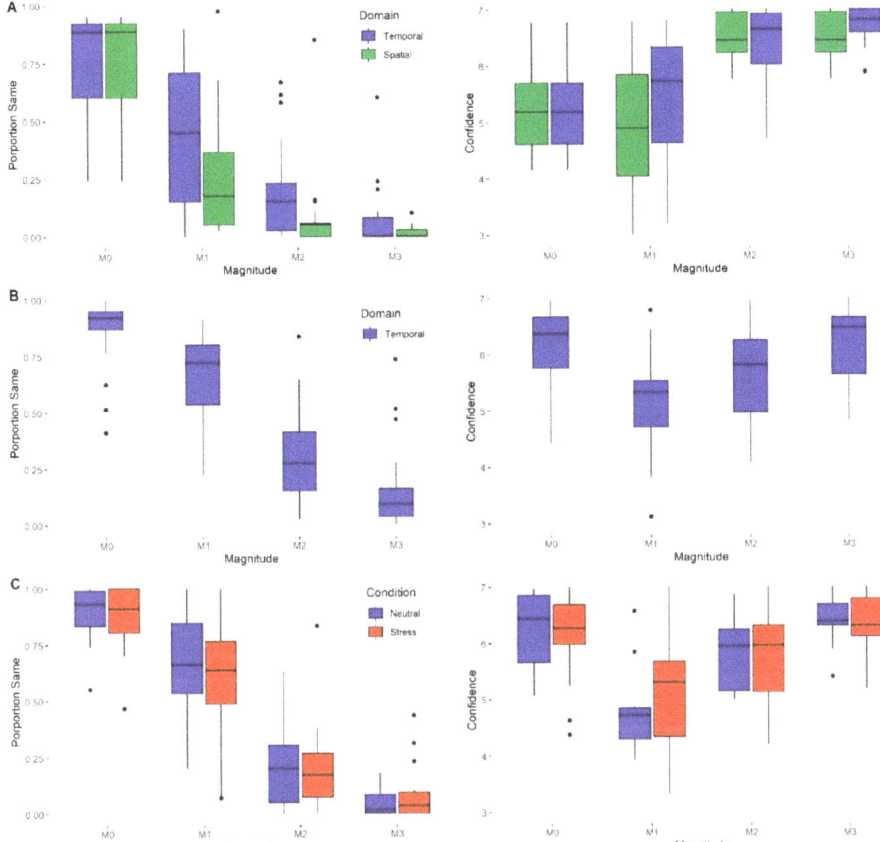

Figure 3. Judgments of SoA (left panels) and confidence (right panels) across three experiments (2–4; A–C). In the left panels, the Y-axis is the proportion of trials in which participants responded that VH's movement was the same as the actual movement, across the different magnitudes of alteration. Importantly, only in M0 (i.e., no alteration) was it correct to respond 'same'. In the right panels, the Y-axis is the participants' mean confidence rating (rated on a scale of 1–7) of their response to the agency question in which their response was correct. Lines within colored boxes are medians. (**A**) Experiment 2. Alterations were introduced in both the spatial (green) and temporal (blue) domain. (**B**) Experiment 3. Alterations were only introduced in the temporal domain. (**C**) Experiment 4. Alterations were introduced only in the temporal domain, and assessed in a neutral (blue) and stress (red) block.

An equivalent repeated-measures ANOVA was used to examine the effects of domain and magnitude of alteration on the confidence of correct trials. A significant main effect of domain was revealed ($F_{1,51} = 6.64$, $p = 0.02$, $\eta^2_p = 0.27$; see Figure 3A), such that participants were more confident in the spatial domain. This finding complements our previous findings that participants were more accurate in the spatial domain. In light of this main effect of domain, in order to examine the effect of magnitude on confidence, we performed a one-way repeated-measures ANOVA with the factor alteration magnitude (0/1/2/3) for each domain separately. In the temporal domain we found a significant main effect of magnitude ($F_{3,51} = 13.89$, $p < 0.001$, $\eta^2_p = 0.45$; see Table S2 in Supplemental Material for summary statistics and pairwise comparisons), as well as in the spatial domain ($F_{3,54} = 25.77$, $p < 0.001$, $\eta^2_p = 0.60$). Contrary to our expectations and findings in subsequent experiments, in the no alteration magnitude, confidence ratings were relatively low. This may be due to the high number of trials with alterations of magnitude zero (i.e., no alteration) and one, that caused participants to be uncertain whether a slight alteration or no alteration occurred.

To further elucidate the relation between SoA in the different domains, we examined the between-subject correlation of sensitivity, criterion and metacognitive confidence between the temporal and spatial domains. For sensitivity, we found a strong correlation between domains ($r = 0.71$, $p < 0.001$). Likewise, for criterion, there was a strong correlation between domains ($r = 0.89$, $p < 0.001$), reflecting that the threshold for evidence used for judgments of agency were related across domains. Finally, for metacognitive confidence we also found a strong correlation between domains ($r = 0.83$, $p < 0.001$). These findings demonstrate that the mechanism underlying embodied SoA and its metacognition are not domain-specific rather rely on a domain-general mechanism perhaps related to the bodily-self. Importantly, these findings are a strong replication of our previous findings concerning across domain correlations for sensitivity and bias [46], and also extend them to the capacity of metacognitive confidence.

Finally, we examined the relation between SoA and APS, assessed via the PQ-B questionnaire. We found a significant negative correlation between APS and sensitivity in the spatial domain ($r = -0.68$, $p = 0.001$) and in the temporal domain ($r = -0.49$, $p = 0.03$). Thus, participants that reported more APS symptoms showed lower sensitivity in both domains. Furthermore, the relation to metacognitive confidence, in both the spatial ($r = -0.65$, $p = 0.003$) and the temporal ($r = -0.57$, $p = 0.01$) domains was significant. Thus, participants that reported higher APS had lower metacognitive confidence.

5.3. Experiment 3

To examine the effect of the magnitude of alteration on SoA a one-way repeated-measures ANOVA with the factor of magnitude (0/1/2/3) was applied. Replicating our finding in experiment 2, a significant main effect of magnitude was found ($F_{3,66} = 121.3$, $p < 0.001$, $\eta^2_p = 0.85$). As the magnitude of alteration increased the proportion of trials judged to be identical decreased (see Figure 3B). Examining the effects of magnitude on the confidence of correct trials, using an equivalent ANOVA, also revealed a significant effect of magnitude ($F_{3,66} = 15.33$, $p < 0.001$, $\eta^2_p = 0.41$). As can be seen in Figure 3B, a U-shaped curve of confidence was observed, with the lowest confidence exhibited in magnitude one of alteration. Presumably, this magnitude of alteration is the most difficult, in line with its high proportions of incorrect responses. As expected, and in contrast to experiment 2, the no alteration condition (i.e., magnitude 0) also exhibited high levels of confidence. Presumably, this reflects the relative ease of correctly identifying movements that are identical.

Examining the correlation between interoceptive accuracy, assessed via the heartbeat counting task, and sensitivity of SoA, assessed via the VH task, we found a significant positive correlation ($r = 0.52$, $p = 0.02$). Similarly, the correlation to metacognitive confidence was also significantly correlated ($r = 0.47$, $p = 0.04$). Thus, individual differences in interoceptive accuracy and both sensitivity and metacognition of embodied SoA were closely linked, as would be expected due to these capacities' close affinity to the bodily-self.

Concerning the relation between the self-reported measures of APS and trait anxiety, and the performance measures of SoA and interoceptive accuracy. Contrary to our hypothesis and the results of experiment 2, the correlation between sensitivity of SoA and APS was not significant ($r = -0.05$, $p = 0.81$), with Bayesian statistics providing anecdotal evidence for lack of a correlation ($BF_{01} = 2.97$). Neither was the correlation between metacognitive confidence and APS significant ($r = -0.17$, $p = 0.45$), with Bayesian statistics providing anecdotal evidence for a lack of correlation ($BF_{01} = 2.94$). Concerning trait anxiety, the sensitivity of SoA was not significantly correlated ($r = -0.15$, $p = 0.52$), with Bayesian statistics providing moderate evidence in favor of a lack of correlation ($BF_{01} = 3.1$). Meanwhile, interoceptive accuracy and anxiety showed a non-significant negative correlation ($r = -0.36$, $p = 0.13$), such that participants with higher levels of anxiety had lower interoceptive accuracy.

5.4. Experiment 4

In this experiment, we examined the effects of experimentally manipulated stress on SoA. First, we assessed the validity of the stress induction both via the subjective experience of stress as reported in the post-experiment interview in which participants rated on a Likert scale ranging from 1–5 how stressful they experienced each block to be, and via the physiological change in HRV between blocks. As expected, the mean rating of stress experienced in the stress block (M = 2.68, SEM = 0.24) was higher than in the neutral block (M = 2.00, SEM = 0.22), and this difference was significant (t_{18} = 3.24, p = 0.005, Cohen's d = 0.74). In contrast, the difference between HRV in the stress block (M = 0.049, SEM = 0.005) and the neutral block (M = 0.052, SEM = 0.005) was not significant (t_{13} = 0.49, p = 0.63). Importantly, the subjective experience of stress was correlated with the change in HRV (r = −0.64, p = 0.014). Thus, changes in HRV reflect individual differences in the subjective experience of stress following its induction. Accordingly, in the analyses concerning the effects of stress, we included HRV as a covariate to capture these individual differences.

We examined the effect of stress on SoA via a repeated-measures ANOVA with the factors block (neutral/stress) and magnitude of alteration (0/1/2/3), and change in HRV as a covariate. There was a significant main effect of magnitude ($F_{3,36}$ = 86.71, p < 0.001, η^2 = 0.87; see Figure 3C), replicating our previous findings concerning the decrease in SoA as magnitude increases. The main effect of block was not significant ($F_{1,12}$ < 1, p = 0.40). Meanwhile, the interaction between block and delay was significant ($F_{3,24}$ = 3.56, p = 0.024, η^2 = 0.20), with participants under stress more likely to misattribute their movement in the largest magnitude of alteration. Yet none of the post-hoc comparisons between blocks across the different magnitudes of alteration were significant (p > 0.12). Comparing sensitivity of SoA between blocks, contrary to our expectation the difference between sensitivity in the stress block (M = 1.78, SEM = 0.22) and the neutral block (M = 1.75, SEM = 0.19), was not significant ($F_{1,12}$ < 1, p = 0.37). The equivalent Bayesian analysis yielded anecdotal evidence in favor of the null effect of the block (BF_{01} = 2.67). Thus, it seems that the stress induction did not affect overall SoA.

Examining the effect of stress on confidence with the equivalent ANOVA used for SoA, we found a significant main effect of magnitude ($F_{3,24}$ = 9.74, p < 0.001, η^2 = 0.54; see Figure 3C). Replicating experiment 3, confidence across magnitudes displayed a U-shaped curve with the lowest confidence in the first magnitude of alteration. The main effect of block was not significant ($F_{1,8}$ = 2.63, p = 0.14), nor was the interaction of block and magnitude ($F_{3,24}$ = 1.1, p = 0.37). Comparing metacognitive confidence between blocks, under stress metacognitive confidence was higher (M = 0.43, SEM = 0.08) in comparison to the neutral block (M = 0.41, SEM = 0.07), and this difference was significant ($F_{1,12}$ = 10.6, p = 0.007, η^2_p = 0.47). Thus, contrary to our hypothesis, stress significantly improved metacognitive confidence.

Finally, examining the correlation between sensitivity of SoA and APS, contrary to our expectation, we did not find a significant correlation (r = −0.07, p = 0.79), with Bayesian analysis providing anecdotal to moderate evidence for lack of a correlation (BF_{01} = 2.98).

5.5. The Relation between APS and SoA across Experiments

To further examine the relation between APS and SoA with increased statistical power, we pooled the participants from the three experiments (i.e., Exp. 2–4) in which the binary judgment of SoA was used and sensitivity could be extracted, and examined only SoA in the temporal domain, because it was measured in all three studies (in experiment 4 we included only the neutral block). APS showed a negative correlation to sensitivity (r = −0.17, p = 0.19; see Figure 4A) and metacognition of SoA (r = −0.20, p = 0.12; see Figure 4B), yet contrary to our expectation these correlations were not significant. Noting that one participant in experiment 4 endorsed an extremely high number of APS symptoms (18 out of 21 items), we reexamined the correlation, excluding this participant as an outlier. There are two justifications for this decision. First, clinical cutoffs of the PQB are typically set at between 3 to 8 items [81,99]; thus the participant's high number of items endorsed likely points to his misunderstanding of the questionnaire or extreme clinical distress that was not evident in his functioning. Second, the number of items endorsed by this participant is more than three standard deviations from the participants' mean number of items endorsed. Excluding this participant, there was a significant correlation between APS and sensitivity ($r = -0.27$, $p = 0.04$) and metacognitive confidence ($r = -0.32$, $p = 0.01$) of SoA. Yet, it should be noted that these correlations were not corrected for multiple comparisons.

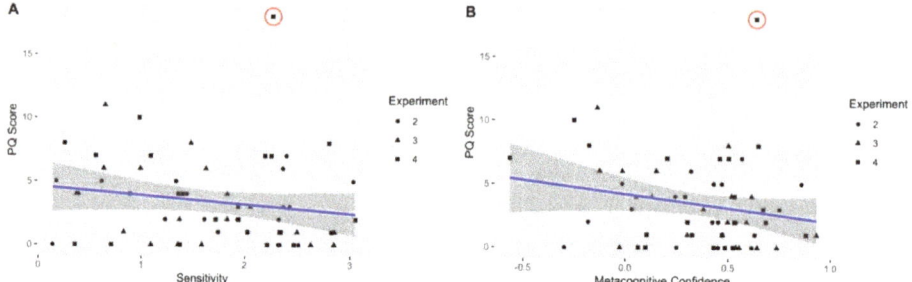

Figure 4. Correlation between APS and sensitivity (**A**) and metacognitive confidence (**B**) across the three experiments (experiment 2–4). The blue line denotes the linear regression fit and the shaded area is 95% confidence interval of fit. A red circle surrounds the participant identified as an outlier.

6. Discussion

Across four experiments, using a virtual reality paradigm, we examined two questions pertaining to embodied SoA. The first question focused on the relationship between embodied SoA and other facets of the bodily-self, such as body ownership and interoception. All of our predictions derived from this question were corroborated. First, we found that increased magnitude of alteration significantly decreased graded subjective ratings of both SoA and body ownership, validating the ecological validity of our experimental paradigm of embodied SoA (prediction1; experiment1). These two measures exhibited strong within-trial correlations, further supporting a unified construct of the bodily-self. This finding is in contrast to theoretical and empirical accounts [26,100] that argue for a dissociation between these two processes and is in line with previous studies that have found the two to be correlated [28,73]. Second, our prediction that sensitivity and criteria would be correlated across temporal and spatial domain (prediction 2; experiment 2) was strongly supported and replicates the findings of our previous study [46]. These correlations support an account of a domain-general processing of embodied SoA, differing between individuals but stable across different sensorimotor prediction domains. The current study also expanded this correlation across domains to the capacity of metacognitive confidence of SoA. Metacognitive confidence, reflecting the degree to which the participant is aware of his performance, bridges between immediate judgments of agency and more reflexive knowledge pertaining to the certainty of these judgments [57]. Correlated metacognition together with correlated criterion point to similar subjective processes inherently related to embodied SoA, lending further support to the existence of a central, domain-general representation of the bodily-self. Future neuroimaging studies may attempt to examine whether embodied SoA across domains involves similar or distinct neural mechanisms and regions. In line with our third prediction and further supporting embodied SoA's connection to the bodily-self [2,52,101–103], we found that interoceptive accuracy was significantly correlated with SoA (prediction 3; experiment 3). Previous studies have found that interoceptive accuracy is linked to body ownership [84] and peripersonal space [85]. The current finding demonstrates the importance of awareness to cardiac signals in influencing enactment, that alongside embodiment, shape our representation of the bodily-self.

A limitation pertaining to our finding that SoA was closely related to the bodily-self is that in the current study (Exp. 2–4) we only examined one aspect of SoA, namely the effect of sensorimotor alterations on SoA. Importantly, it should be noted that SoA entails additional aspects [22], such as agentic authorship (i.e., did I or someone else perform the action [24,31]) as well as the effect of passive as opposed to active actions and the effect of volition on SoA [29,104,105]. Furthermore, the wording of experiment 1's question (i.e., "I felt as if the movement presented was my own") is ambiguous in the sense that it may be interpreted as probing either the sensorimotor congruency or the agentic authorship aspect of SoA. Hence, additional studies are needed in order to disentangle the relationship of these additional aspects of SoA to the bodily-self. Additionally, Exp. 1 only probed the effect of alterations in the temporal domain on SoA. In light of previous findings that have found significant differences between domains and their effect on different aspects of SoA [24], future studies should also examine the effects of spatial alterations on the subjective experience of SoA.

Examining the relation between impaired SoA and APS yielded precarious results (prediction 6). Only in experiment 2 was the correlation to SoA in both domains significant, whereas in both experiments 3 and 4, we did not find significant correlations and Bayesian analyses provided anecdotal to moderate evidence for lack of a correlation. Pooling participants from all three experiments, the correlation was only significant when excluding an outlier. From these mixed findings, we derive two preliminary conclusions that although consistent with existing research, nonetheless need to be replicated in future studies. First, the significant correlations found between self-reported APS and embodied SoA are in line with the 'psychosis continuum' that posits the existence of psychotic-like experiences also in normative functioning populations [106]. Importantly, the current study expands previous studies [70] by showing that APS is related to both impaired sensitivity of embodied SoA and its metacognition. Interestingly, a recent study using VR to manipulate other aspects of the embodied Self (i.e., making the participant bigger or smaller) also showed a correlation between sensitivity to this alteration and APS [107]. Our correlation between self-reported psychotic symptoms and metacognition points to the potential role metacognition may play in attenuating and translating experimentally measured impairments into real-world functioning [108–110]. Second, the precariousness of the correlations highlights the wide range of symptoms endorsed in the general population, which especially affects small sample sizes. To clarify, we fully acknowledge the seminal importance of self-report questionnaires in the early stages of screening for risk of psychosis [81,99,111]. Yet, due to the low specificity of the questionnaires, some individuals endorse a high number of items that may not be indicative of actual APS and introduces additional noise to correlational analyses. Accordingly, we interpret these mixed findings with cautious enthusiasm and believe that they require further replication.

Our second question based on the pivotal role of stress in breakdowns of the self and psychosis examined the effects of stress on SoA. It yielded complex findings that did not corroborate our two predictions. The first prediction (prediction 4; experiment 3) concerning the correlation between trait anxiety and SoA was not corroborated. Although stress and anxiety are closely related concepts [72], a single self-report questionnaire of anxiety may not capture the 'stress-sensitivity' that has been found to be elevated during the early stages of psychosis. It is typically assessed at numerous time points over an extended period, via the experience sampling method that allows us to assess participants' reaction to daily stressors [112–114]. Future studies will use this method, which captures minute fluctuations in both anxiety and subjective stress, as well as obtaining a more stable measure of stress reactivity over an extended period. We also note the small sample size and low statistical power may have impaired the detection of a potential relationship. Furthermore, contrary to our prediction, we found that experimentally manipulating mild psychosocial stress in healthy individuals improved metacognitive confidence and did not affect the sensitivity of SoA (prediction 5; experiment 4). In line with the well-established inverted U-shape effect of stress on performance [115], we hypothesize that the mild stress placed healthy participants in the upward part of the inverted U, as evidenced by their enhanced metacognition. This finding highlights the importance of using a graded manipulation of stress that will allow us to calibrate the effects of the stress manipulation on the participant's subjective experience, allowing us to compare participants' performance at an equated level of subjective stress.

Although stress did not impair SoA in the current experiments, we nonetheless believe that paradigms integrating virtual reality and stress inductions are a promising avenue. It is well recognized that preceding full-blown psychosis and schizophrenia, most individuals undergo a period of heightened APS, in a risk period often coined 'clinical high-risk' [116–118]. Improving our ability to accurately predict which at-risk individuals will eventually convert to full-blown schizophrenia is a pressing goal that holds a potential to improve the harsh prognosis of schizophrenia. This has led to an ongoing search for neurocognitive characteristics and biomarkers specific to the clinical high-risk population in general and convertors in particular [71,119,120]. Yet the correlation between various impairments and the actual prognosis is typically weak at best. In line with the prominent role of stress in the etiology of psychosis and at-risk individual's heightened reactivity to mild daily stressors [112,113], we have recently hypothesized that neurocognitive performance under stress may be of greater predictive value than neurocognitive performance per se [108]. Analogous to cardiac patients that during rest exhibit an electrocardiogram similar to healthy controls and only under cardiac stress (i.e., walking on a treadmill) is their signal differentiable. Neurocognitive deficits during the at-risk phase may only be identifiable in a stressful environment that mimics the environment in which psychosis typically occurs [108,121]. Importantly, experiment 4 served as a pilot study to examine the effect of stress on neurocognitive capacities associated with the bodily-self in at-risk populations. In the hope that performance under stress will yield insight into the etiology of psychosis and improve our ability to predict conversion.

7. Conclusions

The current study examined embodied SoA using a virtual reality paradigm. We found a strong connection between embodied SoA and other facets of the bodily-self, both replicating our previous finding [46] that SoA is highly correlated across different domains of alteration, and finding that it is correlated with interoceptive accuracy and body ownership. In addition, embodied SoA was correlated with self-reported psychotic symptoms, further supporting the disturbance of the bodily-self in the psychosis continuum. Finally, examining how embodied SoA is impacted by stress in a normative population, we found that it was not impaired. Despite this finding, which was contrary to our hypothesis, we believe that examining the effects of stress on embodied SoA in clinical populations holds promise for better understanding the role of stress in the etiology of psychosis.

Supplementary Materials: The following are available online at http://www.mdpi.com/2077-0383/9/9/2931/s1, Supplemental Material Section A: Exclusion Criteria and Number of Participants Excluded from Experiments, Supplemental Material Section B: Description of Brief included in the Stress Induction of Experiment 4, Supplemental Material Section C: Tables of Summary Statistics for VH task, Table S1. Summary statistics of the VH task across the four experiments, Mean (S.E.M), Table S2. Summary statistics of the confidence rating of correct responses in the VH task across the experiments 2–4, Mean (S.E.M).

Author Contributions: Conceptualization and methodology, Y.S., D.K., and R.S.; software, Y.S. and R.S.; data curation, Y.S., R.M. and G.P.; investigation, Y.S., R.M. and G.P.; formal analysis, Y.S. and R.S.; resources and funding acquisition, R.S.; project administration, Y.S.; writing—original draft preparation, Y.S. and R.S.; writing—review and editing, Y.S., D.K. and R.S. All authors have read and agreed to the published version of the manuscript.

Funding: This research was supported by an Israeli Science Foundation grant (#1169/17) to R.S.

Acknowledgments: We wish to thank Amit Regev Krugwasser and Yair Zvilichovsky for their assistance with the technical set-up of the experimental paradigm.

Conflicts of Interest: The authors declare no conflict of interest.

References

1. Blanke, O.; Metzinger, T. Full-body illusions and minimal phenomenal selfhood. *Trends Cogn. Sci.* **2009**, *13*, 7–13. [CrossRef] [PubMed]
2. Blanke, O.; Slater, M.; Serino, A. Behavioral, Neural, and Computational Principles of Bodily Self-Consciousness. *Neuron* **2015**, *88*, 145–166. [CrossRef] [PubMed]
3. Sass, L.A.; Parnas, J. Schizophrenia, consciousness, and the self. *Schizophr. Bull.* **2003**, *29*, 427–444. [CrossRef] [PubMed]
4. Salomon, R. The Assembly of the Self from Sensory and Motor Foundations. *Soc. Cogn.* **2017**, *35*, 87–106. [CrossRef]
5. Gallagher, S. The Natural Philosophy of Agency. *Philos. Compass* **2007**, *2*, 347–357. [CrossRef]
6. Metzinger, T. Self models. *Scholarpedia* **2007**, *2*, 4174. [CrossRef]
7. Botvinick, M.; Cohen, J. Rubber hands 'feel' touch that eyes see. *Nature* **1998**, *391*, 756. [CrossRef]
8. Ehrsson, H.H.; Wiech, K.; Weiskopf, N.; Dolan, R.J.; Passingham, R.E. Threatening a rubber hand that you feel is yours elicits a cortical anxiety response. *Proc. Natl. Acad. Sci. USA* **2007**, *104*, 9828–9833. [CrossRef]
9. Lenggenhager, B.; Tadi, T.; Metzinger, T.; Blanke, O. Video ergo sum: Manipulating bodily self-consciousness. *Science* **2007**, *317*, 1096–1099. [CrossRef]
10. De Vignemont, F.; Fourneret, P. The sense of agency: A philosophical and empirical review of the "Who" system. *Conscious. Cogn.* **2004**, *13*, 1–19. [CrossRef]
11. Haggard, P. Sense of agency in the human brain. *Nat. Rev. Neurosci.* **2017**, *18*, 196. [CrossRef] [PubMed]
12. Kalckert, A.; Ehrsson, H.H. The moving rubber hand illusion revisited: Comparing movements and visuotactile stimulation to induce illusory ownership. *Conscious. Cogn.* **2014**, *26*, 117–132. [CrossRef] [PubMed]
13. Aarts, H.; Custers, R.; Wegner, D.M. On the inference of personal authorship: Enhancing experienced agency by priming effect information. *Conscious. Cogn.* **2005**, *14*, 439–458. [CrossRef]
14. Moore, J.W.; Fletcher, P.C. Sense of agency in health and disease: A review of cue integration approaches. *Conscious. Cogn.* **2012**, *21*, 59–68. [CrossRef]
15. Synofzik, M.; Vosgerau, G.; Lindner, A. Me or not me–An optimal integration of agency cues? *Conscious. Cogn.* **2009**, *18*, 1065–1068. [CrossRef] [PubMed]
16. Wegner, D.M.; Sparrow, B.; Winerman, L. Vicarious agency: Experiencing control over the movements of others. *J. Personal. Soc. Psychol.* **2004**, *86*, 838. [CrossRef] [PubMed]
17. Wegner, D.M. The mind's best trick: How we experience conscious will. *Trends Cogn. Sci.* **2003**, *7*, 65–69. [CrossRef]
18. Frith, C.; Blakemore, S.-J.; Wolpert, D. Abnormalities in the awareness and control of action. *Philos. Trans. R. Soc. Lond. Ser. B Biol. Sci.* **2000**, *355*, 1771–1788. [CrossRef]
19. Wolpert, D.M. Computational approaches to motor control. *Trends Cogn. Sci.* **1997**, *1*, 209–216. [CrossRef]
20. Jeannerod, M. The sense of agency and its disturbances in schizophrenia: A reappraisal. *Exp. Brain Res.* **2009**, *192*, 527. [CrossRef]
21. Christensen, M.S.; Grünbaum, T. Sense of agency for movements. *Conscious. Cogn.* **2018**, *65*, 27–47. [CrossRef] [PubMed]
22. Christensen, M.S.; Grünbaum, T. Sense of moving: Moving closer to the movement. *Sensat. Mov.* **2017**, 64–84. [CrossRef]
23. Anscombe, G.E.M. *Intention*; Harvard University Press: Cambridge, MA, USA, 2000.
24. Farrer, C.; Bouchereau, M.; Jeannerod, M.; Franck, N. Effect of distorted visual feedback on the sense of agency. *Behav. Neurol.* **2008**, *19*, 53–57. [CrossRef] [PubMed]
25. Gentsch, A.; Kathmann, N.; Schütz-Bosbach, S. Reliability of sensory predictions determines the experience of self-agency. *Behav. Brain Res.* **2012**, *228*, 415–422. [CrossRef] [PubMed]
26. Kalckert, A.; Ehrsson, H.H. Moving a rubber hand that feels like your own: A dissociation of ownership and agency. *Front. Hum. Neurosci.* **2012**, *6*, 40. [CrossRef]
27. Ma, K.; Hommel, B. The role of agency for perceived ownership in the virtual hand illusion. *Conscious. Cogn.* **2015**, *36*, 277–288. [CrossRef]
28. Salomon, R.; Fernandez, N.B.; Van Elk, M.; Vachicouras, N.; Sabatier, F.; Tychinskaya, A.; Llobera, J.; Blanke, O. Changing motor perception by sensorimotor conflicts and body ownership. *Sci. Rep.* **2016**, *6*, 1–13. [CrossRef]

29. Salomon, R.; Lim, M.; Kannape, O.; Llobera, J.; Blanke, O. "Self pop-out": Agency enhances self-recognition in visual search. *Exp. Brain Res.* **2013**, *228*, 173–181. [CrossRef]
30. Jeannerod, M. Visual and action cues contribute to the self-other distinction. *Nat. Neurosci.* **2004**, *7*, 422–423. [CrossRef]
31. Sirigu, A.; Daprati, E.; Pradat-Diehl, P.; Franck, N.; Jeannerod, M. Perception of self-generated movement following left parietal lesion. *Brain* **1999**, *122*, 1867–1874. [CrossRef]
32. Caspar, E.A.; Cleeremans, A.; Haggard, P. The relationship between human agency and embodiment. *Conscious. Cogn.* **2015**, *33*, 226–236. [CrossRef]
33. Engbert, K.; Wohlschläger, A.; Haggard, P. Who is causing what? The sense of agency is relational and efferent-triggered. *Cognition* **2008**, *107*, 693–704. [CrossRef] [PubMed]
34. Salomon, R.; Malach, R.; Lamy, D. Involvement of the intrinsic/default system in movement-related self recognition. *PLoS ONE* **2009**, *4*, e7527. [CrossRef] [PubMed]
35. Frith, C.; Done, D. Experiences of alien control in schizophrenia reflect a disorder in the central monitoring of action. *Psychol. Med.* **2009**, *19*, 359–363. [CrossRef] [PubMed]
36. Wolpert, D.M.; Kawato, M. Multiple paired forward and inverse models for motor control. *Neural Netw.* **1998**, *11*, 1317–1329. [CrossRef]
37. Wolpert, D.M.; Ghahramani, Z.; Jordan, M.I. An internal model for sensorimotor integration. *Science* **1995**, *269*, 1880. [CrossRef]
38. Blakemore, S.-J.; Wolpert, D.M.; Frith, C.D. Central cancellation of self-produced tickle sensation. *Nat. Neurosci.* **1998**, *1*, 635–640. [CrossRef]
39. Nielsen, T. Volition: A new experimental approach. *Scand. J. Psychol.* **1963**, *4*, 225–230. [CrossRef]
40. Sato, A.; Yasuda, A. Illusion of sense of self-agency: Discrepancy between the predicted and actual sensory consequences of actions modulates the sense of self-agency, but not the sense of self-ownership. *Cognition* **2005**, *94*, 241–255. [CrossRef]
41. Synofzik, M.; Thier, P.; Lindner, A. Internalizing agency of self-action: Perception of one's own hand movements depends on an adaptable prediction about the sensory action outcome. *J. Neurophysiol.* **2006**, *96*, 1592. [CrossRef]
42. Bergouignan, L.; Nyberg, L.; Ehrsson, H.H. Out-of-body-induced hippocampal amnesia. *Proc. Natl. Acad. Sci. USA* **2014**, *111*, 4421–4426. [CrossRef] [PubMed]
43. Bohil, C.J.; Alicea, B.; Biocca, F.A. Virtual reality in neuroscience research and therapy. *Nat. Rev. Neurosci.* **2011**, *12*, 752. [CrossRef]
44. Debarba, H.G.; Bovet, S.; Salomon, R.; Blanke, O.; Herbelin, B.; Boulic, R. Characterizing first and third person viewpoints and their alternation for embodied interaction in virtual reality. *PLoS ONE* **2017**, *12*, e0190109. [CrossRef] [PubMed]
45. Kannape, O.A.; Schwabe, L.; Tadi, T.; Blanke, O. The limits of agency in walking humans. *Neuropsychologia* **2010**, *48*, 1628–1636. [CrossRef]
46. Krugwasser, A.R.; Harel, E.V.; Salomon, R. The boundaries of the self: The sense of agency across different sensorimotor aspects. *J. Vis.* **2019**, *19*, 14. [CrossRef] [PubMed]
47. Synofzik, M.; Thier, P.; Leube, D.T.; Schlotterbeck, P.; Lindner, A. Misattributions of agency in schizophrenia are based on imprecise predictions about the sensory consequences of one's actions. *Brain* **2010**, *133*, 262–271. [CrossRef]
48. Limanowski, J.; Kirilina, E.; Blankenburg, F. Neuronal correlates of continuous manual tracking under varying visual movement feedback in a virtual reality environment. *NeuroImage* **2017**, *146*, 81–89. [CrossRef]
49. Herbelin, B.; Salomon, R.; Serino, A.; Blanke, O. 5. Neural Mechanisms of Bodily Self-Consciousness and the Experience of Presence in Virtual Reality. *Hum. Comput. Conflu. Transform. Hum. Exp. Symbiotic Technol.* **2015**. [CrossRef]
50. Sanchez-Vives, M.V.; Slater, M. From presence to consciousness through virtual reality. *Nat. Rev. Neurosci.* **2005**, *6*, 332–339. [CrossRef]
51. Park, H.-D.; Bernasconi, F.; Bello-Ruiz, J.; Pfeiffer, C.; Salomon, R.; Blanke, O. Transient Modulations of Neural Responses to Heartbeats Covary with Bodily Self-Consciousness. *J. Neurosci.* **2016**, *36*, 8453–8460. [CrossRef]
52. Park, H.-D.; Blanke, O. Coupling Inner and Outer Body for Self-Consciousness. *Trends Cogn. Sci.* **2019**, *23*, 377–388. [CrossRef] [PubMed]

53. Suzuki, K.; Garfinkel, S.N.; Critchley, H.D.; Seth, A.K. Multisensory integration across exteroceptive and interoceptive domains modulates self-experience in the rubber-hand illusion. *Neuropsychologia* **2013**, *51*, 2909–2917. [CrossRef] [PubMed]
54. Aspell, J.E.; Heydrich, L.; Marillier, G.; Lavanchy, T.; Herbelin, B.; Blanke, O. Turning Body and Self Inside Out: Visualized Heartbeats Alter Bodily Self-Consciousness and Tactile Perception. *Psychol. Sci.* **2013**, *24*, 2445–2453.
55. Bury, G.; García-Huéscar, M.; Bhattacharya, J.; Ruiz, M.H. Cardiac afferent activity modulates early neural signature of error detection during skilled performance. *NeuroImage* **2019**, *199*, 704–717. [CrossRef]
56. Wessel, J.R.; Danielmeier, C.; Ullsperger, M. Error awareness revisited: Accumulation of multimodal evidence from central and autonomic nervous systems. *J. Cogn. Neurosci.* **2011**, *23*, 3021–3036. [CrossRef]
57. Chambon, V.; Filevich, E.; Haggard, P. What is the human sense of agency, and is it Metacognitive? In *The Cognitive Neuroscience of Metacognition*; Springer: Berlin/Heidelberg, Germany, 2014; pp. 321–342.
58. Metcalfe, J.; Van Snellenberg, J.X.; DeRosse, P.; Balsam, P.; Malhotra, A.K. Judgements of agency in schizophrenia: An impairment in autonoetic metacognition. *Philos. Trans. R. Soc. Lond. B Biol. Sci.* **2012**, *367*, 1391–1400. [CrossRef] [PubMed]
59. Carlson, E.B.; Dalenberg, C.; McDade-Montez, E. Dissociation in posttraumatic stress disorder part I: Definitions and review of research. *Psychol. Trauma Theory Res. Pract. Policy* **2012**, *4*, 479–489. [CrossRef]
60. Sass, L.; Pienkos, E.; Nelson, B.; Medford, N. Anomalous self-experience in depersonalization and schizophrenia: A comparative investigation. *Conscious. Cogn.* **2013**, *22*, 430–441. [CrossRef]
61. Schauer, M.; Elbert, T. Dissociation following traumatic stress etiology and treatment. *J. Psychol.* **2010**, *218*, 109–127. [CrossRef]
62. Stein, D.J.; Koenen, K.C.; Friedman, M.J.; Hill, E.; McLaughlin, K.A.; Petukhova, M.; Ruscio, A.M.; Shahly, V.; Spiegel, D.; Borges, G.; et al. Dissociation in posttraumatic stress disorder: Evidence from the world mental health surveys. *Biol. Psychiatry* **2013**, *73*, 302–312. [CrossRef]
63. Fowles, D.C. Schizophrenia: Diathesis-stress revisited. *Annu. Rev. Psychol.* **1992**, *43*, 303–336. [CrossRef] [PubMed]
64. Walker, E.F.; Diforio, D. Schizophrenia: A neural diathesis-stress model. *Psychol. Rev.* **1997**, *104*, 667–685. [CrossRef] [PubMed]
65. Pruessner, M.; Cullen, A.E.; Aas, M.; Walker, E.F. The neural diathesis-stress model of schizophrenia revisited: An update on recent findings considering illness stage and neurobiological and methodological complexities. *Neurosci. Biobehav. Rev.* **2017**, *73*, 191–218. [CrossRef]
66. Croft, J.; Heron, J.; Teufel, C.; Cannon, M.; Wolke, D.; Thompson, A.; Houtepen, L.; Zammit, S. Association of Trauma Type, Age of Exposure, and Frequency in Childhood and Adolescence with Psychotic Experiences in Early Adulthood. *JAMA Psychiatry* **2019**, *76*, 79–86. [CrossRef] [PubMed]
67. McGrath, J.J.; McLaughlin, K.A.; Saha, S.; Aguilar-Gaxiola, S.; Al-Hamzawi, A.; Alonso, J.; Bruffaerts, R.; De Girolamo, G.; De Jonge, P.; Esan, O.; et al. The association between childhood adversities and subsequent first onset of psychotic experiences: A cross-national analysis of 23 998 respondents from 17 countries. *Psychol. Med.* **2017**, *47*, 1230–1245. [CrossRef]
68. Frith, C. *The Cognitive Neuropsychology of Schizophrenia*; Psychology Press: London, UK, 2014.
69. Nelson, B.; Whitford, T.J.; Lavoie, S.; Sass, L.A. What are the neurocognitive correlates of basic self-disturbance in schizophrenia?: Integrating phenomenology and neurocognition. Part 2 (Aberrant salience). *Schizophr. Res.* **2014**, *152*, 20–27. [CrossRef]
70. Asai, T.; Tanno, Y. Highly schizotypal students have a weaker sense of self-agency. *Psychiatry Clin. Neurosci.* **2008**, *62*, 115–119. [CrossRef]
71. Nelson, B.; Lavoie, S.; Li, E.; Sass, L.A.; Koren, D.; McGorry, P.D.; Jack, B.N.; Parnas, J.; Polari, A.; Allott, K.; et al. The neurophenomenology of early psychosis: An integrative empirical study. *Conscious. Cogn.* **2020**, *77*, 102845. [CrossRef]
72. Eysenck, M.W.; Derakshan, N.; Santos, R.; Calvo, M.G. Anxiety and cognitive performance: Attentional control theory. *Emotion* **2007**, *7*, 336–353. [CrossRef]
73. Kalckert, A.; Ehrsson, H.H. The spatial distance rule in the moving and classical rubber hand illusions. *Conscious. Cogn.* **2014**, *30*, 118–132. [CrossRef]
74. Salomon, R.; Lim, M.; Pfeiffer, C.; Gassert, R.; Blanke, O. Full body illusion is associated with widespread skin temperature reduction. *Front. Behav. Neurosci.* **2013**, *7*, 65. [CrossRef] [PubMed]

75. Hara, M.; Pozeg, P.; Rognini, G.; Higuchi, T.; Fukuhara, K.; Yamamoto, A.; Higuchi, T.; Blanke, O.; Salomon, R. Voluntary self-touch increases body ownership. *Front. Psychol.* **2015**, *6*, 1509. [CrossRef] [PubMed]
76. Leube, D.T.; Knoblich, G.; Erb, M.; Grodd, W.; Bartels, M.; Kircher, T.T. The neural correlates of perceiving one's own movements. *Neuroimage* **2003**, *20*, 2084–2090. [CrossRef] [PubMed]
77. Sato, A. Both motor prediction and conceptual congruency between preview and action-effect contribute to explicit judgment of agency. *Cognition* **2009**, *110*, 74–83. [CrossRef] [PubMed]
78. Stanislaw, H.; Todorov, N. Calculation of signal detection theory measures. *Behav. Res. Methods Instrum. Comput.* **1999**, *31*, 137–149. [CrossRef] [PubMed]
79. Goodman, L.A.; Kruskal, W.H. Measures of Association for Cross Classifications. *J. Am. Stat. Assoc.* **1954**, *49*, 732–764.
80. Nelson, T.O. A comparison of current measures of the accuracy of feeling-of-knowing predictions. *Psychol. Bull.* **1984**, *95*, 109. [CrossRef]
81. Loewy, R.L.; Pearson, R.; Vinogradov, S.; Bearden, C.E.; Cannon, T.D. Psychosis risk screening with the Prodromal Questionnaire—Brief Version (PQ-B). *Schizophr. Res.* **2011**, *129*, 42–46. [CrossRef]
82. Schandry, R. Heart beat perception and emotional experience. *Psychophysiology* **1981**, *18*, 483–488. [CrossRef]
83. Garfinkel, S.N.; Seth, A.K.; Barrett, A.B.; Suzuki, K.; Critchley, H.D. Knowing your own heart: Distinguishing interoceptive accuracy from interoceptive awareness. *Biol. Psychol.* **2015**, *104*, 65–74. [CrossRef]
84. Tsakiris, M.; Tajadura-Jiménez, A.; Costantini, M. Just a heartbeat away from one's body:Interoceptive sensitivity predicts malleability of body-representations. *Proc. R. Soc. B Biol. Sci.* **2011**, *278*, 2470–2476. [CrossRef]
85. Ardizzi, M.; Ferri, F. Interoceptive influences on peripersonal space boundary. *Cognition* **2018**, *177*, 79–86. [CrossRef]
86. Spielberger, C.D.; Gorsuch, R.L.; Lushene, R.E. Manual for the State-Trait Anxiety Inventory (Self Evaluation Questionnaire). *Palo Alto Calif. Consult. Psychol.* **1970**, *22*, 1–24.
87. Kirschbaum, C.; Pirke, K.-M.; Hellhammer, D.H. The 'Trier Social Stress Test—A tool for investigating psychobiological stress responses in a laboratory setting. *Neuropsychobiology* **1993**, *28*, 76–81. [CrossRef] [PubMed]
88. Dedovic, K.; Renwick, R.; Mahani, N.K.; Engert, V. The Montreal Imaging Stress Task: Using functional imaging to investigate the effects of perceiving and processing psychosocial stress in the human brain. *J. Psychiatry Neurosci.* **2005**, *30*, 319–325.
89. *G.Nautilus Wireless 64-Channel EEG Acquisition System*; g.tec Medical Engineering GmbH: Schiedlberg, Austria. Available online: https://www.gtec.at/product/gnautilus-pro/ (accessed on 1 August 2019).
90. Thayer, J.F.; Lane, R.D. A model of neurovisceral integration in emotion regulation and dysregulation. *J. Affect. Disord.* **2000**, *61*, 201–216. [CrossRef]
91. Kim, H.G.; Cheon, E.J.; Bai, D.S.; Lee, Y.H.; Koo, B.H. Stress and heart rate variability: A meta-analysis and review of the literature. *Psychiatry Investig.* **2018**, *15*, 235–245. [CrossRef] [PubMed]
92. Quintana, D.S.; Alvares, G.A.; Heathers, J.A.J. Guidelines for Reporting Articles on Psychiatry and Heart rate variability (GRAPH): Recommendations to advance research communication. *Transl. Psychiatry* **2016**, *6*, e803. [CrossRef]
93. Castro, M.N.; Villarreal, M.F.; Bolotinsky, N.; Papávero, E.; Goldschmidt, M.G.; Costanzo, E.Y.; Drucaroff, L.; Wainsztein, A.; de Achával, D.; Pahissa, J.; et al. Brain activation induced by psychological stress in patients with schizophrenia. *Schizophr. Res.* **2015**, *168*, 313–321. [CrossRef] [PubMed]
94. MathWorks, T. *Matlab Version 9.6.0 (R2019a)*; The MathWorks: Natick, MA, USA, 2019.
95. *JASP*, Version 0.9; Computer software; JASP Team: Amsterdam, The Netherlands, 2018.
96. Wagenmakers, E.J.; Marsman, M.; Jamil, T.; Ly, A.; Verhagen, J.; Love, J.; Selker, R.; Gronau, Q.F.; Šmíra, M.; Epskamp, S.; et al. Bayesian inference for psychology. Part I: Theoretical advantages and practical ramifications. *Psychon. Bull. Rev.* **2018**, *25*, 35–57. [CrossRef]
97. Kruschke, J.K.; Liddell, T.M. Bayesian data analysis for newcomers. *Psychon. Bull. Rev.* **2018**, *25*, 155–177. [CrossRef]
98. Keysers, C.; Gazzola, V.; Wagenmakers, E.-J. Using Bayes factor hypothesis testing in neuroscience to establish evidence of absence. *Nat. Neurosci.* **2020**, *23*, 788–799. [CrossRef] [PubMed]

99. Savill, M.; Ambrosio, J.D.; Cannon, T.D.; Loewy, R.L. Psychosis risk screening in different populations using the Prodromal Questionnaire: A systematic review. *Early Interv. Psychiatry* **2017**, *12*, 1–12. [CrossRef] [PubMed]
100. Gallagher, S. Philosophical conceptions of the self: Implications for cognitive science. *Trends Cogn. Sci.* **2000**, *4*, 14–21. [CrossRef]
101. Marshall, A.C.; Gentsch, A.; Schütz-Bosbach, S. The interaction between interoceptive and action states within a framework of predictive coding. *Front. Psychol.* **2018**, *9*, 1–14. [CrossRef] [PubMed]
102. Salomon, R.; Ronchi, R.; Dönz, J.; Bello-Ruiz, J.; Herbelin, B.; Martet, R.; Faivre, N.; Schaller, K.; Blanke, O. The insula mediates access to awareness of visual stimuli presented synchronously to the heartbeat. *J. Neurosci.* **2016**, *36*, 5115–5127. [CrossRef]
103. Seth, A.K. Interoceptive inference, emotion, and the embodied self. *Trends Cogn. Sci.* **2013**, *17*, 565–573. [CrossRef] [PubMed]
104. Haggard, P.; Clark, S.; Kalogeras, J. Voluntary action and conscious awareness. *Nat. Neurosci.* **2002**, *5*, 382–385. [CrossRef]
105. Tsakiris, M.; Prabhu, G.; Haggard, P. Having a body versus moving your body: How agency structures body-ownership. *Conscious. Cogn.* **2006**, *15*, 423–432. [CrossRef]
106. Van Os, J.; Linscott, R.J.; Myin-Germeys, I.; Delespaul, P.; Krabbendam, L. A systematic review and meta-analysis of the psychosis continuum: Evidence for a psychosis proneness–persistence–impairment model of psychotic disorder. *Psychol. Med.* **2009**, *39*, 179–195. [CrossRef]
107. Drori, G.; Bar-Tal, P.; Stern, Y.; Zvilichovsky, Y.; Salomon, R. UnReal? Investigating the Sense of Reality and Psychotic Symptoms with Virtual Reality. *J. Clin. Med.* **2020**, *9*, 1627. [CrossRef] [PubMed]
108. Koren, D.; Scheyer, R.; Reznik, N.; Adres, M.; Apter, A.; Parnas, J.; Seidman, L.J. Basic self-disturbance, neurocognition and metacognition: A pilot study among help-seeking adolescents with and without attenuated psychosis syndrome. *Early Interv. Psychiatry* **2017**. [CrossRef]
109. Koren, D.; Scheyer, R.; Stern, Y.; Adres, M.; Reznik, N.; Apter, A.; Seidman, L.J. Metacognition strengthens the association between neurocognition and attenuated psychosis syndrome: Preliminary evidence from a pilot study among treatment-seeking versus healthy adolescents. *Schizophr. Res.* **2019**, *210*, 207–214. [CrossRef]
110. Koren, D.; Seidman, L.J.; Goldsmith, M.; Harvey, P.D. Real-world cognitive—And metacognitive—Dysfunction in schizophrenia: A new approach for measuring (and remediating) more "right stuff". *Schizophr. Bull.* **2006**, *32*, 310–326. [CrossRef]
111. McDonald, M.; Christoforidou, E.; Van Rijsbergen, N.; Gajwani, R.; Gross, J.; Gumley, A.I.; Lawrie, S.M.; Schwannauer, M.; Schultze-Lutter, F.; Uhlhaas, P.J. Using online screening in the general population to detect participants at clinical high-risk for psychosis. *Schizophr. Bull.* **2018**, *45*, 600–609. [CrossRef] [PubMed]
112. Myin-Germeys, I.; van Os, J. Stress-reactivity in psychosis: Evidence for an affective pathway to psychosis. *Clin. Psychol. Rev.* **2007**, *27*, 409–424. [CrossRef] [PubMed]
113. Klippel, A.; Viechtbauer, W.; Reininghaus, U.; Wigman, J.; van Borkulo, C.; Myin-Germeys, I.; Wichers, M. The Cascade of Stress: A Network Approach to Explore Differential Dynamics in Populations Varying in Risk for Psychosis. *Schizophr. Bull.* **2017**, *44*, 328–337. [CrossRef] [PubMed]
114. Reininghaus, U.; Kempton, M.J.; Valmaggia, L.; Craig, T.K.J.; Garety, P.; Onyejiaka, A.; Gayer-Anderson, C.; So, S.H.; Hubbard, K.; Beards, S.; et al. Stress sensitivity, aberrant salience, and threat anticipation in early psychosis: An experience sampling study. *Schizophr. Bull.* **2016**, *42*, 712–722. [CrossRef] [PubMed]
115. Yerkes, R.M.; Dodson, J.D. The relation of strength of stimulus to rapidity of habit-formation. *J. Comp. Neurol. Psychol.* **1908**, *18*, 459–482. [CrossRef]
116. Fusar-Poli, P.; Borgwardt, S.; Bechdolf, A.; Addington, J.; Riecher-Rössler, A.; Schultze-Lutter, F.; Keshavan, M.; Wood, S.; Ruhrmann, S.; Seidman, L.J.; et al. The psychosis high-risk state: A comprehensive state-of-the-art review. *Arch. Gen. Psychiatry* **2013**, *70*, 107–120. [CrossRef] [PubMed]
117. van der Gaag, M.; Smit, F.; Bechdolf, A.; French, P.; Linszen, D.H.; Yung, A.R.; McGorry, P.; Cuijpers, P. Preventing a first episode of psychosis: Meta-analysis of randomized controlled prevention trials of 12 month and longer-term follow-ups. *Schizophr. Res.* **2013**, *149*, 56–62. [CrossRef] [PubMed]
118. Tsuang, M.T.; Van Os, J.; Tandon, R.; Barch, D.M.; Bustillo, J.; Gaebel, W.; Gur, R.E.; Heckers, S.; Malaspina, D.; Owen, M.J.; et al. Attenuated psychosis syndrome in DSM-5. *Schizophr. Res.* **2013**, *150*, 31–35. [CrossRef] [PubMed]

119. Light, G.A.; Swerdlow, N.R. Bending the curve on psychosis outcomes. *Lancet Psychiatry* **2015**, *2*, 365–367. [CrossRef]
120. Tsuang, M.T.; Shapiro, D.I.; Ronzio, A.; Bearden, C.E.; Cadenhead, K.S.; Addington, J.; McGlashan, T.H.; Walker, E.F.; Stone, W.S.; Perkins, D.O.; et al. Association of Neurocognition with Transition to Psychosis. *JAMA Psychiatry* **2016**, *73*, 1239. [CrossRef]
121. Gupta, S.; Ranganathan, M.; Dsouza, D.C. The early identification of psychosis: Can lessons be learnt from cardiac stress testing? *Psychopharmacology* **2016**, *233*, 19–37. [CrossRef]

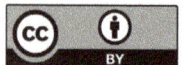

© 2020 by the authors. Licensee MDPI, Basel, Switzerland. This article is an open access article distributed under the terms and conditions of the Creative Commons Attribution (CC BY) license (http://creativecommons.org/licenses/by/4.0/).

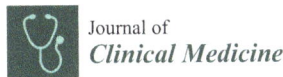

Article

The Equivalence between Virtual and Real Feared Stimuli in a Phobic Adult Sample: A Neuroimaging Study

Wenceslao Peñate [1], Francisco Rivero [1], Conrado Viña [1], Manuel Herrero [1], Moisés Betancort [1], Juan De la Fuente [2], Yolanda Álvarez-Pérez [2] and Ascensión Fumero [1,*]

[1] Universidad de La Laguna, 38200 La Laguna, Spain; wpenate@ull.edu.es (W.P.); friverop@ull.edu.es (F.R.); cmvinalo@ull.edu.es (C.V.); mherrero@ull.edu.es (M.H.); moibemo@ull.edu.es (M.B.)
[2] Servicio Canario de la Salud, 38004 S.C. Tenerife, Spain; jafuente@ull.es (J.D.l.F.); yolanda.alvarezperez@sescs.es (Y.Á.-P.)
* Correspondence: afumero@ull.es

Received: 4 October 2019; Accepted: 2 December 2019; Published: 4 December 2019

Abstract: The clinical use of virtual reality (VR) has proven its efficacy, especially when used as an exposure technique. A prominent property of VR's utility is its equivalence with the reality it represents. In this study, we explored this equivalence in a clinical context using neuroimaging. A sample of 32 adults with specific phobias (i.e., to cockroaches, spiders, or lizards) was divided into two groups: One was exposed to phobic stimuli using VR and the other was exposed to real phobic images (RI). We used brain activations as a dependent measure, focusing specifically on brain areas usually associated with fear processing. Whole-brain analysis detected higher activations for RI in the hippocampus, occipital, and calcarine areas. A specific analysis of the amygdala and insula also detected higher activations and extensions in response to RI, but VR stimuli also activated those areas in a significant manner. These results suggest that even in those cases where RI stimuli activate all of the brain's fear-processing circuits, VR stimuli do so as well. This implies that VR can be useful as an exposure technique similar to RI and applied as more than a mere training mechanism.

Keywords: virtual reality; real phobic images; anxiety disorders; specific phobia; fMRI; neuroimaging

1. Introduction

The use of virtual reality (VR) as a tool for psychological treatment has grown since it was first employed [1] as an exposure procedure for the treatment of phobic disorders. Since then, many studies have been conducted with VR as the main therapeutic resource, which has maintained interest in this topic over the years [2]. Although VR has been employed in several therapeutic approaches, it most often takes the form of "virtual reality exposure therapy" (VRET) [3].

The efficacy and efficiency of VRET have been proven in a considerable number of clinical trials and experimental designs, as shown by several systematic reviews and meta-analyses [3–6]. There are several reasons for this efficacy: VR is an intermediate step in graduated exposure, a safe condition in which to train patients to cope with real stimuli. VR also enhances exposure when VRET is combined with in vivo exposure [5–10]. Interestingly, two processes in the functioning of VR can be inferred from these explanations: VR accurately represents real stimuli (exposure process [8]), and VR is an opportunity to cope with a distressing stimulus (training process [11,12]).

The efficacy of VRET has a prerequisite related to the physical properties of the virtual scenarios used. The key concept here is immersive technology. This concept is related to VR's property of "enveloping" participants and making them feel as if they are "actually there". There are several definitions of immersive technology [13]. These definitions share the idea that the more similar a virtual context is to a real one, the greater its immersive power. Technical characteristics (e.g., environments, distinctness, movements) and the type of presentation (i.e., 3D) are physical attributes that can shape a more immersive and consequently more effective VR [14]. Implicitly, the fact that VR scenarios are "immersive" also means that they are processed similarly to real ones. However, this property of sensation of presence, being a prerequisite, is not sufficient to explain the efficacy of VRET [15]. This efficacy seems to be supported in the property of VR to stimulate a brain representation to create an embodied simulation of the body in the world, including main informational processes: Visceral/autonomic, sensory, and motor information [15]. As a consequence, observed brain activations as a function of VRET need to reflect this embodied simulation.

Functional magnetic resonance imaging (fMRI) studies have shed light on how patients with phobias process phobic stimuli. According to systematic reviews and meta-analyses [16–20], the presence of phobic stimuli is associated with greater activation of the left amygdala and insular cortex than of other brain areas. Other structures involved in phobic responses are the fusiform gyrus, the left dorsolateral prefrontal cortex, and the left cingulate cortex. Compared to the limbic areas, frontal areas have been found to be less consistent and less stable in processing phobic stimuli. These findings are congruent with the existence of a dual-route functional network in processing feared stimuli [21–24]: Wave1, a short/unconscious route that involves a direct link between the thalamus and the amygdala; and Wave2, a long/conscious route that involves the thalamus-sensory and cortex-entorhinal cortex–hippocampus–subiculum–amygdala.

Given that therapeutic exposure is related to how patients process phobic stimuli, the activation of these routes can have direct implications for exposure efficacy: Conscious routes imply more complex processing and a better opportunity for patients to change the significance of a phobic stimulus and develop a more adaptive response. In this regard, the present study was aimed at testing whether exposure to virtual phobic stimuli in a group of patients with specific phobias (i.e., to small animals) could activate the same brain regions as exposure to real image stimuli. We also intended to test whether virtual stimuli could also facilitate the activation of the conscious Wave2 route in processing phobic stimuli (as real image stimuli do) and to consider the implications of these data for the efficacy of exposure techniques. Specifically, we planned to compare activity in empirically supported brain regions associated with phobic stimulus processing.

2. Materials and Methods

2.1. Participants

The sample was composed of 32 adults. There were 26 (real phobic images (RI): 40.6%; VR: 40.6%) female and 6 (RI: 9.4%; VR: 9.4%) male participants. Sixteen participants (mean age 35.25 years, SD 12.17) were exposed to real images of small animals (i.e., cockroaches, spiders, or lizards), and 16 participants (mean age 33.43 years, SD 10.26) watched films of virtual images of such animals. The phobic stimulus matched the individual's phobia.

All participants were right-handed and had normal vision. The main inclusion criterion was being an adult with a diagnosis of specific phobia. The phobia had to be a primary psychological disorder and not be explained by another health condition. Other inclusion criteria for participants included not receiving any treatment for a specific phobia at the time of the study and not having any impediment to undergoing a magnetic resonance imaging session.

2.2. Instruments

The Composite International Diagnostic Interview (CIDI), Version 2.1 (WHO, Geneve, Switzerland) [25] was used to verify the diagnosis of phobia. The CIDI is a structured interview for major mental disorders according to the CIE-10 criteria [26]. For the purposes of this study, questions related to a specific phobia, social phobia, agoraphobia, and panic attacks were selected. Participants diagnosed with a specific small-animal phobia were included (F40.218; [26]).

The S–R Inventory of Anxiousness [27] is a 14-item inventory with a 5-point Likert-type scale that assesses physiological, cognitive, and behavioral anxiety symptoms associated with an anxiety-inducing situation. The phobic stimulus target is pointed out prior to the participant's response. The inventory has shown high internal consistency (0.95) and adequate convergent validity [27,28]. For the current study, Cronbach's alpha was 0.79.

The Beck Anxiety Inventory (BAI) [29] is a 21-item self-report instrument for assessing the severity of anxiety states. Participants are asked to rate the severity of each symptom using a 4-point Likert-type scale ranging from 0 ("Not at all") to 3 ("Severely—I could barely stand it"). Total scores range from 0 to 63. Scores of 26–63 represent severe anxiety [29]. Cronbach's alpha for the current study was high (0.93).

Hand preference was assessed with the Edinburgh Handedness Inventory (EHI) [30]. This inventory consists of ten items: Writing, drawing, throwing, using scissors, toothbrush, knife (without fork), spoon, broom, striking a match, and opening a box. Participants indicated the strength of their hand preference for each of the 10 items by putting one or two ticks in the appropriate column, or one tick in each column if they were indifferent about that item. The EHI provides a Laterality Quotient ranging from +100 (totally right-handed) to −100 (totally left-handed).

2.3. Design

A 2 × 2 factor design was used: The first independent variable was "stimulus format" with two levels (real images and virtual reality), and the second independent variable was "type of stimulus" (phobic and neutral stimulus).

The stimuli consisted of small animals in motion. These were filmed in 3D video for the real images. To control the presentation modality effects, 3D recorded movies were used as the models to create the virtual reality stimuli. The arousal properties of these virtual reality stimuli were tested by measuring activations of the brain regions of interest (ROIs) at the initial fMRI session. Because the virtual stimuli were directly related to each specific phobia (i.e., participants with a spider phobia received only spider stimuli), stimulus valence was not assessed. All participants were informed about the stimulus format (virtual or real images).

Both the real image and virtual reality formats included both phobic stimuli (i.e., cockroaches, spiders, or lizards) and neutral stimuli (i.e., wooden balls). All images were presented before an identical white background. Stimuli were presented in 3D virtual reality video format (VR group) and 3D real image video format (RI group). Figure 1 shows examples of the RI and VR stimuli.

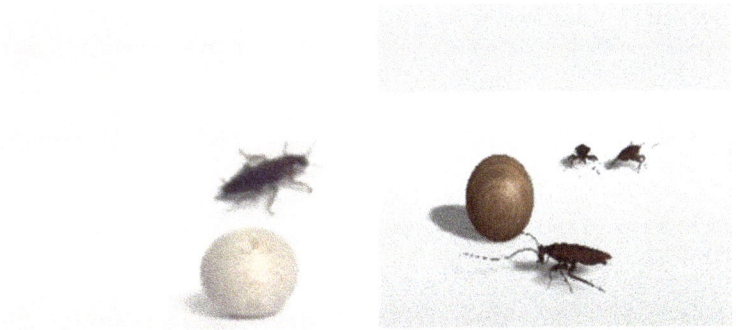

Figure 1. Example of the real image (RI) and virtual reality (VR) stimuli.

Participants were randomly assigned (direct method) to one of two groups: One received the stimuli in virtual reality format (VR group) and the other received them as real images (RI group). Participants were exposed to two different conditions: Phobic stimuli and neutral stimuli (i.e., wooden balls).

We used neuroimaging activations as dependent variables. The images were filtered for ROI, taking into account previous results with patients with phobias [16–20]. Nine regions were selected for both hemispheres: Amygdala, hippocampus, insula, fusiform gyrus, occipital cortex (inferior, medial, and superior), calcarine area, and thalamus.

Stimuli were recorded in 3D and projected in the MRI scanner in stereoscopic 3D video using Visual Stim digital MRI-compatible 3D glasses (graphics card: GeForce 8600GT), (Resonance Technology Inc., Northridge, CA, US). We presented the stimuli using a block design. Each participant was randomly presented with 16 blocks of phobic images and 16 blocks of images of wooden balls. The duration of each block was 20 seconds.

2.4. Procedure

The study was conducted from April to July 2016. Phobic participants were recruited through various media (i.e., website, press, flyers, radio, TV, and newspapers). Next, an e-mail with the inventories was sent to possible participants. The initial diagnosis of specific phobia according to participants' inventory scores was corroborated by a semistructured interview. Those who did not meet the inclusion criteria (or met the exclusion criteria) were excluded. In addition, due to the interference with the fMRI analysis, participants with nonremovable metal devices were excluded. Participants signed an informed consent form included in the study that had been approved by the Ethics Committee for Research and Animal Welfare of the University of La Laguna (CEIBA2012-0033). After their participation, subjects were entitled to receive as payment an eight-session free psychological treatment for specific animal phobia.

2.5. fMRI Data Acquisition

Functional MRI data were collected with a 3T General Electric Signa Excite scan (General Electric, Madrid, Spain). The BOLD signal was measured with an echo planar imaging sequence with 30 ms of echo time, 2000 ms of repetition time, 25.6 of field of view, and 75° of flip angle. The image dimensions were $64 \times 64 \times 32$ mm with $4 \times 4 \times 4$ mm voxel dimensions.

2.6. fMRI and Data Analysis

Brain images were analyzed with Statistical Parametric Mapping (SPM 12) software (London University College, London, UK). Preprocessing procedures included realigning, coregistering, segmenting (with forward deformation fields), normalizing (structural images with a $1 \times 1 \times 1$ mm voxel size and functional images with a $4 \times 4 \times 4$ mm voxel size), and smoothing (Gaussian Kernel of 8 mm, FWHM). Images were rendered and adjusted to the standard brain template of the Montreal Neurological Institute (MNI).

The 2×2 factor design was tested with a two-way ANOVA to compare the main effects of image format and stimuli and the interaction effect between image format and stimuli on the whole-brain activation.

In addition, images were filtered for ROIs (amygdala, hippocampus, insula, fusiform gyrus, occipital cortex, calcarine area, and thalamus). All these ROIs were extracted from the WFU Pickatlas 3.0.5b (Radiology Informatic and Imaging Laboratory, Winston-Salem, NC, US) for SPM 12 with the Automated Anatomical Labeling (AAL2) brain atlas and Brodmann areas atlas.

The Family-Wise Error ($p < 0.05$ FWE corrected) correction was used. However, noncorrected probabilities were admitted when they were congruent with the biological model of phobias (but never higher than 0.001 uncorrected). The error was corrected considering that there was activation when the activated area was equal to or greater than a 3-voxel cluster with a voxel size of $4 \times 4 \times 4$ mm.

3. Results

An initial statistical analysis was performed to test the comparability between the VR group and RI group in anxiety measures (S–R and BAI scores). No significant differences (see Figure 2) were found between the two groups in these variables ((S–R: VR group M = 7.75, SD = 2.7; RI group M = 6.4, SD = 4.22) (BAI: VR group M = 18.0, SD = 14.14; RI group M = 16.3, SD = 11.95)).

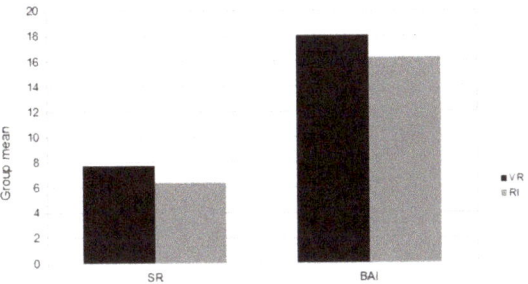

Figure 2. Anxiety measures.

After that, a two-way ANOVA (whole-brain analysis) was conducted with image format (virtual, real) and type of stimulus (phobic, neutral) as independent variables. The whole-brain activations are shown in Figure 3. The interaction effect was significant (F (1.60) = 25.22, $p < 0.05$). This value was considered as the F score threshold. Moreover, an overall main effect was found for type of stimulus (F (1.60) = 26.78, $p < 0.05$). This main effect revealed a significant difference between phobic stimuli and neutral stimuli in brain activity: Fear-related stimuli generated higher brain activation than neutral stimuli. There were no differences in brain activity according to the image format factor (virtual vs. real phobic stimuli).

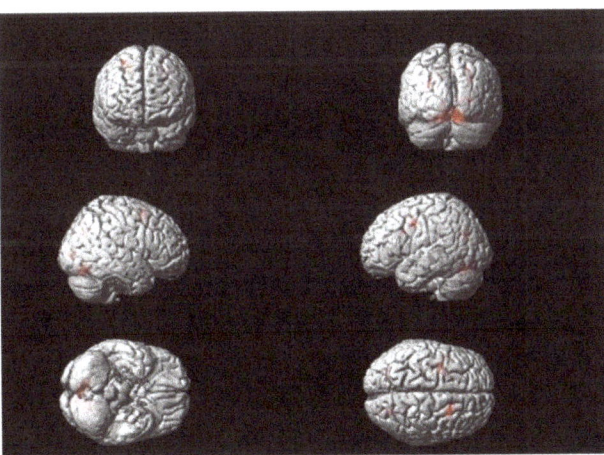

Figure 3. Whole-brain interaction effect. F (1.60) = 25.22, $p < 0.05$ (Family Wise Estimation (FWE)).

The following analyses were performed on the brain areas selected as ROIs. For exploratory reasons, a significance threshold of $p \leq 0.001$, uncorrected $k \geq 3$, was used to detect subtle changes in brain activation. In addition, to reduce the probability of false positive results, we set a contiguity threshold for cluster volumes of at least 20 voxels with a size of 2 × 2 × 2 mm [31] and did not consider clusters with a Z lower than 3.00. The fMRI comparisons between the RI group and the VR group in ROI brain areas are summarized in Table 1. These results showed significantly higher activations with real images in the hippocampus (R: F(1.60) = 25.77, $p < 0.001$; L: F(1.60) = 23.74, $p < 0.001$), fusiform gyrus (F(1.60) = 48.44, $p < 0.000$), bilateral middle occipital cortex (R: F(1.60) = 41.25, $p < 0.000$; L: F(1.60) = 46.09, p < 0.000), bilateral superior occipital cortex (R: F(1.60) = 44.78, $p < 0.000$; L: F(1.60) =

37.34, $p < 0.00$), and bilateral calcarine area (R: $F(1.60) = 32.07$, $p < 0.01$; L: $F(1.60) = 29.53$, $p < 0.01$). No differences were observed in the amygdala, insula, bilateral inferior occipital cortex, or thalamus in RI compared to VR.

Table 1. fMRI comparisons between the RI group and the VR group in brain regions of interest (ROIs).

AREA	Coordinates	Hemisphere	K	Z	P
Real Image > VR Phobics					
Amygdala		Right/Left			n.s.
Hippocampus	22, −28, −6	Right	4	3.4	0.0001
Insula		Right/Left			n.s.
Fusiform gyrus	38, −72, −18	Right	11	4.54	0.0001
	22, −64, 14	Right	3	4.51	0.0001
	−34, -52, −22	Left	18	3.92	0.0001
	−26, −68, −6	Left	-	3.51	0.0001
	34, −48, −14	Right	4	3.37	0.0001
Occipital cortex					
Inferior		Right			n.s.
Middle	26, −88, 6	Right	49	4.29	0.0001
Superior	26, −72,34	Right	28	4.42	0.0001
Inferior		Left			n.s.
Middle	−30, −72, 26	Left	38	4.47	0.0001
Superior		Left			n.s.
Calcarine area	−14, −76, 1	Left	10	3.7	0.0001
Thalamus		Right/Left			n.s.

n.s.: Not significant. RI: Real Image; VR: Virtual Reality; AREA: Brain region, K: Voxel's number, Z: Tipical score.

A new and specific ROI analysis was performed separately for the amygdala and insula as two brain areas usually associated with the processing of anxiety-related stimuli, taking virtual vs. real image phobic stimuli as an independent variable. Figure 4 shows the activation observed in the amygdala. The response to real image stimuli was significant in a cluster in both the right amygdala (18, 0, −14) and left amygdala (−26, −4, −22), which both exhibited intense activity (t mean = 6.21; t SD = 0.20 right side, and t mean = 4.98; t SD = 0.54 left side). For VR stimuli, significant activity occurred in both the right (18, 0, −14) and left clusters (−26, 0, −22), which showed similar intensity (t mean = 4.59; t SD = 0.27 right side, and t mean = 4.40; t SD = 0.19 left side). These data revealed that stimulus processing was greater and more extensive in the real image format than in virtual reality.

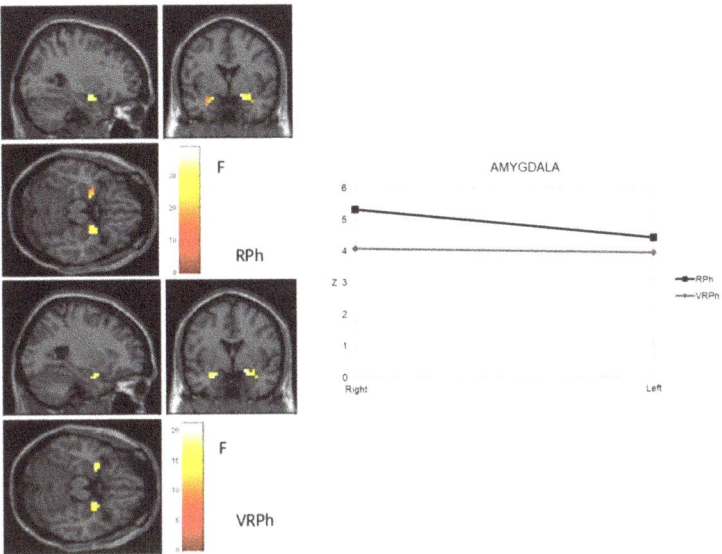

Figure 4. Amygdala activation of phobic stimuli processing (virtual and real format) in an adult sample with a specific phobia. RPh: Phobic real image; VRPh: Phobic virtual reality image.

Figure 5 shows activation of the insula. A similar activation was found in the right insula (42, 24, 2) with both real and virtual images. Yet, in the left insula, real images were associated with greater intensity ($Z = 7.10$; $p < 0.000$; $Z = 6.22$; $p < 0.000$; $Z = 5.47$; $p < 0.000$; $Z = 5.45$; $p < 0.000$) and extension (42, 24, 2; −46, 12, −6; −30, −28, 22; 38, −28, 22). These data suggest that fear-related (compared to neutral) images preferentially activated many of the regions involved in a hierarchical system responsible for organizing defensive behavior in both virtual and real image formats.

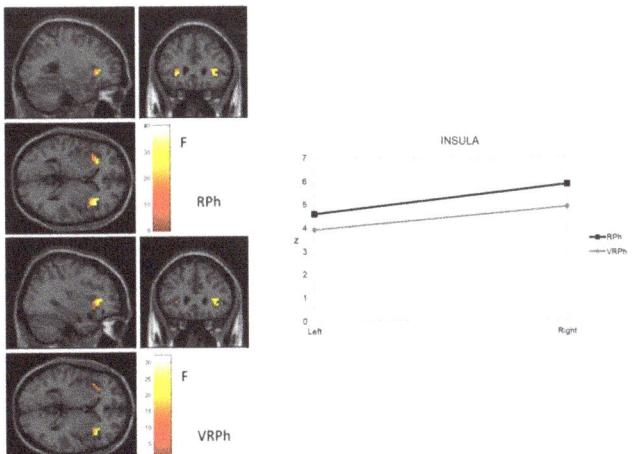

Figure 5. Insula activation of phobic stimuli processing (virtual and real format) in an adult sample with specific phobia.

Finally, to test the research objective related to the functional processing of Wave2 with virtual or real image phobic stimuli, new ROI analyses were performed: We explored the involvement of visual and limbic brain areas and their connectivity, selecting the Brodmann visual area and the amygdala for study. The insula was also selected because of its functional relationship in processing interceptive inputs. Figure 6 shows the results obtained. Initial data showed that visual processing of the stimuli started similarly for both groups. The primary visual activity associated with phobic stimulus processing (BA17) was similar in the RI and VR groups. However, there were differences in the associative visual cortex (BA18 and BA19). Specifically, the real image was significant in a cluster (46, −72, −6) of the right occipital cortex with very extensive (52 BA18 voxels and 59 BA19 voxels) and intense activity (BA18 t mean = 4.75; t SD = 2.85 and BA19 t mean = 5.72; t SD = 3.82). In the VR group, significant activity occurred in both right and left clusters. In the right cluster (46, −72, −6), it was observed in the same coordinate with similar intensity (BA18 t mean = 5.71; t SD = 2.02 and BA19 t mean = 4.90; t SD = 3.33), but was less extensive (4 BA18 voxels and 11 BA19 voxels). In the left cluster (−30, −88, −18), significant activity was observed in the associative visual areas with the same extension in BA18 and BA19 (15 voxels) and stronger intensity (BA18 t mean = 5.51; t SD = 2.96 and BA19 t mean = 4.44; t SD = 1.80). These results suggested differential Wave2 phobic stimulus processing according to the image format.

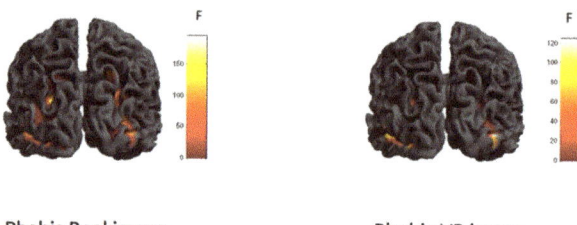

Phobic Real image   Phobic VR image

Figure 6. Visual activation of phobic stimuli processing (virtual and real format) in an adult sample with a specific phobia.

4. Discussion

In the present study, we attempted to test whether exposure to virtual phobic stimuli activated the same brain areas as exposure to real image stimuli in a group of patients with phobias to small animals. This was explored specifically in regions usually associated with phobic stimulus processing: Amygdala, hippocampus, insula, fusiform gyrus, occipital cortex, calcarine area, and thalamus.

As pointed out by previous systematic reviews and meta-analyses, greater activations were found in the areas traditionally involved in fear processing [16–20]. These activations were found regardless of whether participants were exposed to virtual stimuli or real image stimuli. The absence of a main effect of image format supports the idea that virtual reality activates similar brain areas to those that real images do, including the regions involved in both Wave1 and Wave2 phobic stimulus processing. Main differences between VR and RI phobic stimuli were observed in activation intensity: Real images generated greater intensity in the hemodynamic response than virtual images. These data support an idea that is simple, but has clear implications for exposure technique: Real phobic images produce higher anxiety responses, but virtual stimuli also produce significant levels of anxiety [32]. These results can be understood as an initial endorsement of the use of VR as an exposure procedure [8] and not as a mere training opportunity [11,12].

As mentioned above, both VR and RI activated the two fear processing routes, but greater activation of the visual areas (inferior, medial, and superior occipital cortex and calcarine area) was observed with RI stimuli. The differences between real and virtual images were not found in the primary visual area (BA17), but in the associative visual areas (BA18 and BA19). The calcarine area has been found to play a main role in the visual network associated with the conditioning of fear [33,34]. These data indicate a greater activation of the Wave2/conscious route when participants are exposed to real image phobic stimuli. This greater involvement of associative visual processing has also been observed when the stimulus resembles the experience of the individual, as happens with in vivo exposure to the phobic stimulus [35,36]. These results support the idea that real images activate more areas from the Wave2 processing of phobic stimuli than VR and could be a therapeutic resource. Brain activation with feared stimuli produces higher levels of distress, and maintaining exposure to real images eventually starts to reduce anxiety. Consequently, the more patients become accustomed to facing the feared stimulus, the less anxious they will be when they face it again and, therefore, the less they will associate it with the expected negative response.

The study of the interaction between the independent variables in the various brain areas selected for their involvement in phobia processing, as shown by the ANOVA, revealed differences in the brain activation of cortical perceptual regions, but not in the limbic system regions. However, the differences in the ROI analysis observed in the amygdala and insula indicate that fear-related stimuli produced higher and more extensive brain activation when real images were processed compared to images presented in virtual reality. As shown by the data, there was also a greater activation (and extension) in the left insula when participants were exposed to RI compared to VR stimuli. It has been proposed that the insula integrates bottom-up interoceptive signals with top-down information [37]. Specifically, a signal is activated when affective visual stimuli are processed and this signal is guided by certain top-down requirements. The presence of feared stimuli represents an excellent opportunity for these requirements. Subsequently, this signal can be conveyed to control regions such as the prefrontal cortex for appropriate behavioral output. This "appropriate" behavior may take the form of an escape behavior for patients with phobias. In fact, the higher intensity of insula activation during real phobic stimulus presentation can be associated with more escape behaviors [38]. In addition, VR stimuli may be more suitable for the exposure procedure because they are less likely to activate escape behaviors.

As virtual stimuli affect ROIs that are usually related to brain responses to phobias, VR produces a significant subjective experience and generates a sense of presence. Thus, virtual phobic stimuli can produce a significant level of anxiety. Yet, as shown by the differences in brain activation, the immersive properties of virtual stimuli are lower than those of real images, but VR also activates a complex neural connectivity, including several associative areas, far from a mere activation of fear circuitry. Does this imply that VR can initiate an embodied simulation, aside from a rigorous representation of fear stimuli? As cited [15], embodied simulation is being proposed as the key mechanism for why VRET is effective, because VR provides a mental internal model, as a predictive coding regulating the body in its context effectively. As a result, more thorough experimental designs (with precise brain measures regarding embodiment) are needed.

Meanwhile, in practice, exposure to real phobic images produces higher activations and it also may require a greater effort to voluntarily inhibit emotional activation than exposure to virtual stimuli and consequently may lead to more escape behaviors. Although there are no conclusive data on this [39], given that VR phobic stimulus exposure activates fewer escape behaviors, lower attrition rates and more therapeutic adherence can be expected, as reported by other studies [7,9,39,40]. For this, according to our data, virtual phobic stimuli require two paradoxical properties: They must be as similar as possible to real stimuli to activate the mechanisms associated with fear responses, but at the same time, participants need to be able to identify them as virtual.

This study has several limitations. First, the small sample size may have affected the reliability of the results [41]. In addition, also due to sample size, sex differences could not be taken into account. Furthermore, this study only used one type of specific phobia (i.e., small animal phobia) with few experimental stimulation conditions: Data about comorbid phobias and evolution time were not taken into account, and these data can affect results. Moreover, we did not assess participants' level of disgust as an emotional state different to fear/phobia [42], nor did we measure their escape behavior. However, the role of neural activity with escape/avoidance behavior is well established [43]. To add, we used 3D filmed real phobic stimuli as a representative condition to in vivo exposure, but this equivalence was not tested. Finally, we did not establish if the results were due to a phobic condition or could also be observed in anxious nonphobic individuals.

5. Conclusions

In short, the small animal images filmed in both real image and virtual reality formats generated the functional activation of the brain regions involved in the emotional processing of fear—thalamus, amygdala, hippocampus, fusiform gyrus, insula and occipital cingulate, and prefrontal cortices—in phobic individuals. However, real images produced more intense brain activations and a different pattern of hemodynamic responses than those elicited by virtual reality stimuli. This notwithstanding, these differences do not preclude the use of VR as an exposure resource, as the virtual images provided a sufficiently intense distress response in phobic individuals, activated a conscious process pathway, and, furthermore, led to fewer escape behaviors. These data support the use of virtual reality as an exposure procedure in the treatment of phobia disorders with similar properties to activate underlying mechanisms of exposure techniques.

Author Contributions: Conceptualization, methodology, formal analysis, and original draft preparation: W.P., F.R., C.V., M.H., M.B., J.D.L.F., and A.F.; writing—review and editing, W.P., F.R., Y.A.-P. and A.F.; Editing the final version, W.P, F.R., Y.A.-P. and A.F.

Funding: This study was carried out thanks to the financial support provided by the Ministry of Science, Innovation and Universities of Spain (projects PSI2013-42912-R and PSI2017-83222-R).

Acknowledgments: Thank you to the Servicio General de Apoyo a la Investigación de la Universidad de La Laguna (SEGAI).

Conflicts of Interest: The authors declare no conflict of interest.

References

1. North, M.; North, S. Virtual environments and psychological disorders. *Electron. J. Virtual Cult.* **1994**, *2*, 37–42.
2. Powers, M.B.; Rothbaum, B.O. Recent advances in virtual reality therapy for anxiety and related disorders: Introduction to the special issue. *J. Anxiety Disord.* **2019**, *61*, 1–2. [CrossRef] [PubMed]
3. Krijn, M.; Emmelkamp, P.M.G.; Olafsson, R.P.; Biemond, R. Virtual reality exposure therapy of anxiety disorders: A review. *Clin. Psychol. Rev.* **2004**, *24*, 259–281. [CrossRef] [PubMed]
4. De Carvalho, M.R.; Freire, R.C.; Nardi, A.E. Virtual reality as a mechanism for exposure therapy. *World J. Biol. Psychiat.* **2010**, *11*, 220–230. [CrossRef]
5. Opriş, D.; Pintea, S.; García-Palacios, A.; Botella, C.; Szamosközi, Ş.; David, D. Virtual reality exposure therapy in anxiety disorders: A quantitative meta-analysis. *Depress. Anxiety* **2012**, *29*, 85–93. [CrossRef]
6. Powers, M.B.; Emmelkamp, P.M.G. Virtual reality exposure therapy for anxiety disorders: A meta-analysis. *J. Anxiety Disord.* **2008**, *22*, 561–569. [CrossRef]
7. Carl, E.; Stein, A.T.; Levihn-Coon, A.; Pogue, J.R.; Rothbaum, B.; Emmelkamp, P.; Asmundson, G.J.G.; Carlbring, P.; Powers, M.B. Virtual reality exposure therapy for anxiety and related disorders: A meta-analysis of randomized controlled trials. *J. Anxiety Disord.* **2019**, *61*, 27–36. [CrossRef]
8. Botella, C.; Fernández-Álvarez, J.; Guillén, V.; García-Palacios, A.; Baños, R. Recent progress in virtual reality exposure therapy for phobias: A systematic review. *Curr. Psychiat. Rep.* **2017**, *19*, 42. [CrossRef]
9. Fernández-Álvarez, J.; Rozental, A.; Carlbring, P.; Colombo, D.; Riva, G.; Anderson, P.L.; Baños, R.M.; Benbow, A.A.; Bouchard, S.; Bretón-López, J.M.; et al. Deterioration rates in Virtual Reality Therapy: An individual patient data level meta-analysis. *J. Anxiety Disord.* **2019**, *61*, 3–17. [CrossRef]
10. Morina, N.; Ijntema, H.; Meyerbröker, K.; Emmelkamp, P.M.G. Can virtual reality exposure therapy gains be generalized to real-life? A meta-analysis of studies applying behavioral assessments. *Behav. Res. Ther.* **2015**, *74*, 18–24. [CrossRef]
11. Pasco, D. The potential of using virtual reality technology in physical activity settings. *Quest* **2013**, *65*, 429–441. [CrossRef]
12. Zeng, N.; Pope, Z.; Lee, J.E.; Gao, Z. Virtual Reality Exercise for anxiety and depression: A preliminary review of current research in an emerging field. *J. Clin. Med.* **2018**, *7*, 42. [CrossRef]
13. Suh, A.; Prophet, J. The state of immersive technology research: A literature analysis. *Comput. Hum. Behav.* **2018**, *86*, 77–90. [CrossRef]

14. Rubio-Tamayo, J.L.; Gertrudix-Barrio, M.; García-García, F. Immersive environments and virtual reality: Systematic review and advances in communication, interaction and simulation. *Multimodal Technol. Interact.* **2017**, *1*, 21. [CrossRef]
15. Riva, G.; Wiederhold, B.K.; Mantovani, F. Neuroscience of virtual reality: From virtual exposure to embodied medicine. *Cyberpsychol. Behav. Soc. Netw.* **2019**, *22*, 82–96. [CrossRef] [PubMed]
16. Del Casale, A.; Ferracuti, S.; Rapinesi, C.; Serata, D.; Piccirilli, M.; Savoja, V.; Kotzalidis, G.D.; Manfredi, G.; Angeletti, G.; Tatarelli, R.; et al. Functional neuroimaging in specific phobia. *Psychiatr. Res. Neuroimaging* **2012**, *202*, 181–197. [CrossRef]
17. Fullana, M.A.; Harrison, B.J.; Soriano-Mas, C.; Vervliet, B.; Cardoner, N.; Ávila-Parcet, A.; Radua, J. Neural signatures of human fear conditioning: An updated and extended meta-analysis of fMRI studies. *Mol. Psychiatr.* **2016**, *21*, 500–508. [CrossRef]
18. Peñate, W.; Fumero, A.; Viña, C.; Herrero, M.; Marrero, R.J.; Rivero, F. A meta-analytic review of neuroimaging studies of specific phobia to small animals. *Eur. J. Psychiat.* **2017**, *31*, 23–36. [CrossRef]
19. Linares, I.M.P.; Trzesniak, C.; Chagas, M.H.N.; Hallak, J.E.C.; Nardi, A.E.; Crippa, J.A.S. Neuroimaging in specific phobia disorder: A systematic review of the literature. *Rev. Bras. Psiquiatr.* **2012**, *34*, 101–111. [CrossRef]
20. Ipser, J.C.; Singh, L.; Stein, D.J. Meta-analysis of functional brain imaging in specific phobia. *Psychiat. Clin. Neurosci.* **2013**, *67*, 311–322. [CrossRef]
21. Das, T.; Padakannaya, P.; Pugh, K.R.; Singh, N.C. Neuroimaging reveals dual routes to reading in simultaneous proficient readers of two orthographies. *Neuroimage* **2011**, *54*, 1476–1487. [CrossRef] [PubMed]
22. Granziera, C.; Hadjikhani, N.; Arzy, S.; Seeck, M.; Meuli, R.; Krueger, G. In-vivo magnetic resonance imaging of the structural core of the Papez circuit in humans. *Neuroreport* **2011**, *22*, 227–231. [CrossRef] [PubMed]
23. Papez, J.W. A proposed mechanism of emotion. 1937. *J. Neuropsychi. Clin. N.* **1995**, *7*, 103–112. [CrossRef]
24. Rivero, R.; Herrero, M.; Viña, C.; Álvarez-Pérez, Y.; Peñate, W. Neuroimaging in cockroach phobia: An experimental study. *Int. J. Clin. Health Psych.* **2017**, *17*, 207–215. [CrossRef]
25. Kessler, R.C.; Üstün, T.B. The world mental health (WMH) survey initiative version of the world health organization (WHO) composite international diagnostic interview (CIDI). *Int. J. Meth. Psych. Res.* **2004**, *13*, 93–121. [CrossRef] [PubMed]
26. World Health Organization. *The ICD-10 Classification of Mental and Behavioural Disorders: Clinical Descriptions and Diagnostic Guidelines*; WHO: Geneva, Switzerland, 1992.
27. Endler, N.S.; Hunt, J.M.C.V.; Rosenstein, A.J. An S-R Inventory of Anxiousness. *Psychol. Monogr.* **1962**, *76*, 143–146. [CrossRef]
28. Kameoka, V.A.; Tanaka-Matsumi, J. The appropriateness of using the S-R Inventory of Anxiousness to measure sources of behavioral variability. *Appl. Psych. Meas.* **1981**, *5*, 229–235. [CrossRef]
29. Beck, A.T.; Epstein, N.; Brown, G.; Steer, R.A. An inventory for measuring clinical anxiety: Psychometric properties. *J. Consult. Clin. Psych.* **1988**, *56*, 893. [CrossRef]
30. Oldfield, R.C. The assessment and analysis of handedness: The Edinburgh inventory. *Neuropsychologia* **1971**, *9*, 97–113. [CrossRef]
31. Forman, S.D.; Cohen, J.D.; Fitzgerald, M.; Eddy, W.F.; Mintun, M.A.; Noll, D.C. Improved assessment of significant activation in functional magnetic resonance imaging (fMRI): Use of a cluster-size threshold. *Magn. Reson. Med.* **1995**, *33*, 636–647. [CrossRef]
32. Juan, M.C.; Baños, R.; Botella, C.; Pérez, D.; Alcañíz, M.; Monserrat, C. An augmented reality system for the treatment of acrophobia: The sense of presence using immersive photography. *Presence Teleop. Virt.* **2006**, *15*, 393–402. [CrossRef]
33. Lithari, C.; Moratti, S.; Weisz, N. Limbic areas are functionally decoupled and visual cortex takes a more central role during fear conditioning in humans. *Sci. Rep.* **2016**, *6*, 29220. [CrossRef] [PubMed]
34. Silverstein, D.N.; Ingvar, M. A multi-pathway hypothesis for human visual fear signaling. *Front. Syst. Neurosci.* **2015**, *9*, 101. [CrossRef] [PubMed]
35. Paquette, V.; Lévesque, J.; Mensour, B.; Leroux, J.M.; Beaudoin, G.; Bourgouin, P.; Beauregard, M. Change the mind and you change the brain: Effects of cognitive-behavioral therapy on the neural correlates of spider phobia. *NeuroImage* **2003**, *18*, 401–409. [CrossRef]
36. Weiner, K.S.; Zilles, K. The anatomical and functional specialization of the fusiform gyrus. *Neuropsychologia* **2016**, *83*, 48–62. [CrossRef]

37. Gu, X.; Hof, P.R.; Friston, K.J.; Fan, J. Anterior insular cortex and emotional awareness. *J. Comp. Neurol.* **2013**, *521*, 3371–3388. [CrossRef]
38. Palminteri, S.; Justo, D.; Jauffret, C.; Pavlicek, B.; Dauta, A.; Delmaire, C.; Czernecki, V.; Karachi, C.; Capelle, L.; Durr, A.; et al. Critical roles for anterior insula and dorsal striatum in punishment-based avoidance learning. *Neuron* **2012**, *76*, 998–1009. [CrossRef]
39. Benbow, A.A.; Anderson, P.L. A meta-analytic examination of attrition in virtual reality exposure therapy for anxiety disorders. *J. Anxiety Disord.* **2019**, *61*, 18–26. [CrossRef]
40. Peñate, W.; Roca, M.J.R.; Pitti, C.T.; Bethencourt, J.M.; de la Fuente, J.A.; Gracia, R.G. Cognitive-behavioral treatment and antidepressants combined with virtual reality exposure for patients with chronic agoraphobia. *Int. J. Clin. Hlth. Psych.* **2014**, *14*, 9–17. [CrossRef]
41. Button, K.S.; Ioannidis, J.P.; Mokrysz, C.; Nosek, B.A.; Flint, J.; Robinson, E.S.; Munafò, M.R. Power failure: Why small sample size undermines the reliability of neuroscience. *Nat. Rev. Neurosci.* **2013**, *14*, 365. [CrossRef]
42. Bareither, I.; Hasler, F.; Strasser, A. Nueve ideas para mejorar la neurociencia. *Mente Cereb.* **2015**, *73*, 48–51.
43. Gogolla, N. The insular cortex. *Curr. Biol.* **2017**, *27*, R580–R586. [CrossRef] [PubMed]

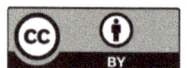

© 2019 by the authors. Licensee MDPI, Basel, Switzerland. This article is an open access article distributed under the terms and conditions of the Creative Commons Attribution (CC BY) license (http://creativecommons.org/licenses/by/4.0/).

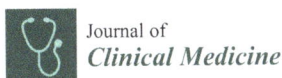

Article

Exposure to a Standardized Catastrophic Scenario in Virtual Reality or a Personalized Scenario in Imagination for Generalized Anxiety Disorder

Tanya Guitard [1], Stéphane Bouchard [2,3,*], Claude Bélanger [1] and Maxine Berthiaume [3]

[1] Département de Psychologie, Université du Québec à Montréal, Montréal, QC H3C 3P8, Canada; tanya.guitard@videotron.ca (T.G.); belanger.claude@uqam.ca (C.B.)
[2] Département de Psychoéducation et de Psychologie, Université du Québec en Outaouais, Gatineau, QC J8X 3X7, Canada
[3] School of Psychology, University of Ottawa, Ottawa, ON K1N 6N5, Canada; mbert094@uottawa.ca
* Correspondence: stephane.bouchard@uqo.ca

Received: 19 January 2019; Accepted: 26 February 2019; Published: 5 March 2019

Abstract: The cognitive behavioral treatment of generalized anxiety disorder (GAD) often involves exposing patients to a catastrophic scenario depicting their most feared worry. The aim of this study was to examine whether a standardized scenario recreated in virtual reality (VR) would elicit anxiety and negative affect and how it compared to the traditional method of imagining a personalized catastrophic scenario. A sample of 28 participants were first exposed to a neutral non-catastrophic scenario and then to a personalized scenario in imagination or a standardized virtual scenario presented in a counterbalanced order. The participants completed questionnaires before and after each immersion. The results suggest that the standardized virtual scenario induced significant anxiety. No difference was found when comparing exposure to the standardized scenario in VR and exposure to the personalized scenario in imagination. These findings were specific to anxiety and not to the broader measure of negative affect. Individual differences in susceptibility to feel present in VR was a significant predictor of increase in anxiety and negative affect. Future research could use these scenarios to conduct a randomized control trial to test the efficacy and cost/benefits of using VR in the treatment of GAD.

Keywords: Generalized Anxiety Disorder (GAD); virtual reality; exposure in virtual reality; cognitive exposure; standardized scenario; personalized scenario

1. Introduction

In the treatment of anxiety disorders, exposure is defined as "any procedure that confronts the person with a stimulus which typically elicits an undesirable behavior or an unwanted emotional response" [1] (p. 121). This stimulus can take an animate form (animal, insect), inanimate (heights, storms), a situation (public speaking), or even a thought (memories of a traumatic event, anticipation of a catastrophe). Regardless of the stimulus, the purpose of exposure is to learn new mental associations between the stimuli and lack of threat [2,3]. Considering that exposure requires confronting feared stimuli, the confrontation is associated with an increase in anxiety [4]. Studies have demonstrated that, compared to people who do not suffer from an anxiety disorder, immersions in virtual reality (VR) can elicit anxiety in people suffering from specific phobia [5], and from obsessive-compulsive disorder characterized by fear of contamination [6] or by checking behaviors [7]. Several studies, summarized in literature reviews (e.g., [8]) and meta-analyses (e.g., [9–11]), have documented the relevance and efficacy of using VR to conduct exposure (also called *in virtuo* exposure, [12]) in the treatment of anxiety disorders.

VR is defined as the product of using computer and behavioral interfaces to simulate the behavior of 3D entities that interact in real time with each other and with a user immersed via sensorimotor channels [13]. VR systems are designed so images viewed in a head mounted display (HMD) change according to the user's head movements. When immersed in VR, individuals can explore different environments, allowing them to feel as if they are physically in this synthetic environment [14]. This feeling of being "in" the virtual environment is called "presence" [15] and is considered an important feature of VR.

Conducting exposure *in virtuo* in the context of cognitive behavior therapy (CBT) has several benefits when compared to in vivo exposure. First, *in virtuo* exposure allows a greater control over the environment, which can be practical for both therapists and patients [16]. Unanticipated events (e.g., poor conditions during an airplane flight or unexpected animal/insect reactions) are less likely, allowing a more controlled exposure session. *In virtuo* exposure also provides greater standardization of the exposure cues, which can be useful for researchers as well as clinicians. Finally, using VR is considered more attractive than in vivo exposure for some patients [17].

However, creating virtual environments for *in virtuo* exposure for the treatment of generalized anxiety disorder (GAD) could be more complex than with other anxiety disorders. GAD is defined by excessive anxiety or worries almost every day for at least six months and concerning a variety of themes. It is characterized by fear of negative and uncertain future events [18–20]. As opposed to other anxiety disorders, people suffering from GAD are not essentially afraid of specific and concrete stimuli. They are afraid of uncertainty accompanied with a broad range of situations. In the cognitive-behavioral treatment of GAD, exposure is often conducted in the imagination, where patients have to repeat mentally or write down a scenario depicting one of their worst catastrophic worries [21,22].

Using VR for exposure with GAD has its share of advantages [23]. For example, not all patients are good at imagining or visualizing feared situations, yet exposure in imagination is often used with GAD patients. It may be difficult to know what patients are thinking about, if they are engaged in avoidance or neutralization behaviors while doing exposure, or if the right stimuli are included in the scenario. With respect to neutralization, subtle avoidance and safety seeking behaviors, using standardized scenarios reduces the risks of avoidance because the content of the scenario is known and visible to the therapist during the immersion in VR.

Previous work has been conducted to identify common ingredients in the exposure scenarios of actual GAD patients [24] and to proposed standardized scenarios that can be used for exposure [25]. Empirical data collected with GAD patients exposed in imagination to their personal worry scenarios or to the standardized ones showed that standardized scenarios can elicit anxiety (as measured with self-report and heart rate) and negative affect [25]. In their research, Guitard and her colleagues [25] demonstrated that the effect size of exposure in imagination to the individualized scenarios was slightly higher than the standardized ones on the measure of heart rate but, nevertheless, the results were positive enough to warrant transposing the scenarios used in imagination into VR scenarios and testing them with people suffering from GAD.

Accordingly, the goal of the current study is to document the potential of virtual environments adapted from catastrophic scenarios to induce the anxiety necessary to eventually use VR as an exposure strategy in the treatment of GAD. Three exposure scenarios are compared: (a) exposure to a neutral virtual environment; (b) exposure in imagination to a personalized scenario (IM-Exp); and (3) exposure in VR to a standardized scenario (VR-Exp). Each participant was exposed to all three conditions, first to the neutral environment and then to exposure in imagination or in VR, in random order. The hypothesis was that exposure in VR will induce more anxiety than the neutral scenario. Power estimations were performed before the study, with medium to large effect sizes expected for this hyposhesis based on results from other studies [5,6,25]. To prevent having to prove the null hypothesis (i.e., *in virtuo* being as effective as in vivo) without justification, no formal hypothesis was expressed for the comparison between exposure in VR and in imagination, and no power estimation was conducted a priori.

2. Materials and Methods

2.1. Participants

Inclusion criteria for this study were as follows: (a) primary diagnosis of GAD, (b) aged between 18 and 65, and (c) never having experienced VR before. The Randot Stereo™ test from Western Ophtalmics was used to assess if participants have stereoscopic vision. Exclusion criteria consisted of: (a) suffering from an anxiety disorder other than GAD as primary diagnosis; (b) suffering from claustrophobia, because the experimentation was held in an immersive CAVE-Like system, a rather confined area; (c) use of benzodiazepines, because of the impact this type of medication might have on the variables measured; and (d) suffering from any of the following health issues (due to potential interactions with VR): diseases related to the inner ear or vestibular system, cardiovascular diseases or circulatory disorders, migraines, blood pressure disorders or diabetes. The final sample included a total of 28 participants who all met the criteria.

2.2. Procedure

Participants were recruited through the Université du Québec en Outaouais (UQO) via email and posters. The project, conducted in concordance with the Declaration of Helsinki and the Canadian Tri-Council policy statement for ethical conduct for research involving humans, was approved by the Ethics Committee of UQO and participants signed a free and informed consent form. All individuals who wanted to participate in the study were first briefly screened by phone in order to assess whether or not excessive worry seemed present. In cases where anxiety was caused by another disorder, they were referred to another service. When GAD seemed probable and exclusion criteria were screened, a first meeting was scheduled to proceed to the complete evaluation using the ADIS-IV. The participants included in the study were randomly assigned to one of the two conditions: (a) exposure to a standardized scenario in VR followed by exposure to an individualized scenario in imagination (VR-Exp/IM-Exp; $n = 13$) or (b) exposure to an individualized scenario in imagination followed by exposure to standardized scenario in VR (IM-Exp/VR-Exp.; $n = 15$). At the end of the assessment session, all participants were given a battery of questionnaires to complete alone at home (without consulting other people) and return at the following meeting. In session 2, participants were asked to identify a worry theme and write a catastrophic scenario based on their worst fear. The writing of the scenario began during the session to allow time for the therapist to review the content and give feedback to the participant. Following this, participants were asked to further improve their scenario, if needed. They were told not to read their scenario at home to avoid habituation. A third and final session was scheduled in which the exposures took place. Each participant was first immersed in a neutral non-catastrophic virtual environment for 5 min that consisted of a quiet and empty room with a glass door and the sun shining in from large windows. Participants were asked to physically walk around the room to familiarize themselves with VR. Following the first experimental exposure scenario (either in VR or in imagination), a distraction task was performed where participants were asked to dash the A letter each time it occurred in a random and incomprehensible text. Following the distraction task, the other experimental exposure session took place. At the end of the third session, debriefing was completed to ensure the well-being of the participants following the brief exposure to the anxiety provoking scenarios and offer relevant clinical referrals, if necessary.

2.3. Virtual Environments (VE)

The three standardized exposure scenarios used in imagination by Guitard et al. [25] were recreated in VR and the experimenter selected one based on the main worry theme as reported by the participant: (a) VE 1: an emergency room (used with 11 participants), (b) VE 2: an apartment (used with 15 participants), or (c) VE 3: a student room (used with 2 participants).

2.3.1. VE 1: Emergency Room

This environment was created with the intention of eliciting worry in participants suffering mostly from worries related to health. The participant was immersed in a hospital emergency waiting room. Other patients are nearby and display symptoms of sickness (coughing) or fatigue. One is wearing a disposable face mask. Sounds are heard, such as a mother crying after receiving bad news concerning her child, and a wife is told that nothing can be done to save her husband, etc. Other patients are called to see the doctor, but not the participant. At some point, doctors come into the waiting room and discuss a case while looking at the participant, who cannot, however, understand what they are saying.

2.3.2. VE 2: Apartment

The setting for this scenario is an apartment that participants are invited to visit. Participants first overhear a conversation taking place behind closed doors suggesting that an accident has occurred. Afterwards, a special announcement is made on the radio regarding recent burglaries in the neighborhood. At the same time, a rock is thrown at the window, and when the participant looks out the window, a group of men is seen roughing up another individual. Finally, a brief message is left on the answering machine. Seven message options are available to choose from: (a) the police calling because a loved one was involved in an accident, (b) the doctor calling regarding test results that were previously overlooked, (c) the participant's spouse, either male or female, is saying that they have met a new lover and are leaving, (d) the bank needs to be called back regarding several late payments and is threatening to take action, (e) a receptionist from work calling regarding recent budget cuts and a problem involving the participant, (f) the university calling regarding unpaid tuition fees and the impossibility of registering for the semester, or (g) the school is calling regarding the participant's child's recent behavior and academic problems.

2.3.3. VE 3: Student Room

The third environment, created for students, alludes to both academic difficulties and social isolation. The participant is in his or her room having to study for upcoming exams. Scattered unpaid bills are visible and suggest financial difficulties. Voices are heard coming from the hall, talking about a student who is failing out of the program. Roommates heard from another room are planning a party to which the participant is not invited and that might, furthermore, disrupt his or her study time.

2.4. Measures

2.4.1. Diagnostic and Clinical Measures of Severity

An initial diagnosis of GAD was made using the ADIS-IV at the first session. Questionnaires were then given to each participant to be filled out at home and brought back at the next session. Those questionnaires were used to further assess each participant and assess the clinical severity of the sample as well as describe VR factors that may influence the results.

Diagnostic Measure: Anxiety Disorders Interview Schedule for DSM-IV (ADIS-IV)

This semi-structured interview allows for a thorough evaluation of anxiety disorders as well as mood disorders, substance-abuse disorders, and somatoform disorders as they hold the higher comorbidity rates with anxiety disorders. The ADIS-IV [26] was used for diagnostic purposes and the severity score on the diagnosis of GAD is reported to describe the sample.

Clinical Measure: Penn State Worry Questionnaire (PSWQ)

The French translation of this questionnaire [27] comes from Ladouceur et al. [28]. This 16-item questionnaire measures the level of worry typical to GAD on a scale of 1 to 5. The psychometric properties of the English version are very good, with good internal consistency (Cronbach's alpha ranging from 0.86 to 0.95) and test retest reliability (ranging from 0.74 to 0.93) [29,30]. The same was found for the French version (see [30]) indicate equally good validity and internal consistency. The PSWQ was used to describe the sample.

Clinical Measure: Cognitive Avoidance Questionnaire (CAQ; Original French Version)

Cognitive avoidance plays an important role in maintaining excessive worry in GAD. This measure [31] was therefore used to evaluate the degree of cognitive avoidance in the sample. Studies have indicated good psychometric features for this scale with a Cronbach's alpha of 0.95 for the totality of the items on an adult sample and of 0.92 on a sample of adolescents, both non-clinical samples.

2.4.2. Measures of Users' Experience in Virtual Reality

These questionnaires measure important concepts in clinical applications of VR. They allow comparing reactions of participants from one study to another.

Users' Experience: Presence Questionnaire (PQ)

The PQ is a French-Canadian translation (validated by the Cyberpsychology Laboratory of UQO [32]) of the Witmer and Singer Presence Questionnaire [33]. This questionnaire contains 24 items in the form of closed-ended questions, on a scale of 1 ("not at all") to 7 ("completely"), and as a measure of presence it is useful to describe how participants perceive the properties of the virtual environments and the technology used. Cronbach's alpha reaches 0.84. The duration of administration was approximately 7 min.

Users' Experience: Gatineau Presence Questionnaire (GPQ)

This questionnaire was created by the Cyberpsychology Laboratory as a brief supplement to the PQ to address the experience felt by the users while immersed [6]. It includes four questions, on a scale of 0–100. The GPQ has a Cronbach's alpha of 0.69.

Users' Experience: Simulator Sickness Questionnaire (SSQ)

This questionnaire is a French-Canadian translation (validated by the Cyberpsychology Laboratory of UQO [34]) of the Simulator Sickness Questionnaire [35] designed to measure the level of unwanted negative effects induced by the immersions in VR. It consists of 16 items, rated on a four-point scale. This questionnaire was administered to participants for the first time at the beginning of the meeting involving virtual reality, in order to know their physical state well before the first immersion (results not shown) and after the immersion in VR. Cronbach's alpha reaches 0.87. The SSQ was scored according to guidelines from Bouchard et al. [34] and the raw total score is reported.

2.4.3. Dependent Variables

The following questionnaires were used as dependent variables to assess the level of anxiety and negative affect throughout the experimentation process of the third session. Participants had to fill out these questionnaires after each exposure session.

Dependent Variable: State Scale of the State Trait Anxiety Inventory—Form Y1 (STAI-Y1)

The French version of this questionnaire [36,37] was used. Only the Y-1 version (state form) was retained for the present study because the goal of the project was to assess anxiety levels at different times during the experimentation rather than evaluate anxiety traits in the participants. The French version of this measure has excellent psychometric values, with a Cronbach's alpha of 0.94 and 0.86 for men and women, respectively [36].

Dependent Variable: Negative Affect Scale of the Positive and Negative Affect Schedule (PANAS)

The French-Canadian version [38] of the questionnaire developed by Watson, Clark and Tellegen [39] was used. It consists of two scales; one measuring positive affect and the other negative affect. Only the negative affect subscale is reported here, given the study's focus on anxiety. Items represent different feelings and emotions that are rated on a 5-point scale ranging from 1 ("very slightly or not at all") to 5 ("extremely"). Internal consistency of the negative affect subscale is adequate, with a Cronbach's alpha ranging from 0.80 to 0.84.

2.4.4. Predictors of Levels of Anxiety and Negative Affect During the Immersion in VR

Predictor: Intolerance of Uncertainty Scale (IUS; Original French Version)

This questionnaire [20] rates the degree of intolerance to uncertainty using 27 items that describe uncertainty as negative and something to be avoided. Participants have to rate each item on a 5-point Likert scale ranging from 1 ("not at all characteristic of me") to 5 ("entirely characteristic of me"). This measure possesses very good internal consistency (Cronbach's alpha of 0.91) and good convergent validity with the PSWQ. Also, the main advantage of this measure is its good sensibility and specificity to excessive worry that allows it to be administered more than once during treatment to assess progress [21]. The IUS, and the following two questionnaires, were used to describe the sample and explore potential predictors of patient's reactions in VR.

Predictor: Why Worry-II (WW-II)

This questionnaire is a revised version of the original Why Worry [31]. It assesses positive beliefs about worry with five different subscales: (1) worry as a problem solving tool; (2) worry helps motivate; (3) worrying protects and prepares in the face of a negative outcome; (4) worrying can, in itself, prevent a negative outcome and (5) worry is a positive personality trait. This self-reported measure contains 25 items ranging from 1 ("not at all true") to 5 ("absolutely true"). This questionnaire possesses good test-retest reliability ($r = 0.81$) and internal consistency (Cronbach's alpha of 0.93) [40].

Predictor: Immersive Tendencies Questionnaire (ITQ)

This questionnaire is a French-Canadian translation (validated by the Cyberpsychology Laboratory of UQO [32]) of the Immersion Tendencies Questionnaire [33] and contains 18 items calculated on a scale of 1 ("never") to 7 ("often"). This questionnaire aims to measure the predisposition of the individual to experience presence. It was administered only once. Cronbach's alpha reaches 0.78.

2.5. Experimenters and Hardware

Four experimenters, all doctorate students with training in CBT for anxiety disorders, conducted the study. Supervision was made available to them and provided by a licensed psychologist. The immersions in VR were conducted in a 6-side CAVE-Like system using retro projected stereoscopic displays and wireless motion tracking (see Laforest et al. [6] for a technical description and a picture).

3. Results

3.1. Sample Description

The sample ($N = 28$) consisted of 24 women and 4 men with a primary diagnosis of GAD. They were all francophone with a mean age of 38.33 (SD = 12.78). According to the PSWQ, participants scored within the range of adults suffering from GAD. Comorbid disorders were diagnosed in 64.3% of the sample—social anxiety being the most frequent ($n = 8$) while others were specific phobias ($n = 4$), panic disorder ($n = 3$), obsessive-compulsive disorder ($n = 1$), and other diagnosis ($n = 2$). Further description of the sample is provided in Table 1. No differences were found between the two conditions on the GAD severity (as assessed with the ADIS-IV and the PSWQ), on how they perceived the quality of the VR system (PQ), and in unwanted negative side effects induced by the immersion in VR (SSQ).

Table 1. General description of the sample.

Variable	N	%	Mean (SD)
Nationality			
Canadian	25	89.3	
Senegalese	1	3.6	
Level of education			
University (some or completed)	18	64.3	
College or professional diploma	5	17.9	
High school diploma	3	10.7	
Some high school	2	7.1	
Socioeconomic status			
High	9	32.1	
Middle	15	53.6	
Low	4	14.3	
Marital status			
Married	10	35.7	
Single	8	28.6	
Common-law partner	8	28.6	
Divorced	2	7.1	
Descriptive clinical measures of generalized anxiety disorder			
Anxiety Disorders Interview Schedule-IV severity of GAD			5.7 (0.93)
Penn State Worry Questionnaire			59.88 (8.89)
Cognitive Avoidance Questionnaire			68.32 (20.35)
Descriptive measures of users' experience in virtual reality			
Presence Questionnaire after the VR-Exp scenario			61.17 (19.05)
Gatineau Presence Questionnaire after the VR-Exp scenario			89.90 (14.32)
Simulator Sickness Questionnaire after the VR-Exp scenario			9.57 (6.65)
Predictive measures selected for exploratory analyses			
Intolerance of Uncertainty Scale			68.61 (21.62)
Why Worry-II Questionnaire			47.29 (17.93)
Immersive Tendencies Questionnaire			70.88 (16.81)

3.2. Statistical Analyses

Prior to analyses, all variables to be used in further analyses were examined for accuracy of data entry, missing values, normality of distribution, and univariate outliers. After ensuring that there were no errors in data entry or missing values, we screened for extreme kurtosis and skewness values (below 1.5 or above -1.5), which would indicate non-normal distributions. The negative affect scale of the PANAS (neutral scenario and second exposure) had extreme kurtosis values. We also screened for univariate outliers on the state anxiety scale of the STAI and the negative affect scale of the PANAS. When univariate outliers were found, they were winsorized to the next most extreme but acceptable value in that condition (with a z-score less than 1.96 or above -1.96). To do so, z-scores were first obtained for all variables to be used in further analyses. When a z-score was greater than 1.96 or less than -1.96, the next most extreme but acceptable value in the same condition was found and replaced the extreme value that needed to be winsorized. This procedure eliminated all outliers and extreme skewness and kurtosis values. Parametric analyses were then performed, with descriptive results reported in Table 2 (note that results were similar if the data is not corrected for outliers).

Table 2. Means and standard deviations of dependent variables in each experimental condition for the three scenarios.

Measure and Scenario	Condition			
	IM-Exp/VR-Exp		VR-Exp/IM-Exp	
	M	(SD)	M	(SD)
STAI-Y1				
Neutral environment	39.67	(10.83)	41.92	(13.12)
Exposure scenario 1	50.20	(12.81)	46.00	(12.91)
Exposure scenario 2	47.00	(12.66)	51.00	(14.74)
PANAS_NA				
Neutral environment	15.47	(5.14)	15.08	(4.25)
Exposure scenario 1	18.33	(6.23)	17.23	(5.12)
Exposure scenario 2	15.67	(3.60)	19.46	(8.61)

Note: IM-Exp = exposure to a personalized scenario in imagination, VR-Exp = exposure to a standardized scenario in virtual reality.

Following data screening, variables were analyzed with repeated measures ANOVAs, followed by a priori orthogonal within-subjects contrasts. Contrasts focused on the impact of the neutral scenario and first exposure and of the first and second exposures on the cognitive exposure group compared to the virtual exposure group. All Mauchly's (sphericity) values were non-significant, therefore the non-corrected values were used. To control for Type-I error rate, Bonferroni corrections were applied. Controlling with ANCOVAs for the use of three standardized scenarios did not change the interpretation of the results. When results were not significant, the expected number of participants required to detect a significant difference at alpha = 0.05 with a power of 0.80 is reported based on Cohen [41] to illustrate the magnitude of the differences.

Descriptive information and results for all dependent variables following the ANOVAs are reported in Tables 2 and 3 respectively. For the main effect of Time, a repeated measures ANOVA showed a significant increase in anxiety as measured with the STAI-Y1, when comparing exposure to the neutral VE and exposure to either a catastrophic scenario (traditional personalized scenario or VR scenario, see Figure 1 for illustration). The interaction was non-significant, indicating that exposure to the traditional personalized scenario over time did not elicit more anxiety than exposure to the virtual scenario. The first contrast revealed that the first exposure to either the traditional personalized scenario or the virtual scenario was significantly more anxiety provoking than exposure to the neutral scenario [$t(26) = 3.82, p < 0.001$, eta-squared = 0.22, effect size = large, power = 0.96]. The interaction contrast was non-significant [$t(26) = -0.58, p > 0.05$, eta-squared = 0.006, effect-size = very small, power = 0.10, expected N to detect a significant difference with a power of 0.80 > 2000], showing that both scenarios induced anxiety. The contrast from the first exposure to the second exposure was non-significant [$t(26) = 0.48, p > 0.05$. eta-squared -0.004, effect-size = very small, power = 0.07, expected N to detect a significant difference with a power of 0.80 > 2000], suggesting that the first exposure was not more anxiety provoking than the second exposure, regardless of the scenario. However, the interaction contrast was significant [$t(26) = 2.20, p < 0.05$, partial eta-squared = 0.09, effect-size = medium, power = 0.65], indicating that the traditional personalized scenario elicited more anxiety than the VR scenario. The interaction did not remain significant when applying the Bonferroni correction.

Results on the negative affect scale of the PANAS were somewhat different (see Figure 2 for illustration). In the group first exposed to traditional cognitive exposure, negative affect decreased in the second exposure whereas the second group, first exposed to VR, shows an increase in negative affect when exposed to the traditional personalized scenario. The results for the main effect of Time from the ANOVA revealed non-significant increase in negative affect overall. The first a priori contrast indicated that negative affect did significantly increase from the neutral scenario to the first exposure in both scenarios [$t(26) = 2.59$, $p < 0.05$, eta-squared = 0.11, effect-size = medium, power = 0.78], although the increase did not remain significant when applying the Bonferroni correction. The interaction contrast was non-significant [$t(26) = 0.94$, $p > 0.05$, eta-squared = 0.02, effect-size = small, power = 0.20, expected N to detect a significant difference with a power of 0.80 = 344], revealing a similar and only slight increase in negative affect. The second a priori interaction contrast was non-significant [$t(26) = 2.03$, $p > 0.05$ eta-squared = 0.07, effect-size = medium, power = 0.60, expected N to detect a significant difference with a power of 0.80 = 120], although the effect size was close to significance.

Table 3. Results of main effects of repeated measures ANOVAs for the comparative effect of cognitive exposure generalized anxiety disorder (GAD) scenarios presented in imagination and in virtual reality.

Effect	MS	df	F	p	ηp^2
STAI-Y1					
Time	564.10	2	9.03	< 0.001	0.258
Time × Condition	129.96	2	2.08	0.135	0.074
Condition	4.06	1	0.01	0.92	0.000
PANAS_NA					
Time	53.87	2	2.97	0.60	0.102
Time × Condition	48.75	2	2.69	0.078	0.094
Condition	56.38	1	0.61	0.44	0.023

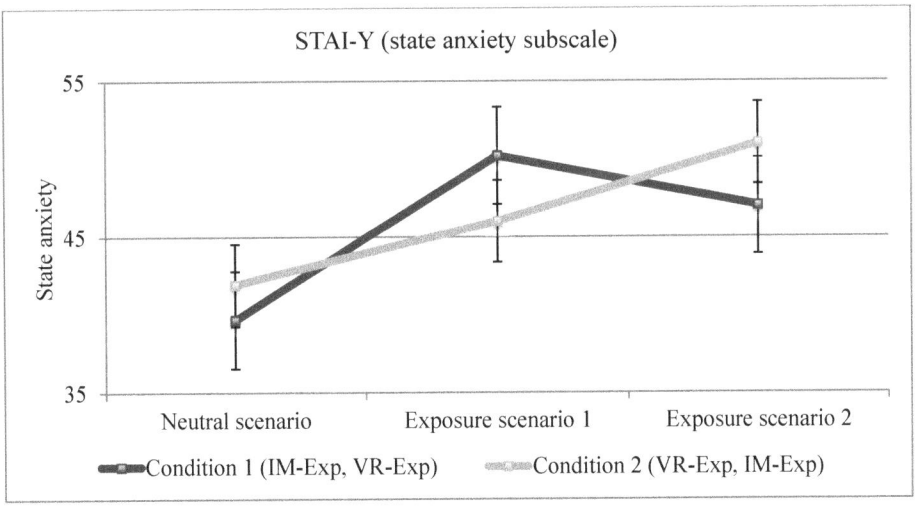

Figure 1. Illustration of the differential impact of exposure to a neutral scenario in virtual reality, a personalized scenario in imagination (IM-Exp) and a standardized scenario in virtual reality (VR-Exp) on the self-report measure of anxiety.

Further exploratory analyses were conducted to study predictors of the impact of the exposure to the standardized catastrophic scenarios in VR. To respect a subject-to-variable ratio that minimizes parameter inflation and maximizes replicability, only three predictors were selected: two variables related to GAD (intolerance of uncertainty—IUS, and beliefs about worry—WW-II) and one related to VR (immersive tendencies - ITQ). Prior to performing the analyses, data were screened for linearity (by examining a scatterplot), multicollinearity (by verifying the tolerance and VIF values), autocorrelation among the residuals (by verifying the Durbin-Watson values and examining a scatterplot), multivariate normality (by examining a histogram), and homoscedasticity (by examining a scatterplot). All assumptions were met.

In the exploratory predictor analyses of state anxiety during exposure to the standardized scenario in VR, the main regression was significant [adjR^2 = 0.44, $F_{(3, 24)}$ = 7.29, $p < 0.01$]. Two predictors were significant, the usefulness of worrying (WW-II; t = 2.99, partial r = 0.46, $p < 0.01$) and the immersive tendency (ITQ; t = 4.14, partial r = 0.63, $p < 0.001$). Intolerance of uncertainty was not a significant predictor (IUS; t = −0.9, partial r = −0.15, p = 0.35 ns). The exploratory predictor analyses of negative affect was significant [adjR^2 = 0.32, $F_{(3, 24)}$ = 4.79, $p < 0.05$], with only the immersive tendency standing out as a significant predictor (ITQ; t = 3.54, partial r = 0.6, $p < 0.01$). Regression parameters were not significant for the WW-II (t = 1.62, partial r = 0.27, p = 0.12 ns) and the IUS (t = −0.22, partial r = −0.04, p = 0.83 ns). The scaterplots in Figure 3 illustrate the tendecy, and individial differences, for higher predispositions to feel present in VR to be associated with more anxiety and negative affect.

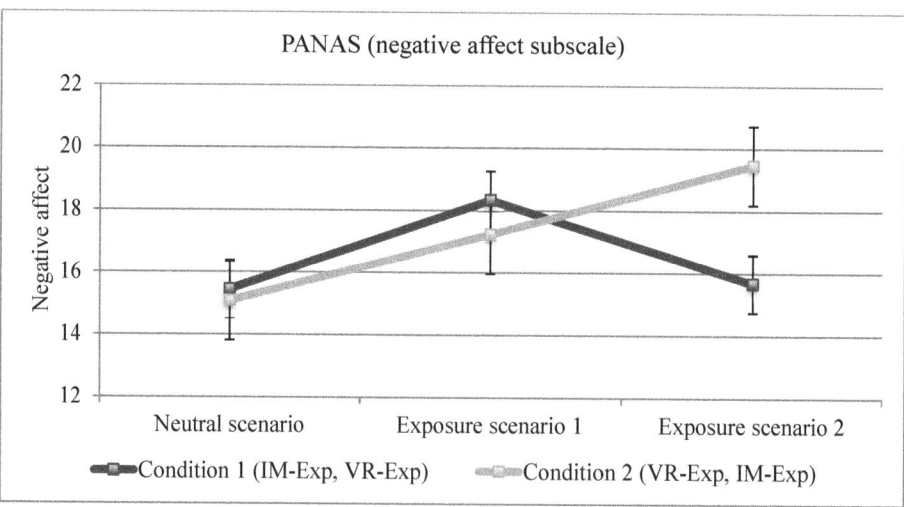

Figure 2. Illustration of the differential impact of exposure to a neutral scenario in virtual reality, a personalized scenario in imagination (IM-Exp) and a standardized scenario in virtual reality (VR-Exp) on the self-report measure of negative affect.

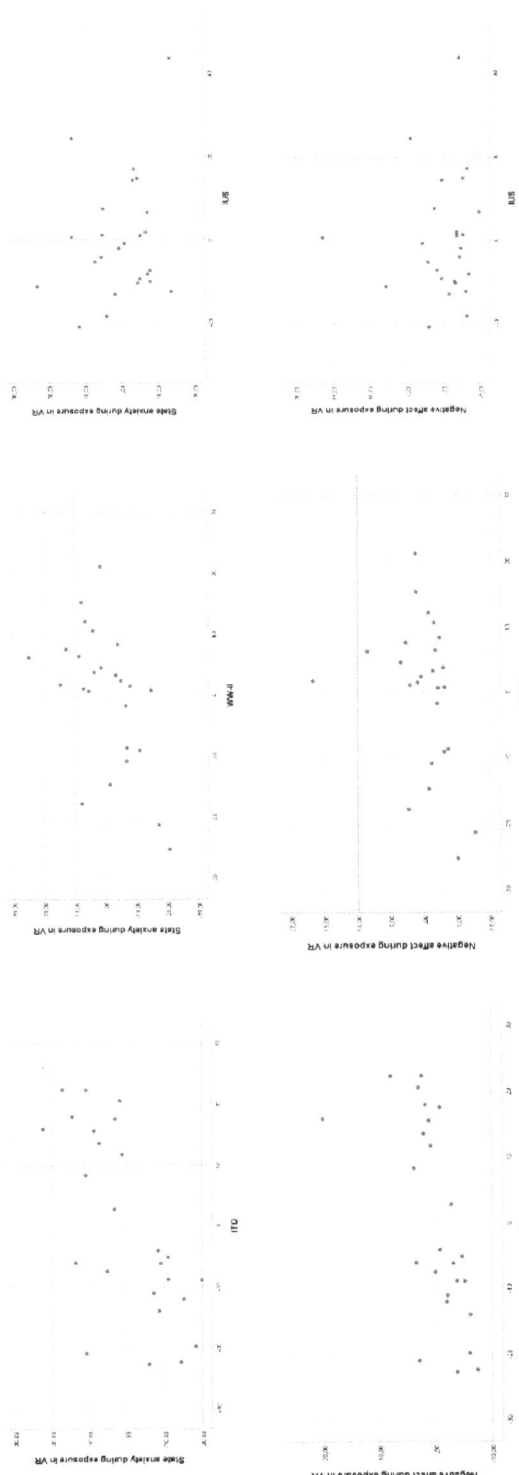

Figure 3. Scatterplots for the three predictors of state anxiety (**top** three) and negative affect (**bottom** three): immersive tendency (ITQ, **left** plot), positive beliefs about worry (WW-II, **center** plot), and intolerance of uncertainty (IUS, **right** plot).

4. Discussion

The goal of the current study was to assess the potential of VR scenarios to elicit anxiety in GAD patients, with the long-term research goal of facilitating cognitive exposure in CBT. The current study compared a standardized scenario in VR and a traditional personalized scenario. More precisely, we compared traditional exposure in imagination using a personalized catastrophic scenario to exposure in VR to a standardized scenario. Exposure to a neutral scenario was used as a baseline for comparisons. We hypothesized that exposure in VR to the standardized scenario would be significantly more anxiety provoking than the neutral scenario. No specific hypothesis was formulated for the comparison between the modalities of exposure.

Our first hypothesis was supported. The state anxiety scores during exposure in VR and in imagination were significantly higher than the baseline. Results were also in the same range than in the Guitard et al. [25] study, where participants had to imagine the scenarios instead of being exposed to them in VR, and to studies using VR for other anxiety disorders (e.g., [6,7]). The actual difference between exposure to standardized scenarios in VR and personalized scenarios in imagination was significant only when the sequence of exposure sessions was counterbalanced and it did not remain significant after controlling for the number of comparisons. The effect size and statistical power of the comparisons between the two exposure modalities deserve attention. When compared to the neutral scenario, the increase in anxiety experience in the personalized scenario in imagination versus the standardized scenario in VR is associated with a small effect size and more than 2 000 participants would be required to detect a significant difference in the two exposure modalities. This is supporting the potential of VR with GAD patients. However, the direct comparison of the two modalities with each other (i.e., the interaction contrast between the exposure scenarios) is associated with a medium effect size and a lack of power explains why the difference does not remain significant after controlling for the number of comparisons. Overall, this suggests that personalized scenarios may be more anxiety provoking. Based on the multiple regression analysis, we can speculate this may be especially relevant for people who have a strong susceptibility to be immersed in VR. Nevertheless, the potential of using standardized scenarios in VR remains promising because it did elicit anxiety in GAD patients.

The findings are even more interesting because they were observed on the anxiety measure, but not on the less specific measure of negative affect. To be more precise, the impact of the exposure sessions mirror those of the anxiety measure on the a priori contrasts, but the differences do not remain statistically significant after controlling for the number of comparisons. Readers relying more on effect sizes than probability levels, or on power analyses, would consider the finding meaningful, consistent with Guitard et al. [25] and actually revealing more specificity to fear and anxiety than to diffuse negative emotions.

A pilot and independent clinical trial based on our results support our interest in the use of VR with GAD patients. Labbé, Thibault, Côté, and Gosselin [42] assessed the effectiveness of conducting only exposure to one standardized scenario (the emergency waiting room) in VR with people diagnosed with GAD. Participants were exposed three times to the scenario. Results showed a significant improvement on all measures related to GAD post-treatment, including the tendency to worry, symptoms of GAD, and anxiety. Treatment gains were maintained at the two-month follow-up. In addition, the changes were specific to health-related worries, which is consistent with the content of the scenario used for exposure. Results from Labbé et al. [42] are in line with the pioneering paper from Repetto et al. [43] on GAD, although they are the first to address the core fear of GAD.

Some limitations of the current study must be pointed out and discussed. First, the sample is relatively small. The provision of effect sizes should help gauge the magnitude of the experimental manipulations and plan larger studies. The effect of repeated exposure to standardized versus personalized scenarios should also be documented. The sociodemographic and clinical characteristics of the sample are typical of a study sample of GAD patients, with the exception of slightly more women than what is found in the general population, where women are usually three times more likely than men to have GAD [44]. A larger proportion of males would allow comparing the potential impact of gender differences. Documenting sex, economic, marital, and educational status in research articles is important for clinicians and researchers in order to appraise the sample and generalize the results. Reviews have been conducted on the power of immersions in VR to induce anxiety responses (e.g., [45]), but the impact of these variables has not yet been examined. Because these variables are frequently associated with anxiety disorders, their impact on the effect of VR deserve to be explored. The addition of physiological measures of anxiety would have documented and complemented our findings with objective measures [25]. However, heart rate or skin conductance would have been biased and unreliable given implicit differences in the exposure sessions. Participants were seated in the session of exposure in imagination. But in VR, participants were standing up and were physically moving when exploring the virtual environment. The intensity of the anxiety response also deserves attention. The research protocol was not designed to show how much an experience in VR could be frightening to GAD patients, but to show the potential of scenarios with a feeling of uncertainty to elicit anxiety in a population that is known to perceive uncertainty as threatening [18]. Finally, to increase generalization of the results to the psychotherapy contexts, it would have been interesting to conduct the study while patients are already in therapy and ready to proceed with exposure. Such a study comes with methodological challenges and it was considered better to first show that scenarios that are not individualized and presented in VR bear some potential.

Furthermore, the choice of three different VEs instead of only one could be argued as another limitation. However, the drawback of using only one scenario would be not targeting the main worry themes of the participants. This would be far more detrimental than comparing only three slightly different generic scenarios to 28 totally different and individualized ones. A replication study with a sample selected on the basis of the main worry theme would allow a more direct comparison of the exposure modalities with similar themes, or a larger sample would allow comparisons between virtual scenarios. Comparisons with people suffering from other anxiety disorders and with non-anxious participants would help document the specificity of the reactions to GAD.

The results from the exploratory analyses revealed that immersive tendencies, or individual predispositions to feel present, significantly predicted the increase in emotional reactions of participants. The predictive importance of the ITQ was significant when predicting anxiety and negative affect during exposure *in virtuo*. Perceived usefulness of worrying was another significant predictor of state anxiety in VR, but not intolerance of uncertainty. Presenting the neutral immersion in VR to all participants at the beginning of the experiment may have protected against the elements of novelty in the task [25], leaving room for other variables to stand out, such as the severity of dysfunctional thoughts about the usefulness of worry in predicting state anxiety. Future research should document with a larger sample, more predictors, better control for the different VR scenarios and planned hypotheses, and predictors of emotional reactions of patients in VR.

5. Conclusions

Because uncertainty is the core fear underlying GAD [18,19], the current study examined if immersion in virtual standardized scenarios that were developed based on the feeling of uncertainty and typical GAD worry themes may be relevant to be used in CBT. The increase in anxiety during immersion support the potential of VR for exposure, even in the case where feared stimuli are not as specific as in phobias and other anxiety disorders. This paves the way for the development of psychotherapy protocols that would integrate *in virtuo* exposure to test in randomized control trials.

Author Contributions: Conceptualization, T.G., S.B., and C.B.; methodology, T.G., S.B., and C.B.; software, S.B.; validation, S.B. and C.B.; formal analysis, S.B. and M.B.; investigation, T.G.; resources, S.B.; data curation, T.G.; writing—original draft preparation, T.G. and M.B.; writing—review and editing, T.G., S.B., C.B., and M.B.; visualization, T.G., S.B., C.B., and M.B.; supervision, S.B. and C.B.; project administration, T.G.; funding acquisition, S.B.

Funding: This research was funded by Canada Research Chairs, grant number 950-205582.

Conflicts of Interest: Stéphane Bouchard is president and part owner of *In Virtuo*, a company that distributes virtual environments, and conflicts of interest are managed under UQO's conflict of interest policy.

References

1. Marshall, W.L. Exposure. In *Dictionary of Behavior Therapy Techniques*; Bellack, A.S., Herson, M., Eds.; Pergamon Press: New York, NY, USA, 1986; pp. 121–124.
2. Craske, M.G.; Treanor, M.; Conway, C.C.; Zbozinek, T.; Vervliet, B. Maximizing exposure therapy: An inhibitory learning approach. *Behav. Res. Ther.* **2014**, *58*, 10–23. [CrossRef] [PubMed]
3. Richard, D.C.S.; Lauterbach, D.; Gloster, A.T. Description, mechanisms of action, and assessment. In *Handbook of Exposure Therapies*; Richard, D.C.S., Lauterbach, D., Eds.; Academic Press: Cambridge, MA, USA, 2007; pp. 1–28.
4. Bouchard, S.; Robillard, G.; Larouche, S.; Loranger, C. Description of a treatment manual for *in virtuo* exposure with specific phobia. In *Virtual Reality in Psychological, Medical and Pedagogical Applications*; Eichenberg, C., Ed.; InTech: Rijeka, Croatia, 2012; pp. 82–108.
5. Robillard, G.; Bouchard, S.; Fournier, T.; Renaud, P. Anxiety and presence during VR immersion: A comparative study of the reactions of phobic and non-phobic participants in therapeutic virtual environments derived from computer games. *Cyberpsychol. Behav.* **2003**, *6*, 467–476. [CrossRef] [PubMed]
6. Laforest, M.; Bouchard, S.; Crétu, A.-M.; Mesly, O. Inducing an anxiety response using a contaminated virtual environment: Validation of a therapeutic tool for obsessive-compulsive disorder. *Front. ICT* **2016**, *3*, 18. [CrossRef]
7. Kim, K.; Roh, D.; Kim, C.H.; Cha, K.R.; Rosenthal, M.Z.; Kim, S.I. Comparison of checking behavior in adults with or without checking symptoms of obsessive-compulsive disorder using a novel computer-based measure. *Comput. Methods Programs Biomed.* **2012**, *108*, 434–441. [CrossRef] [PubMed]
8. McCann, R.A.; Armstrong, C.M.; Skopp, N.A.; Edwards-Stewart, A.; Smolenski, D.J.; June, J.D.; Metzger-Abamukong, M.; Reger, G.M. Virtual reality exposure therapy for the treatment of anxiety disorders: An evaluation of research quality. *J. Anxiety Disord.* **2014**, *28*, 625–631. [CrossRef] [PubMed]
9. Chesham, R.K.; Malouff, J.M.; Schutte, N.S. Meta-analysis of the efficacy of virtual reality exposure therapy for social anxiety. *Behav. Chang.* **2018**, *35*, 1–15. [CrossRef]
10. Fernández-Alvarez, J.; Rozental, A.; Carlbring, P.; Colombo, D.; Riva, G.; Anderson, P.L.; Baños, R.M.; Benbow, A.A.; Bouchard, S.; Bretón López, J.M.; et al. Deterioration rates in virtual reality exposure therapy: An individual patient data level meta-analysis. *J. Anxiety Disord.* **2018**, in press. [CrossRef]
11. Morina, N.; Ijntema, H.; Meyerbroker, K.; Emmelkamp, P.M.G. Can virtual reality exposure therapy gains be generalized to real-life? A meta-analysis of studies applying behavioral assessments. *Behav. Res. Ther.* **2015**, *74*, 18–24. [CrossRef] [PubMed]
12. Tisseau, J. In vivo, in vitro, in silico, in virtuo. In Proceedings of the 1st Workshop on SMA in Biology at Meso or Macroscopic Scales, Paris, France, 2 July 2008; pp. 1–17.
13. Fuchs, P.; Moreau, G.; Guitton, P. *Virtual Reality: Concepts and Technologies*; CRC Press: New York, NY, USA, 2011.
14. Wiederhold, B. Virtual Reality in the 1990s: What Did We Learn? *Cyberpsychol. Behav.* **2004**, *3*, 311–314. [CrossRef]
15. Blade, R.A.; Padgett, M.L. Virtual Environments Standards and Terminology. In *Handbook of Virtual Environments: Design, Implementation, and Applications*; Stanney, K., Ed.; Lawrence Erlbaum Associates Publishers: Mahwah, NJ, USA, 2002; pp. 21–33.
16. Hirai, M.; Vernon, L.L.; Cochran, H. Exposure for phobias. In *Handbook of Exposure Therapies*; Richard, D.C.S., Lauterbach, D., Eds.; Academic Press: San Diego, CA, USA, 2007; pp. 247–270.
17. Garcia-Palacios, A.; Hoffman, H.G.; Kwon See, S.; Tsai, A.; Botella, C. Redefining therapeutic success with VR exposure therapy. *Cyberpsychol. Behav.* **2001**, *4*, 341–348. [CrossRef] [PubMed]
18. Dugas, M.J.; Gagnon, F.; Ladouceur, R.; Freeston, M.H. Generalized anxiety disorder: A preliminary test of a conceptual model. *Behav. Res. Ther.* **1998**, *36*, 215–226. [CrossRef]
19. Dugas, M.; Ladouceur, R. Treatment of GAD. Targeting intolerance of uncertainty in two types of worry. *Bheav. Modif.* **2000**, *24*, 635–657. [CrossRef] [PubMed]
20. Freeston, M.H.; Rhéaume, J.; Letarte, H.; Dugas, M.J.; Ladouceur, R. Why do people worry? *Personal. Individ. Differ.* **1994**, *17*, 791–802. [CrossRef]
21. Dugas, M.J.; Robichaud, M. *Cognitive-Behavioral Treatment for Generalized Anxiety Disorder*; Routledge: New York, NY, USA, 2007.

22. Goldman, N.; Dugas, M.J.; Sexton, K.A.; Gervais, N.J. The impact of written exposure on worry. *Behav. Modif.* **2007**, *31*, 512–538. [CrossRef] [PubMed]
23. Bouchard, S.; Côté, S.; Richard, D.C.S. Virtual reality applications for exposure. In *Handbook of Exposure Therapies*; Richard, D.C.S., Lauterbach, D., Eds.; Academic Press: Cambridge, MA, USA, 2007; pp. 347–388.
24. Dallaire, L.; Bouchard, S. Identification des thèmes récurrents d'exposition dans le cadre du traitement cognitif du TAG. Unpublished Manuscript. 2007.
25. Guitard, T.; Bouchard, S.; Bélanger, C. Exposure to standardized catastrophic scenarios with patients suffering from GAD. Presented at the 45th Annual Convention of the Association for Behavioral and Cognitive Therapy (ABCT), Toronto, ON, Canada, 10–13 November 2011.
26. Brown, T.A.; DiNardo, P.A.; Barlow, D.H. *Anxiety Disorders Interview Schedule for DSM-IV (ADIS-IV)*; Psychological Corporation: San Antonio, TX, USA, 1994.
27. Meyer, T.J.; Miller, M.L.; Metzger, R.L.; Borkovec, T.D. Development and validation of the Penn State Worry Questionnaire. *Behav. Res. Ther.* **1990**, *28*, 487–495. [CrossRef]
28. Ladouceur, R.; Freeston, M.H.; Dumont, J.; Letarte, H.; Rhéaume, J.; Gagnon, F.; Thibodeau, N. Penn State Worry Questionnaire: Validity and reliability of a French translation. *Can. Psychol.* **1992**, *33*, 236.
29. Molina, S.; Borkovec, T.D. The Penn State Worry Questionnaire: Psychometric properties and associated characteristics. In *Worrying: Perspectives on Theory, Assessment and Treatment*; Davey, G.C.L., Tallis, F., Eds.; John Wiley & Sons: New York, NY, USA, 1994; pp. 265–283.
30. Gosselin, P.; Langlois, F.; Freeston, M.H.; Ladouceur, R.; Dugas, M.J.; Pelletier, O. Le questionnaire d'évitement cognitif: Développement et validation auprès d'adultes et d'adolescents. *Journal de thérapie comportementale et cognitive* **2002**, *12*, 24–37.
31. Gosselin, P.; Dugas, M.J.; Ladouceur, R.; Freeston, M.H. Évaluation des inquiétudes: Validation d'une traduction française du Penn State Worry Questionnaire. *L'Encéphale* **2001**, *27*, 475–484. [PubMed]
32. Robillard, G.; Bouchard, S.; Renaud, P.; Cournoyer, L.G. Validation canadienne-française de deux mesures importantes en réalité virtuelle: l'Immersive Tendencies Questionnaire et le Presence Questionnaire. In Proceedings of the 25ième congrès de la Société Québécoise pour la Recherche en Psychologie (SQRP), Trois-Rivières, QC, Canada, 1–3 November 2002.
33. Witmer, B.G.; Singer, M.J. Measuring presence in virtual environments: A presence questionnaire. *Presence* **1998**, *7*, 225–240. [CrossRef]
34. Bouchard, S.; Robillard, G.; Renaud, P. Revising the factor structure of the Simulator Sickness Questionnaire. *Annu. Rev. Cyberther. Telemed.* **2007**, *5*, 117–122.
35. Kennedy, R.S.; Lane, N.E.; Berbaum, K.S.; Lilienthal, M.G. Simulator sickness questionnaire: An enhanced method for quantifying simulator sickness. *Int. J. Aviat. Psychol.* **1993**, *3*, 203–220. [CrossRef]
36. Gauthier, J.; Bouchard, S. Adaptation canadienne-française de la forme révisée du State-Trait Anxiety Inventory de Spielberger. *Revue Canadienne des Sciences du Comportement* **1993**, *25*, 559–578. [CrossRef]
37. Spielberger, C.D.; Gorsuch, R.L.; Lushene, R.; Vagg, P.R.; Jacobs, G.A. *Manual for the State-Trait Anxiety Inventory*; Consulting Psychologists Press: Palo Alto, CA, USA, 1983.
38. Gaudreau, P.; Sanchez, X.; Blondin, J.P. Positive and negative affective states in a performance-related setting: Testing the factorial structure of the PANAS across two samples of French-Canadian participants. *Eur. J. Psychol. Assess.* **2006**, *22*, 240–249. [CrossRef]
39. Watson, D.; Clark, L.; Tellegen, A. Development and validation of brief measures of positive and negative affect: The PANAS scales. *J. Personal. Soc. Psychol.* **1988**, *54*, 1063–1070. [CrossRef]
40. Bouvard, M. *Questionnaires et échelles d'évaluation de la personnalité*, 3rd ed.; Elsevier Masson: Paris, France, 2009.
41. Cohen, J. *Statistical Power Analysis for the Behavioral Sciences*; Lawrence Erlbaum Associates: London, UK, 1988.
42. Labbé Thibault, P.; Côté, G.; Gosselin, P. Effet de l'exposition en réalité virtuelle sur les symptômes du trouble d'anxiété généralisée. Ph.D. Thesis, Université de Sherbrooke, Sherbrooke, QC, Canada, 2017.
43. Repetto, C.; Gaggioli, A.; Pallavicini, F.; Cipresso, P.; Raspelli, S.; Riva, G. Virtual reality and mobile phones in the treatment of generalized anxiety disorders: A phase-2 clinical trial. *Pers. Ubiquitous Comput.* **2013**, *17*, 253–260. [CrossRef]

44. Katzman, M.; Bleau, P.; Blier, P.; Chokka, P.; Kjernisted, K.; Van Ameringen, M.; Antony, M.; Bouchard, S.; Brunet, A.; Flament, M.; et al. Canadian clinical practice guidelines for the management of anxiety, posttraumatic stress and obsessive-compulsive disorders. *BMC Psychiatry* **2014**, *14* (Suppl. 1), S1. [CrossRef] [PubMed]
45. Diemer, J.; Mühlberger, A.; Pauli, P.; Zwanzger, P. Virtual reality exposure in anxiety disorders: Impact on psychophysiological reactivity. *World J. Biol. Psychiatry* **2014**, *15*, 427–442. [CrossRef] [PubMed]

© 2019 by the authors. Licensee MDPI, Basel, Switzerland. This article is an open access article distributed under the terms and conditions of the Creative Commons Attribution (CC BY) license (http://creativecommons.org/licenses/by/4.0/).

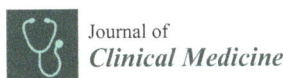

Review

The Benefits of emotion Regulation Interventions in Virtual Reality for the Improvement of Wellbeing in Adults and Older Adults: A Systematic Review

Jessica Isbely Montana [1,*], Marta Matamala-Gomez [1], Marta Maisto [1], Petar Aleksandrov Mavrodiev [1], Cesare Massimo Cavalera [2], Barbara Diana [1], Fabrizia Mantovani [1] and Olivia Realdon [1]

[1] Department of Human Sciences for Education, University of Milano-Bicocca, Piazza dell'Ateneo Nuovo 1, 20126 Milano, Italy; marta.matamalagomez@unimib.it (M.M.-G.); marta.maisto@unimib.it (M.M.); p.mavrodiev@campus.unimib.it (P.A.M.); barbara.diana@unimib.it (B.D.); fabrizia.mantovani@unimib.it (F.M.); olivia.realdon@unimib.it (O.R.)
[2] Department of Psychology, Catholic University of the Sacred Heart, Largo Gemelli 1, 20100 Milan, Italy; cesarem.cavalera@unicatt.it
* Correspondence: jessica.montana@unimib.it

Received: 24 December 2019; Accepted: 5 February 2020; Published: 12 February 2020

Abstract: The impact of emotion regulation interventions on wellbeing has been extensively documented in literature, although only in recent years virtual reality (VR) technologies have been incorporated in the design of such interventions, in both clinical and non-clinical settings. A systematic search, following the Preferred Reporting Items for Systematic Reviews and Meta-Analysis (PRISMA) guidelines, was therefore carried out to explore the state of the art in emotion regulation interventions for wellbeing using virtual reality. The literature on this topic was queried, 414 papers were screened, and 11 studies were included, covering adults and older adults. Our findings offer an overview of the current use of VR technologies for the enhancement of emotion regulation (ER) and wellbeing. The results are promising and suggest that VR-based emotion regulation training can facilitate the promotion of wellbeing. An overview of VR-based training interventions is crucial for better understanding how to use these tools in the clinical settings. This review offers a critical debate on the structure of such intervention protocols. It also analyzes and highlights the crucial role played by the selection of the objective and subjective wellbeing assessment measures of said intervention protocols.

Keywords: emotion regulation; treatment; wellbeing intervention; adults; virtual reality; systematic review

1. Introduction

Emotion is a cultural and psychobiological adaptation mechanism that allows each individual to react flexibly and dynamically to environmental contingencies [1]. Emotions give meaning to our lives, intensify our connection with others, inform us about our needs and feelings and motivate us to make changes [2]. Emotions are multidimensional phenomena. A single emotion comprises of: a cognitive appraisal, a physical sensation, an intention, a subjective "feeling", a motor response and, in most cases, an interpersonal component [1,3]. Emotion Regulation (ER) denotes a set of mental processes that influences which emotions we have when we have them and how we experience and express them [4,5]. It is a dynamic process inherent to the mental functioning of human beings, aimed at down or up-regulating positive or negative emotions in order to reach desirable states [6,7]. Emotion dysregulation denotes the undesired intensification or deactivation given by the person's inability to manage or process emotions effectively [8,9]. Hence, dealing with emotionally rich experience is part of emotional regulation. A priori assumptions as to whether any particular form of emotion regulation is necessarily good or bad do not exist [10]. This is important because it aims to avoid a type of distinction that is made, for example, between coping strategies, as more or less adaptive regardless of the context [11,12]. The emotion regulation process is a mechanism may be used to make things either better or worse, depending on the context. Furthermore, in line with a functionalist perspective, regulatory strategies may accomplish desired goals but still be perceived by others as maladaptive [13], such as when a child cries loudly in order to get attention [7]. A notable contextually adaptive ER strategies is reappraisal. It changes the way one thinks about a potential emotion-eliciting event. Another one is suppression, which changes the behavioral response to an emotion-eliciting event [14]. Thus, an effective situation-based regulation of emotions is necessary for permanent and enduring change in a person's growth and their social functioning [14] and subjective wellbeing [15–17].

The growing development of new technologies and the interest in applying them in the field of psychology have led to the development of novel virtual reality (VR) systems for neuro-rehabilitation [18], or the treatment of different mental health disorders [19–22] with the aim of generating an engaging and realistic virtual world in line with the needs of the person [23]. Applying virtual reality in psychology has one major advantage. It allows researchers and clinicians to create life-like experiences in a safe environment such as a laboratory or a clinical setting [24,25]. VR-based assessment and treatment allows to keep complex variables under control while preserving the complexity of real-life experiences [26]. In this regard, the use of virtual reality is promising, because it allows real-time measurement of cognitive, emotional, physiological, and behavioral responses in a variety of "real-life" situations while allow for full experimental control [27,28]. In particular, concerning the application of VR in clinical psychology, virtual environments have been widely used to enhance the use of successful ER strategies [29]. Since we know that effective ER strategies have led to several important outcomes regarding mental health, subjective and psychological wellbeing, and relationship satisfaction [30]. Hence, positive changes in emotion regulation are an important outcome in the mental health interventions and the development of new technologies such as VR systems could facilitate and increase the positive outcomes of such ER strategies [29,31]. It has been demonstrated that VR systems can evoke emotional experiences that lead to psychologically valuable changes through an enhanced sense of presence in a virtual environment [32–34]. Hence, it is possible to create a sense of 'being there' in a virtual world by designing highly immersive VR experiences, which rely on multisensory feedback mechanisms [35].

Health and wellbeing are considered as indispensable resources for societies and human development [36]. The World Health Organization (WHO) has placed wellbeing on the "Health 2020: the European policy for health and well-being" agenda as an objective for social progress [37]. Following the WHO, the purpose of the present review is to investigate whether wellbeing can be enhanced using new technologies, such as virtual reality. Specifically, the present systematic review aims to better understand the efficacy of emotion regulation interventions for wellbeing, by using virtual reality systems in adults and older adults without psychopathological conditions.

2. Method

A systematic review of the scientific literature has been performed to identify studies that reported VR-based ER interventions for wellbeing in healthy and clinical adults and examined the structure of their protocols. The methodology is presented in the following paragraphs.

2.1. Search Methodology

Preferred Reporting Items for Systematic Reviews and Meta-Analysis (PRISMA) guidelines were followed [38]. Four high-profile databases (PubMed, Embase, Scopus, and Web of Science) were used to perform the computer-based research on the 30th of September 2019 (see Table 1 and Figure 1). According to the PICO format, we defined the review question as, "is VR training for emotion regulation, compared to treatment as usual, effective in improving wellbeing in adults (with psychological distress)." We then proceeded with the definition of keywords for the search strategy.

The string used to carry out the search strategy was ("virtual reality" OR "virtual environment*" OR "digital intervention*" OR "digital technologies") AND ("emotion regulation" OR "affect regulation" OR "wellbeing"). The initial searches on the databases yielded 530 results. Duplicates were removed leaving 414 articles for further evaluation. Table 1 shows the details of the results for each keyword on each database used.

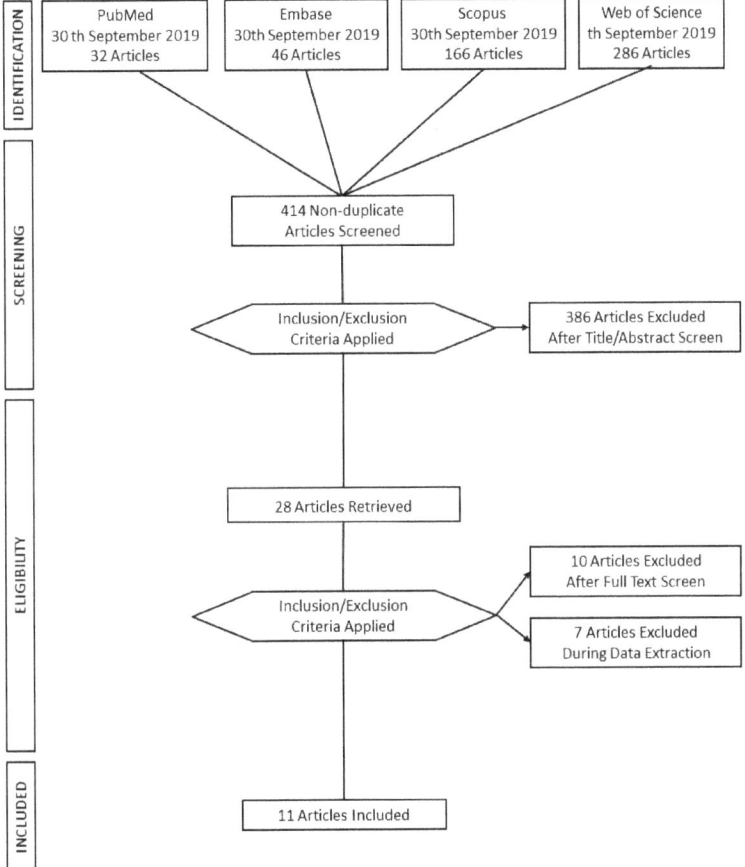

Figure 1. Flow Chart.

Table 1. Detailed search strategy.

"virtual reality" OR "virtual environment*" OR "digital intervention*" OR "digital technologies."						
AND	PubMed	Embase	Scopus	Web of Science		
"emotion regulation"	17	20	40	54		
"affect regulation"	1	1	2	104		
"wellbeing"	14	25	124	128		
Sub total	32	46	166	286	Total	530
					Without duplicates	414

2.2. Study Selection and Inclusion Criteria

This systematic review aims to evaluate the wellbeing and emotion regulation outcome of VR-based interventions in adults and older adults without psychopathological conditions. Given that the interest in VR continues to grow, researchers must focus on how the characteristics of VR systems and the different aspects of the training tasks could influence the intervention outcomes. The aim of this review is to provide knowledge and guide researchers in the selection of the most appropriate VR experience for ER interventions. The flow chart of the search strategy results, according to the PRISMA flow diagram, is shown in Figure 1.

The present systematic review considered randomized control trials, nonrandomized control trials, intervention studies, and case-control studies. Studies on emotion regulation for wellbeing with virtual reality (VR) devices in healthy or pathological adults and older adults presenting the following clinical conditions: traumatic brain injury, motor disabilities, tumor, chronic conditions (heart failure and chronic pain), were included. The review only includes studies in the English language, and which satisfied strict criteria for eligibility (research studies, interventions for adults and older adults, VR non-/semi-/immersive and immersive interventions, interventions for emotion regulation, interventions for wellbeing, healthy population and clinical patients but not psychopathological, wellbeing outcomes). Articles that treat psychopathological disorders such as post-traumatic stress disorder, phobias, substance abuse or psychosis, or lacked necessary information for review in the full-text or the abstract were excluded. Reviews, meeting abstracts, proceedings, poster presentations, notes, case reports, letters to the editor, assessment protocols, editorials, and other editorial materials were also excluded. Retrospective studies were not included because the area of interest requires post-intervention outcomes.

2.3. Risk of Bias Assessment

To assess the risk of bias, the reviewers followed the methods recommended by The Cochrane Collaboration Risk of Bias Tool [39] and the STROBE Statement [40]. Three reviewers (J.I.M., M.M.-G., and M.M.) independently assessed the risk of bias of each included study against key criteria: random sequence generation, allocation concealment, blinding of participants, personnel, and outcomes, incomplete outcome data, selective outcome reporting, and other sources of bias. The following judgments were used: low risk, high risk, or unclear (either lack of information or uncertainty over the potential for bias). Disagreements were resolved through consensus, and another author was consulted to resolve disagreements if necessary. In particular, the selected studies followed strict criteria in the methods, including presenting critical elements of study design, clearly defining all outcomes, describing the setting and relevant dates, including periods of recruitment and exposure, giving sources of data and details of methods of assessment (measurement).

3. Results

Of 414 non-duplicate studies, 386 did not fit the preliminary inclusion criteria; specifically, they did not present ER interventions for wellbeing using VR systems in adult and older adult populations. Subsequently, the full text of 28 articles was retrieved and the studies were evaluated for the specific inclusion criteria. Of 28 studies, only 11 passed the full-text screening phase, while 17 studies were excluded for the reasons that follow: Not interventions (= 4); Results not reported (= 7); Qualitative/descriptive study (= 6).

3.1. Flow Chart of the Results

The present flow chart (Figure 1) shows a summary of the research strategy (presented previously in Table 1), the methodology followed during the study selection process, and the final included studies according to PRISMA Guidelines.

3.2. Risk of Bias

The majority of the studies except one [41] exhibited a medium and high risk of bias across multiple dimensions. Table 2 shows the results for the risk of bias assessment. All the studies included in this review reported the sampling method [41–51], although the performance and the detection biases during blinding phase were unclear for all but one [41]. Concerning the outcomes, only two studies [45,47] presented high risk of bias for missing data handled appropriately or for missing a match between methods and results. Among other risks, we reported a high risk of bias for a small sample size with a range from eight to fifteen participants in three studies [44,47,51]. We considered important to report also a high risk of bias for lacking a control group for an experimental comparison [44,45,47–51]. Lastly, only one study addressed to patients have reported a high risk for no homogeneous clinical sample due to differences in clinical diseases and their specific characteristics [44] that might affect the interpretation of the outcomes. A clean sample is crucial for the comprehension of the ramification of disease on emotional functioning.

Table 2. Risk of bias assessment.

		Random Sequence Generation (Selection Bias)	Allocation Concealment (Selection Bias)	Blinding of Participants and Personal (Performance Bias)	Blinding of Outcome Assessment (Detection Bias)	Incomplete Outcome Data (Attrition Bias)	Selective Reporting (Reporting Bias)	Other Bias
Villani and Riva	2008	low	unclear	unclear	low	low	low	low
Tong et al.	2015	low	unclear	low	unclear	low	low	low
Cikajlo et al.	2016	high	high	unclear	unclear	low	low	high: small sample size/no control group/\no homogeneous clinical sample
Hasan et al.	2016	high	high	unclear	unclear	high	high	high: no control group
Konrad et al.	2016	low	low	low	low	low	low	low
Baez et al.	2017	low	low	unclear	low	low	low	low
Singh et al.	2017	high	high	unclear	unclear	high	high	high: small sample size/no control group
Weerdmeester et al.	2017	high	high	unclear	unclear	low	low	high: no control group
Bornioli et al.	2018	high	high	unclear	unclear	low	low	high: no control group
Lorenzetti et al.	2018	low	low	unclear	unclear	low	low	high: small sample size/no control group
Bornioli et al.	2019	high	high	unclear	unclear	low	low	high: no control group

NOTE: low (risk of bias); unclear (risk of bias); high (risk of bias).

3.3. Study Characteristics

Table 3 shows the studies' characteristics according to extraction parameters. Eleven studies were analyzed to understand the usefulness of interventions for emotion regulation and wellbeing using virtual reality (VR) systems. In order to accomplish the aims of the systematic review and to facilitate the understanding of the selected studies, the following clusters in Table 3 were considered: (1) Authors; (2) Year; (3) Sample (N); (4) Sample characteristics; (5) Mean age (SD or range); (6) VR Task; (7) VR Set-Up; (8) emotion regulation and/or wellbeing assessment; (9) Primary Outcomes.

Table 3. Study characteristics.

	Authors	Year	Sample (N)	Sample Characteristics	Mean Age (SD or Range)	VR Task	VR Set-Up	Emotion Regulation/Wellbeing Assessment	Primary Outcomes
1	Villani & Riva [42]	2008	60 healthy adults	Experimental Group (EG) for three conditions 45 persons (15 for each condition) Control Group (CG) without treatment 15 persons	Range 21–28 years old	relaxation environment + relaxing narrative	Immersive VR Condition: Sony Glastron PLM S-700 with a head-tracker: Intersense Intertrax2 and Semi-immersive DVD Condition: pc (Fujitsu Siemens AMILO Processor, Pentium 4	State-Trait Anxiety Inventory (STAI) and Positive And Negative Affect Scale (PANAS), Visual Analogue Scale (VAS), Coping Orientation to Problems Experienced Questionnaire (COPE) + Physiological Parameters: Respiration Rate, Respiration amplitude, Heart Rate, Heart Amplitude, Skin Conductance, Electromyography	Results show a significant reduction of anxiety and a significant improvement of positive emotional states—in particular, relaxation—measured through self-report questionnaires in all conditions. Physiological parameters showed some good changes related to respiration rate, heart rate, and skin conductance parameters, but less than expected.
2	Tong et al. [43]	2015	13 patients with chronic pain	EG, 7 patients (3 male, 4 female) CG, 6 patients (3 male, 3 female)	Range 35–55 years old (mean = 49, SD = 8.2)	The Virtual Meditative Walk (VMW) + biofeedback	Immersive environment stereoscopic VR display	Numerical Rating Scale (NRS) for Self-Report Pain Levels (values 0–10)	These findings indicate that the VMW (VR paired with biofeedback for MBSR training) was significantly more effective than MBSR alone at reducing reported pain levels among participants.
3	Cikajlo et al. [44]	2016	8 healthy adults and patients	EG, all participants (of which 4 patients with TBI, one with a brain tumor and 4 workers)	Healthy participants Range 27–40 years old; Patients participants Range 24–48 years old	Mindfulness-Based Stress Reduction VR	Immersive head-mounted display Samsung Gear + Samsung Smartphone S6 and Note4	Mindfulness Attention Awareness Scale (MASS) Satisfaction With Life Scale (SWLS) Mini-Mental State Examination Test (MMSE)	Patients achieved very high level of satisfaction (SWLS) at the end of the study. A slight increase in MASS score is also noticeable. All patients had MMSE score 30, except one; his score was 19 at the beginning, 29 at midterm and 26 at the end of the study.
4	Hasan et al. [45]	2016	27 older adults	Elderly group Seniors group	Older Range 70–98 years old; Seniors Range 50–70 years old	Weekly classes for developing ICT skills in aged-care facilities for 2 years	Non-immersive laptops and tablet	Social Care-Related Quality of Life (SCRQoL)	During the 2-year study, the participants developed various computing capabilities. The use of ICT appears to contribute positively to the wellbeing of the elderly: connection, self-worth/ esteem and personal development, productivity, occupation, self-sufficiency, being in control, and enjoyment.

Table 3. Cont.

	Authors	Year	Sample (N)	Sample Characteristics	Mean Age (SD or Range)	VR Task	VR Set-Up	Emotion Regulation/Wellbeing Assessment	Primary Outcomes
5	Konrad et al. [41]	2016	128 healthy adults	34 in the Incongruent Negative group, 34 in the Congruent Negative group, 30 in the Incongruent Positive and 30 in the Congruent Positive group	Range 18–62 years old (M = 24.56, SD = 8.87); 91 female and 37 male	MoodAdaptor—a technology-mediated reflection (TMR) application	Non-immersive mobile app	Subjective Happiness Scale, Satisfaction With Life Scale, Ryff Scales of Psychological Well-Being and Personal Emotion Scale Participants.	Autobiographical memory enhances positive mood through well-documented self-enhancement biases. Negative thoughts when in a positive mood reduced current mood, while positive thoughts, when in a negative mood, enhances it. Selecting incongruent memories is useful for mood-regulation and consequently for improving wellbeing.
6	Baez et al. [46]	2017	40 older adults	EG, 20 participants CG, 20 participants	Range 65–87 years old	OTAGO personalized exercise program for fall prevention	Non-immersive tablet-based application (10.1 inch Sony Xperia tablet)	Physical Activity Enjoyment Scale (PACES), Wellbeing Scale of the Multidimensional Personality Questionnaire (MPQ), Trans Theoretical Model of Behavior Change (TTM), R-UCLA Loneliness Scale	In virtual group exercising, people with lesser physical skills improve to the level of the more fit participants. These results suggest that: the online group could overcome some of the major issues reported in the literature in terms of the negative effect of group-exercising in the motivation of heterogeneous groups; and it helped reduce the effect of the initial skill level and motivation levels of participants in comparison to the trainees complying with the group norm.
7	Singh et al. [47]	2017	15 patients with motor disabilities	EG	Mean age = 22.7, SD = 4.2	Physical activity task	Non-immersive Nintendo® Wii Fit	Depressive, Anxiety and Stress Scales (DASS)	The results of this study demonstrated that there was a significant difference in psychological well-being and reaction time after intervention using interactive VR games.
8	Weerdmeester et al. [48]	2017	72 healthy adults	EG	Range 18–30 (M = 21.5, SD = 2.7); 31% male, 69% female	DEEP VR a virtual reality biofeedback game	Immersive VR game + biofeedback	Trier Social Stress Test	These results provide a promising outlook for using biofeedback video games such as DEEP to help individuals learn how to regulate their physiological arousal engagingly.

Table 3. *Cont.*

	Authors	Year	Sample (N)	Sample Characteristics	Mean Age (SD or Range)	VR Task	VR Set-Up	Emotion Regulation/Wellbeing Assessment	Primary Outcomes
9	Bornioli et al. [49]	2018	269 healthy adults and older adults	EG, all participants see five different environments	Range 18–67 years old (M = 31.69, SD = 13.63; 30.9% male, 69.1% females	exposure urban walking task	Non-immersive laptop	University of Wales Institute of Science and Technology Mood Adjective Checklist (UWIST MACL scale), Russell's circumplex model of affect, Perceived Restorativeness Scale—Short Version (PRS scale)	This study sets out to investigate the immediate psychological wellbeing benefits of virtual exposure to different urban walking settings. The results suggest that walking in high-quality urban settings can have positive outcomes and highlight the negative role of traffic and the potential benefits of historical elements in the affective walking experience.
10	Lorenzetti et al. [5]	2018	8 healthy adults	EG	Range 23–28 years old	exposure to an autumnal nature environment	Non-Immersive virtual environments in a brain-computer interface (BCI) + rtfMRI-NFB	Beck Depression Inventory (BDI), Trait Anxiety Inventory (STAI) and Positive And Negative Affect Scale (PANAS), Emotion Regulation Questionnaire (ERQ) and Satisfaction with Life Scale (SLS)	The study provides a novel proof of concept and demonstrates the feasibility of the implementation of rtfMRI-NFB using virtual environment and music to elicit the neural activity and measure the neural correlates of specific, complex emotional states. Real-time up-regulation of tenderness engaged the hypothalamic septum area and other regions previously implicated in positive affiliative emotions (i.e., medial frontal cortex and temporal pole, precuneus).
11	Bornioli et al. [50]	2019	384 healthy adults and older adults	EG, all participants see five different environments	Range 18–67 years old (M = 35.01, SD = 13.89)	exposure urban walking task	Non-immersive laptop	University of Wales Institute of Science and Technology Mood Adjective Checklist (UWIST MACL scale), Russell's Circumplex Model of Affect, Perceived Restorativeness Scale—Short Version (PRS scale)	Results show the crucial features that make walking positive for psychological wellbeing and encourage walking intentions are perceived safety, comfort, and moderate stimulation.

3.4. Interventions for Adults and Older Adults

3.4.1. Age Differences in Emotional Experience

Several investigations suggest that VR-based ER interventions in adults and older adults could improve quality of life, physical and mental health and delay the onset of health disorders [29,30]. We considered it appropriate to divide the discussion of the results according to the age of the participants. This choice was based on two reasons. Firstly, studies in the adult and elderly populations have different objectives. Secondly, emotional experience, expression and regulation, like all psychological phenomena, depend on physiological functioning [52]. In regard to the former, Gross et al. examine age differences in participants' reactions to negative events, showing that older people report better control over emotions compared to younger people [53]. In regard to the latter, studies observe how heart rate increases and epithelial cells lining the vasculature either constrict or dilate in response to an arousing stimulus. This overall pattern of reactivity is reduced among older adults [54,55].

In the following paragraphs we discuss the characteristics of the selected VR interventions. The examined studies focus on the use of virtual environments for intervening on emotion regulation processes, and for improving the wellbeing of healthy and clinical populations.

3.4.2. Interventions for Adults

The evaluated interventions for adults and older adults (specifically the VR characteristics, the VE content, and the aims) are summarized in Tables 4 and 5 respectively.

Table 4. Interventions for adults.

Study	Sample (Type of)	VE Characteristics	VE Content	Aim of the VR Task
Virtual Environments for Healthy Participants				
Villani and Riva (2008) [42]	Healthy	Immersive	A waterfall and a beach of an island	Relaxation and enhancement of wellbeing
Konrad et al. (2016) [41]	Healthy	Non-immersive	Mood survey	Mood regulation and improvement wellbeing
Weerdmester et al. (2017) [48]	Healthy	Immersive	Underwater world	Regulation of physiological arousal
Bornioli et al. (2018) [49]	Healthy	Non-immersive	Five different pedestrian areas of a town	Enhancement of behavioral activation for wellbeing
Lorenzetti et al. (2018) [51]	Healthy	Non-immersive	A landscape of hills and cornfields	Regulation of physiological arousal
Bornioli et al. (2019) [50]	Healthy	Non-immersive	Five different pedestrian areas of a town	Enhancement of behavioral activation for wellbeing
Virtual Environments for Patients				
Tong et al. (2015) [43]	Clinical	Immersive	Walk in the forest	Mindfulness-based stress reduction
Cikajlo et al. (2016) [44]	Clinical	Immersive	A river and a mountain landscape	Mindfulness-based stress reduction
Singh et al. (2017) [47]	Clinical	Non-immersive	Three different sports: tennis, bowling, and boxing	Enhancement of behavioral activation for wellbeing

Table 5. Interventions for older adults.

Study	Sample (Type of)	VE Characteristics	VE Content	Aim of the VR Task
Virtual Environments for healthy participants				
Hasan et al. (2016) [45]	Healthy	Non-immersive	Social networks, emails	Enhancement of ICT-skills for the improvement of social functioning and wellbeing
Baez et al. (2017) [46]	Healthy	Non-immersive	A gymnasium	Enhancement of behavioral activation for fall prevention and wellbeing
Bornioli et al. (2018) [49]	Healthy	Non-immersive	Five different pedestrian areas of a town	Enhancement of behavioral activation for wellbeing
Bornioli et al. (2019) [50]	Healthy	Non-immersive	Five different pedestrian areas of a town	Enhancement of behavioral activation for wellbeing

3.4.3. Virtual Environments (VE) for Healthy Participants

In what follows we examine studies conducted in a healthy population (see Table 4). Villani and Riva's used two virtual environments, one depicting a waterfall zone, and another an island, to induce relaxation and to enhance the wellbeing of participants [42]. The authors employed these scenarios in a way that maximizes the sense of presence in the virtual world, which enhances the quality of the relaxation experience [42]. Konrad et al. [41] used a web-based technology-mediated reflection (TMR) application, called the "Mood Adaptor," to enhance ER. It is a systematic process that reviews rich digital records of past personal experiences. According to the authors, such autobiographical memory approach increases general wellbeing. In their intervention, participants were instructed to write down a positive thought while experiencing a negative mood and, vice versa, write down a negative thought while in a positive mood [41]. Their explanation relies on the fact that recalling negative experiences while in a positive mood can update the emotional appraisal of the past experience and generate more adaptive perspectives of the past [41].

Weerdmeester et al. [48] have examined the role of self-efficacy in the context of biofeedback video games for ER. A pilot study was conducted with a VR videogame, called DEEP, which uses respiratory-based biofeedback to help individuals cope with stress and anxiety. Self-efficacy was found to be a significant predictor of physiological regulation, and a key factor in the improvement of mental wellbeing [48]. The biofeedback paradigm has been defined as a system in which physiological activity is continuously measured and fed back to the user in real-time [48]. In fact, in Weerdmeester's study, deep, calm breathing allows the player to stay afloat and move smoothly through the underwater world [48]. Lorenzetti et al. [51] have developed a neurofeedback game using a virtual environment as a medium to convey a real-time sensory feedback to participants, in association with ongoing tenderness, anguish, and neutral emotional states. Lorenzetti et al., used a BCI-based neurofeedback system in which neural activity was linked to the color of the virtual environment which allowed the real-time visualization of the fluctuation of emotional states. Orange denoted tenderness, purple—anguish, and natural light tones—neutral disposition [51]. Participants were instructed to experience tenderness or anguish as intensely as possible in the respective trials and to volitionally increase the intensity of their emotions [51].

Bornioli et al. [49,50] support the large amount of evidence concerning the benefits of walking in natural areas. In their two studies, participants had to walk, in five different, virtually recreate, sites: a pedestrianized historic environment in Bristol's Old Town, characterized by neoclassical buildings and cobbled paving; a pedestrianized modern environment in a complex of concrete and glass-fronted buildings; a pedestrianized environment with a mix of greenery and historic elements, framed by the Bristol Cathedral; a commercial road with high street retail outlets and cafés and a single-lane road with moderate moving traffic, constituted by cars and buses; and an urban park. The outcomes underline the crucial features that make walking positive for psychological wellbeing and encourage this activity [49,50].

3.4.4. Virtual Environments for Patients

Other studies have used interventions on patients with specific pathologies (see Table 4) using virtual environments to enhance ER and wellbeing. Two of these used Mindfulness-based Stress Reduction (MBSR) Meditation through virtual environments as a non-pharmacological approach to treating chronic disorders, such as chronic pain [43], and patients with traumatic brain injuries [44]. In both studies, virtual meditation was significantly more effective than MBSR alone in reducing reported levels of pain [43], and at making participants experience a higher level of satisfaction [44]. Singh et al. have examined the impact of VR games on psychological wellbeing, upper limb motor function and reaction time in adults with physical disabilities. In the latter study, wellbeing was a secondary outcome, as a positive consequence of the physical reactivation of the patient through the use of motor task games [47].

3.4.5. Virtual Reality Set-Up

The examined studies have used different types of virtual reality systems. Among the studies that have used immersive VR systems, two have selected a head-mounted display in combination with a smartphone and a head-tracker [42,44]. However, in the study conducted by Tong et al. [43], the authors used a Virtual Meditative Walk system that requires the use of a stereoscopic VR display. The display was mounted on a movable arm to ensure flexibility and to ease patient comfort. Furthermore, the authors used a sensor in order to track changing arousal levels, which are small clips put onto two of the patient's fingertips [43]. In the DEEP biofeedback game study, participants had to use deep diaphragmatic breathing in order to navigate in an immersive virtual environment through an enchanted underwater world [48]. The game used a customized controller belt that measures the expansion of the player's diaphragm and a head-mounted device. Other studies have used non-immersive devices, such as mobile applications [41]; Nintendo® Wii Fit [47]; tablet and laptop [45,46,49,50]; and computer-based interface (BCI) [51].

3.4.6. VR Interventions for Older Adults

Positive emotions have a significant influence on mental and physical health [56,57]. Their role in the wellbeing of the elderly has been established in numerous studies, so it is worthwhile exploring how older adults can improve the number of positive experiences in their daily lives [58]. Digital technologies are a powerful tool to enhance social inclusion [59], to support a more active and independent life in older adults and consequently to facilitate their wellbeing [60]. Among the presently investigated studies (see Table 5), Hasan et al. [45] and Baez et al. [46] proposed VR interventions focused on enhancing abilities for the maintenance of autonomy in older adults. Hasan et al. have carried out a two-year project on the social use of information and communications technologies (ICT) in older adults. The interventions consisted in the establishment of computer kiosks in aged-care facilities and weekly classes for developing ICT skills and enhancing wellbeing [45]. The study conducted by Baez et al. was a home-based intervention program to promote physical activity in older adults [46]. In this study, a web and a tablet application have been delivered to participants in order to enable and motivate them to participate in a home-based group training session, under the supervision of a human coach. After a period of eight weeks of training, participants presented a significant improvement of subjective wellbeing [46]. Moreover, in two studies conducted by Bornioli's and co-authors with older adults, the authors used a virtual walk intervention to enhance physical activity intentions and psychological wellbeing [49,50].

3.5. Outcome Measures for Wellbeing

3.5.1. Physiological Markers

A large number of studies among those evaluated in this systematic review use physiological markers as an objective measure to assess the effectiveness of VR interventions for ER. In this regard, the appraisal theory of Scherer allows us to explain the link between emotional states experienced by participants during interventions and their physiological responses [61,62]. In particular, this occurs due to the direct connections between stimulus evaluation check units and response modalities in the neuroendocrine system, autonomic nervous system, and somatic nervous system, independently from action tendencies [61]. A study by Villani and Riva (2008) [42] shows a significant reduction of anxiety, as well as a significant improvement of positive emotional states, in particular, relaxation, measured through physiological parameters that demonstrate good fluctuations of respiration rate, heart rate, and skin conductance. Tong et al. use a VR system that incorporates biofeedback mechanisms to support the learning of mindfulness practice [43]. This technological intervention may be an effective and long term non-pharmacological alternative to traditional pain management [43]. Furthermore, a biofeedback system has been used through the implementation of a belt for tracking the breathing rhythm of the participant during a VR relaxation-based game [48]. Biofeedback is an interesting mind-body therapy using electronic instruments to help individuals gain awareness and control over physiological processes [63]. Biofeedback is the process of measuring an individual's physiological activity such as brain activity, heart rate or breathing, and subsequently provide real-time information about this activity to the individual [64]. Through this feedback component, participants become more aware of their physiological activity, so they can learn how to gain control over it and improve their wellbeing [65,66].

In addition to the studies examined above, a neurofeedback (NFB) system had been used to enable the participants to regulate their brain activity, to enhance and recover emotional and cognitive capacity and to improve their underlying neurobiology [51]. Neurofeedback makes use of electroencephalography (EEG) biofeedback to guide participants in modifying their cortical activity, alter their states of consciousness, and affect cortically mediated physical and psychological functioning [67]. Novel forms of NFB, such as ones based on real-time functional magnetic resonance imaging (rtfMRI), hold a still vastly unexplored potential for complex technological applications, such as the currently discussed VR-based ER interventions [68].

3.5.2. Wellbeing Scales Outcomes

Given the primary objective of the present manuscript, in Table 6 we summarized an overview of the main wellbeing measures used in the evaluated studies. Several wellbeing measures were used as pre- and post-intervention measures: the State and Trait Anxiety Inventory (STAI) to evaluate anxiety levels [42,51]; the Beck Depression Inventory (BDI) to assess depression levels [51]; the Depressive, Anxiety and Stress Scales (DASS) to assess state anxiety and depression levels [47]; the Positive And Negative Affect Scale (PANAS) to measure the positive and negative affect through 10 positive and 10 negative moods/emotion adjectives [42,51]; the Coping Orientation to Problems Experienced Questionnaire (COPE) assessed the different strategies commonly activated in daily problem solving [42]. Results show a significant reduction of anxiety [42,47,51], and a significant improvement of positive emotional states [42,51]. Given that there is no universal measure of wellbeing, Konrad et al. include both hedonic (e.g., pleasure, satisfaction), and eudaimonic (e.g., meaning, personal growth) scales to triangulate different measurement perspectives: Subjective Happiness Scale, Satisfaction With Life Scale, and Ryff Scales of Psychological Wellbeing [41]. Moreover, positive intervention outcomes have been measured in both clinical and healthy populations with the Mindfulness Attention Awareness Scale (MASS), and the Satisfaction With Life Scale (SWLS) [44]. Tong et al., did not use a scale to monitor changes in mindfulness awareness, rather, they used the pain level and biofeedback data as an objective wellbeing measure [43]. However, there are no subjective wellbeing measures in that study [43]. Another interesting measure that has been used in the reviewed studies is the wellbeing scale of the Multidimensional Personality Questionnaire (MPQ) that underlined improvements in both groups with no significant difference between groups in social wellbeing outcomes [46].

Table 6. Wellbeing Measure Scales Description.

Scale	Description of Measure
State-Trait Anxiety Inventory (STAI)	A commonly used measure of trait and state anxiety. It can be used in clinical settings to diagnose anxiety and to distinguish it from depressive syndromes. Form Y, is its most popular version. It has 20 items for assessing trait anxiety and 20 for state anxiety. All items are rated on a 4-point scale (e.g., from "Almost Never" to "Almost Always"). Higher scores indicate greater anxiety.
Positive And Negative Affect Scale (PANAS)	A self-report questionnaire that consists of two 10-item scales to measure both positive and negative affect. Each item is rated on a 5-point scale of 1 (not at all) to 5 (very much).
Coping Orientation to Problems Experienced Questionnaire (COPE)	A self-reported questionnaire developed to assess a broad range of coping responses with a score on a 4-point scale (e.g., from "I usually don't do this at all" to "I usually do this a lot"). There are two main components to the COPE inventory: problem-focused coping and emotion-focused coping.
Mindfulness Attention Awareness Scale (MASS)	A 15-item scale designed to assess a core characteristic of mindfulness, namely, a receptive state of mind in which attention, informed by a sensitive awareness of what is occurring in the present, simply observes what is taking place.
Satisfaction With Life Scale (SWLS)	A 5-item scale designed to measure global cognitive judgments of one's life satisfaction (not a measure of either positive or negative affect). Participants indicate how much they agree or disagree with items on a 7-point scale (e.g., from 1 "strongly disagree" to 7 "strongly agree").
Subjective Happiness Scale	A 4-item self-report measure developed to assess an individual's overall happiness as measured through self-evaluation on a 7-point Likert-type scale.
Ryff Scales of Psychological Well-Being	A psychometric inventory in which respondents rate statements on a scale of 1 to 6 (e.g., from 1 "strong disagreement" to 6 "strong agreement"). It is based on six factors: autonomy, environmental mastery, personal growth, positive relations with others, purpose in life, and self-acceptance. Higher total scores indicate higher psychological well-being.
Wellbeing scale of the Multidimensional Personality Questionnaire (MPQ)	A personality test meant to measure personality that gives ratings on four broad traits: Positive Emotional Temperament, Negative Emotional Temperament, Constraint, and Absorption. High scorers on the specific wellbeing scale describe: having a cheerful happy disposition; feeling good about themselves; seeing a bright future ahead; being optimists; living interesting, exciting lives; enjoying the things they are doing.
Depressive, Anxiety and Stress Scales (DASS)	A 42-item self report instrument designed to measure the three related negative emotional states of depression, anxiety and tension/stress. The rating is based on a 0-3 point scale (e.g., from 0 "Did not apply to me at all" to 1 "Applied to me very much or most of the time").
Emotion Regulation Questionnaire (ERQ)	A 10-item scale designed to measure respondents' tendency to regulate their emotions in two ways: (1) Cognitive Reappraisal and (2) Expressive Suppression. Respondents answer each item on a 7-point Likert-type scale (e.g., from 1 "strongly disagree" to 7 "strongly agree").
University of Wales Institute of Science and Technology Mood Adjective Checklist (UWIST MACL scale)	A scale that measures self-reported mood in the dimensions of energetic arousal, tense arousal, and hedonic tone.

The Social Care-Related Quality of Life (SCRQoL) Scale was administered to track changes in the quality of life of older users to their daily routines, based on the outcome domains of social care-related quality of life identified in the Adult Social Care Outcomes Toolkit (ASCOT) [45]. Moreover, Weerdmester and colleagues selected the Trier Social Stress Test, a tool for investigating psychobiological stress responses [48]. Pre- and post-wellbeing assessments used the stress and hedonic tone measures based on the University of Wales Institute of Science and Technology Mood Adjective Checklist scale (UWIST MACL), to measure different stress-related states (nervous, tense, relaxed, calm), and the hedonic tone (happy, content, sad, sorry) [49,50].

4. Discussion

This review aimed to investigate how emotion regulation interventions using virtual reality (VR) systems can enhance the wellbeing in healthy and clinical adults and older adults, without presenting psychopathological conditions. In recent years there is a growing interest in the use of advanced technologies in supporting wellbeing and promoting health [34], following emerging evidence that technology can increase emotional, psychological and social wellbeing [69]. Technological approaches appear to be more advantageous in terms of intensity and duration of treatment, costs, and usefulness in the continuity-of-care [70,71]. Considering the multifaceted construct of wellbeing, in what follows, we strive to unpack the complex picture provided by the results of the hereby examined studies. This complexity emerges from the different functional aims of the studies, employed in pursuit of wellbeing enhancement. Three studies (27%) were developed for relaxation or following the Mindfulness-Based Stress Reduction (MBSR) protocol [42–44]; two studies (18%) used biofeedback or neurofeedback as peripherical technique for the regulation of physiological arousal [48,51]; one study (9%) used survey forms for a mood regulation and improvement wellbeing [41]; four studies (37%) intended to encourage a participants' behavioral and physical activation in order to enhance their subjective wellbeing through outdoor [49,50] or indoor activities [46,47]; one study (9%) aimed to enhance ICT-skills of elderly people in support of their social functioning and wellbeing [45].

In the examined studies, virtual reality has been used in different ways to promote wellbeing in healthy and clinical populations. Some authors used mindfulness as a non-pharmacological approach to manage participant's emotion regulation abilities and to enhance their wellbeing [43,44]. It has been demonstrated that immersive VR can be used as a powerful pain control technique to manage and modulate pain in healthy and clinical populations [72–75]. This is in line with the study conducted by Tong et al., in which the authors found that the use of an immersive VR combined with a biofeedback system, can be a helpful approach for managing chronic pain on a long-term scale [43].

In the present review, the combination of VR with biofeedback systems was particularly interesting. In recent years the development and use of game-based biofeedback to promote physical and mental wellbeing is growing [76–78]. An example, is the study of Weerdmester et al., in which an intervention based on the VR game "Deep", combined with a biofeedback system, highlighted positive and promising outcomes to help individuals cope with stress and anxiety [48]. This technique relies on visual and auditory feedback to guide participants in becoming more aware of their breathing and incentivizes the adoption of a more calm and relaxed breathing pattern [66,79,80]. Furthermore, promising results of game-based biofeedback have been found for emotion regulation and the treatment of stress and anxiety [81].

Neurofeedback (NFB) is a type of biofeedback which facilitates the real-time voluntary regulation of brain activity through a brain-computer interface [67,68]. Lorenzetti et al. [51] showed that NFB has promising effects on enhancing behavior, cognitive and emotional processes in healthy subjects. Performing exercises in an immersive VR environment is shown to decrease depression, anxiety, and stress [82]. Intervention outcomes, are in accordance with the literature, highlight a reduction in anxiety scales [42,47,51], and an improvement of positive emotional states [41,42,44,49–51].

For instance, Singh et al. [47] suggest that interactive VR games can be used as an exercise tool to improve psychological wellbeing and reaction time among adults with physical disabilities, for whom the use of technology may promote adherence, motivation, and participation in physical activity and exercise programs [46,47,49,50]. Positive results can also be seen in older adults, as demonstrated in the intervention program proposed by Baez et al. [46]. This intervention program was designed to promote physical activity in older adults, either in a group or in a home-based setting, showing equivalent health outcomes for both groups, but different results when considering adherence [46]. These interventions point out the importance of immediate wellbeing responses, in that, positive affect can be beneficial to long-term health [57,83]. A large number of studies have demonstrated the association of regular physical activity with positive outcomes for improving health and wellbeing conditions [84,85]. Moreover, home-based intervention programs aimed at promoting physical activity in older adults, either in a group or individually, have demonstrated the potential to improve health and functional performance [86]. The social wellbeing in the elderly is another issue that requires attention. Hasan et al. identified the complexity of this problem domain and engaged older adults through activities aimed at enhancing their ability to remain productive [45].

These results are an important outcome for wellbeing. The literature demonstrates that VR-based interventions are as effective as traditional ones in the treatment of different mental disorders, but can achieve positive outcomes in less time [87]. The difference between VR-based interventions and treatment as usual (TAU) remains to be clarified. Some of the currently examined studies, highlights a significative difference between the experimental and the control group [43,46], but further randomized controlled trials are required to achieve a better understanding of the effectiveness of VR compared to non-VR interventions.

Why are VR-based ER interventions important for wellbeing? To address this question, we have to consider several things. Emotions can be transient phenomena which emerge from momentary situational goals and subside with the short-term achievement of such goals [88]. Emotions can also derive from long-term goals and enduring values concerning health, close relationships, and important work-related projects [89]. Hence, knowing the specific antecedents of specific emotions is crucial to better understand the complexity and potential of technological ER interventions.

The present review underlines that virtual reality systems evoke a general positive emotion and could promote a healthy life [90] and an optimal state of functioning such as flow [91]. The sense of flow in VR is evoked when the user is immersed in a highly rewarding activity, accompanied by a high sense of control [92,93]. Flow can subsequently promote the feeling of immersion in the virtual environment [94]. Four studies among those investigated, have used an immersive VR system and have emphasized the importance of the immersion degree in a virtual environment. These studies used a head-mounted display (HMD) through which participants can be immersed in an interactive virtual reality scenario [19]. Through the HMD, the experimenter may provide different sensory input, as well as synchronize participants' movements with the generated virtual feedback (e.g., avatar movements, or reaching virtual objects) [20]. In order to increase the sense of immersion, feedback across different sensory channels is provided, such as, visual, acoustic, and tactile. This can also be achieved through the use of input tools such as trackers, gloves and other controllers, that allow to continuously monitor the position and movements of the users, and synchronize them with the VR interactions [32,95]. From a psychological point of view, at the basis of the feeling of immersion in VR is the sense of "presence," defined as the psychological sensation of "being there" in the virtual scene instead of in the physical and real environment [28,35,96]. The sense of presence has also been defined as the "feeling of being in a world that exists outside of self" [93,94]. The sense of presence in a virtual environment is given not only by the realism of its graphics but also by subjective characteristics, such as the potential of a given virtual scenario to elicit certain emotional responses [42]. In this way, a VR-based intervention can modify personal experiences by inspiring users to try new things [97] and allow them to modify habitual emotional responses to specific situations [7,98]. A VR system has the potential for a laboratory vs. everyday functioning rapprochement. Virtual environments allow to immerse participants in digitally recreated real-world activities which can be enacted in the safety of the laboratory setting [99]. The ability of VR systems to reproduce the complexity of real-life situations is a peculiar element for ER interventions. Due to this peculiarity, the user can be immersed in a complex virtual environment that requires the use of a complex set of ER strategies that form a dynamic pattern. An ER strategy does not have to be unique and universal, but in order to be useful and transferable to daily life, it must be adaptive and generalizable across situations [6,100]. In this sense, the use of virtual reality is promising, because it allows the user to learn complex ER strategies and, potentially, experience them in different environments similar to the real world. Lastly, a VR system provides experimental control and dynamic presentation of stimuli in ecologically valid scenarios [18,26,27,71,101]. This can be done by measuring the real-time cognitive, emotional, physiological and behavioural responses in a variety of life-like virtual situations [28].

The obtained results show that interventions using virtual reality systems allow people to change or improve their ER strategies. One such strategy is "situation selection" [4]. It is an antecedent-focused strategy that examines all the actions that we execute before the emotional response has become fully active and has modified behavioral or physiological responses and selects the best action [55]. Furthermore, technology can provide different options to appraise emotional stimuli, hence different cognitive appraisals pertaining to the same potential trigger and eventually different emotional responses [7]. In regard to patients with specific disorders, VR interventions can facilitate the approach to rehabilitation therapy by training more contextually adaptive ER strategies such as "reappraisal", which lead to better short-term affective, cognitive, and social consequences, compared to less adaptive strategies such as "suppression" [14]. VR systems improve patients ability to regulate the emotions that accompany their everyday experiences with their health condition [29]. Such targeted interventions that facilitate a reappraisal, can elicit a subsequent "cognitive change" [7,55]. This change refers to selecting what meaning people attach to the specific intervention [4,7]. External variables that are properties of the stimulus can influence the choice of emotion regulation strategy; in fact, reappraisal affordances, defined as the opportunities for re-interpretating a stimulus, which are inherent to the stimulus itself, can greatly shape such choices [13]. The personal meaning assigned to a specific situation is crucial for establishing habitual experiential, behavioral and physiological responses which repeat in that same situation [5].

One of the main aims of emotion regulation interventions is to modify the emotional responses of the subjects to one specific situation [102]. The outcome of the interventions reviewed in this article could be interpreted according to "The process model of emotion regulation" of Gross. According to Gross reappraisal-like processes could influence emotional responses. Efforts to down-regulate emotion through reappraisal alters the trajectory of the entire emotional response, leading to lesser experiential, behavioral, and physiological responses [7,102]. An example of this process is found in the studies that used Mindfulness-Based Stress Reduction (MBSR) protocol in virtual reality to minimize the negative emotional impact in patients with traumatic brain injuries [44] and the Meditative Virtual Walk for patients with chronic pain [43]. Mindfulness is a core skill of Dialectical Behavioral Therapy employed in the treatment of emotion dysregulation. It consists in observing, describing, and "allowing" emotions to flow without judging them or trying to inhibit them. Mindfulness is hypothesized to influence the habitual or automatic response to emotional behaviors and their associated appraisals. Hence, in comparison to Gross's Model, mindfulness may alter automatic response tendencies by altering the habitual approach or avoidance response to that of a non-judgemental awareness of the emerging emotions [103]. During the interventions the individual can reappraise the emotional responses to their health conditions. This type of reappraisal can also be seen in the intervention conducted by Konrad et al. [41]. In this intervention, subjects were asked to describe a negatively appraised past experience while in a positive mood. This was proven to update their emotional response to the past experience, encouraging the emergence of more adaptive perspectives [104,105]. Finally, virtual reality tools promote the sense of environmental mastery and the continued development of competence and self-knowledge, both in clinical and non-clinical populations [106,107]. However, there is a major difference between both populations. In a healthy population, an ER intervention can cultivate more adaptive, for daily life, ER strategies. In a clinical population, ER interventions are useful for increasing the patient's ability to handle their specific pathology.

In conclusion, the choice of wellbeing measures is essential to assessing the efficacy of the intervention. Humans do not act mechanically, but rather according to their subjective interpretation of the world. Hence, objective indicators alone may not be sufficient to hedge the several conceptualizations of wellbeing [108]. It is fundamental to gain knowledge about the subjective interpretations of emotional states. This can happen by directly asking people about their emotions, perceptions, and evaluations [108]. Currently, wellbeing is not a clearly defined concept and the present review shows that several ways to measure wellbeing exist [36]. Despite that difficulty, it is important for studies to clarify the theoretical framework of wellbeing in which the intervention intends to operate. The choice of the theoretical framework can better guide the design of the intervention and the choice of more adequate wellbeing measures.

5. Conclusions

In conclusion, the results of this systematic review show that technology can improve the ability of people to handle emotionally-rich life situations by training more contextually adaptive emotion regulation strategies.

The use of virtual reality in this sense is promising because it allows the user to learn complex ER strategies in the context of life-like digital environments. VR interventions can modify the user's ER by inspiring new actions, allowing for the modification of the emotional response across a reappraisal of emotional stimuli, and subsequently, memorizing the re-evaluated experience. Finally, virtual reality is a tool that fosters a sense of environmental mastery, and, a feeling of personal growth and autonomy.

The literature in this field is going in an interesting direction, and we recommend some future steps based on the findings of this systematic review, for future design, implementation, and evaluation of VR-based ER interventions in healthy adults and older adults. The results of this systematic review underly the importance of an appropriate assessment and highlight the positive effects of assessing both subjective and objective measures in future studies to fully evaluate the efficacy of VR interventions for ER. The results from both subjective and objective measures will provide an overall and complete frame of the efficacy of VR interventions for ER. Finally, future research should aim to investigate the underlying mechanisms and factors that may contribute to the effectiveness of biofeedback systems when using VR interventions for ER in order to maximize their positive therapeutic outcomes.

Author Contributions: Conceptualization O.R. and J.I.M.; methodology, J.I.M. and M.M.-G.; studies selection, J.I.M., M.M.-G. and M.M.; data curation, J.I.M., M.M.-G. and M.M.; writing—original draft preparation, J.I.M.; writing—review and editing, O.R., M.M.-G., B.D., C.M.C. and P.A.M.; final editing of English P.A.M.; supervision, O.R. and F.M.; project management F.M. All authors were involved in a critical revision of the manuscript for important intellectual content. All the authors approved the final version of the manuscript for submission. All authors have read and agreed to the published version of the manuscript.

Funding: The study was co-funded by Lombardy Region within the Project named SIDERA^B "Sistema Integrato DomiciliarE e Riabilitazione Assistita al Benessere" (Announcement POR-FESR 2014–2020).

Conflicts of Interest: The authors declare no conflict of interest.

References

1. Scherer, K.R. Emotions are emergent processes: They require a dynamic computational architecture. *Philos. Trans. R. Soc. B Biol. Sci.* **2009**, *364*, 3459–3474. [CrossRef] [PubMed]
2. Leahy, R.; Tirch, D.; Napolitano, L. Why is emotion regulation important? *Psychother. Aust.* **2012**, *19*, 68–81.
3. Beck, A.T. *Cognitive Therapy and the Emotional Disorders*, 1st ed.; International Universities Press: Madison, CT, USA, 1976.
4. Gross, J.J. The Emerging Field of Emotion Regulation: An Integrative Review. *Rev. Gen. Psychol.* **1998**, *2*, 271–299. [CrossRef]
5. Gross, J.J. Emotion regulation: Affective, cognitive, and social consequences. *Psychophysiology* **2002**, *39*, 281–291. [CrossRef] [PubMed]
6. Gross, J.J. Emotion regulation: Current status and future prospects. *Psychol. Inq.* **2015**, *26*, 1–26. [CrossRef]
7. Gross, J.J.; Thompson, R.A. Emotion Regulation: Conceptual Foundations. In *Handbook of Emotion Regulation*; The Guilford Press: New York, NY, USA, 2007; pp. 3–24.
8. Cole, P.M.; Michel, M.K.; Teti, L.O.D. The Development of Emotion Regulation and Dysregulation: A Clinical Perspective. *Monogr. Soc. Res. Child Dev. Dev. Emot. Regul. Biol. Behav. Consid.* **1994**, *59*, 73–100. [CrossRef]
9. Lazarus, R.S.; Folkman, S. *Stress, Appraisal, and Coping*; Springer Publishing Company: Berlin/Heidelberg, Germany, 1984.
10. Thompson, R.A.; Calkins, S.D. The double-edged sword: Emotional regulation for children at risk. *Dev. Psychopathol.* **1996**, *8*, 163–182. [CrossRef]
11. Parker, J.D.A.; Endler, N.S. Coping and defense: A historical overview. In *Handbook of Coping: Theory, Research, Applications*; John Wiley & Sons: Oxford, UK, 1996; pp. 3–23.
12. Folkman, S.; Lazarus, R.S. Coping as a Mediator of Emotion. *J. Personal. Soc. Psychol.* **1988**, *54*, 466–475. [CrossRef]
13. Suri, G.; Sheppes, G.; Young, G.; Abraham, D.; McRae, K.; Gross, J.J. Emotion regulation choice: The role of environmental affordances. *Cogn. Emot.* **2018**, *32*, 963–971. [CrossRef]
14. John, O.P.; Gross, J.J. Healthy and unhealthy emotion regulation: Personality processes, individual differences, and life span development. *J. Personal.* **2004**, *72*, 1301–1334. [CrossRef]

15. Greenberg, L.S. *Emotion-Focused Therapy*; Theories of Psychotherapy; American Psychological Association: Worcester, MA, USA, 2011.
16. Lucas, R.E.; Diener, E. Subjective Well-Being. In *Handbook of Emotion*; T.G. Press: New York, NY, USA, 2008; pp. 471–484.
17. Diener, E.; Suh, E.M.; Lucas, R.E.; Smith, H.L. Subjective Well-Being: Three Decades of Progress. *Psychol. Bull.* **1999**, *125*, 276–302. [CrossRef]
18. Montana, J.I.; Tuena, C.; Serino, S.; Cipresso, P.; Riva, G. Neurorehabilitation of Spatial Memory Using Virtual Environments: A Systematic Review. *J. Clin. Med.* **2019**, *8*, 1516. [CrossRef] [PubMed]
19. Mishkind, M.C.; Norr, A.M.; Katz, A.C.; Reger, G.M. Review of Virtual Reality Treatment in Psychiatry: Evidence Versus Current Diffusion and Use. *Curr. Psychiatry Rep.* **2017**, *19*. [CrossRef] [PubMed]
20. Clus, D.; Larsen, M.E.; Lemey, C.; Berrouiguet, S. The use of virtual reality in patients with eating disorders: Systematic review. *J. Med. Internet Res.* **2018**, *20*, 1–9. [CrossRef]
21. Wiederhold, B.K.; Riva, G.; Gutiérrez-Maldonado, J. Virtual Reality in the Assessment and Treatment of Weight-Related Disorders. *Cyberpsychol. Behav. Soc. Netw.* **2016**, *19*, 67–73. [CrossRef]
22. Rus-Calafell, M.; Garety, P.; Sason, E.; Craig, T.J.K.; Valmaggia, L.R. Virtual reality in the assessment and treatment of psychosis: A systematic review of its utility, acceptability and effectiveness. *Psychol. Med.* **2018**, *48*, 362–391. [CrossRef]
23. Riva, G.; Gaggioli, A.; Villani, D.; Preziosa, A.; Morganti, F.; Corsi, R.; Faletti, G.; Vezzadini, L. NeuroVR: An open source virtual reality platform for clinical psychology and behavioral neurosciences. *Stud. Health Technol. Inf.* **2007**, *125*, 394–399.
24. Riches, S.; Garety, P.; Rus-Calafell, M.; Stahl, D.; Evans, C.; Sarras, N.; Yeboah, K.; Valmaggia, L. Using Virtual Reality to Assess Associations Between Paranoid Ideation and Components of Social Performance: A Pilot Validation Study. *Cyberpsychol. Behav. Soc. Netw.* **2019**, *22*, 51–59. [CrossRef]
25. Valmaggia, L. The use of virtual reality in psychosis research and treatment. *World Psychiatry* **2017**, *16*, 245–246. [CrossRef]
26. Parsons, T.D.; Carlew, A.R.; Magtoto, J.; Stonecipher, K. The potential of function-led virtual environments for ecologically valid measures of executive function in experimental and clinical neuropsychology. *Neuropsychol. Rehabil.* **2017**, *27*, 777–807. [CrossRef]
27. Serino, S.; Baglio, F.; Rossetto, F.; Realdon, O.; Cipresso, P.; Parsons, T.D.; Cappellini, G.; Mantovani, F.; De Leo, G.; Nemni, R.; et al. Picture Interpretation Test (PIT) 360°: An Innovative Measure of Executive Functions. *Sci. Rep.* **2017**, *7*, 1–10. [CrossRef] [PubMed]
28. Bohil, C.J.; Alicea, B.; Biocca, F.A. Virtual reality in neuroscience research and therapy. *Nat. Rev. Neurosci.* **2011**, *12*. [CrossRef]
29. Colombo, D.; Fernández-álvarez, J.; Palacios, A.G.; Cipresso, P.; Botella, C.; Riva, G. New technologies for the understanding, assessment, and intervention of emotion regulation. *Front. Psychol.* **2019**, *10*. [CrossRef]
30. Villani, D.; Carissoli, C.; Triberti, S.; Marchetti, A.; Gilli, G.; Riva, G. Videogames for Emotion Regulation: A Systematic Review. *Games Health J.* **2018**, *7*, 85–99. [CrossRef] [PubMed]
31. Kompus, K. Virtual-reality-assisted therapy in patients with psychosis Title. *Lancet Psychiatry* **2018**, *5*, 189–191. [CrossRef]
32. Riva, G.; Baños, R.M.; Botella, C.; Mantovani, F.; Gaggioli, A. Transforming experience: The potential of augmented reality and virtual reality for enhancing personal and clinical change. *Front. Psychiatry* **2016**, *7*, 1–14. [CrossRef] [PubMed]
33. Baños, R.M.; Etchemendy, E.; Mira, A.; Riva, G.; Gaggioli, A.; Botella, C. Online positive interventions to promote well-being and resilience in the adolescent population: A narrative review. *Front. Psychiatry* **2017**, *8*. [CrossRef]
34. Schek, E.J.; Mantovani, F.; Realdon, O.; Dias, J.; Paiva, A.; Schramm-Yavin, R.; Pat-Horenczyk, S. Positive Technologies for Promoting Emotion Regulation Abilities in Adolescents. In *Lecture Notes of the Institute for Computer Sciences, Social Informatics and Telecommunications Engineering*; Springer: Berlin/Heidelberg, Germany, 2016; pp. 169–174.
35. Sanchez-Vives, M.V.; Slater, M. Opinion: From presence to consciousness through virtual reality. *Nat. Rev. Neurosci.* **2005**, *6*, 332–339. [CrossRef]

36. Feller, S.C.; Castillo, E.G.; Greenberg, J.M.; Abascal, P.; Van Horn, R.; Wells, K.B.; University of California, Los Angeles Community Translational Science Team. Emotional well-being and public health: Proposal for a model national initiative. *Public Health Rep.* **2018**, *133*, 136–141. [CrossRef]
37. Vik, M.H. Measuring subjective well-being for policy purposes: The example of well-being indicators in the WHO 'Health 2020' framework. *J. Scand. Public Health* **2018**, *46*, 279–286. [CrossRef]
38. Moher, D.; Liberati, A.; Tetzlaff, J.; Altman, D.G.; Grp, P. Preferred Reporting Items for Systematic Reviews and Meta-Analyses: The PRISMA Statement (Reprinted from Annals of Internal Medicine). *Phys. Ther.* **2009**, *89*, 873–880. [CrossRef] [PubMed]
39. Higgins, J.; Green, S. *Cochrane Handbook for Systematic Reviews of Interventions*; Version 5; John Wiley & Sons: Hoboken, NJ, USA, 2011.
40. Von Elm, E.; Altman, D.G.; Egger, M.; Pocock, S.J.; Gøtzsche, P.C.; Vandenbroucke, J.P. The Strengthening the Reporting of Observational Studies in Epidemiology (STROBE) statement: Guidelines for reporting observational studies. *Lancet* **2007**, *370*, 1453–1457. [CrossRef]
41. Konrad, A.; Tucker, S.; Crane, J.; Whittaker, S. Technology and Reflection: Mood and Memory Mechanisms for Well-Being. *Psychol. Well Being* **2016**, *6*. [CrossRef] [PubMed]
42. Villani, D.; Riva, G. Presence and relaxation: A preliminary controlled study. *PsychNol. J.* **2008**, *6*, 7–26.
43. Tong, X.; Gromala, D.; Choo, A.; Amin, A.; Shaw, C. The Virtual Meditative Walk: An Immersive Virtual Environment for Pain Self-modulation Through Mindfulness-Based Stress Reduction Meditation. In Proceedings of the 7th International Conference, VAMR 2015, Held as Part of HCI International 2015, Los Angeles, CA, USA, 2–7 August 2015; Lecture Notes in Computer Science. Springer Int. Publ.: Cham, Switzerland, 2015; pp. 388–397. [CrossRef]
44. Cikajlo, I.; Čižman-Štaba, U.; Vrhovac, S.; Larkin, F.; Roddy, M. Recovr: Realising collaborative virtual reality for wellbeing and self-healing. In Proceedings of the 3rd IASTED International Conference Telehealth Assistive Technology TAT 2016, Zurich, Switzerland, 5–7 October 2016; pp. 11–17. [CrossRef]
45. Hasan, H.; Linger, H. Enhancing the wellbeing of the elderly: Social use of digital technologies in aged care. *Educ. Gerontol.* **2016**, *42*, 749–757. [CrossRef]
46. Baez, M.; Far, I.K.; Ibarra, F.; Ferron, M.; Didino, D.; Casati, F. Effects of online group exercises for older adults on physical, psychological and social wellbeing: A pilot trial Marcos. *J. Chem. Inf. Model.* **2017**, *53*, 1689–1699. [CrossRef]
47. Singh, D.K.A.; Rahman, N.N.A.; Seffiyah, R.; Chang, S.Y.; Zainura, A.K.; Aida, S.R.; Rajwinder, K.H.S. Impact of virtual reality games on psychological well-being and upper limb performance in adults with physical disabilities: A pilot study. *Med. J. Malays.* **2017**, *72*, 119–121.
48. Weerdmeester, J.; van Rooij, M.; Harris, O.; Smit, N.; Engels, R.C.M.E.; Granic, I. Exploring the role of self-efficacy in biofeedback video games. In Proceedings of the CHI Play 2017 Ext. Abstr.—Ext. Abstr. Publ. Annu. Symp. Comput. Interact. Play, Amsterdam, The Netherlands, 15–18 October 2017; pp. 453–461. [CrossRef]
49. Bornioli, A. Psychological Wellbeing Benefits of Simulated Exposure to Five Urban Settings: An Experimental Study from the Pedestrian's Perspective. *Transp. Res. Part A Policy Pract.* **2019**, *123*, 200–215. [CrossRef]
50. Bornioli, A.; Parkhurst, G.; Morgan, P.L. Affective experiences of built environments and the promotion of urban walking. *Transp. Res. Part. A Policy Pract.* **2019**, *123*, 200–215. [CrossRef]
51. Lorenzetti, V.; Bruno, M.; Rodrigo, B.; Chao, S.; Murat, Y.; Carlos, J.T.-C.; Jorge, M. Emotion regulation using virtual environments and real-time fMRI neurofeedback. *Front. Neurol.* **2018**, *9*, 1–15. [CrossRef]
52. Turk, C.S.; Carstensen, L.L. Emotion Regulation and Aging. In *Handbook of Emotion Regulation*; Guilford: New York, NY, USA, 2007; pp. 307–325.
53. Gross, J.J.; Carstensen, L.L.; Pasupathi, M.; Tsai, J.; Skorpen, C.G.; Hsu, A.Y.C. Emotion and aging: Experience, expression, and control. *Psychol. Aging* **1997**, *12*, 590–599. [CrossRef] [PubMed]
54. Cacioppo, J.T.; Berntson, G.G.; Klein, D.J.; Poehlmann, K.M. The psychophysiology of emotion across the lifespan. *Annu. Rev. Gerontol. Geriatr.* **1998**, *17*, 27–65.
55. Gross, J.J. Antecedent- and Response-Focused Emotion Regulation: Divergent Consequences for Experience, Expression, and Physiology. *J. Personal. Soc. Psychol.* **1998**, *74*, 224–237. [CrossRef]
56. Singh, V.; Padmanabhan, B.; de Vreede, T.; de Vreede, G.-J.; Andel, S.; Spector, P.E.; Benfield, S.; Aslami, A. A content engagement score for online learning platforms. In Proceedings of the Fifth Annual ACM Conference Learning Scale—L@S '18, London, UK, 26–28 June 2018; pp. 1–4. [CrossRef]

57. Consedine, N.S.; Moskowitz, J.T. The role of discrete emotions in health outcomes: A critical review. *Appl. Prev. Psychol.* **2007**, *12*, 59–75. [CrossRef]
58. Baños, R.M.; Castilla, D.; Etchemendy, E.; Garcia-Palacios, A. Positive mood induction procedures for virtual environments designed for elderly people. *Interact. Comput.* **2012**, *24*, 131–138. [CrossRef]
59. Choi, N.G.; DiNitto, D.M. Internet Use Among Older Adults: Association with Health Needs, Psychological Capital, and Social Capital. *J. Med. Internet Res.* **2013**, *15*, e97. [CrossRef]
60. Winstead, V.; Yost, E.A.; Cotten, S.R.; Berkowsky, R.W.; Anderson, W.A. The Impact of Activity Interventions on the Well-Being of Older Adults in Continuing Care Com. *J. Appl. Gerontol.* **2014**, *33*, 888–911. [CrossRef]
61. Sander, D.; Grandjean, D.; Scherer, K.R. A systems approach to appraisal mechanisms in emotion. *Neural Netw.* **2005**, *18*, 317–352. [CrossRef]
62. Scherer, K.R.; Schorr, A.; Johnstone, T. Appraisal Processes in Emotion: Theory, Methods, Research. In *Handbook of Affective Sciences*; Oxford University Press: Oxford, UK, 2003; pp. 92–120.
63. Frank, D.L.; Khorshid, L.; Kiffer, J.; Moravec, C.S.; McKee Michael, G. Biofeedback in medicine: Who, when, why and how? *Mental Health in Family Medicine*. **2010**, *7*, 85–91.
64. Wheat, A.L.; Larkin, K.T. Biofeedback of heart rate variability and related physiology: A critical review. *Appl. Psychophysiol. Biofeedback* **2010**, *35*, 229–242. [CrossRef]
65. Gevirtz, R. The Promise of Heart Rate Variability Biofeedback: Evidence-Based Applications. *Biofeedback* **2013**, *41*, 110–120. [CrossRef]
66. Gilbert, C.; Moss, D. Biofeedback and Biological Monitoring. In *Handbook of Mind-Body Medicine for Primary Care: Behavioral and Physiological Tools*; Sage Publications: Thousand Oaks, CA, USA, 2003; pp. 109–122.
67. La Vaque, T.J. Neurofeedback, Neurotherapy, and Quantitative EEG. In *Handbook of Mind-Body Medicine for Primary Care*; Sage Publications: Thousand Oaks, CA, USA, 2003; pp. 123–136.
68. Yucha, C.B.; Montgomery, D. *Evidence-Based Practice in Biofeedback and Neurofeedback*; Association for Applied Psychophysiology and Biofeedback: Wheat Ridge, CO, USA, 2008.
69. Serino, S.; Cipresso, P.; Gaggioli, A.; Riva, G. The potential of pervasive sensors and computing for positive technology. In *Pervasive and Mobile Sensing and Computing for Healthcare: Smart Sensors, Measurement and Instrumentation*; Mukhopadhyay, S.C., Postolache, O.A., Eds.; Springer: New York, NY, USA, 2013.
70. Realdon, O.; Rossetto, F.; Nalin, M.; Baroni, I.; Cabinio, M.; Fioravanti, R.; Saibene, F.L.; Alberoni, M.; Mantovani, F.; Romano, M.; et al. Technology-enhanced multi-domain at home continuum of care program with respect to usual care for people with cognitive impairment: The Ability- TelerehABILITation study protocol for a randomized controlled trial. *BMC Psychiatry* **2016**, 1–9. [CrossRef] [PubMed]
71. Realdon, O.; Rossetto, F.; Nalin, M.; Baroni, I.; Romano, M.; Catania, F.; Frontini, D.; Mancastroppa, S.; Alberoni, M.; Zurloni, V.; et al. The Technology-Enhanced Ability Continuum-of-Care Home Program. for People with Cognitive Disorders: Concept Design and Scenario of Use. In Proceedings of the International Symposium on Pervasive Computing Paradigms for Mental Health, Buenos Aires, Argentina, 23–24 April 2018.
72. Matamala-Gomez, M.; Donegan, T.; Bottiroli, S.; Sandrini, G.; Sanchez-Vives, M.V.; Tassorelli, C. Immersive virtual reality and virtual embodiment for pain relief. *Front. Hum. Neurosci.* **2019**, *13*, 279. [CrossRef] [PubMed]
73. Matamala-Gomez, M.; Gonzalez, A.M.D.; Slater, M.; Sanchez-Vives, M.V. Decreasing Pain Ratings in Chronic Arm Pain Through Changing a Virtual Body: Different Strategies for Different Pain Types. *J. Pain* **2019**, *20*. [CrossRef] [PubMed]
74. Hoffman, H.G.; Patterson, D.R.; Carrougher, G.J.; Sharar, S.R. Effectiveness of virtual reality-based pain control with multiple treatments. *Clin. J. Pain* **2001**, *17*, 229–235. [CrossRef] [PubMed]
75. Baer, R.A. Mindfulness training as a clinical intervention: A conceptual and empirical review. *Clin. Psychol. Pract.* **2003**, *10*, 125–143. [CrossRef]
76. Bingham, P.; Bates, J.H.T.; Thompson-Figueroa, T.; Lahiri, J. A breath biofeedback computer game for children with cystic fibrosis. *Clin. Paediatr.* **2010**, *49*, 337–342. [CrossRef]
77. Fernández-Aranda, F.; Jiménez-Murcia, S.; Penelo, E. Video games as a complementary therapy tool in mental disorders: PlayMancer, a European multicentre study. *J. Ment. Health* **2012**, *21*, 364–374. [CrossRef]
78. Lobel, A.; Gotsis, M.; Reynolds, E.; Annetta, M.; Engels, I.; Granic, R.C.M.E. Designing and utilizing biofeedback games for emotion regulation: The case of nevermind. In Proceedings of the 2016 CHI Conference Extended Abst, San Jose, CA, USA, 7–12 May 2016.
79. Schwartz, M.S. *Biofeedback: A Practitioner's Guide*, 2nd ed.; The Guilford Press: New York, NY, USA, 1995.

80. Peper, E.; Harvey, R.; Takebayashi, N. Biofeedback an evidence based approach inclinical practice. *Jpn. J. Biofeedback Res.* **2009**, *36*, 3–10.
81. Pham, Q.; Khatib, Y.; Fox, S.; Green, T. Feasibility and efficacy of an mHealth game for managing anxiety: 'Flowy' randomized controlled pilot trial and design evaluation. *Games Health J.* **2016**, *5*, 50–67. [CrossRef]
82. Tyson, S.; Selley, A. A content analysis of physiotherapy for postural control in people with stroke: An observational study. *Disabil. Rehabil.* **2006**, *28*, 865–872. [CrossRef] [PubMed]
83. Ryan, R.M.; Deci, E.L. On happiness and human potentials: A review of research on hedonic and eudaimonic well-being. *Annu. Rev. Psychol.* **2001**, *52*, 141–166. [CrossRef] [PubMed]
84. Thibaud, M.; Bloch, F.; Tournoux-Facon, C.; Brèque, C.; Rigaud, A.S.; Dugué, B.; Kemoun, G. Impact of physical activity and sedentary behaviour on fall risks in older people: A systematic review and meta-analysis of observational studies. *Eur. Rev. Aging Phys. Act.* **2012**, *9*, 5–15. [CrossRef]
85. Stuart, M.; Chard, S.; Benvenuti, F.; Steinwachs, S. Community Exercise: A Vital Component to Healthy Aging. *Healthcarepapers* **2009**, *10*, 23–28. [CrossRef] [PubMed]
86. El Khoury, F. The effect of fall prevention exercise programmes on fall induced injuries in community dwelling older adults: Systematic review and meta-analysis of randomised controlled trials. *BMJ Res.* **2013**. [CrossRef]
87. Mohr, D.C.; Cheung, K.; Schueller, S.M.; Brown, H.; Duan, N. Continuous Evaluation of Evolving Behavioral Intervention Technologies. *Am. J. Prev. Med.* **2013**, *45*, 1–11. [CrossRef] [PubMed]
88. Clore, G. Why emotions vary in intensity. In *The Nature of Emotion: Fundamental Questions*; Ekman, P., Davidson, R.J., Eds.; Oxford University Press: Oxford, UK, 1994; pp. 386–393.
89. Richards, J.M.; Gross, J.J. Emotion regulation and memory: The cognitive costs of keeping one's cool. *J. Personal. Soc. Psychol.* **2000**, *79*, 410–424. [CrossRef]
90. Granic, I.; Lobel, A.; Engels, R.C.M.E. The Benefits of Playing Video Games. *Am. Psychol.* **2014**, *69*, 66–78. [CrossRef]
91. Sherry, J.L. Flow and Media Enjoyment. *Commun. Theory* **2004**, *14*, 328–347. [CrossRef]
92. Nakamura, J.; Csikszentmihalyi, M. The Concept of Flow. In *Oxford Handbook of Positive Psychology*; Snyder, U., Ed.; Oxford University Press: Oxford, UK, 2009; pp. 89–105.
93. Riva, G.; Castelnuovo, G.; Mantovani, F. Transformation of flow in rehabilitation: The role of advanced communication technologies. *Behav. Res. Methods* **2006**, *38*, 237–244. [CrossRef]
94. Riva, G.; Waterworth, J.A.; Waterworth, E.L. The layers of presence: A bio-cultural approach to understanding presence in natural and mediated environments. *Cyberpsychol. Behav. Soc. Netw.* **2004**, *7*, 405–419. [CrossRef] [PubMed]
95. Riva, G. From Virtual to Real Body. *J. Cyberther. Rehabil.* **2008**, *1*, 7–22.
96. Steuer, J. Defining Virtual Reality: Characteristics Determining Telepresence. *J. Commun.* **1992**, *42*, 73–94. [CrossRef]
97. Valmaggia, L.R.; Latifa, L.; Kempton, M.J.; Rus-Calafell, M. Virtual reality in the psychological treatment for mental health problems: An systematic review of recent evidence. *Psychiatry Res.* **2016**, *236*, 189–195. [CrossRef] [PubMed]
98. Slater, M.; Steed, A. Depth of Presence in Virtual Environments. *Presence Teleoper. Virtual Environ.* **1994**. [CrossRef]
99. Parsons, T.D. Virtual Reality for Enhanced Ecological Validity and Experimental Control in the Clinical, Affective and Social Neurosciences. *Front. Hum. Neurosci.* **2015**, *9*, 1–19. [CrossRef]
100. Gross, J.J. Emotion regulation: Conceptual and empirical foundations. In *Handbook of emotion regulation*; Gross, J.J., Ed.; Guilford Press: New York, NY, USA, 2014; pp. 3–20.
101. Realdon, O.; Serino, S.; Savazzi, F.; Rossetto, F.; Cipresso, P.; Parsons, T.D.; Cappellini, G.; Mantovani, F.; Mendozzi, L.; Nemni, R.; et al. An ecological measure to screen executive functioning in MS: The Picture Interpretation Test (PIT). *Sci. Rep.* **2019**, 1–8. [CrossRef]
102. Ochsner, K.N.; Gross, J.J. The Neural Architecture of Emotion Regulation. In *Handbook of Emotion Regulation*; Guilford: New York, NY, USA, 2007; pp. 87–109.
103. Linehan, M.M.; Bohus, M.; Lynch, T.R. Dialectical Behavior Therapy for Pervasive Emotion Dysregulation: Theoretical and Practical Underpinnings. In *Handbook of Emotion Regulation*; Guilford: New York, NY, USA, 2007; pp. 581–606.

104. Boals, A.; Klein, K. Word Use in Emotional Narratives about Failed Romantic Relationships and Subsequent Mental Health. *J. Lang. Soc. Psychol.* **2005**, *24*, 252–268. [CrossRef]
105. Petrie, K.J.; Booth, R.J.; Pennebaker, J.W. The Immunological Effects of Thought Suppression. *J. Personal. Soc. Psychol.* **1998**, *75*, 1264–1272. [CrossRef]
106. Ryff, C.D.; Singer, B.H.; Love, G.D. Positive health: Connecting well-being with biology. *Philos. Trans. R. Soc. B Biol. Sci.* **2004**, *359*, 1383–1394. [CrossRef]
107. Ryff, C.D. Psychological Well-Being in Adult Life. *Curr. Dir. Psychol. Sci.* **1995**, *4*, 99–104. [CrossRef]
108. Kroll, C.; Kroll, C.; Delhey, J. A Happy Nation? Opportunities and Challenges of Using Subjective Indicators in Policymaking. *Soc. Indic. Res.* **2013**, *114*, 13–28. [CrossRef]

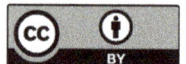

© 2020 by the authors. Licensee MDPI, Basel, Switzerland. This article is an open access article distributed under the terms and conditions of the Creative Commons Attribution (CC BY) license (http://creativecommons.org/licenses/by/4.0/).

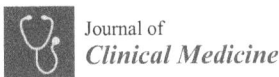

Review

Use of Virtual Reality for the Management of Anxiety and Pain in Dental Treatments: Systematic Review and Meta-Analysis

Nansi López-Valverde [1], Jorge Muriel Fernández [1], Antonio López-Valverde [1,*], Luis F. Valero Juan [2], Juan Manuel Ramírez [3], Javier Flores Fraile [1], Julio Herrero Payo [1], Leticia A. Blanco Antona [1], Bruno Macedo de Sousa [4] and Manuel Bravo [5]

[1] Department of Surgery, University of Salamanca, Instituto de Investigación Biomédica de Salamanca (IBSAL), 37007 Salamanca, Spain; nlovalher@usal.es (N.L.-V.); murimuriel@gmail.com (J.M.F.); j.flores@usal.es (J.F.F.); jhpayo@usal.es (J.H.P.); lesablantona@gmail.com (L.A.B.A.)
[2] Department of Biomedical and Diagnostic Sciences, University of Salamanca, Avda. Alfonso X El Sabio S/N, 37007 Salamanca, Spain; luva@usal.es
[3] Department of Morphological Sciences, University of Cordoba, Avenida Menéndez Pidal s/n, 14071 Cordoba, Spain; jmramirez@uco.es
[4] Institute for Occlusion and Orofacial Pain Faculty of Medicine, University of Coimbra, Polo I - Edifício Central Rua Larga, 3004-504 Coimbra, Portugal; brunomsousa@usal.es
[5] Department of Preventive and Community Dentistry, Facultad de Odontología, Campus de Cartuja s/n, 18071 Granada, Spain; mbravo@ugr.es
* Correspondence: anlopezvalverde@gmail.com

Received: 26 February 2020; Accepted: 27 March 2020; Published: 5 April 2020

Abstract: Background: Dental treatments often cause pain and anxiety in patients. Virtual reality (VR) is a novel procedure that can provide distraction during dental procedures or prepare patients to receive such type of treatments. This meta-analysis is the first to gather evidence on the effectiveness of VR on the reduction of pain (P) and dental anxiety (DA) in patients undergoing dental treatment, regardless of age. Methods: MEDLINE, CENTRAL, PubMed, EMBASE, Wiley Library and Web of Science were searched for scientific articles in November 2019. The keywords used were: "virtual reality", "distraction systems", "dental anxiety" and "pain". Studies where VR was used for children and adults as a measure against anxiety and pain during dental treatments were included. VR was defined as a three-dimensional environment that provides patients with a sense of immersion, transporting them to appealing and interactive settings. Anxiety and pain results were assessed during dental treatments where VR was used, and in standard care situations. Results: 31 studies were identified, of which 14 met the inclusion criteria. Pain levels were evaluated in four studies ($n = 4$), anxiety levels in three ($n = 3$) and anxiety and pain together in seven ($n = 7$). Our meta-analysis was based on ten studies ($n = 10$). The effect of VR was studied mainly in the pediatric population (for pain SMD = −0.82). In the adult population, only two studies (not significant) were considered. Conclusions: The findings of the meta-analysis show that VR is an effective distraction method to reduce pain and anxiety in patients undergoing a variety of dental treatments; however, further research on VR as a tool to prepare patients for dental treatment is required because of the scarcity of studies in this area.

Keywords: virtual reality; distraction systems; dental anxiety; pain

1. Introduction

Pain suppression during dental interventions has been a major accomplishment for humankind. In 1842, William E. Clarke gave ether to a patient for the removal of a tooth; later, in 1844, a dentist named Horace Wells used nitrous oxide as an anesthetic for dental extractions; and in 1846, another dentist, William T. G. Morton, became a pioneer in the use of inhaled ether as an anaesthetic at the Massachusetts General Hospital [1].

Patient anxiety when facing dental procedures is determined by two circumstances: on the one hand, the prior act of anesthetizing, which in itself frequently causes a state of phobia [2] and, on the other hand, the subsequent dental treatment. The number of studies on this pathology has exponentially increased over the last few years, growing from a very low number in the 1940s to the more than 6000 papers that are currently available, according to the U.S. National Library of Medicine (Figure 1).

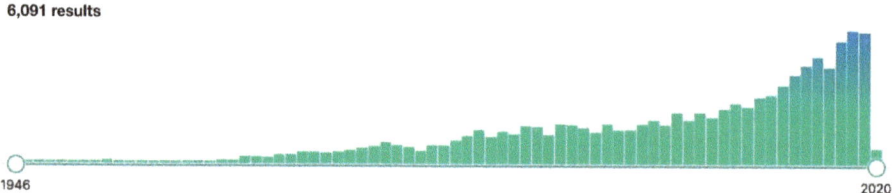

Figure 1. Increasing tendency of publications, according the U.S. National Library of Medicine database, using "dental phobia" as the keyword.

Different therapies have been proposed for the prevention and treatment of P and DA, among them virtual reality (VR) distraction techniques [3].

Although it is a concept that is difficult to define, VR is generally accepted as a three-dimensional environment generated by means of computer technology that creates a sense of immersion in the user, transporting the individual to appealing and interactive settings [4].

The benefits of using VR for the reduction of dental anxiety (DA) and pain (P) levels during dental procedures has been extensively addressed in scientific literature [5–9], and its usefulness as a distraction tool is receiving increasing attention in medical contexts [9]. During aversive experiences, VR can improve pain management [10] and reduce the perceived duration of the procedure [11]. Moreover, a recent systematic review examined the effectiveness of virtual reality distraction in reducing pain [12]. This could be an advantage for many patients who reject DA control using anti-anxiety drugs because of their disadvantages or side effects, which can be, among others, impaired cognitive function and coordination, since they act as depressants on specific areas of the central nervous system [13–15].

The purpose of this study was to conduct a systematic review of literature comparing the effectiveness of the use of VR as a method for reducing anxiety and pain levels during dental treatment. This systematic review constitutes an essential tool to synthesize the scientific information available, increasing the validity of the conclusions and of individual studies, and identifying areas of uncertainty, where research is necessary. Meta-analysis (when possible) provides very useful information, to facilitate understanding of the effect of a treatment or intervention, both in general and in specific groups of patients. In addition, it allows us to increase the precision in the estimation of the effect, detecting effects of moderate magnitude, but of clinical importance, that could go unnoticed in primary studies.

2. Methods

The study selection process was carried out according to the Preferred Reporting Items for Systematic Review and Meta-Analyses (PRISMA) guidelines for systematic reviews and meta-analysis [16].

2.1. Protocol

The search strategy was conducted using the population, intervention, comparison and outcome (PICO) framework, based on the following question:

"Are distraction techniques using VR effective against the anxiety and pain caused by dental procedures?"

To answer this question, a population of patients undergoing dental treatment, with no age limit, were selected. The intervention consisted in using audio–visual or VR distraction methods. Controls were patients who were not subjected to audio–visual or VR distraction methods. The results revised in the literature were the DA or P values obtained using different validated scales:

- For pain: Visual Analogic Scale (VAS), Wong–Baker Faces Scale (W–BFS) and Faces Pain Scale-Revise (FPS-R).
- For anxiety: Consolability Scale (FLACC), Verbal Rating Scale (VRS), Modified Dental Anxiety Scale (MDAS), (Norman Corah's anxiety questionnaire (NCAQ) and Venham's Clinical Anxiety Rating Scale (VCARS).

2.2. Search Method for the Identification of Studies

A search of the MEDLINE, CENTRAL, PubMed, EMBASE, Wiley Library and Web of Science electronic databases was conducted in November 2019 to identify relevant scientific articles. The search terms used were: "virtual reality", "distraction systems", "dental anxiety", "pain".

2.3. Inclusion and Exclusion Criteria

Inclusion criteria:

(a) Articles published in English.
(b) Randomized controlled clinical trials related to dental anxiety and pain associated with dental procedures in children and adults.
(c) Studies assessing anxiety in said procedures.

Exclusion criteria:

(a) Non-randomized studies or non-controlled clinical trials.
(b) Comparative studies.
(c) Narrative reviews and systematic reviews.
(d) Case studies.
(e) Irrelevant and duplicate studies and those that did not meet the established inclusion criteria.

2.4. Data Extraction and Analysis

Studies that made no reference to the research question were removed, and the titles and abstracts of the articles selected were obtained and entered in an Excel spreadsheet. Two reviewers (NL-V and JMF) selected the titles and abstracts independently. Discrepancies in terms of study inclusion were discussed between the two mentioned reviewers until consensus was reached. Subsequently, the full texts of the selected studies were obtained for their review and inclusion.

2.5. Risk of Bias (RoB) of Included Articles

The Cochrane Collaboration, London, UK, tool was used to assess the methodology of the scientific evidence in all the selected studies [17].

2.6. Quality of the Reports of the Included Studies

This was assessed according to the modified Strengthening the Reporting of Observational studies in Epidemiology (STROBE) statement [18], which includes a total of 22 items. Each item was assessed by reviewers NL-V and JMF, who attributed scores of 0 (not reported) or 1 (reported), carrying out a complete count of all the studies included (Table 1).

Table 1. Checklist of Reporting of Observational studies in Epidemiology (STROBE) criteria reported by the included studies. Each item was judged as "0" (not reported) or "1" (reported). The total score of each of included studies was also recorded.

Authors	Asl Aminabadi et al. [22]	Tanja-Dijkstra et al. [9]	Nunna et al. [23]	Gujjar et al. [6]	Niharika et al. [24]	Al-Halabi et al. [20]	Raghav et al. [7]	Tanja-Dijkstra et al. [19]	Shetty et al. [25]	Al-Khotani et al. [26]	Mitrakul et al. [27]	Asvanund et al. [28]	Bentsen et al. [21]	Sweta et al. [2]
Section and item														
1. Title and Abstract	1	1	1	1	1	1	1	1	1	1	1	1	1	1
Introduction														
2. Background	1	1	1	1	1	1	1	1	1	1	1	1	1	1
3. Objectives	1	1	1	1	1	1	1	1	1	1	1	1	1	1
Methods														
4. Study design	1	1	1	1	1	1	1	1	1	1	1	1	1	1
5. Setting	1	1	1	1	1	1	1	0	1	1	1	1	1	1
6. Participants	1	1	1	1	1	1	1	1	1	1	1	1	1	1
7. Variables	1	1	1	1	1	1	1	1	1	1	1	1	1	1
8. Data sources/ Measurement	1	1	1	1	1	1	1	1	1	1	1	1	1	1
9. Bias	1	0	0	0	0	1	0	0	0	1	1	0	1	0
10. Study Size	1	1	1	1	1	1	1	1	1	1	1	1	1	1
11. Quantitative variables	1	1	1	1	1	1	1	1	1	1	1	1	1	1
12. Statistical Methods	1	1	1	1	1	1	1	1	1	1	1	1	1	1
Results														
13. Participants	1	1	1	1	1	1	1	1	1	1	1	1	1	1
14. Descriptive data	1	1	1	1	1	1	1	1	1	1	1	1	1	1
15. Outcome data	1	1	1	1	1	1	1	1	1	1	1	1	1	1
16. Main results	1	1	1	1	1	1	1	1	1	1	1	1	1	1
17. Other analyses	0	0	1	1	1	1	1	0	1	0	1	1	0	1
Discussion														
18. Key results	1	1	1	1	1	1	1	1	1	1	1	1	1	1
19. Limitations	1	0	0	0	0	1	0	0	0	1	1	0	1	0
20. Interpretation	1	1	1	1	1	1	1	1	1	1	1	1	1	1
21. Generalisability	1	1	1	1	1	1	1	1	1	1	1	1	1	1
Other information														
22. Funding	1	1	1	1	1	1	1	1	1	1	1	1	1	1
Total score	21	19	20	20	20	22	20	18	20	21	22	20	21	20

Mode Value: 27.4 (± 0.85).

2.7. Statistical Analysis

In the meta-analysis, four studies were excluded on the grounds that two of them [7,19] did not present results and the other two [20,21] presented confusing results at the time of their assessment. Physiological data, such as pulse rate, degree of oxygen saturation, blood pressure and more were not included, incorporating data related to pain and anxiety only, during dental treatments. Pain and anxiety were analyzed separately in children and adults. The mean scores and SDs (standard deviations) for pain and anxiety, during the procedure with VR and control, were extracted from the selected articles, using mean scores and interquartile ranges, or reported, directly, by the authors of the studies. Other information not related to VR was not taken into consideration in our meta-analysis. The different measurement scales and VR devices used were not considered. The meta-analysis was performed using Stata v.14.2 (StataCorp LP, College Station, TX, USA) and closely followed the methods proposed by the Cochrane collaboration [17]. The methods can be observed in the different tables and figures. The standardized difference of means (SMD) was used as a measure of effect to account for different measurement scales both for anxiety and pain. Statistical heterogeneity among studies was assessed using the Q test according to Dersimonian and Laird and the I2 index (heterogeneity: I2 > 30% being moderate, >50% substantial and >75% considerable [17]). We decided to pool the study-specific estimates with the random effects model to protect our composite estimates (for anxiety and pain) from heterogeneity in the context of a relatively limited number of studies. We also decided a priori to present the results not only for all the studies together, but also as a subgroup analysis according to age group (children and adults) derived from the different clinical usefulness and interpretation. Finally, funnel graphs (not shown) and p-value calculation (Egger test) were used to assess the publication bias.

3. Results

3.1. Characteristics of the Studies

Until November 2019, a total of 31 studies were gathered and subsequently assessed by the reviewers. Three duplicate studies were removed after an initial detection. A second detection led to the removal of 14 studies, which left a total of 14 full-text studies for the final selection [2,6,7,9,19–28] (Figure 2). Pain levels were assessed in four studies, two in children [20,28] and two in adults [2,21]; anxiety levels in three, two in adults [9,19] and one in children [26]; and anxiety and pain together in seven studies, five in children [22–25,27] and two in adults [6,7].

Table 2 provides a general description of the details of each study. The risk of bias (RoB Cochrane Collaboration Tool) in the studies considered is shown in Figure 3. All the studies complied with random sequence. Two of the studies included [25,28] did not comply with allocation concealment and only 35% complied with blinding of participants and personnel. It should be noted that none of the studies included complied with blinding of outcome assessment.

Table 2. Details of each study.

Study (Year)	Journal	Children Values (Ma, n, Ar)	Adult Values (Ma, n, Ar)	Dental Procedure	VR Device Equipment	Measuring Scales DA	Measuring Scales P	Outcomes
Asl Aminabadi et al. 2012 [22]	J Dent Res Dent Clin Dent Prospect	Ma = 5.4, n = 120, Ar = 4–6		Restorative treatment in primary molars.	I-glasses 920HR Ilixco, Inc. Menlo Park, CA, USA.	MDAS	W-BFS	There was a significant decrease in pain perception and anxiety scores with the use of VR eyeglasses during dental treatment.
Tanja-Dijkstra et al 2014 [9]	Plos One J		Ma = 33.1, n = 69, Ar = Nr	A simulated dental treatment.	Eyeglasses EVuzix iWear VR920 headset. Dual-core, 1.3GHz Intel processor with Nvidia GT 540 M graphics card.	MDAS		Participants with higher dental anxiety showed more interested in using VR during real dental treatment than those with lower levels of dental anxiety. Dental patients who have a positive dental treatment experience thanks to VR, might have fewer unpleasant memories and thus be less likely to postpone a future dental visit.
Nunna et al 2019 [23]	J Dent Anesth Pain Med	Ma = Nr, n = 70, Ar = 7–11		- Counter-stimulation. - Local anaesthesia administration with virtual reality distraction.	Lenovo smartphone, Sennheiser earphones, and ANTVR glasses.	VCARS	W-BFS	Assessment of mean anxiety scores showed a significant difference in girls belonging to the VR group.
Gujjar et al. 2019 [6]	Journal of Anxiety Disorders		Ma = group 1, 25.3, group 2, 23, n = 30, Ar = Nr	Routine dental treatment.	Eyeglasses: Dell XPS-8700 desktop with 4th Generation Intel Core i7-4790 processor (8M Cache, up to 4.0 GHz) and ASUS NVIDIA GEFORCE GTX 750 TI OC 2CB GDDR5 graphic card.	MDAS	VAS	The results of this study provide evidence to support the efficacy of VR in the treatment of dental phobia. Study limitations: - No blinding of patients or therapist in the interventions. - VR compared with pamphlet information.
Niharika et al. 2018 [24]	J Indian Soc Pedod Prev Dent	Ma = Group A (7.17 ± 0.316) Group B (7.28 ± 0.300), n = 40, Ar = 4–8		Routine dental care (pulp therapy in mandibular primary molars). Local anaesthetic.	Google VR Box and Anti-Tank Virtual Reality 3D Glasses	MDAS	W-BFS	Two groups. Childhood Anxiety-Related Disorders scores did not differ significantly between the two groups. In both groups, a statistically significant difference was detected between the two treatment sessions (with and without VR).
Al-Halabi et al. 2018 [21]	Anaesth Pain & Intensive Care	Ma = 7.4, n = 102, Ar = 7–10		Local anaesthesia in mandibular arch (inferior alveolar nerve block).	Eyeglasses (BlackBug™ Virtual Reality Glasses 3D VR Box Headsets, China)	MDAS	W-BFS	Three groups. There was no significant difference in the anxiety of groups. There was a statistically significant difference in the anxiety and pain level in pulse rate. Limitations: - No blinding of the external investigator. - The size of the VR Box was a little too big.
Raghav et al. 2016 [7]	BMC Oral Health J		Ma = Nr, n = 30, Ar = 19–45	1. Restorative dental procedure which may or may not be requiring local anaesthesia. 2. Extraction procedure requiring local anaesthesia.	Oculus development kit 2HMD, with a resolution of 960 × 1080 per eye and with a 100 degree field of view.	MDAS	VAS	Two groups, VR (Idle, Mirror, Syringe, Soundless Drill, Drill with Sound, 35-second exposures) and informational pamphlet control groups. Efficacy of VR in the treatment of dental phobia in the setting of the dental procedure. A limitation of the present study is the absence of in vivo exposure therapy as gold standard control group.

Table 2. Cont.

Study (Year)	Journal	Children Values (Ma, n, Ar)	Adult Values (Ma, n, Ar)	Dental Procedure	VR Device Equipment	Measuring Scales DA	Measuring Scales P	Outcomes
Tanja-Dijkstra et al. 2014 [34]	Trials J		Ma = Nr, n = 90, Ar = Nr	Dental treatment	Eyeglasses. A Sony personal 3D viewer, connected to an Alienware gaming laptop. Participants can walk around in the virtual environment by using a Zeemote JS1 thumb stick controller.	MDAS		This study compared two types of VR, natural environment and urban environment. It included both referred patients and inhouse patients from a dental clinic and two separate procedures are described, one for each type of patient.
Shetty et al. 2019 [25]	The Journal of Clinical Paediatric Dentistry	Ma = Nr, n = 120, Ar = 5–8		Dental treatment (vital pulp therapy)	Eyeglasses. VR device (i-glasses 920HR, Iiixco Inc., Menlo Park, CA, USA)	MDAS	W-BFS	Two groups. The group with VR distraction, reported a decrease in the severity of anxiety. Lower pain scores were observed in the VR group.
Al-Khotani et al. 2016 [26]	Acta Odontologica Scandinavica	Ma = 8.2, n = 56, Ar = 7–9		Dental examination, oral hygiene information, prophylaxis, restorative treatment.	Eyeglasses. DVD Players, gaming systems like Sony Play Station Pro, Microsoft X-BOX, Nintendo WII	MDAS		Two groups. VR and control group. Significant reduction in anxiety throughout the restorative procedure (including injection with local anaesthesia) in VR group.
Mitrakul et al. 2015 [27]	European Journal of Paediatric Dentistry	Ma = 6.9 ± 0.9, n = 42, Ar = 5–8		Restorative dental treatment in maxilla or mandible under local anaesthetic injection.	Eyeglasses. (Shenzhen Longway Vision Technology Co. Ltd, Shenzhen, China).	FPS-R	FLACC	Two groups. Group 1 received treatment without wearing VR in the first visit and wearing VR in a second visit. In Group 2, VR was used vice versa.
Asvanund et al. 2015 [28]	Quintessence International	Ma = 7 ± 0.8, n = 49, Ar = 5–8		Restorative dental treatment (local anaesthetic injection in the maxillary arch or mandibular block).	Eyeglasses (Shenzhen Longway Vision Technology Co. Ltd, Shenzhen, China).	FPS-R	FLACC	The study assesses pain and anxiety without making a distinction. The limitation of this study is that the FLACC score was assessed by playing back the video recording of each visit, which was done by two paediatric dentists who could not be blinded to the child's use of VR.
Bentsen et al. 2001 [1]	Eur J of Pain-London		Ma = Nr, n = 23, Ar = 20–49	Dental treatment	Video glasses (NV-HD 660 PanasonicTM)		VAS	The study was a split-mouth, randomized design (2 dental filling). Dental treatments were performed without anaesthesia. 74% of patients would prefer VR if they were to receive a second dental filling.
Sweta et al. 2019 [2]	Ann Maxillofac Surgery		Ma = 39.72 ± 15.93, n = 50, Ar = Nr	Local anaesthesia in patients undergoing a dental procedure.	Nr	NCAQ		Local anaesthesia and extractions reported the highest anxiety levels among the patients. Limitations of this study: - Small sample size. - Patients were not in control of their VR environment.

n (Participant number); Ma (Mean age years); Ar (Age range years); Nr (Not reported); VAS (Visual Analogic Scale); W-BFS (Wong–Baker Faces Scale); FPS-R (Faces Pain Scale-Revised); FLACC (Consolability Scale); VRS (Verbal Rating Scale); MDAS (Modified Dental Anxiety Scale); NCAQ (Norman Corah's anxiety questionnaire); VCARS (Venham's Clinical Anxiety Rating Scale). DA (Dental Anxiety); P (Pain).

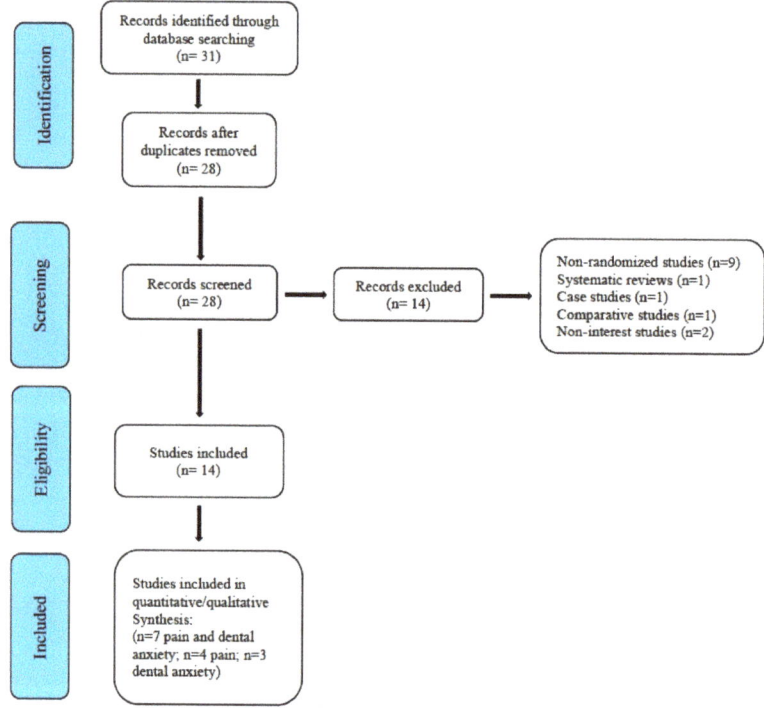

Figure 2. Flow chart of the study selection process. PRISMA (Preferred Reporting Items for Systematic Review and meta Analyses) [16].

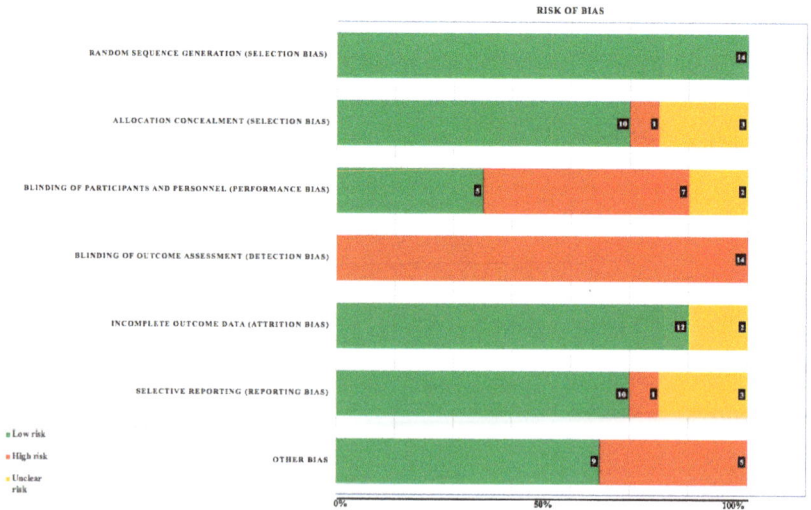

Figure 3. Risk of bias.

The STROBE criteria reported an average score of 27.4 (± 0.85), the maximum scores corresponding to the studies by Al-Halabi et al. [20] and Mitrakul et al. [27]. It is also noteworthy that Item 9 (Bias) was only reported in five studies [21,22,24,26,27], which is also the case with Item 19 (Limitations) [20–22,26,27] (Table 1).

3.2. VR and Anxiety Management

Regarding anxiety, the composite measure is not significant, neither for all together (children + adults) ($p = 0.302$), nor for children ($p = 0.243$) (Figure 4) nor adults ($p = 0.567$) (Figure 5). The heterogeneity seems to be moderate (Table 3).

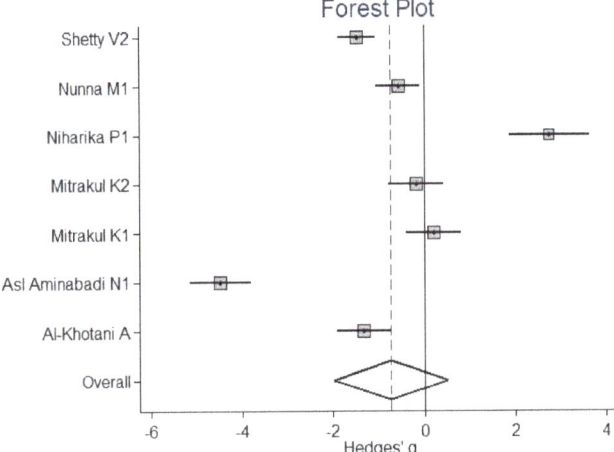

Figure 4. Forest plot for anxiety in Children.

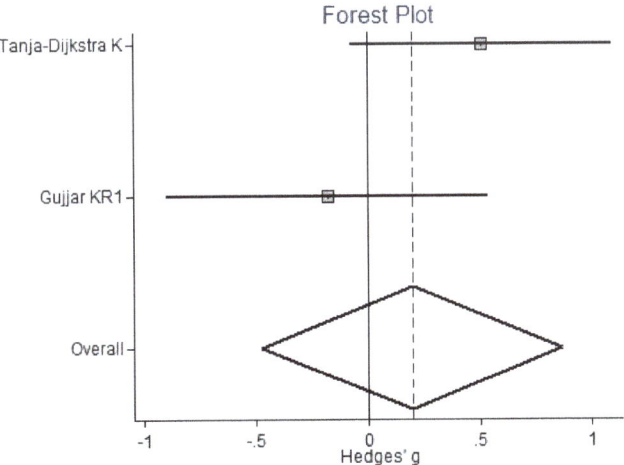

Figure 5. Forest plot for Anxiety in Adults.

Table 3. Meta-analysis of anxiety. Characteristics of individual studies and meta-analysis. a: Standardized difference of means.

Age group/Study	Year	Scale	Test		Control				SMD[a]		Heterogeneity I² (p-Value)	Public.bias p-Value (Egger Test)
			n	Mean ± sd	n	Mean ± sd	Weight	Mean	95%-CI	p-Value		
Children + Adults (n = 9)			282		284			−0.54	−1.58 to 0.49	0.302	31% (p = 0.169)	p = 0.399
Children (n = 7) (see Figure 5)												
Shetty V2 [25]	2019	MDAS	60	11.3 ± 3.5	60	16.5 ± 3.5	14.6%	−1.48	−1.88 to −1.07			
Nunna M1 [23]	2019	VCARS	35	0.57 ± 0.61	35	1.00 ± 0.84	14.5%	−0.58	−1.06 to −0.10			
Niharika P1 [24]	2018	MDAS	20	19.6 ± 0.9	20	17.3 ± 0.8	13.8%	2.74	1.86 to 3.63			
Mitrakul K2 [27]	2015	FLACC	21	26.0 ± 9.1	21	28.0 ± 12.0	14.3%	−0.18	−0.79 to 0.43			
Mitrakul K1 [27]	2015	FLACC	21	29.5 ± 11.3	21	27.3 ± 10.6	14.3%	0.20	−0.41 to 0.80			
Asl Aminabadi N1 [22]	2012	MDAS	60	12.6 ± 1.0	60	17.7 ± 1.2	14.2%	−4.46	−5.14 to −3.78			
Al-Khotani A [26]	2016	MDAS	28	0.14 ± 0.36	28	0.75 ± 0.52	14.3%	−1.34	−1.93 to −0.76			
Total			245		245		100%	−0.74	−1.99 to 0.51	0.243	38% (p = 0.139)	p = 0.536
Adults (n = 2) (see Figure 6)												
Tanja-Dijkstra K [9]	2014	MDAS	22	3.73 ± 0.65	24	3.33 ± 0.87	54.6%	0.51	−0.08 to 1.10			
Gujjar KR1 [6]	2019	MDAS	15	18.3 ± 2.6	15	18.8 ± 2.8	45.4%	−0.18	−0.90 to 0.54			
Total			37		39			0.20	−0.48 to 0.87	0.567	0% (p = 0.317)	-

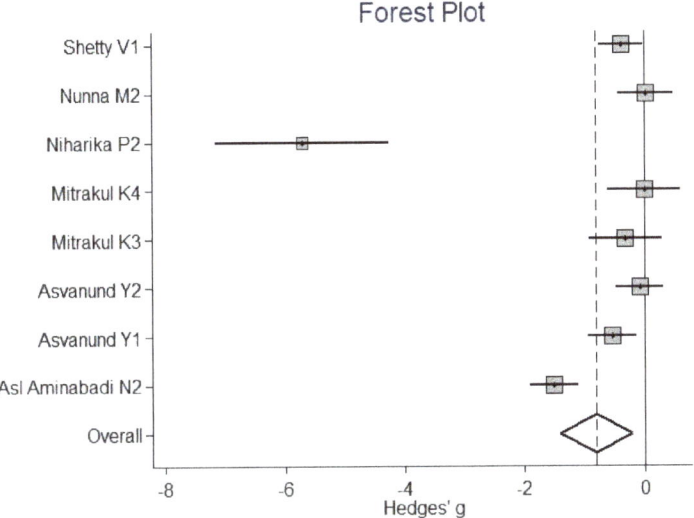

Figure 6. Forest plot for pain in Children.

3.3. VR and Pain Management

For pain, there is a significant protection for children (SMD = −0.82, i.e., a substantial effect according to Cohen's scale [29]) (Figure 6), but not for adults (Figure 7), since the 95%-confidence interval (CI) includes the null value 0 (Table 4). Neverhterless, it is based only on two studies.

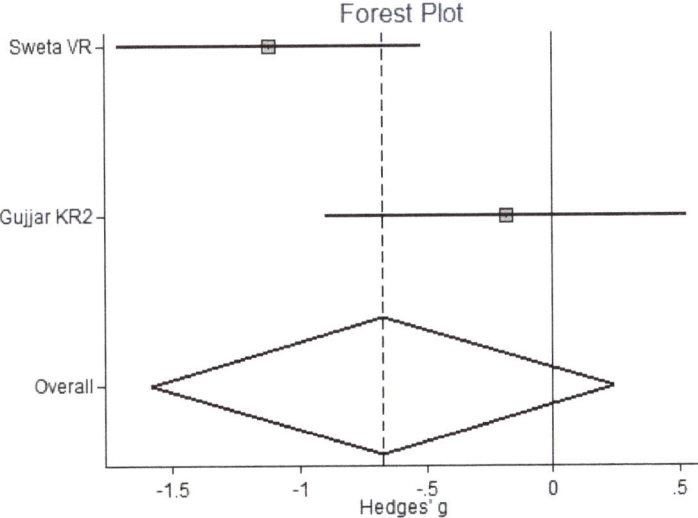

Figure 7. Forest plot for Pain in Adults.

Table 4. Meta-analysis of pain according to random effect models. Characteristics of individual studies and meta-analysis. a: Standardized difference of means.

Age group/Study	Year	Scale	Test		Control		Weight	Mean	SMD[a]		Heterogeneity I² (p-Value)	Public.bias p-Value (Egger Test)
			n	Mean ± sd	n	Mean ± sd			95%-CI	p-Value		
Children + Adults (n = 10)			355		355			−0.77	−1.28 to −0.26	0.003	65.8% (0.002)	0.173
Children (n = 8) (see Figure 7)												
Shetty V1 [25]	2019	W-BFS	60	2.00 ± 0.50	60	2.42 ± 1.47	13.6%	−0.38	−0.74 to −0.0			
Nurma M2 [23]	2019	W-BFS	35	3.03 ± 2.22	35	2.97 ± 2.49	13.2%	0.03	−0.44 to 0.49			
Niharika P2 [24]	2018	W-BFS	20	2.56 ± 0.39	20	5.22 ± 0.51	7.8%	−5.71	−7.16 to −4.25			
Mitrakul K4 [27]	2015	FPS-R	21	1.90 ± 2.93	21	1.90 ± 3.32	12.5%	0.00	−0.60 to 0.60			
Mitrakul K3 [27]	2015	FPS-R	21	0.86 ± 1.49	21	1.62 ± 2.94	12.5%	−0.32	−0.93 to 0.29			
Asvanund Y2 [28]	2015	FPS-R	49	2.23 ± 2.29	49	2.46 ± 3.46	13.5%	−0.08	−0.47 to 0.32			
Asvanund Y1 [28]	2015	FPS-R	49	1.57 ± 2.29	49	3.04 ± 3.08	13.5%	−0.54	−0.94 to −0.13			
Asl Aminabadi N2 [22]	2012	W-BFS	60	1.89 ± 0.65	60	3.00 ± 0.81	13.4%	−1.50	−1.91 to −1.10			
Total			315		315		100%	−0.82	−1.42 to −0.22	0.008	71% (p = 0.001)	p = 0.180
Adults (n = 2) (see Figure 7)												
Sweta VR [2]	2019	VAS	25	1.28 ± 0.89	25	2.60 ± 1.38	52.3%	−1.12	−1.72 to −0.52			
Gujjar KR2 [6]	2019	VAS	15	68 ± 10	15	70 ± 14	47.7%	−0.18	−0.90 to 0.53			
Total			40		40			−0.67	−1.58 to 0.24	0.149	0% (p = 0.317)	-

3.4. Publication Bias and Heterogeneity

All estimates seem not to be affected by publication bias, according to the Egger test (Tables 1 and 2), but heterogeneity seems to be substantial.

4. Discussion

While anxiety and pain are usually associated with dental treatments, the number of studies addressing their management, especially during anesthetic block, which is one of the procedures that usually causes great anxiety among patients, is very limited [2,30].

Although most studies are based on pediatric population, fear of dental treatment affects 15%–20% of the population, being recognized by the World Health Organization (WHO) as a real pathology [3,31,32] that leads those who are affected by it to reject even the most basic dental treatments, such as simple dental check-ups or cleanings [33]; thus, its management is essential to improve the patient's quality of life [34].

Despite the existence of rigorous reviews of literature [5], we believe that this is the first systematic review and meta-analysis focused on the efficacy of VR in patients, regardless of age, who suffer from anxiety triggered by dental treatments.

Our meta-analysis is based on 10 studies: two on pain, two on DA and six on DA and P together, and has proved that VR is an effective tool for reducing pain (SMD = −0.82), as reported by child patients during a variety of dental procedures.

Some studies proved that, both for pain and anxiety, the use of VR was more effective in children than in adults. A possible reason for this could be that VR is especially appealing to children, since they become more engaged in whimsical thinking and are fascinated by imaginative play [35].

Nevertheless, regarding age, it should be noted that the differences in the efficacy of VR, in each study, could be due to the interpretive problems to which these analyses are susceptible; such phenomenon, known as ecological fallacies, could be associated either to the heterogeneity of the study's characteristics (methodological diversity), or to the study populations (clinical diversity) [36].

VR was found to be more effective for treating P and DA than conventional treatments; however, it is difficult to assess its efficacy as compared to other types of distraction. Klassen and colleagues [37] conducted a meta-analysis on distraction using music therapy as an alternative method to reduce anxiety and pain in different medical and dental procedures, finding a significant reduction, with an effect size of 0.35. A Cochrane review of psychological interventions using different types of distraction to relieve pain in children and adolescents, published in 2006 and updated in 2013 and 2018 [38–40], reported different distraction techniques such as musical therapy, reading, watching films, hypnosis, breathing techniques and combined cognitive-behavioral strategies, as effective tools to reduce pain and anxiety during needle procedures. However, the reviewers considered the level of certainty of the review to be low, since in most of these studies there was no blinding of participants and assessors. This is consistent with our meta-analysis, according to which only 35% of the studies included met this requirement.

The heterogeneity of VR software and hardware is also relevant to the immersive approach, which is influenced by the interaction with the virtual environment, either through translation or change of position, rotation or change of direction, viewpoint or perspective and visual field. This aspect is difficult to analyze when referred to patients who are undergoing dental treatment (especially in children), since adequate patient immersion is hindered by the fact that they are expected to remain with their heads as still as possible to facilitate the professional's work [41].

Large devices (hardware), also hinder the dentist's work, limiting vision of and access to the dental operation area [42].

Another interesting aspect that has not been given due regard by researchers is gender difference and its significance in terms of fear of dental treatment. Patients who suffer from dental phobia are characterized by a gender-specific brain structure. Such differences have not been sufficiently addressed by researchers and clinicians, and could contribute to greater effectiveness in the management of dental phobia [43].

Likewise, patients' different personality traits were not considered in the studies included, either. Patients with dental fear and a high predisposition to anxiety magnify their pain expectations when they are exposed to critical situations. When patients with dental anxiety undergo dental treatment, their beliefs about the negative consequences of bodily excitement can negatively influence their assessment of pain linked to such treatment [44]. DA as a predisposing factor is associated with a state of anxiety, which has a constant impact on pain during the patient's entire dental treatment; hence, anxiety should be assessed as a critical step not only towards anxiety management in patients with high DA, but also towards P management in all dental patients [45].

On the other hand, the studies included used different pain and DA assessment scales: VAS, W-BFS, FPS-R FLACC, VRS, MDAS, NCAQ and VCARS. Likewise, none of the studies included single scales for joint assessment by dentist and patient. Vital signs as emotional state indicators were also assessed in some of the studies, thus it would be convenient and appropriate to find validated scales that might be used to adequately assess all of these aspects [46].

Eijlers and colleagues [5,47] presented two preparatory studies for pediatric surgery based on VR training programs; however, the use of this type of preparatory program before certain dental procedures is yet to be explored by researchers and, therefore, it is currently not possible to compare effects with and without preparation.

Moreover, none of the studies drew attention to factors that could moderate VR's effectiveness, such as a subject's sensitivity to anxiety or their temperament. Shy and emotional temperaments could be associated with dental anxiety [48–51].

For all these reasons, we believe that this systematic review has certain limitations in terms of number, quality and methodology of the studies included: only three studies in adults were included [2,6,9], which is too scarce to consider them significant in our analysis, the authors themselves even acknowledge the limited sample size in one of them [2], and the existence of major limitations with regard to participant and assessor blinding, in another [6].

Hence, to determine the effects of VR on anxiety and pain in dental treatments, it would be necessary to reduce the risk of bias, to remove confusion factors and to establish a clear definition of the adequate parameters, all with the purpose of obtaining results that can be translated into broad clinical applications, so that the evidence can effectively support the practice of clinical dentistry.

5. Conclusions

This systematic review and meta-analysis leads to the conclusion that VR is a useful tool to reduce P in children undergoing dental treatment. No significant effect was found for DA. Studies in adults are scarce. On the other hand, most of the studies chose to focus on immersion in the pediatric population, neglecting a series of aspects that should be considered, such as training programs, the different types of software and hardware of virtual reality devices, the temperament and patient personality, gender difference and more. Due to all this, the role of virtual reality in the control of anxiety and dental pain in children and adults should be considered as a topic for future research.

Author Contributions: Study concept and design: N.L.-V., A.L.-V., J.M.F.; Acquisition of data (Literature search and Study Selection): N.L.-V., J.F.F., J.M.R.; Analysis and interpretation of data (literature): M.B., L.F.V.J., J.H.P., L.A.B.A.; Drafting of the manuscript: N.L.-V.; A.L.-V., B.M.d.S.; Critical revision of the manuscript for important intellectual content: A.L.-V., M.B. All authors have read and agreed to the published version of the manuscript.

Conflicts of Interest: The authors declare no conflict of interest.

Abbreviations

VR	Virtual Reality
DA	Dental Anxiety
VAS	Visual Analogic Scale
W–BFS	Wong–Baker Faces Scale
FPS-R	Faces Pain Scale-Revise
FLACC	Consolability Scale
VRS	Verbal Rating Scale
MDAS	Modified Dental Anxiety Scale
NCAQ	Norman Corah's anxiety questionnaire
VCARS	Venham's Clinical Anxiety Rating Scale
RoB	Risk of Bias
SDs	Standard Deviation
SMD	Standard Mean Deviation
CI	Confidence Interval

References

1. López-Valverde, A.; Montero, J.; Albaladejo, A.; Gómez de Diego, R. The discovery of surgical anesthesia: Discrepancies regarding its authorship. *J. Dent. Res.* **2011**, *90*, 31–34. [CrossRef] [PubMed]
2. Sweta, V.R.; Abhinav, R.P.; Asha, R. Role of Virtual Reality in Pain Perception of Patients Following the Administration of Local Anesthesia. *Ann. Maxillofac. Surg.* **2019**, *9*, 110–113. [PubMed]
3. Ougradar, A.; Ahmed, B. Patients' perceptions of the benefits of virtual reality during dental extractions. *Br. Dent. J.* **2019**, *227*, 813–816. [CrossRef] [PubMed]
4. Carl, E.; Stein, A.T.; Levihn-Coon, A.; Pogue, J.R.; Rothbaum, B.; Emmelkamp, P.; Asmundson, G.; Carlbring, P.; Powers, M.B. Virtual reality exposure therapy for anxiety and related disorders: A meta-analysis of randomized controlled trials. *J. Anxiety Disord.* **2019**, *61*, 27–36. [CrossRef]
5. Eijlers, R.; Utens, E.; Staals, L.M.; de Nijs, P.F.A.; Berghmans, J.M.; Wijnen, R.M.H.; Hillegers, M.H.J.; Dierckx, B.; Legerstee, J.S. Systematic Review and Meta-analysis of Virtual Reality in Pediatrics: Effects on Pain and Anxiety. *Anesth. Analg.* **2019**, *129*, 1344–1353. [CrossRef]
6. Gujjar, K.R.; van Wijk, A.; Kumar, R.; de Jongh, A. Efficacy of virtual reality exposure therapy for the treatment of dental phobia in adults: A randomized controlled trial. *J. Anxiety Disord.* **2019**, *62*, 100–108. [CrossRef]
7. Raghav, K.; Van Wijk, A.J.; Abdullah, F.; Islam, M.N.; Bernatchez, M.; De Jongh, A. Efficacy of virtual reality exposure therapy for treatment of dental phobia: A randomized control trial. *BMC Oral Health* **2016**, *27*, 25. [CrossRef]
8. Wiederhold, M.D.; Gao, K.; Wiederhold, B.K. Clinical use of virtual reality distraction system to reduce anxiety and pain in dental procedures. *Cyberpsychol. Behav. Soc. Netw.* **2014**, *17*, 359–365. [CrossRef]
9. Tanja-Dijkstra, K.; Pahl, S.; White, M.P.; Andrade, J.; Qian, C.; Bruce, M.; May, J.; Moles, D.R. Improving dental experiences by using virtual reality distraction: A simulation study. *PLoS ONE* **2014**, *2*, e91276. [CrossRef]
10. Dahlquist, L.M.; McKenna, K.D.; Jones, K.K.; Dillinger, L.; Weiss, K.E.; Ackerman, C.S. Active and passive distraction using a head-mounted display helmet: Effects on cold pressor pain in children. *Health Psychol.* **2014**, *26*, 794–801. [CrossRef]
11. Schneider, S.M.; Hood, L.E. Virtual reality: A distraction intervention for chemotherapy. *Oncol. Nurs. Forum* **2007**, *34*, 39–46. [CrossRef] [PubMed]
12. Malloy, K.M.; Milling, L.S. The effectiveness of virtual reality distraction for pain reduction: A systematic review. *Clin. Psychol. Rev.* **2010**, *30*, 1011–1018. [CrossRef] [PubMed]
13. American Society of Anesthesiologists Task Force on Sedation and Analgesia by Non-Anesthesiologists. Practice guidelines for sedation and analgesia by non-anesthesiologists. *Anesthesiology* **2002**, *96*, 1004–1017. [CrossRef] [PubMed]
14. Dixon, R.A.; Kenyon, C.; Marsh, D.R.; Thornton, J.A. Midazolam in conservative dentistry. A cross-over trial. *Anaesthesia* **1986**, *41*, 276–281. [CrossRef]
15. Foley, J. The way forward for dental sedation and primary cares? *Br. Dent. J.* **2002**, *193*, 161–164. [CrossRef]

16. Hutton, B.; Ferrán Catalá-López, F.; Moher, D. The PRISMA statement extension for systematic reviews incorporating network meta-analysis: PRISMA-NMA. *Med. Clin.* **2016**, *16*, 262–266. [CrossRef]
17. Higgins, J.P.T.; Altman, D.G.; Sterne, J.A.C. *Cochrane Handbook for Systematic Reviews of Interventions*, version 5.1.0; Higgins, J.P.T., Green, S., Eds.; The Cochrane Collaboration: London, UK, 2006; Chapter 8; Available online: http://www.cochrane-handbook.org (accessed on 20 October 2019).
18. Vandenbroucke, J.P.; von Elm, E.; Altman, D.G.; Gøtzsche, P.C.; Mulrow, C.D.; Pocock, S.J.; Charles, P.; James, J.S.; Matthias, E. STROBE Initiative. Strengthening the reporting of observational studies in epidemiology (STROBE): Explanation and elaboration. *PLoS Med.* **2007**, *4*, e297. [CrossRef]
19. Tanja-Dijkstra, K.; Pahl, S.; White, M.P.; Andrade, J.; May, J.; Stone, R.J.; Bruce, M.; Mills, I.; Auvray, M.; Gabe, R.; et al. Can virtual nature improve patient experiences and memories of dental treatment? A study protocol for a randomized controlled trial. *Trials* **2014**, *22*, 90. [CrossRef]
20. Al-Halabi, M.N.; Bshara, N.; AlNerabieah, Z. Effectiveness of audio visual distraction using virtual reality eyeglasses versus tablet device in child behavioral management during inferior alveolar nerve block. *Anaesth. Pain Intensive Care* **2018**, *22*, 55–61.
21. Bentsen, B.; Svensson, P.; Wenzel, A. Evaluation of effect of 3D video glasses on perceived pain and unpleasantness induced by restorative dental treatment. *Eur. J. Pain* **2001**, *5*, 373–378. [CrossRef]
22. Asl Aminabadi, N.; Erfanparast, L.; Sohrabi, A.; Ghertasi Oskouei, S.; Naghili, A. The Impact of Virtual Reality Distraction on Pain and Anxiety during Dental Treatment in 4-6 Year-Old Children: A Randomized Controlled Clinical Trial. *J. Dent. Res. Dent. Clin. Dent. Prospect.* **2012**, *6*, 117–124.
23. Nunna, M.; Dasaraju, R.K.; Kamatham, R.; Mallineni, S.K.; Nuvvula, S. Comparative evaluation of virtual reality distraction and counter-stimulation on dental anxiety and pain perception in children. *J. Dent. Anesth. Pain Med.* **2019**, *19*, 277–288. [CrossRef] [PubMed]
24. Niharika, P.; Reddy, N.V.; Srujana, P.; Srikanth, K.; Daneswari, V.; Geetha, K.S. Effects of distraction using virtual reality technology on pain perception and anxiety levels in children during pulp therapy of primary molars. *J. Indian Soc. Pedod. Prev. Dent.* **2018**, *36*, 364–369. [CrossRef] [PubMed]
25. Shetty, V.; Suresh, L.R.; Hegde, A.M. Effect of Virtual Reality Distraction on Pain and Anxiety during Dental Treatment in 5 to 8 Year Old Children. *J. Clin. Pediatr. Dent.* **2019**, *43*, 97–102. [CrossRef]
26. Al-Khotani, A.; Bello, L.A.; Christidis, N. Effects of audiovisual distraction on children's behaviour during dental treatment: A randomized controlled clinical trial. *Acta Odontol. Scand.* **2016**, *74*, 494–501. [CrossRef] [PubMed]
27. Mitrakul, K.; Asvanund, Y.; Arunakul, M.; Paka-Akekaphat, S. Effect of audiovisual eyeglasses during dental treatment in 5–8 year-old children. *Eur. J. Paediatr. Dent.* **2015**, *16*, 239–245. [PubMed]
28. Asvanund, Y.; Mitrakul, K.; Juhong, R.O.; Arunakul, M. Effect of audiovisual eyeglasses during local anesthesia injections in 5- to 8-year-old children. *Quintessence Int.* **2015**, *46*, 513–521.
29. Cohen, J. *Statistical Power Analysis for the Behavioral Sciences*, 2nd ed.; Lawrence Erlbaum Associates: New York, NY, USA, 1988.
30. Yamashita, Y.; Shimohira, D.; Aijima, R.; Mori, K.; Danjo, A. Clinical Effect of Virtual Reality to Relieve Anxiety During Impacted Mandibular Third Molar Extraction Under Local Anesthesia. *J. Oral Maxillofac. Surg.* **2019**, *26*, 31343–31346. [CrossRef]
31. Hill, K.B.; Chadwick, B.; Freeman, R.; O'Sullivan, I.; Murray, J.J. Adult Dental Health Survey 2009: Relationships between dental attendance patterns, oral health behaviour and the current barriers to dental care. *Br. Dent. J.* **2013**, *214*, 25–32. [CrossRef]
32. Seligman, L.D.; Hovey, J.D.; Chacon, K.; Ollendick, T.H. Dental anxiety: An understudied problem in youth. *Clin. Psychol. Rev.* **2017**, *55*, 25–40. [CrossRef]
33. De Stefano, R. Psychological Factors in Dental Patient Care: Odontophobia. *Medicina* **2019**, *8*, 55. [CrossRef] [PubMed]
34. Fiorillo, L. Oral Health: The First Step to Well-Being. *Medicina* **2019**, *7*, 55. [CrossRef] [PubMed]
35. Bolton, D.; Dearsley, P.; Madronal-Luque, R.; Baron-Cohen, S. Magical thinking in childhood and adolescence: Development and relation to obsessive compulsion. *Br. J. Dev. Psychol.* **2002**, *20*, 479–494. [CrossRef]
36. Thompson, S.G.; Higgins, J.P. How should meta-regression analyses be undertaken and interpreted? *Stat. Med.* **2002**, *21*, 559–573. [CrossRef]

37. Klassen, J.A.; Liang, Y.; Tjosvold, L.; Klassen, T.P.; Hartling, L. Music for pain and anxiety in children undergoing medical procedures: A systematic review of randomized controlled trials. *Ambul. Pediatr.* **2008**, *8*, 117–128. [CrossRef]
38. Uman, L.S.; Chambers, C.T.; McGrath, P.J.; Kisely, S. Psychological interventions for needle-related procedural pain and distress in children and adolescents. *Cochrane Database Syst. Rev.* **2006**, *18*. [CrossRef]
39. Uman, S.L.; Birnie, K.A.; Noel, M.; Parker, J.A.; Chambers, C.T.; McGrath, P.J.; Kisely, S.R. Psychological interventions for needle-related procedural pain and distress in children and adolescents. *Cochrane Database Syst. Rev.* **2013**, *10*. [CrossRef]
40. Birnie, K.A.; Noel, M.; Chambers, C.T.; Uman, L.S.; Parker, J.A. Psychological interventions for needle-related procedural pain and distress in children and adolescents. *Cochrane Database Syst. Rev.* **2018**, *10*. [CrossRef]
41. Hoffman, H.G.; Sharar, S.R.; Coda, B.; Everett, J.J.; Ciol, M.; Richards, T.; Patterson, D.R. Manipulating presence influences the magnitude of virtual reality analgesia. *Pain* **2004**, *111*, 162–168. [CrossRef]
42. Yu, M.; Zhou, R.; Wang, H.; Zhao, W. An evaluation for VR glasses system user experience: The influence factors of interactive operation and motion sickness. *Appl. Ergon.* **2019**, *74*, 206–213. [CrossRef]
43. Schienle, A.; Scharmüller, W.; Leutgeb, V.; Schäfer, A.; Stark, R. Sex differences in the functional and structural neuroanatomy of dental phobia. *Brain Struct. Funct.* **2013**, *218*, 779–787. [CrossRef]
44. Klages, U.; Kianifard, S.; Ulusoy, O.; Wehrbein, H. Anxiety sensitivity as predictor of pain in patients undergoing restorative dentalprocedures. *Community Dent. Oral Epidemiol.* **2006**, *34*, 139–145. [CrossRef] [PubMed]
45. Lin, C.S.; Wu, S.Y.; Yi, C.A. Association between Anxiety and Pain in Dental Treatment: A Systematic Review and Meta-analysis. *J. Dent. Res.* **2017**, *96*, 153–162. [CrossRef] [PubMed]
46. Astramskaitė, I.; Juodžbalys, G. Scales used to rate adult patients' psycho-emotional status in tooth extraction procedures: A systematic review. *Int. J. Oral Maxillofac. Surg.* **2017**, *46*, 886–898. [CrossRef] [PubMed]
47. Eijlers, R.; Legerstee, J.S.; Dierckx, B.; Staals, L.M.; Berghmans, J.; van der Schroeff, M.P.; Wijnen, R.M.; Utens, E.M. Development of a Virtual Reality Exposure Tool as Psychological Preparation for Elective Pediatric Day Care Surgery: Methodological Approach for a Randomized Controlled Trial. *JMIR Res. Protoc.* **2017**, *6*, e174. [CrossRef] [PubMed]
48. Jain, A.; Suprabha, B.S.; Shenoy, R.; Rao, A. Association of temperament with dental anxiety and behaviour of the preschool child during the initial dental visit. *Eur. J. Oral Sci.* **2019**, *127*, 147–155. [CrossRef] [PubMed]
49. Stenebrand, A.; Wide Boman, U.; Hakeberg, M. Dental anxiety and temperament in 15-year olds. *Acta Odontol. Scand.* **2013**, *71*, 15–21. [CrossRef]
50. Lundgren, J.; Elfström, M.L.; Berggren, U. The relationship between temperament and fearfulness in adult dental phobic patients. *Int. J. Paediatr. Dent.* **2007**, *17*, 460–468. [CrossRef]
51. Bergdahl, M.; Bergdahl, J. Temperament and character personality dimensions in patients with dental anxiety. *Eur. J. Oral. Sci.* **2003**, *111*, 93–98. [CrossRef]

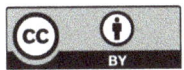

© 2020 by the authors. Licensee MDPI, Basel, Switzerland. This article is an open access article distributed under the terms and conditions of the Creative Commons Attribution (CC BY) license (http://creativecommons.org/licenses/by/4.0/).

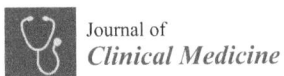

Retraction

Retraction: Lopez-Valverde, N.; et al. Use of Virtual Reality for the Management of Anxiety and Pain in Dental Treatments: Systematic Review and Meta-Analysis. *J. Clin. Med.* 2020, 9, 1025

Nansi López-Valverde [1], Jorge Muriel Fernández [1], Antonio López-Valverde [1,*], Luis F. Valero Juan [2], Juan Manuel Ramírez [3], Javier Flores Fraile [1], Julio Herrero Payo [1], Leticia A. Blanco Antona [1], Bruno Macedo de Sousa [4] and Manuel Bravo [5]

1. Department of Surgery, University of Salamanca, Instituto de Investigación Biomédica de Salamanca (IBSAL), 37007 Salamanca, Spain; nlovalher@usal.es (N.L.-V.); murimuriel@gmail.com (J.M.F.); j.flores@usal.es (J.F.F.); jhpayo@usal.es (J.H.P.); lesablantona@gmail.com (L.A.B.A.)
2. Department of Biomedical and Diagnostic Sciences, University of Salamanca, Avda. Alfonso X El Sabio S/N, 37007 Salamanca, Spain; luva@usal.es
3. Department of Morphological Sciences, University of Cordoba, Avenida Menéndez Pidal s/n, 14071 Cordoba, Spain; jmramirez@uco.es
4. Institute for Occlusion and Orofacial Pain Faculty of Medicine, University of Coimbra, Polo I - Edifício Central Rua Larga, 3004-504 Coimbra, Portugal; brunomsousa@usal.es
5. Department of Preventive and Community Dentistry, Facultad de Odontología, Campus de Cartuja s/n, 18071 Granada, Spain; mbravo@ugr.es
* Correspondence: anlopezvalverde@gmail.com

Received: 22 July 2020; Accepted: 23 July 2020; Published: 28 July 2020

The authors of a recent published paper [1] in the *Journal of Clinical Medicine* retract their paper due to the serious flaws in the study design and data presentation. These errors were reported by two readers of the journal. The authors would like to acknowledge both readers pointing out such important mistakes. The authors apologize for not using the final data to conduct the analysis, resulting in unreliable results. The editor-in-chief and academic editors of the *Journal of Clinical Medicine* have checked this case. The editor-in-chief has approved the retraction. Both readers have been informed about the retraction decision.

The authors apologize to readers of the *Journal of Clinical Medicine* for any inconvenience this may have caused. MDPI is a member of the Committee on Publication Ethics and takes the responsibility to uphold strict ethical policies and standards very seriously.

Reference

1. López-Valverde, N.; Muriel Fernández, J.; López-Valverde, A.; Valero Juan, L.F.; Ramírez, J.M.; Flores Fraile, J.; Herrero Payo, J.; Blanco Antona, L.A.; Macedo de Sousa, B.; Bravo, M. Use of Virtual Reality for the Management of Anxiety and Pain in Dental Treatments: Systematic Review and Meta-Analysis. *J. Clin. Med.* **2020**, *9*, 1025.

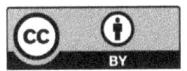 © 2020 by the authors. Licensee MDPI, Basel, Switzerland. This article is an open access article distributed under the terms and conditions of the Creative Commons Attribution (CC BY) license (http://creativecommons.org/licenses/by/4.0/).

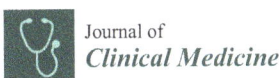

Article

The Use of a Virtual Reality Platform for the Assessment of the Memory Decline and the Hippocampal Neural Injury in Subjects with Mild Cognitive Impairment: The Validity of Smart Aging Serious Game (SASG)

Monia Cabinio [1], Federica Rossetto [1], Sara Isernia [1], Francesca Lea Saibene [1], Monica Di Cesare [1], Francesca Borgnis [1], Stefania Pazzi [2], Tommaso Migliazza [2], Margherita Alberoni [1], Valeria Blasi [1,*] and Francesca Baglio [1]

1. IRCCS Fondazione Don Carlo Gnocchi ONLUS, via Capecelatro 66, 20148 Milan, Italy; mcabinio@dongnocchi.it (M.C.); frossetto@dongnocchi.it (F.R.); sisernia@dongnocchi.it (S.I.); fsaibene@dongnocchi.it (F.L.S.); mdicesare@dongnocchi.it (M.D.C.); fborgnis@dongnocchi.it (F.B.); malberoni@dongnocchi.it (M.A.); fbaglio@dongnocchi.it (F.B.)
2. Consorzio di Bioingegneria e Informatica medica (CBIM), 27100 Pavia, Italy; s.pazzi@cbim.it (S.P.); t.migliazza@cbim.it (T.M.)
* Correspondence: vblasi@dongnocchi.it; Tel.: +39-0240308069

Received: 31 March 2020; Accepted: 1 May 2020; Published: 6 May 2020

Abstract: Due to the lack of pharmacological treatment for dementia, timely detection of subjects at risk can be of seminal importance for preemptive rehabilitation interventions. The aim of the study was to determine the usability of the smart aging serious game (SASG), a virtual reality platform, in assessing the cognitive profile of an amnestic mild cognitive impairment (aMCI) population, its validity in discriminating aMCI from healthy controls (HC), and in detecting hippocampal degeneration, a biomarker of clinical progression towards dementia. Thirty-six aMCI and 107 HC subjects were recruited and administered the SASG together with a neuropsychological evaluation. All aMCI and 30 HC subjects performed also an MRI for hippocampal volume measurement. Results showed good usability of the SASG despite the low familiarity with technology in both groups. ROC curve analyses showed similar discriminating abilities for SASG and gold standard tests, and a greater discrimination ability compared to non-specific neuropsychological tests. Finally, linear regression analysis revealed that the SASG outperformed the Montreal cognitive assessment test (MoCA) in the ability to detect neuronal degeneration in the hippocampus on the right side. These data show that SASG is an ecological task, that can be considered a digital biomarker providing objective and clinically meaningful data about the cognitive profile of aMCI subjects.

Keywords: virtual reality; serious game; mild cognitive impairment; dementia; Alzheimer disease; digital biomarker; hippocampus; MRI; cognitive rehabilitation; computerized assessment

1. Introduction

Virtual reality (VR) has been defined as an application that allows users to navigate and interact with a three-dimensional computer-generated environment in real time [1]. Paralleling the advancements of information technology (IT) in the implementation of multi-dimensional platforms for the care of patients [2–4], VR gives the opportunity to improve cognitive assessment allowing more ecological and smart instruments of evaluation [5–10]. In particular, serious games (SGs), defined as "digital applications specialized for purposes other than entertaining" [11,12], with their capacity to implement

VR environments can represent an easily-accessible method to assess cognitive functions in a more ecological way, since they can host complex environments resembling real-life context with different levels of complexity [7,9,10,13].

Although the field of SGs is quite young, digital applications for clinical purposes are becoming more and more available, and some of them have been validly used in healthy subjects [10,14,15] as well as in clinical populations, particularly in Parkinson's disease [9,16] and in subjects with amnestic mild cognitive impairment (aMCI) and dementia [17–22]. Data from the literature confirm that SGs are not only appropriate but also recommended for the assessment and stimulation of elderly people with MCI and dementia [23].

Faced with the increasing number of new evaluation instruments, the need to implement scientifically valid, reliable and smart instruments to detect clinical and pre-clinical conditions in the early stages is of pivotal importance.

MCI is a "mild neurocognitive disorder" [24,25] lying on the continuum between normal aging and cognitive decline [26,27], affecting approximately 10% to 20% of adults over 65 years of age [26]. MCI is defined as a symptomatic pre-dementia stage in which the cognitive impairment does not affect the functional activities of daily living [26]. The incidence for the development of dementia in individuals with MCI older than 65 years of age is approximately 4.9% in two years [28]. Among the different forms of MCI, the amnestic form (aMCI) refers to a condition in which the memory dysfunction predominates [29] and that is associated with specific brain changes, such as reduction of hippocampal volume [30,31] and cortical thinning in medial temporal [30] and parietal [32,33] cortices. These abnormalities are specific for aMCI and represent biomarker of neuronal degeneration [34]. In particular, the reduction of the hippocampal volume is currently considered a biomarker to detect the subjects with aMCI at higher risk of cognitive decline [35,36]. Consequently, with their brain changes aMCI subjects have a higher risk of developing Alzheimer's disease (AD), when compared to non-amnestic MCI [37]. This strong association with dementia makes aMCI an important target for early pharmacological and rehabilitation interventions such as cognitive and physical exercise training [38,39]. In this line, at the beginning of 2018 the American Academy of Neurology published the new practice guidelines, underlying the importance to assess people in this pre-clinical condition using validated tools, detecting both functional impairment and cognitive status in a longitudinal way [28]. For large scale and timely screening for aMCI, more ecological tools, mimicking everyday activities, are becoming a cardinal issue. In this line, an ecological, virtual 3D environment-based tool named "smart aging" (smart aging serious game, SASG-http://www.cbim.it/en_new/serious-games-en/index.html [7,10]), aimed at evaluating multiple cognitive domains, was developed. The SASG integrates five cognitive tasks in a setting resembling a real house. Subjects are asked to play the tasks of the game following simple instructions while moving through the rooms, while the software evaluates performance accuracy and reaction times. When tested in a large cohort of aged cognitively-preserved subjects, SASG was demonstrated to be a valid tool for assessing cognitive functions [10]. The interface of SASG is specifically designed to be easily accessible to older or non-expert computer users by means of a touchscreen, a first-person perspective, and an automatic navigation system.

According to these premises, the present study had a three-fold aim: 1. to evaluate the usability of SASG in a cohort of aMCI patients and healthy controls (HC), taking into account the familiarity with the used technology; 2. to investigate the validity of SASG in discriminating between aMCI and healthy control subjects in comparison with gold standard pencil paper neuropsychological tests; and 3. to determine the validity of the SASG in detecting hippocampal degeneration as a neuroimaging marker of neuronal injury in comparison to gold standard pencil paper neuropsychological tests.

2. Materials and Methods

2.1. Recruited Sample

A total sample of 139 subjects participated in the study. Subjects with a diagnosis of aMCI ($n = 32$) were consecutively recruited from the outpatient memory clinic at the IRCCS Fondazione Don Carlo Gnocchi ONLUS (FDG, Milan, Italy). The inclusion criteria were: (1) aMCI diagnosis according to the recommendations of the National Institute on Aging [27] and the DSM 5 diagnostic criteria [24]; (2) presence of a mini-mental state examination [40] score ≥ 24, corrected for age and years of education according to Italian normative data [41]; (3) age ≥ 65 years and school attendance ≥ 3 years; (4) abnormal memory function confirmed by an informant and documented by the neuropsychological examination; (5) no impairment in functional activities of daily living as determined by a clinical interview with both the patient and the caregiver; (6) absence of psychiatric illnesses, with particular attention to depressive symptoms (Hamilton depression rating scale score ≤ 12 [42]) and severe behavioral disturbance; (7) absence of severe auditory/visual loss that can prevent from the use of technological device and from the execution of the serious game; (8) absence of major brain abnormalities at MRI scan or significant cerebral vascular diseases (Hachinski score above 4) [43].

A sample of age-, gender- and education-matched HC ($n = 107$) was also included. HC were obtained from the CBIM repository and from volunteers recruited from FDG. In more detail, HC were recruited from universities of the third age, social clubs and among volunteers working in the FDG and caregivers of outpatients. All the HC lived independently, had active social and cognitive lives and were native Italian speakers. They underwent an in-clinic neuropsychological evaluation including MMSE score and a neurological interview to exclude major neurological complaint. They fit the inclusion criteria number 3, 5, 6 and 7 of the above listing and presented a MMSE ≥ 28. The study was approved by the Ethics Committee of the Don Gnocchi Foundation and all subjects signed a written and informed consent.

2.2. Neuropsychological Evaluation

All subjects performed in a clinical setting and in close proximity with SASG completion, a neuropsychological evaluation. This was conducted by a trained neuropsychologist using conventional pencil–paper test including:

[i] the Montreal cognitive assessment test (MoCA): an established rapid cognitive screening tool able to differentiate MCI from normal aging and from AD patients, with a high sensitivity and specificity [44,45]. Raw data were corrected according to Italian normative data [46].

[ii] the immediate and delayed recall scores obtained from the free and cued selective reminding test (FCSRT, [47]), a widely used memory test that provides details on the encoding and retrieval phases of the memorization processes. Data were corrected according to [48].

[iii] the trail making test (TMT, [49]), versions A and B, for the assessment of executive functions and mental flexibility, as well as visual search, and processing speed. Data were corrected according to [50].

2.3. Serious Game Task: The Smart Aging Serious Game (SASG)

Each subject was asked to complete, in a clinical setting, a single SASG (http://www.cbim.it/en_new/serious-games-en/index.html) session, extensively described elsewhere [6,7,10]. Shortly, the SASG was administered in presence of a neuropsychologist and was performed using a touch-screen monitor, in a first-person perspective. SAGS is an ecological serious game based on a virtual house, in which subjects are asked to interact with the different parts of the scenario and to perform specific tasks. All the actions performed by the subjects within the SAGS are recorded and measured, allowing the assessment of memory, executive functions, working memory, and visual spatial processes [10] through the execution of five tasks. Task 1 (T1), named "Object search", investigates memory, spatial orientation and attention; task 2 (T2), called "Water the flowers while listening to the radio", assesses executive functions and divided attention; task 3 (T3), "Make a phone call", evaluates executive functions, selective attention, working and perspective memory; task 4 (T4), "Choose the right object", investigates memory and task 5 (T5), "Find the objects", assesses long-term memory (recall), spatial orientation and attention.

In order to familiarize with the virtual environment and the use of the touch screen before the actual evaluative session, subjects naïve in the use of ICT and touch screens, were presented with a 10-min interactive demo. Successively, no other feedback was provided while the subjects were performing the serious games.

In line with Bottiroli (2017) [10], we collected accuracy (accuracy index, AI) and time (time index, TI) measurements for each SAGS task. AI and TI were then converted into z-scores considering the mean and standard deviation of the HC sample. For each task a total score was computed (as the difference between AI and TI, in line with [10] and the sum of the total scores of all tasks was computed to calculate the Smart Aging Total Score (SASG-Total).

Computer familiarity measures were collected with an ad hoc questionnaire according to [51]. Specifically, each subject was asked to fill out a computer questionnaire concerning its familiarity with computers and touch-screen use, expressed in terms of frequency of use, before SASG session.

2.4. MRI Acquisition and Analysis

All of the aMCI performed a single brain MRI acquisition (1.5 T Siemens Magnetom Avanto, Erlangen, Germany) within two weeks from the neuropsychological evaluation, to collect a high-resolution 3D-T1 image (MPRAGE; TR/TE = 1900/3.37 ms, FoV = 192 mm × 256 mm, in-plane resolution 1 mm × 1 mm, slice thickness = 1 mm, number of axial slices = 176) in order to measure hippocampal volumes. The MRI protocol included a dual-echo turbo spin echo proton density PD/T2-weighted image (repetition time (TR) = 5550 ms, echo time (TE) = 23/103 ms, matrix size = 320 × 320 × 45, resolution 0.8 × 0.8 × 3 mm^3) for the evaluation of the white matter hyperintensities.

High-resolution T1 images have been analyzed using Freesurfer's recon-all pipeline (https://surfer.nmr.mgh.harvard.edu/, [52]) and total hippocampal volumes have been segmented using the hippocampal subfield segmentation tool of Freesurfer (v.6.0) [53], basing on a statistical postmortem atlas built primarily upon ultra-high resolution (~0.1 mm isotropic) MRI data. Quality checks were performed at each step of the pipeline, and at the end of the cortical parcellation according to ENIGMA guidelines (http://enigma.ini.usc.edu). Total intracranial volume (TIV) has been computed using Freesurfer automatic subcortical segmentation, on the basis of the probabilistic aseg atlas [54]. Hippocampal volumes were then normalized for the total intracranial volume obtaining a normalized value (n-Hipp), using a proportional approach [55].

2.5. Statistical Analyses

Statistical analyses have been performed using MedCalc 18.5 (http://www.medcalc.org). Descriptive statistics included relative and absolute frequencies for categorical variables, median and IQ range for non-normally distributed continuous measures and means and standard deviation (SD) for continuous measures. The normality of data distribution was assessed considering the skewness and kurtosis coefficients and an appropriate parametric/non-parametric test was used for statistical analyses. When appropriate, data were corrected for multiple comparison using the Bonferroni correction, dividing the α-value (0.05) by the number of statistical tests on dependent variables.

Direct comparisons (one-way ANOVA or Mann–Whitney) on age, gender and educational level were performed to assess the between-groups matching for these variables. In order to assess the presence of hippocampal degeneration, n-Hipp volume of aMCI group was compared to an internal dataset of 30 healthy subjects with comparable age, gender and education and with the same inclusion criteria defined in the Section 2.1.

For aim 1, i.e., evaluating the usability of SASG, a between-groups comparison was performed on the results of the computer and touch screen familiarity questionnaire with a chi-squared analysis.

The key performance indicator considered for the usability of the platform was the percentage of subjects that completed the SASG evaluation (all 5 tasks). Moreover, in order to test the influence of the familiarity with computers and the SASG score, a 2 × 2 ANOVA with clinical group (aMCI vs HC) and frequency of computer use factor (infrequent vs. frequent) on SASG total score data was performed.

For aim 2, that is, determining the validity of SASG in discriminating between aMCI and HC, we performed between groups direct comparisons (one-way ANOVA or Mann–Whitney) for SASG, for the conventional pencil–paper test used to detect aMCI (MoCA total score, FCSRT scores), and for pencil paper–tests not focused on mnemonic functions (TMT-A and B). To further investigate the validity of SASG, a ROC (Receiver Operating Characteristics) curve analysis was performed to determine differences in the sensitivity and specificity of SASG in comparison with MoCA, FCSRT, TMT A and B. On the basis of our ROC curves, the best cut-off score for SASG in discriminating between HC and MCI was also investigated (Youden J index).

Finally, for aim 3, i.e., determining the ability of SASG to detect the hippocampal neuronal loss, a partial correlation analysis was performed between SASG Task total score (SASG-Total) and n-Hipp and between MoCA test and n-Hipp. Age, gender and years of education were included as a covariate of no interest. Only tasks that resulted significantly correlated with n-Hipp volume were entered into a linear regression analysis.

3. Results

3.1. Demographics and SASG Usability

Demographics of the recruited sample are detailed in Table 1. No between-group differences in age, education and gender were found. As expected, the two groups differed in the MMSE score. Moreover, aMCI subjects showed significantly lower n-Hipp volume bilaterally compared to the HC group belonging to the MRI internal database ($n = 27$; mean age 73.59 ± 4.88 years; nine males, mean education 11.59 ± 3.81 years; MMSE 29.33 ± 0.89). Due to movement artifacts, two subjects with aMCI were excluded from MRI data analyses ($n = 30$; mean age 76.07 ± 4.73 years, 15 males, mean education 10.87 ± 3.80; MMSE 27.69 ± 1.76).

Table 1. Group comparison to compare healthy controls (HC) and amnestic mild cognitive impairment (aMCI) groups for demographic variables.

	aMCI	HC	p-Value [η2; Observed Power]
n	32	107	
Age, yrs (mean ± SD)	76.75 ± 5.31	76.47 ± 3.03	n.s.
Gender (M:F)	17:15	54:53	n.s. #
Education, yrs (mean ± SD)	10.75 ± 3.84	10.95 ± 4.09	n.s.
MMSE	27.65 ± 1.79	28.74 ± 1.27	0.0027
N-Hipp volume	n = 30	n = 27	
Left n-Hipp (mean ± SD)	0.001710 ± 0.0000	0.002055 ± 0.0000	<0.001 ** [0.22; 0.96]
Right n-Hipp (mean ± SD)	0.001783 ± 0.0000	0.002099 ± 0.0000	<0.001 ** [0.26; 0.99]

n: number of subjects; yrs: years; SD: standard deviation; M: male; F: female; MMSE: mini mental state examination; N-Hipp volume: normalized hippocampal volume; # Chi-squared Test; ** ANOVA = age and education as covariates and (η2 partial value; observed power).

Results from the computer familiarity scale (Table 2) shows no differences between groups in the frequency of computer use, with 53.12% of aMCI and 60.38% of HC subjects who never used a PC, while the remaining had a frequent use (at least weekly). The frequency of use of a touch screen was comparable between groups: 62.5% of aMCI and 72.65% of HC who had never used a touch screen before the participation in the study; 18.75% of aMCI and 20.75% of HC who used it unfrequently (not more than once a month); and 18.75% of aMCI and 6.60% of HC who had a frequent (at least weekly) use. All the subjects from both groups completed the five tasks of the SASG session indicating an appropriate level of usability of the digital tool also for a population of aMCI. Testing the influence of familiarity on SASG score our ANOVA 2 × 2 results shows significant group effect ($F(1134) = 64.109$,

$p < 0.001$), however, the effect of frequency of use factor was not significant (F(1134) = 2.975, $p = 0.087$) and no significant interactions were found (F(1134) = 0.74, $p = 0.391$), indicating that familiarity with the use of the PC did not influence SASG score.

Table 2. Frequency of use for technological devices in our sample.

	aMCI	HC	p-Value
n	32	106	
Frequency of computer use			
Infrequent % (n)	53.12% (17)	60.38% (64)	n.s. #
Frequent (at least once a week) % (n)	46.88% (15)	39.62% (42)	
Frequency of use of a touch screen (last year)			
Never % (n)	62.5% (20)	72.64% (77)	n.s. #
Infrequent % (n)	18.75% (6)	20.76% (22)	
Frequent (at least once a week) % (n)	18.75% (6)	6.60% (7)	

n: number of subjects; # Chi-squared test; n.s.: not significant.

3.2. Neuropsychological Assessment Results

Data relative to the neuropsychological evaluation (Table 3) reveal that for the MoCA test total score the aMCI group performance was within the normal range (see cut-off values in Table 3) but significantly worse than the HC. As for the memory performances, assessed with the FCSRT test, the aMCI group performed worse than controls and below the cut-off value in all four indices assessing immediate and delayed free and total recall memory. On the contrary, the performances at the TMT A and B test were in the normal range and comparable between groups.

Table 3. Neuropsychological evaluation. ES = Equivalent Score. ES = 0 pathological score; ES = 1 borderline range.

Test	aMCI	HC	Cut-off (ES = 0)	ES = 1	p-Value
n	32	107			
MoCA (mean ± SD)	22.26 ± 2.84	26.97 ± 2.35	≤15.50	15.51–18.28	<0.001 *
FCSRT (median, IQ range)					
IFR adjusted	19.59 (15.79 to 23.80)	27.38 (25.38 to 29.42)	≤19.59	19.60–22.53	<0.0001 §
ITR	36 (33.5 to 36.00)	36 (36.0 to 36)	<35	–	0.0005 §
DFR adjusted	6.12 (2.67 to 10.16)	9.67 (8.67 to 10.89)	≤6.31	6.32–7.66	<0.0001 §
DTR	12 (9.5 to 12.0)	12 (12 to 12)	<11	–	<0.0001 §
TMT (median, IQ range)					
TMT-A	39 (21.5 to 64.0)	40 (28.0 to 59.0)	>93	93–69	n.s §
TMT-B	91 (55.0 to 182.75)	77.5 (49 to 115)	>282	282–178	n.s. §

n: number of subjects; MoCA: Montreal cognitive assessment—adjusted total scores [46]; FCSRT: free and cued selective reminding test [48]; IFR: immediate free recall; ITR: immediate total recall; DFR: delayed free recall; DTR: delayed total recall; TMT: trail making test [49]; in bold = p-values surviving Bonferroni's correction ($p < 0.007$) * One-Way ANOVA; § Mann–Whitney test.

3.3. SASG Results

Results of the SASG (Table 4) show significant differences between groups in the accuracy of all SASG tasks, with the exception of T2 and T3, and in the time indices of all subtests except the T4. SASG-total is significantly lower in the aMCI group.

ROC curves were computed to evaluate the diagnostic sensitivity and specificity of SASG-total and all the pencil–paper neuropsychological tests (Figure 1, Table 5). The results show high values for both parameters for all tests except the TMT A and B. Moreover, the ROC comparison analysis reveals that SASG-total is comparable to MoCA and FCSRT in the ability to discriminate between groups, while the comparison with TMT A and B reveals significantly higher ability for the SASG-total.

Table 4. Smart aging serious game (SASG) evaluation, expressed in z-scores. Mann–Whitney test. Effect size (d) and power are also included for each statistic.

Test	aMCI (Mean, IQ)	HC (Mean, IQ)	p-Value	Effect Size (d)	Power (1-β err prob)
SASG Accuracy Index (AI)					
Task 1	−0.96 (−1.60 to −0.31)	0.12 (−0.31 to 0.55)	**<0.0001**	1.04	0.99
Task 2	0.48 (0.10 to 0.74)	0.23 (−0.28 to 0.68)	0.040	0.33	0.36
Task 3	−0.78 (−0.78 to 0.83)	0.83 (−0.78 to 0.83)	0.026	0.45	0.59
Task 4	−0.99 (−2.39 to 0.15)	0.41 (−0.15 to 0.98)	**<0.0001**	0.94	0.99
Task 5	−1.75 (−2.51 to −0.63)	0.50 (−0.06 to 0.50)	**<0.0001**	1.28	0.99
SASG Time index (TI)					
Task 1	1.02 (0.72 to 1.53)	−0.06 (−0.70 to 0.65)	**<0.0001**	1.26	0.99
Task 2	0.63 (0.28 to 1.40)	−0.01 (−0.57 to 0.50)	**<0.0001**	0.90	0.99
Task 3	1.03 (0.69 to 1.46)	−0.19 (−0.78 to 0.77)	**<0.0001**	1.19	0.99
Task 4	0.45 (−0.20 to 0.69)	0.15 (−0.78 to 0.74)	n.s.	0.34	0.37
Task 5	1.33 (1.28 to 1.38)	−0.30 (−0.90 to 1.19)	**<0.0001**	1.81	0.99
SASG–Total	−8.29 (−12.04 to −4.90)	0.84 (−3.07 to 3.71)	**<0.0001**	1.61	0.99

SASG-total: smart aging serious game total score; in bold = p-values surviving Bonferroni correction ($p < 0.005$).

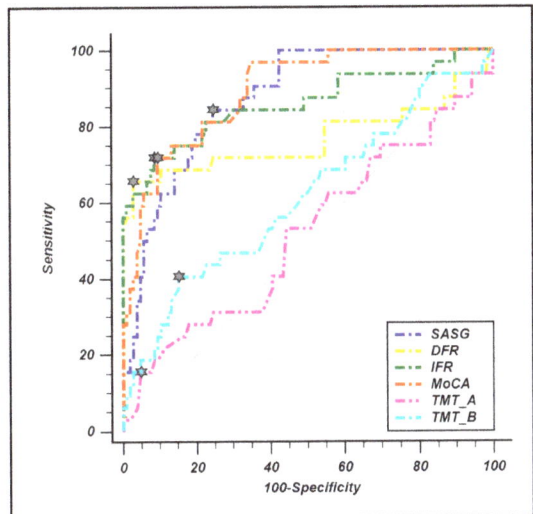

Figure 1. ROC curve comparison between smart aging total score and conventional paper-and-pencil test. Little stars indicate the criterion associated to Youden J statistic.

Table 5. Statistical comparison between the SASG ROC curve and other tests in terms of sensitivity, specificity, AUC, SE and confidence intervals.

Test	Sensitivity	Specificity	AUC	SE	95% CI	p-Value	Criterion Value (J Index)
SASG-Total	84.4	75.5	0.88	0.03	0.81 to 0.92	–	≤−3.28 (0.60)
MoCA (adj)	71.9	90.6	0.89	0.03	0.81 to 0.94	n.s.	≤23.44 (0.62)
FCSRT – DFR (adj)	65.6	97.2	0.76	0.06	0.67 to 0.83	n.s.	≤6.78 (0.63)
FCSRT – IFR (adj)	71.9	91.5	0.85	0.05	0.79 to 0.91	n.s.	≤22.35 (0.63)
TMT-A (adj)	15.6	95.3	0.52	0.06	0.43 to 0.60	<0.0001	≤14 (0.11)
TMT-B (adj)	40.63	84.91	0.61	0.06	0.53 to 0.70	0.0001	>130 (0.25)

Results have been considered as statistically significant when surviving Bonferroni corrected threshold, $p < 0.01$. p-value = comparison with SASG-Total. AOC: area under the curve; SE: standard error; CI: confidence interval; J: Youden J statistic; SASG-total: smart aging serious game total score; MoCA: Montreal cognitive assessment; FCSRT: free and cued selective reminding test; DFR: delayed free recall; IFR: immediate free recall; TMT: trail making test; adj: adjusted.

3.4. SASG, MoCA and Hippocampal Volume

When investigating the presence of neuronal degeneration through n-Hipp volume, we found a significant volumetric reduction in aMCI compared to HC subjects bilaterally (Table 1). Moreover, results of the partial correlations between SASG-total and neuropsychological variables (MoCA, FCSRT and TMT) with hippocampal volume reveal significant correlation between right n-Hipp volume and the serious game. No significant relation is present with MoCA score FCSRT and TMT after Bonferroni correction (Table 6).

Table 6. Partial correlations between test and normalized hippocampal volume. Age, gender and education have been included as covariates of no interest. Results have been considered as statistically significant when surviving Bonferroni-corrected threshold ($p < 0.008$).

		Left n-Hipp	Right n-Hipp
n		30	30
SASG-Total			
	Corr	0.28	0.50
	p-value	n.s.	0.0076
MoCA			
	Corr	−0.08	0.06
	p-value	n.s.	n.s.
FCSRT-IFR/DFR			
	Corr	0.30/0.4673	0.39/0.48
	p-value	n.s./0.0140	0.046/0.011
TMT-A/B			
	Corr	0.29/0.24	0.15/0.08
	p-value	n.s./n.s.	n.s./n.s.

n-Hipp: normalized hippocampal volume; SASG-total: smart aging serious game total score; Corr: correlation coefficient r; MoCA: Montreal cognitive assessment; FCSRT: free and cued selective reminding test; DFR: delayed free recall; IFR: immediate free recall; TMT: trail making test; n.s.: not significant.

Finally, a linear regression analysis to evaluate the predictive value of SASG to determine hippocampal volume reveals a significant relationship between right n-Hipp and SASG-total (R^2: 0.14; p-value: 0.042).

4. Discussion

The recent technological advancements in digital medicine have fostered the development of innovative tools for a better care of people's health and wellbeing [56]. In the last years, several lines of research have led to the development of innovative ICT solutions to perform cognitive evaluation with the use of SGs, virtually reality based instruments able to reproduce more ecological environments, in both healthy and neurological populations [5,7–10,16,23]. Recent data demonstrated the usability and efficacy of SG for the early detection and monitoring of cognitive impairment in neurodegenerative disorders [57].

The first aim of the present study was to test the usability of an innovative virtual reality tool, the smart aging serious game (SASG) platform, in a cohort of aMCI subjects.

In our sample, the majority of subjects (whether aMCI or HC) had never used a PC and a touch screen before performing the SASG session. Despite this finding, no effects of familiarity were found on the SASG score and all the participants were able to go through the whole SASG session in a clinical setting, indicating a good level of usability. This result confirms the good usability of the platform for our sample. Indeed, SASG interface was specifically implemented for older and non-expert users and did not necessitate skilled abilities [6,10]. All the aspects of the usability of the platform were considered in a previous work [6] and several technical precautions were considered. For instance, to overcome the difficulties in navigating through 3D scenarios, the touch screen was found to be more usable than the mouse. Moreover, these data suggest the possibility to also use the SASG platform remotely from the patient's home. This last use, though, will require a dedicated validation.

The second aim of the study was to determine the validity of the SASG in discriminating between a preclinical population with aMCI and successful aging subjects. Data on well-established pencil–paper tests confirmed the amnestic profile of the aMCI population that showed reduced scores in the MoCA test, and in the immediate and delayed FCSRT subtests and relative total scores [58]. On the contrary, as expected no differences between groups were found in the TMT tests, a task specifically targeted to measure visual–motor skills, mental flexibility, processing speed and sequencing [59]. This confirms the specificity of the amnestic impairment of the aMCI a preclinical condition with a high risk to develop AD type of dementia. The cognitive profile using SASG depicts a picture similar to the one observed with conventional paper-and-pencil tests. In detail, considering only the accuracy (i.e., independently from the time of execution), aMCI have a reduced performance in all tasks involving mnemonic functions (T1, T4 and T5) with preserved competences in tasks involving mainly executive functions and attention (T2 and T3). When considering the time of execution (i.e., independently from the accuracy), results show a slowdown in aMCI in all tasks except task 4, the only one presenting with a reduced visual complexity due to the bi-dimensional aspect of the scenario and thus not requesting an increased cognitive effort to deal with the greater graphical complexity of a 3D-environment [7,10]. Given the comparable unfamiliarity with technology in both groups, the reduced performances in the aMCI versus HC subjects can be reasonably interpreted as the result of the different neuropsychological profile. Taken together, these data highlight the validity of SASG in discriminating aMCI from HC.

To further investigate this issue, we calculated the specificity and sensitivity of SASG and compared them to those of gold standard tests for aMCI detection, the MoCA test and the immediate and delayed recall of the FCSRT. Results of these analyses show that SASG has a very good performance (AUC: 0.879) in discriminating between groups, and these are statistically comparable to immediate and delayed recall of the FCSRT and to MoCA test, as shown with the ROC analysis. This is in agreement with data demonstrating the validity of the FCSRT in detecting memory deficits in subjects at risk of AD, making the use of this test recommended by the International Working Group (IWG) [11]. Finally, SASG results in a significantly higher sensitivity and specificity when compared to the TMT. This result was expected due to lack of involvement of mnemonic abilities in the TMT. Taken together these data demonstrate the validity of SASG in detecting mild neurocognitive deficits involving the memory domain that do not impact the functionality of everyday life such as in the aMCI condition [26].

Finally, the third aim was to test the relationship between the SASG tasks and the hippocampal volumes. Results show that SGSA is comparable to FCSRT and outperforms MoCA in the ability to detect the reduction in the hippocampal volume. This datum is very important since pre-morbid hippocampal volume is predictive of a subsequent clinical progression towards AD and it is thus considered a biomarker [35,36]. In a previous study by Sarazin et al. [60], the FCSRT was proved to be correlated with left hippocampal volume, particularly in the CA1 region in AD patients [60]. In our study we found a significant relationship between SASG performance and right hippocampus volume. Interestingly, this asymmetric relationship can be due to the visual–spatial nature of the task. The right hippocampus has been indeed demonstrated to be involved in memory for locations within an environment, and this corresponds to some of the tasks involved in the SASG evaluation (see [61] for a review).

5. Conclusions

In conclusion, this virtual-based tool constitutes an ecological and clinically meaningful task, useful to assess the cognitive profile in subjects with subtle and selective memory complaints such as aMCI subjects. SASG has substantial advantages that make it useful even in a clinical context: it is user friendly, ecological and motivating for the users [10,62]. The integration of technology into cognitive assessment practices provides a new ground for a modern approach to neuropsychology, making it able to digitally collect and combine a higher number of variables in a better evaluation of the behavioral profile. This aspect is of seminal importance and, in this perspective, the SASG represents an ecological tool for the timely detection of the functional impairment of this clinical condition, as recommended in the practical guidelines on MCI of the American Academy of Neurology [28]. Moreover, the significant relationship of SASG performance with the right hippocampal volume demonstrates how results on this task hold the potential to offer a putative digital biomarker able to capture the aMCI condition. The herein presented data are relevant because they show the efficacy of SASG in recognition of patients at risk to develop AD in a pre-clinical stage. Considering the lack of pharmacological treatments for this condition, early detection of subjects at risk is decisive for the implementation of timely and effective rehabilitation interventions as the only opportunity to reduce the risk and the impact of the cognitive decline.

Author Contributions: Conceptualization, F.B. (Francesca Baglio) and V.B. Recruitment of subjects, M.A. and S.P. Software, S.P. and T.M. Data collection, F.R., S.I., F.L.S., M.D.C. and F.B. (Francesca Borgnis). Statistical analyses and data interpretation, M.C., V.B., and F.B. (Francesca Baglio). Writing first draft, M.C., V.B., F.B. (Francesca Baglio). Writing—review and editing, all authors. All authors have read and agreed to the published version of the manuscript.

Funding: This research was funded by the ITALIAN MINISTRY OF HEALTH, Ricerca Corrente 2018–2020.

Acknowledgments: In memoriam of Professor Massimo Musicco, an eminent scientist in the field of Dementia. The authors are grateful for his help in data analyses and interpretation.

Conflicts of Interest: The authors declare no conflict of interest.

References

1. Pratt, D.R.; Zyda, M.; Kelleher, K. Virtual reality: In the mind of the beholder. *IEEE Computer* **1995**, *7*, 17–19.
2. Realdon, O.; Rossetto, F.; Nalin, M.; Baroni, I.; Cabinio, M.; Fioravanti, R.; Saibene, F.L.; Alberoni, M.; Mantovani, F.; Romano, M.; et al. Technology-enhanced multi-domain at home continuum of care program with respect to usual care for people with cognitive impairment: The Ability-TelerehABILITation study protocol for a randomized controlled trial. *BMC Psychiatry* **2016**, *16*, 425. [CrossRef] [PubMed]
3. Wiederhold, B.K.; Riva, G. Virtual reality therapy: emerging topics and future challenges. *Cyberpsychol. Behav. Soc. Netw.* **2019**, *22*, 3–6. [CrossRef] [PubMed]
4. Colombo, D.; Fernandez-Alvarez, J.; Patane, A.; Semonella, M.; Kwiatkowska, M.; Garcia-Palacios, A.; Cipresso, P.; Riva, G.; Botella, C. Current state and future directions of technology-based ecological momentary assessment and intervention for major depressive disorder: A systematic review. *J. Clin. Med.* **2019**, *8*, 465. [CrossRef]
5. Realdon, O.; Serino, S.; Savazzi, F.; Rossetto, F.; Cipresso, P.; Parsons, T.D.; Cappellini, G.; Mantovani, F.; Mendozzi, L.; Nemni, R.; et al. An ecological measure to screen executive functioning in MS: The Picture interpretation test (PIT) 360 degrees. *Sci. Rep.* **2019**, *9*, 1–8. [CrossRef]
6. Zucchella, C.; Capone, A.; Codella, V.; Vecchione, C.; Buccino, G.; Sandrini, G.; Pierelli, F.; Bartolo, M. Assessing and restoring cognitive functions early after stroke. *Funct. Neurol.* **2014**, *29*, 255–262. [CrossRef]
7. Zucchella, C.; Sinforiani, E.; Tassorelli, C.; Cavallini, E.; Tost-Pardell, D.; Grau, S.; Pazzi, S.; Puricelli, S.; Bernini, S.; Bottiroli, S.; et al. Serious games for screening pre-dementia conditions: From virtuality to reality? A pilot project. *Funct. Neurol.* **2014**, *29*, 153–158.
8. Fabbri, L.; Mosca, I.E.; Gerli, F.; Martini, L.; Pancani, S.; Lucidi, G.; Savazzi, F.; Baglio, F.; Vannetti, F.; Macchi, C. GOAL working group the games for older adults active life (GOAL) project for people with mild cognitive impairment and vascular cognitive impairment: A study protocol for a randomized controlled trial. *Front. Neurol.* **2019**, *9*, 1040. [CrossRef]
9. Serino, S.; Baglio, F.; Rossetto, F.; Realdon, O.; Cipresso, P.; Parsons, T.D.; Cappellini, G.; Mantovani, F.; De Leo, G.; Nemni, R.; et al. Picture interpretation test (PIT) 360 degrees: An innovative measure of executive functions. *Sci. Rep.* **2017**, *7*, 1–10. [CrossRef]
10. Bottiroli, S.; Tassorelli, C.; Lamonica, M.; Zucchella, C.; Cavallini, E.; Bernini, S.; Sinforiani, E.; Pazzi, S.; Cristiani, P.; Vecchi, T.; et al. Smart aging platform for evaluating cognitive functions in aging: A comparison with the MoCA in a normal population. *Front. Aging Neurosci.* **2017**, *9*, 1–14. [CrossRef]
11. Dubois, B.; Feldman, H.H.; Jacova, C.; Hampel, H.; Molinuevo, J.L.; Blennow, K.; DeKosky, S.T.; Gauthier, S.; Selkoe, D.; Bateman, R.; et al. Advancing research diagnostic criteria for Alzheimer's disease: The IWG-2 criteria. *Lancet Neurol.* **2014**, *13*, 614–629. [CrossRef]

12. Robert, P.H.; Konig, A.; Amieva, H.; Andrieu, S.; Bremond, F.; Bullock, R.; Ceccaldi, M.; Dubois, B.; Gauthier, S.; Kenigsberg, P.A.; et al. Recommendations for the use of serious games in people with alzheimer's disease, related disorders and frailty. *Front. Aging Neurosci.* **2014**, *6*, 54. [CrossRef] [PubMed]
13. Valladares-Rodriguez, S.; Perez-Rodriguez, R.; Anido-Rifon, L.; Fernandez-Iglesias, M. Trends on the application of serious games to neuropsychological evaluation: A scoping review. *J. Biomed. Inform.* **2016**, *64*, 296–319. [CrossRef] [PubMed]
14. Savazzi, F.; Isernia, S.; Jonsdottir, J.; Di Tella, S.; Pazzi, S.; Baglio, F. Design and implementation of a serious game on neurorehabilitation: Data on modifications of functionalities along implementation releases. *Data Brief.* **2018**, *20*, 864–869. [CrossRef]
15. Savazzi, F.; Isernia, S.; Jonsdottir, J.; Di Tella, S.; Pazzi, S.; Baglio, F. Engaged in learning neurorehabilitation: Development and validation of a serious game with user-centered design. *Comput. Educ.* **2018**, *125*, 53–61. [CrossRef]
16. Cipresso, P.; Albani, G.; Serino, S.; Pedroli, E.; Pallavicini, F.; Mauro, A.; Riva, G. Virtual multiple errands test (VMET): A virtual reality-based tool to detect early executive functions deficit in Parkinson's disease. *Front. Behav. Neurosci.* **2014**, *8*, 405. [CrossRef]
17. Plancher, G.; Tirard, A.; Gyselinck, V.; Nicolas, S.; Piolino, P. Using virtual reality to characterize episodic memory profiles in amnestic mild cognitive impairment and Alzheimer's disease: Influence of active and passive encoding. *Neuropsychologia* **2012**, *50*, 592–602. [CrossRef]
18. Lee, J.Y.; Kho, S.; Yoo, H.B.; Park, S.; Choi, J.S.; Kwon, J.S.; Cha, K.R.; Jung, H.Y. Spatial memory impairments in amnestic mild cognitive impairment in a virtual radial arm maze. *Neuropsychiatr. Dis. Treat.* **2014**, *10*, 653–660. [CrossRef]
19. Manera, V.; Petit, P.D.; Derreumaux, A.; Orvieto, I.; Romagnoli, M.; Lyttle, G.; David, R.; Robert, P.H. 'Kitchen and cooking,' a serious game for mild cognitive impairment and Alzheimer's disease: A pilot study. *Front. Aging Neurosci.* **2015**, *7*, 24. [CrossRef]
20. Fukui, Y.; Yamashita, T.; Hishikawa, N.; Kurata, T.; Sato, K.; Omote, Y.; Kono, S.; Yunoki, T.; Kawahara, Y.; Hatanaka, N.; et al. Computerized touch-panel screening tests for detecting mild cognitive impairment and Alzheimer's disease. *Intern. Med.* **2015**, *54*, 895–902. [CrossRef]
21. Zygouris, S.; Giakoumis, D.; Votis, K.; Doumpoulakis, S.; Ntovas, K.; Segkouli, S.; Karagiannidis, C.; Tzovaras, D.; Tsolaki, M. Can a virtual reality cognitive training application fulfill a dual role? Using the virtual supermarket cognitive training application as a screening tool for mild cognitive impairment. *J. Alzheimers Dis.* **2015**, *44*, 1333–1347. [CrossRef] [PubMed]
22. Allain, P.; Foloppe, D.A.; Besnard, J.; Yamaguchi, T.; Etcharry-Bouyx, F.; Le Gall, D.; Nolin, P.; Richard, P. Detecting everyday action deficits in Alzheimer's disease using a nonimmersive virtual reality kitchen. *J. Int. Neuropsychol. Soc.* **2014**, *20*, 468–477. [CrossRef] [PubMed]
23. Manera, V.; Ben-Sadoun, G.; Aalbers, T.; Agopyan, H.; Askenazy, F.; Benoit, M.; Bensamoun, D.; Bourgeois, J.; Bredin, J.; Bremond, F.; et al. Recommendations for the use of serious games in neurodegenerative disorders: 2016 Delphi panel. *Front. Psychol.* **2017**, *8*, 1243. [CrossRef] [PubMed]
24. American Psychiatric Association (APA). *Diagnostic and Statistical Manual of Mental Disorders (DSM V)*; American Psychiatric: Washington, DC, USA, 2013.
25. Stokin, G.B.; Krell-Roesch, J.; Petersen, R.C.; Geda, Y.E. Mild neurocognitive disorder: An old wine in a new bottle. *Harv. Rev. Psychiatry* **2015**, *23*, 368–376. [CrossRef] [PubMed]
26. Langa, K.M.; Levine, D.A. The diagnosis and management of mild cognitive impairment: A clinical review. *JAMA* **2014**, *312*, 2551–2561. [CrossRef] [PubMed]
27. Albert, M.S.; DeKosky, S.T.; Dickson, D.; Dubois, B.; Feldman, H.H.; Fox, N.C.; Gamst, A.; Holtzman, D.M.; Jagust, W.J.; Petersen, R.C.; et al. The diagnosis of mild cognitive impairment due to Alzheimer's disease: Recommendations from the national institute on Aging-Alzheimer's association workgroups on diagnostic guidelines for Alzheimer's disease. *Alzheimers Dement.* **2011**, *7*, 270–279. [CrossRef]
28. Petersen, R.C.; Lopez, O.; Armstrong, M.J.; Getchius, T.S.D.; Ganguli, M.; Gloss, D.; Gronseth, G.S.; Marson, D.; Pringsheim, T.; Day, G.S.; et al. Author response: Practice guideline update summary: Mild cognitive impairment: Report of the guideline development, dissemination, and implementation subcommittee of the American academy of neurology. *Neurology* **2018**, *91*, 373–374. [CrossRef]

29. Petersen, R.C.; Lopez, O.; Armstrong, M.J.; Getchius, T.S.D.; Ganguli, M.; Gloss, D.; Gronseth, G.S.; Marson, D.; Pringsheim, T.; Day, G.S.; et al. Practice guideline update summary: Mild cognitive impairment: Report of the guideline development, dissemination, and implementation subcommittee of the American academy of neurology. *Neurology* **2018**, *90*, 126–135. [CrossRef]
30. Martin, S.B.; Smith, C.D.; Collins, H.R.; Schmitt, F.A.; Gold, B.T. Evidence that volume of anterior medial temporal lobe is reduced in seniors destined for mild cognitive impairment. *Neurobiol. Aging.* **2010**, *31*, 1099–1106. [CrossRef]
31. Apostolova, L.G.; Mosconi, L.; Thompson, P.M.; Green, A.E.; Hwang, K.S.; Ramirez, A.; Mistur, R.; Tsui, W.H.; de Leon, M.J. Subregional hippocampal atrophy predicts Alzheimer's dementia in the cognitively normal. *Neurobiol. Aging.* **2010**, *31*, 1077–1088. [CrossRef]
32. Smith, S.M.; Nichols, T.E. Threshold-free cluster enhancement: Addressing problems of smoothing, threshold dependence and localisation in cluster inference. *Neuroimage* **2009**, *44*, 83–98. [CrossRef] [PubMed]
33. Smith, C.D.; Chebrolu, H.; Wekstein, D.R.; Schmitt, F.A.; Jicha, G.A.; Cooper, G.; Markesbery, W.R. Brain structural alterations before mild cognitive impairment. *Neurology* **2007**, *68*, 1268–1273. [CrossRef] [PubMed]
34. Whitwell, J.L.; Petersen, R.C.; Negash, S.; Weigand, S.D.; Kantarci, K.; Ivnik, R.J.; Knopman, D.S.; Boeve, B.F.; Smith, G.E.; Jack, C.R., Jr. Patterns of atrophy differ among specific subtypes of mild cognitive impairment. *Arch. Neurol.* **2007**, *64*, 1130–1138. [CrossRef]
35. Devanand, D.P.; Pradhaban, G.; Liu, X.; Khandji, A.; De Santi, S.; Segal, S.; Rusinek, H.; Pelton, G.H.; Honig, L.S.; Mayeux, R.; et al. Hippocampal and entorhinal atrophy in mild cognitive impairment: Prediction of Alzheimer disease. *Neurology* **2007**, *68*, 828–836. [CrossRef]
36. Jack, C.R. Jr.; Petersen, R.C.; Xu, Y.C.; O'Brien, P.C.; Smith, G.E.; Ivnik, R.J.; Boeve, B.F.; Waring, S.C.; Tangalos, E.G.; Kokmen, E. Prediction of AD with MRI-based hippocampal volume in mild cognitive impairment. *Neurology* **1999**, *52*, 1397–1403. [CrossRef] [PubMed]
37. Michaud, T.L.; Su, D.; Siahpush, M.; Murman, D.L. The risk of incident mild cognitive impairment and progression to dementia considering mild cognitive impairment subtypes. *Dement. Geriatr. Cogn. Dis. Extra* **2017**, *7*, 15–29. [CrossRef]
38. Nagamatsu, L.S.; Handy, T.C.; Hsu, C.L.; Voss, M.; Liu-Ambrose, T. Resistance training promotes cognitive and functional brain plasticity in seniors with probable mild cognitive impairment. *Arch. Intern. Med.* **2012**, *172*, 666–668. [CrossRef]
39. Suzuki, T.; Shimada, H.; Makizako, H.; Doi, T.; Yoshida, D.; Ito, K.; Shimokata, H.; Washimi, Y.; Endo, H.; Kato, T. A randomized controlled trial of multicomponent exercise in older adults with mild cognitive impairment. *PLoS ONE* **2013**, *8*, e61483. [CrossRef]
40. Folstein, M.F.; Folstein, S.E.; McHugh, P.R. "Mini-mental state". A practical method for grading the cognitive state of patients for the clinician. *J. Psychiatr. Res.* **1975**, *12*, 189–198. [CrossRef]
41. Measso, G.; Cavarzeran, F.; Zappalà, G.; Lebowitz, B.D.; Crook, T.H.; Pirozzolo, F.J.; Amaducci, F.A.; Massari, D.; Grigoletto, F. The mini mental state examination: Normative study of an Italian random sample. *Dev. Neuropsychol.* **1993**, *9*, 77–85. [CrossRef]
42. Hamilton, M. A rating scale for depression. *J. Neurol. Neurosurg. Psychiatry* **1960**, *23*, 56–62. [CrossRef] [PubMed]
43. Rosen, W.G.; Terry, R.D.; Fuld, P.A.; Katzman, R.; Peck, A. Pathological verification of ischemic score in differentiation of dementias. *Ann. Neurol.* **1980**, *7*, 486–488. [CrossRef] [PubMed]
44. Nasreddine, Z.S.; Phillips, N.A.; Bedirian, V.; Charbonneau, S.; Whitehead, V.; Collin, I.; Cummings, J.L.; Chertkow, H. The montreal cognitive assessment, MoCA: A brief screening tool for mild cognitive impairment. *J. Am. Geriatr. Soc.* **2005**, *53*, 695–699. [CrossRef] [PubMed]
45. Conti, S.; Bonazzi, S.; Laiacona, M.; Masina, M.; Coralli, M.V. Montreal cognitive assessment (MoCA)-Italian version: Regression based norms and equivalent scores. *Neurol. Sci.* **2015**, *36*, 209–214. [CrossRef] [PubMed]
46. Santangelo, G.; Siciliano, M.; Pedone, R.; Vitale, C.; Falco, F.; Bisogno, R.; Siano, P.; Barone, P.; Grossi, D.; Santangelo, F.; et al. Normative data for the montreal cognitive assessment in an Italian population sample. *Neurol. Sci.* **2015**, *36*, 585–591. [CrossRef]
47. Grober, E.; Buschke, H. Genuine memory deficits in dementia. *Dev. Neuropsychol.* **1987**, *3*, 13–16. [CrossRef]
48. Frasson, P.; Ghiretti, R.; Catricala, E.; Pomati, S.; Marcone, A.; Parisi, L.; Rossini, P.M.; Cappa, S.F.; Mariani, C.; Vanacore, N.; et al. Free and cued selective reminding test: An Italian normative study. *Neurol. Sci.* **2011**, *32*, 1057–1062. [CrossRef]

49. Reitan, R.M. Validity of the trail making test as an indicator of organic brain damage. *Percept. Mot. Skills* **1958**, *8*, 271–276. [CrossRef]
50. Giovagnoli, A.R.; Del Pesce, M.; Mascheroni, S.; Simoncelli, M.; Laiacona, M.; Capitani, E. Trail making test: Normative values from 287 normal adult controls. *Ital. J. Neurol. Sci.* **1996**, *17*, 305–309. [CrossRef]
51. Bottiroli, S.; Cavallini, E. Can computer familiarity regulate the benefits of computer-based memory training in normal aging? A study with an Italian sample of older adults. *Neuropsychol. Dev. Cogn. B Aging Neuropsychol. Cogn.* **2009**, *16*, 401–418. [CrossRef]
52. Dale, A.M.; Fischl, B.; Sereno, M.I. Cortical surface-based analysis. I. Segmentation and surface reconstruction. *Neuroimage* **1999**, *9*, 179–194. [CrossRef] [PubMed]
53. Iglesias, J.E.; Augustinack, J.C.; Nguyen, K.; Player, C.M.; Player, A.; Wright, M.; Roy, N.; Frosch, M.P.; McKee, A.C.; Wald, L.L.; et al. Alzheimer's disease neuroimaging initiative. A computational atlas of the hippocampal formation using ex vivo, ultra-high resolution MRI: Application to adaptive segmentation of in vivo MRI. *Neuroimage* **2015**, *115*, 117–137. [CrossRef] [PubMed]
54. Fischl, B.; Salat, D.H.; Busa, E.; Albert, M.; Dieterich, M.; Haselgrove, C.; van der Kouwe, A.; Killiany, R.; Kennedy, D.; Klaveness, S; et al. Whole brain segmentation: Automated labeling of neuroanatomical structures in the human brain. *Neuron* **2002**, *33*, 341–355. [CrossRef]
55. Voevodskaya, O.; Simmons, A.; Nordenskjold, R.; Kullberg, J.; Ahlstrom, H.; Lind, L.; Wahlund, L.O.; Larsson, E.M.; Westman, E. Alzheimer's disease neuroimaging initiative. The effects of intracranial volume adjustment approaches on multiple regional MRI volumes in healthy aging and Alzheimer's disease. *Front. Aging Neurosci.* **2014**, *6*, 264. [CrossRef]
56. Topol, E. *Preparing the Healthcare Workforce to Deliver the Digital Future the Topol Review: An Independent Report on Behalf of the Secretary of State for Health and Social Care*; NHS Health Education: London, UK, 2019.
57. Tarnanas, I.; Schlee, W.; Tsolaki, M.; Muri, R.; Mosimann, U.; Nef, T. Ecological validity of virtual reality daily living activities screening for early dementia: Longitudinal study. *JMIR Serious Games* **2013**, *1*, e1. [CrossRef]
58. Grober, E.; Sanders, A.E.; Hall, C.; Lipton, R.B. Free and cued selective reminding identifies very mild dementia in primary care. *Alzheimer Dis. Assoc. Disord.* **2010**, *24*, 284–290. [CrossRef]
59. Bowie, C.R.; Harvey, P.D. Administration and interpretation of the trail making test. *Nat. Protoc.* **2006**, *1*, 2277–2281. [CrossRef]
60. Sarazin, M.; Chauvire, V.; Gerardin, E.; Colliot, O.; Kinkingnehun, S.; de Souza, L.C.; Hugonot-Diener, L.; Garnero, L.; Lehericy, S.; Chupin, M.; et al. The amnestic syndrome of hippocampal type in Alzheimer's disease: An MRI study. *J. Alzheimers Dis.* **2010**, *22*, 285–294. [CrossRef]
61. Burgess, N.; Maguire, E.A.; O'Keefe, J. The human hippocampus and spatial and episodic memory. *Neuron* **2002**, *35*, 625–641. [CrossRef]
62. Matamala-Gomez, M.; Maisto, M.; Montana, J.; Mavrodiev, P.; Baglio, F.; Rossetto, F.; Mantovani, F.; Riva, G.; Realdon, O. The role of engagement in teleneurorehabilitation: A systematic review. *Front. Neurol.* **2020**. [CrossRef]

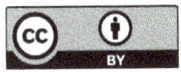

© 2020 by the authors. Licensee MDPI, Basel, Switzerland. This article is an open access article distributed under the terms and conditions of the Creative Commons Attribution (CC BY) license (http://creativecommons.org/licenses/by/4.0/).

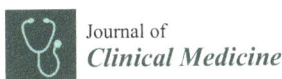

Article

The Effect of a Virtual Reality-Based Intervention Program on Cognition in Older Adults with Mild Cognitive Impairment: A Randomized Control Trial

Ngeemasara Thapa [1,2], Hye Jin Park [1,2], Ja-Gyeong Yang [1,2], Haeun Son [1,2], Minwoo Jang [1,2], Jihyeon Lee [1], Seung Wan Kang [3], Kyung Won Park [4] and Hyuntae Park [1,2,*]

1. Department of Health Sciences, Graduate School, Dong-A University, Busan 49315, Korea; ngeemasara@gmail.com (N.T.); mihd3987@hanmail.net (H.J.P.); sky940702@naver.com (J.-G.Y.); haundl123@naver.com (H.S.); mtow0620@gmail.com (M.J.); lose0918@naver.com (J.L.)
2. Laboratory of Smart Healthcare, Dong-A University, Busan 49315, Korea
3. Data Center for Korean EEG, College of Nursing, Seoul National University, Seoul 03080, Korea; drdemian@snu.ac.kr
4. Department of Neurology, Dong-A University College of Medicine, Busan 49201, Korea; neuropark@dau.ac.kr
* Correspondence: htpark@dau.ac.kr; Tel.: +82-10-8876-4221

Received: 31 March 2020; Accepted: 27 April 2020; Published: 29 April 2020

Abstract: This study aimed to investigate the association between a virtual reality (VR) intervention program and cognitive, brain and physical functions in high-risk older adults. In a randomized controlled trial, we enrolled 68 individuals with mild cognitive impairment (MCI). The MCI diagnosis was based on medical evaluations through a clinical interview conducted by a dementia specialist. Cognitive assessments were performed by neuropsychologists according to standardized methods, including the Mini-Mental State Examination (MMSE) and frontal cognitive function: trail making test (TMT) A & B, and symbol digit substitute test (SDST). Resting state electroencephalogram (EEG) was measured in eyes open and eyes closed conditions for 5 minutes each, with a 19-channel wireless EEG device. The VR intervention program (3 times/week, 100 min each session) comprised four types of VR game-based content to improve the attention, memory and processing speed. Analysis of the subjects for group–time interactions revealed that the intervention group exhibited a significantly improved executive function and brain function at the resting state. Additionally, gait speed and mobility were also significantly improved between and after the follow-up. The VR-based training program improved cognitive and physical function in patients with MCI relative to controls. Encouraging patients to perform VR and game-based training may be beneficial to prevent cognitive decline.

Keywords: virtual reality; dementia; mild cognitive impairment; electroencephalogram

1. Introduction

Dementia is a syndrome characterized by global cognitive impairment [1] and an estimated 50 million people worldwide have dementia [2]. It is most prevalent in individuals aged > 65 years and is considered as the greatest health challenge in the 21st century [3]. The pharmacological treatments have not yet led to an important breakthrough in the treatment of dementia, resulting in gravitation toward non-pharmacological approaches to alter the progressive course of the disease [4]. Mild cognitive impairment (MCI) is the prodromal stage of dementia [5], with around 46% progressing to dementia within 3 years [6]. Some MCI patients are stable or return to a normal state over time [7]. Thus, MCI serves as an ideal stage for preventive interventions.

The most promising non-pharmacological interventions for delaying the progression of MCI to dementia are exercise, cognitive training [8] and multicomponent intervention [9], and recently, virtual reality (VR) has also been explored for treatment and prevention of dementia [10]. A randomized control trial in normal older adults comparing physical exercise, cognitive exercise and VR exercise demonstrated that VR exercise showed significant improvements in cognitive as well as physical function, and VR exercise was more favored than physical exercise by the elderly [11]. In older adults with MCI, VR intervention has been reported to improve memory function [12]. VR is a computer-simulated environment, closely resembling real-life situations and scenarios, which provides the user with the sensation of physically "being there" [13,14]. VR can be divided into non- immersion, semi-immersion, and full immersion, based on the levels of immersion. Immersive VR provides enhanced ecological validity and the possibility to personalize the activity and environment to the needs of individuals, making VR-based training more engaging [15]. The higher level of immersion corresponds to a more realistic VR environment to the user [16]. The immersive VR has been used mostly for neurophysiological assessment, cognitive rehabilitation and the effect of VR on different cognitive domains such as executive function, attention, memory and spatial orientation is being investigated [17].

Immersive VR-based cognitive training has recently attracted attention in the research filed of MCI and dementia [18]. A recent meta-analytic study has also reported the positive effect of semi-immersive VR on cognition and physical function in individuals with MCI and dementia [19]. A fully immersive VR-based cognitive intervention study on older adults with and without dementia reported significantly higher cognitive progress in those without dementia compared to those with dementia [20]. A feasibility study using fully immersive VR cognitive training in MCI and dementia patients showed a high feeling of safety, satisfaction, reduced anxiety fatigue and low discomfort compared to pen-paper training [15]. This advantage of VR over pen-paper cognitive training can be beneficial to ensure adherence to cognitive training and when performed with caution, it has the potential to be an efficient intervention for dementia patients [15,21].

Nevertheless, immersive VR is increasingly used in health-related fields and interventions and has the potential to be a powerful tool in delaying the onset of degenerative brain and mental diseases. However, the evidence regarding the effectiveness of immersive VR in MCI and dementia is limited [22], especially the fully immersive type of VR. Several studies still rely mostly on non- and semi-immersive VR [23] and the advantages of VR with full immersion and interaction on prevention of dementia have not yet been explored to their full potential. Therefore, we aimed to investigate the effect of the fully immersive virtual reality intervention on cognitive, brain and physical function in older adults with MCI. In addition to the neurocognitive tests, we also used electroencephalography (EEG) to assess the effect of VR intervention on cognition in our study. EEG is the least invasive measure of brain electrical activity. EEG power measures are associated with memory, executive function and global cognition in patients with MCI [24].

2. Materials and Methods

2.1. Subjects

The study was announced through three regional health care centers in Busan metropolitan city, South Korea. A total of 234 participants applied and all of them underwent a screening process. The inclusion criteria were: (i) >55 and <85 years and (ii) individuals diagnosed with MCI based on medical evaluations consisting of neurological examinations and detailed neuropsychological assessments conducted by a dementia specialist. MCI was defined by the Consortium to Establish a Registry for Alzheimer's Disease Assessment Packet (CERAD) with the cut-off score developed by Chandler et al. [25]. Following some exclusion criteria, 100 out of 234 subjects were recruited to be part of this study. The exclusion criteria are explained in Figure 1. Thirty-two subjects out of 100 did not participate in the study due to personal reasons, hence our study included a total of 68 subjects who were then randomly allocated to either the control (n = 34) or VR-intervention (n = 34) group. To avoid selection bias, the random allocation was assigned via a computer-generated, fixed block randomization procedure to either the intervention or control group, generating blocks stratified by age, gender, education level, and participating center. The participants' mean age was 72.5 ± 5.32 years (mean ± standard deviation (SD)).

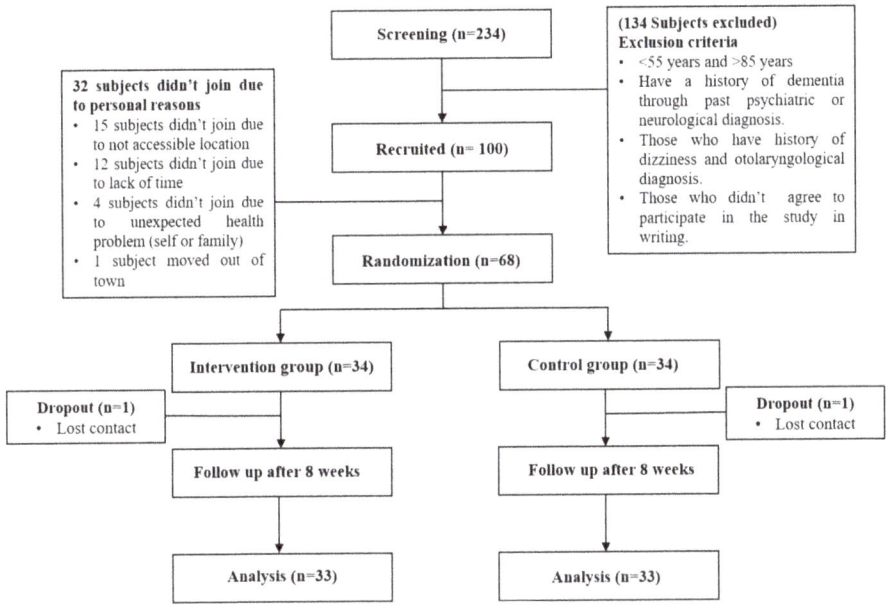

Figure 1. Flowchart of study design.

The study procedure was approved by Dong-A University Institutional Review Board on 24 October 2019 (IRB No. 2-1040709-AB-N-01-201909-HR-036-04) and all participants provided signed informed consent at the beginning of the study. This study is registered in the University Hospital Medical Information Network (UMIN) Clinical Trials Registry (Registration No. UMIN000040107).

2.2. Intervention

The intervention group performed a total of 24 sessions of VR-based cognitive training for eight weeks. Three sessions were held per week and each VR training session lasted for 100 minutes, which also included instruction regarding VR training and eye stretching exercises in between VR training, as described in Figure 2. On the other hand, the control group participated in an educational program on general health care once a week during the study intervention period (8 sessions). Each session was 30 to 50 minutes. The program was led by health professionals, an exercise specialist, a physical therapist and a nutritionist, and subjects were given information such as nutrition regarding proper diet and foods, and exercise tips to prevent geriatric diseases such as frailty, sarcopenia and dementia. In addition to VR training, the intervention group was also provided with an educational program following the same protocol as the control group.

The VR training consisted of 4 series of games. All the VR training game contents were developed by SY Innotech Inc., Busan, South Korea. The VR training was performed with an Oculus VR headset (Oculus quest headset) and two wireless hand controllers, one for each hand. The virtual reality program consists of four types (Figure 2): Juice making: This game requires the subject to pick a recipe for making a given juice in a virtual reality space, memorize the listed fruits, select the memorized material from the shelf and toss it into a container. The container is vigorously shaken until juice is made and then poured into the cup. Crow Shooting: The shooting game is set up on the beachside where the subjects are asked to shoot flying black birds. The right controller turns into a gun and the left controller into a shield. Fireworks (find the fireworks number): Three numbers are shown on the screen when the game starts and fireworks burst in a random order from the numbers. When the firework display is over, the subjects need to click the numbers in the order of which the firework exploded. Love house (d: memory object at the house): In this particular game, subjects are placed in a virtually simulated house where they were given 30 seconds to memorize the location of objects in the shelf and around the living area. The items are then misplaced, and the subjects are required to reorganize the objects in the correct location with the help of a VR hand controller.

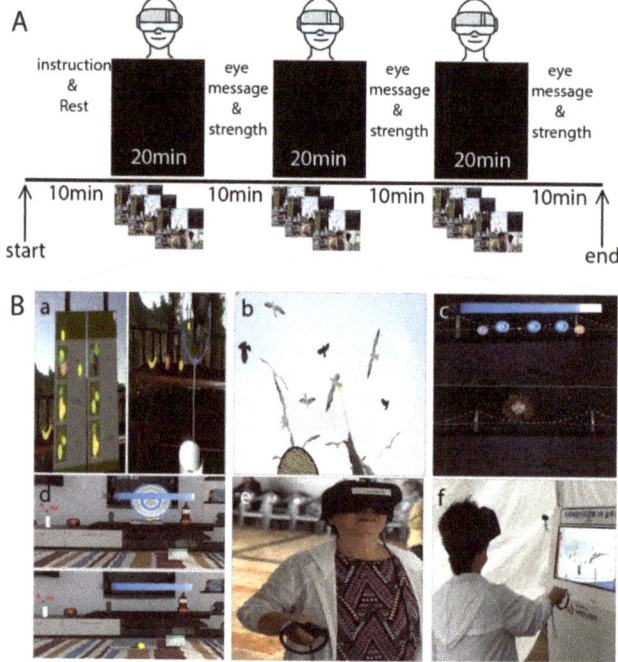

Figure 2. (**A**) This figure illustrates the design for the virtual reality (VR) training design and game contents. The total training duration was 100 minutes (three 20 min VR training sessions, and three 10 min eye massage and stretching sessions) held three times a week for 8 weeks. (**B**) The contents of the VR training games: (a) juice making, (b) crow shooting, (c) find the fireworks number, (d) memory object at the house, (e) and (f) example of subject.

2.3. Cognitive Function

Cognitive assessments were performed by neuropsychologists according to standardized methods. Global cognitive function was assessed with the Korean version of the Mini-Mental State Examination-Dementia screening test (MMSE-DS) [26]. From the National Center for Geriatrics and Gerontology Functional Assessment Tool (NCGG-FAT), the trail making test (TMT) A & B, and symbol digit substitution test (SDST) in the form of an electronic tablet were used to assess cognitive function [27]. In TMT A, the subjects were instructed to touch the target number in consecutive order of 1–15 shown in the tablet as quickly as possible. In TMT B, the subjects were instructed to touch numbers and letters alternatively in consecutive order. In SDST, 9 pairs of numbers and symbols were shown in the top half of the tablet display, and the subjects were asked to match the symbols to their corresponding numbers displayed in the bottom half of the display. TMT and SDST were both timed, and shorter time taken to complete the test indicated better cognitive function.

2.4. EEG Recording and Data Acquisition

The EEG was recorded in a dimly lit and quiet room with a Cognionics Quick-20 (Cognionics Inc., San Diego, CA, USA) dry EEG headset. The EEG headset had a built-in design based on the international 10–20 system (Fp1, Fp2, F7, F3, Fz, F4, F8, T3, C3, Cz, C4, T4, T5, P3, Pz, P4, T6, O1 and O2) positioned according to the international 10–20 system [28]. The resting state EEG data of 5 minutes was recorded with the eyes closed condition. The subjects were instructed to keep their eyes closed but stay awake during EEG recordings. The EEG was recorded at a sampling rate of 500 Hz and filtered through a band-pass of 0.53–120 Hz. The electrodes impedance was kept under 500 kΩ. The artifact removal was conducted with independent component analysis (ICA) individually for each channel. The EEG brain power ratio-theta/beta ratio (TBR), theta/alpha ratio (TAR) and delta/alpha ratio (DAR) between baseline and follow-up data (within the VR intervention and control groups) were analyzed in iSyncBrain software, v.2.1, 2018 (iMediSync, Inc., Seoul, South Korea) and the difference was observed with paired t-test. The EEG band power was shown in a topographic map (Topo map) plotted with the built-in sLoreta function in iSyncBrain software v.2.1. The differences were observed with paired t-test.

2.5. Physical Function

Physical function was assessed by gait speed test, mobility test and handgrip strength. The gait speed test was 7 m long, which included a 1.5 m acceleration distance, a 4 m "preferred walking speed" followed by a 1.5 m deceleration distance. Only the 4 m walk was timed. The 8-feet Up and Go test of 2.44 m was used to assess mobility. Handgrip strength (HGS) of the non-dominant hand was measured with a digital hand dynamometer (TKK 5101 Grip-D Takei, Tokyo, Japan). The HGS was measured twice and the mean value was used for statistical analysis. During the test, participants were instructed to maintain their shoulders slightly apart from their body, and hold the dynamometer pointing to the ground.

Socio-demographic variables such as education, age, medication intake and smoking were acquired through interviews by trained researchers.

2.6. Statistical Analysis

All comparisons were two-sided, with an alpha level of 0.05. All statistical analyses were analyzed using the IBM SPSS Statistics, version 25.0, 2017 software package for Windows (SPSS Inc., Chicago, IL, USA). The Shapiro–Wilk test was used to determine the normality of the data distribution. The independent t-test or the chi-square test was used to assess differences in the baseline (beginning of the intervention) variables. We used the intention-to-treat approach, and between-group comparisons of continuous variables were conducted using a repeated measures analysis of variance (ANOVA) model after adjusting for the potential covariates (age, sex and years of education) for primary and secondary endpoint outcome. Time was treated as a categorical variable, and the models included group, time and group-by-time interaction as fixed effects. The conclusions about the effectiveness of the VR intervention were based on between-group comparisons of change in global and prefrontal cognitive function (working memory, processing and executive function) from baseline to 8 weeks after, as assessed with the MMSE, TMT A & B, SDST and other physical function determined by the time-by-group interaction of the model.

3. Result

In Table 1, the demographics of the study population along with baseline physical functions and global cognitive functions are described. There are no significant differences in parameters between the intervention and control groups at the baseline.

Table 1. Selected anthropometric, cognitive and physical function characteristics of the subjects at the baseline.

Variables	VR Intervention	Control
n (male)	34 (6)	34 (10)
Age (years)	72.6 ± 5.4	72.7 ± 5.6
Education (years)	9.3 ± 4.0	8.4 ± 3.5
Height (m)	1.58 ± 0.08	1.58 ± 0.08
No. of medication intake (n)	2.3 ± 1.4	2.12 ± 1.4
Weight (kg)	60.7 ± 9.8	61.3 ± 9.1
BMI (kg/m^2)	24.3 ± 3.0	24.5 ± 2.7
SBP (mg/hg)	129.6 ± 15.8	129.6 ± 17.9
DBP (mg/hg)	74.8 ± 11.3	69.5 ± 11.8
Grip strength (kg)	22.2 ± 6.3	23.4 ± 5.7
Gait speed (s)	1.15 ± 0.33	1.18 ± 0.21
8-feet Up and Go (s)	6.27 ± 1.48	7.04 ± 2.02
MMSE (score)	26.0 ± 1.8	26.3 ± 3.3
TMT A (s)	26.3 ± 7.3	27.9 ± 9.2
TMT B (s)	56.6 ± 25.0	58.5 ± 28.1
SDST (score)	33.4 ± 9.0	32.4 ± 8.2

BMI: Body mass index, SPB: Systolic blood pressure, DBP: Diastolic blood pressure, MMSE: Mini mental state examination, TMT A: Trail making test A, TMT B: Trail making test B, SDST: Symbol digit substitution test. The values are expressed in mean and standard deviation (mean ± SD). All variables have no significant differences measured by independent t- test or chi-square test.

In Table 2, TMT B time decreased significantly in the intervention group compared to the control group (p = 0.03). Similarly, small, but not significant, positive changes were observed in MMSE and SDST. The physical function such as gait speed (p =0.02) and 8-feet Up and Go were significantly improved (p = 0.03) in the intervention group.

Table 2. The comparison of physical function and global cognitive function between baseline and post intervention in the VR intervention and the control groups.

Variables	VR Intervention			Control			Group x Time Interaction	
	Baseline	Follow Up	p-Value [a]	Baseline	Follow Up	p-Value [a]	p-Value [b]	Effect Size
Grip strength (kg)	22.2 ± 6.3	24.4 ± 5.3	0.03	23.4 ± 5.7	23.9 ± 5.7	n.s.	n.s.	-
Gait speed (m/s)	1.15 ± 0.33	1.19 ± 0.37	0.04	1.18 ± 0.21	1.12 ± 0.26 *	0.01	0.02	0.143
8-feet Up and go (s)	6.77 ± 1.48	6.32 ± 1.92	0.02	7.04 ± 2.02	7.06 ± 1.87 *	n.s.	0.03	0.107
MMSE (score)	26.0 ± 1.8	26.9 ± 2.0	n.s.	26.3 ± 3.3	26.4 ± 2.7	n.s.	n.s.	-
TMT A (s)	26.3 ±7.3	24.2 ± 5.3	0.04	27.9 ± 9.2	27.8 ± 8.1	n.s.	n.s.	-
TMT B (s)	56.6 ± 25.0	51.3 ± 24.8	0.03	58.5 ± 28.1	63.2 ± 25.1 *	0.01	0.03	0.208
SDST (score)	33.4 ± 9.0	39.6 ± 9.5	0.02	32.4 ± 8.2	21.8 ± 8.2	< 0.01	0.03	0.264

The values are expressed in mean and standard deviation (mean ± SD). [a] Paired t-test between baseline and follow-up assessment. [b] Repeated-measures analysis of variance (ANOVA) testing interaction of intervention (VR intervention versus control) by time (baseline versus follow-up) for each outcome, adjusted for age, gender and years of education. Effect size is partial eta squared for group by time. * Represents a significant difference between the intervention and control group. n.s. = not significant, MMSE: Mini mental state examination, TMT A: Trail making test A, TMT B: Trail making test B, SDST: Symbol digit substitution test.

3.1. EEG

3.1.1. Band Power

In the elderly, increased Theta wave (>3.5 to <8 Hz) is associated with the risk of developing cognitive impairment [29,30]. The theta has been observed to be significantly decreased around the parietal (p = 0.013) and temporal (p = 0.036) regions at follow up (G2) compared to baseline (G1) in the VR intervention group (Figure 3).

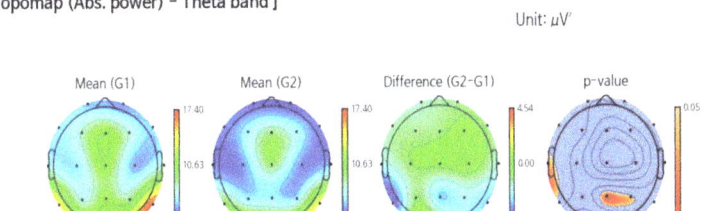

Figure 3. This figure shows a significant decrease in Theta power in the parietal ($p = 0.013$) and temporal areas ($p = 0.036$) at follow up (G2) compared to baseline (G1) in the VR intervention group.

3.1.2. Power Ratio

The higher TBR is related to mind wandering, which is considered to be associated with reduced attention [31]. In the VR intervention group, the Theta/Beta ratio (TBR) is decreased in the temporal ($p = 0.035$) and parietal ($p = 0.027$) regions at follow up (Figure 4). In the control group, all power ratios did not show any changes.

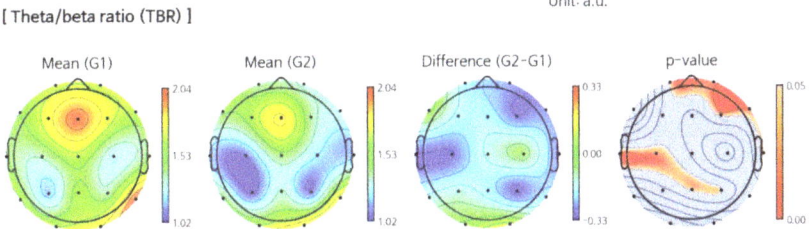

Figure 4. This figure shows a significant decrease in the Theta/Beta power ratio ($p = 0.027$) at follow up (G2) compared to baseline (G1) in the VR intervention group.

4. Discussion

Our study examined the effect of a VR game intervention on cognitive and brain activity in older adults with MCI. Our findings show that the VR game intervention is an effective way to improve cognitive and frontal brain function in MCI patients. The improvements in the 8-feet Up and Go test and gait speed were also observed in the intervention group.

Over the past decade, technology-based cognitive interventions have gained immense interest worldwide. Our study results show positive effects for the VR intervention on key outcome variables, such as cognitive and physical function. The VR intervention effect in the cognition category is consistent with the result of a systematic review by Coyle et al. [32]. Coyle and colleagues showed that the VR intervention moderately improved the cognitive function of participants with cognitive impairment. A recent VR study has reported improvements in executive functions [33] after the VR intervention, similar to our study results. TMT is often used as a measure of executive function [34]. TMT A measures psychomotor speed and visual scanning, while TMT B reflects working memory [35–37]. However, our results showed significant positive improvements in TMT B but not in TMT A. The contents of our VR training consisted of games such as love home, juice making and fireworks, which required subjects to memorize objects, recipes and numbers respectively, highly involving use of working memory along with other cognitive functions, such as attention and processing speed. This could explain the significant change in TMT B score. In addition, we also measured brain electrical activity during the resting state of mind. The theta power was observed to be decreased in the VR intervention at follow up. Increased theta, in the elderly, is associated with the risk of developing cognitive impairment [29,30]. Our study also a showed significant decrease in TBR in the temporal and parietal regions of the brain. The higher TBR was observed to be related to mind wandering, which is considered to be associated with reduced attention [31]. However, detailed studies over a longer period on each EEG rhythm are required to draw its strong relationship with VR training.

Studies have also shown that VR intervention is effective to improve physical function and walking speed of community-dwelling patients who had a stroke [38–40]. Our study results further expand this data as significant improvements in physical function, especially gait speed and the 8-feet Up and Go test, in MCI patients were observed after 8 weeks of VR training. Several studies have found physical functions such as handgrip strength [41–43] and gait speed [44] to be associated with cognitive decline in older adults. Gait speed has been reported to rely on motor function and cognitive processes, which includes executive function and attention [45], which may explain the relationship between gait speed and cognition. Furthermore, improved brain function may be due to health promoting behaviors, such as physical activity and nutrition, and health literacy [46]. However, further studies are needed in order to evaluate the bidirectional relationship between the improvement of cognition and physical function.

VR provides an artificial interactive environment closely representing reality. Older adults with dementia can experience various sensory stimulation in a comfortable and safe virtually simulated environment, which could lead to a boost in functional learning and transfer of learned functions [47]. Unlike computerized computer training, VR is immersive and closely mimics reality, intensifying ecological legitimacy, offering greater potential for transfer to activities of daily life (ADL) [48]. We performed fully immersive VR training in order to examine the effectiveness of using VR intervention on cognitive, brain and physical function in MCI patients. The VR contents in our study used real life locations. Fully immersive VR corresponds more to feeling like the individual is experiencing real-life scenarios [23]. A functional magnetic resonance imaging study showed that the virtual reality-generated environment activates the associated brain areas, similar to the real environment [49].

Our study yielded a positive effect of fully immersive VR training on cognitive as well as physical function in older adults with MCI. The subjects in the VR intervention group strongly adhered to the training and the dropout number was low (n = 1). One of the limitations of our study was that there was no follow up in the middle of the intervention period or some period after the study was over, due to which the short- and long-term effect of the VR intervention on cognition and physical function were not observed. Secondly, the VR intervention program group had more sessions (n = 24) compared to the control group (n = 8) and hence, the intervention group had more interaction with each other and their supervising health professionals. The increased social interaction has been associated with preventing cognitive decline [50,51]. This could have somewhat contributed to positive results in the intervention group. The participants of our study were predominantly women (n = 52), compared to men (n = 16), and future studies regarding gender differences on the effect of the VR intervention are necessary.

5. Conclusions

In summary, our results show that VR-based cognitive training has a positive effect on cognition in MCI patients. Although the global cognitive function did not change significantly, we observed significant improvement in executive function, and some physical functions such as gait speed and the 8-feet Up and Go test. Moreover, the EEG test showed a positive change in brain activity related to attention after the intervention period. Nevertheless, further work is needed in this area to confirm the long-term effectiveness and feasibility.

Author Contributions: Conceptualization, H.P.; methodology, J.-G.Y., H.J.P. and M.J.; software, N.T., J.-G.Y., S.W.K. and J.L.; formal analysis, H.S., K.W.P. and N.T.; investigation, N.T., M.J., J.L., H.J.P. and J.-G.Y.; writing—original draft preparation, N.T. and H.P.; writing—review and editing, N.T., H.P.; visualization, N.T. and H.P.; supervision, H.P.; project administration, H.P.; funding acquisition, H.P. All authors have read and agreed to the published version of the manuscript.

Funding: This research was funded by the Dong-A University research grant.

Acknowledgments: The authors would like to thank the CEO Yeanhwa Lee and Sujin Seo of SY Inotech Inc., who provided VR contents for this study and helped us in operating the program. We thank the patients for participating in the Busan Metropolitan HealthCare Center. We also thank Dave (DaeKeun) Kim and other technical staff of iMediSync Inc. for the support in EEG data analysis and data filtering. We would also like to thank Hansol Kim for providing the administrative support.

Conflicts of Interest: The authors declare no conflict of interest.

References

1. National Collaborating Centre for Mental Health (UK). Dementia. In *Dementia: A NICE-SCIE Guideline on Supporting People With Dementia and Their Carers in Health and Social Care*; British Psychological Society: Lester, UK, 2007.
2. World Health Organization. Dementia. Available online: https://www.who.int/news-room/fact-sheets/detail/dementia (accessed on 26 February 2020).
3. Livingston, G.; Sommerlad, A.; Orgeta, V.; Costafreda, S.G.; Huntley, J.; Ames, D.; Ballard, C.; Banerjee, S.; Burns, A.; Cohen-Mansfield, J. Dementia prevention, intervention, and care. *Lancet* **2017**, *390*, 2673–2734. [CrossRef]
4. D'Cunha, N.M.; Georgousopoulou, E.N.; Dadigamuwage, L.; Kellett, J.; Panagiotakos, D.B.; Thomas, J.; McKune, A.J.; Mellor, D.D.; Naumovski, N. Effect of long-term nutraceutical and dietary supplement use on cognition in the elderly: A 10-year systematic review of randomised controlled trials. *Br. J. Nutr.* **2018**, *119*, 280–298. [CrossRef]
5. Albert, M.S.; DeKosky, S.T.; Dickson, D.; Dubois, B.; Feldman, H.H.; Fox, N.C.; Gamst, A.; Holtzman, D.M.; Jagust, W.J.; Petersen, R.C. The diagnosis of mild cognitive impairment due to Alzheimer's disease: Recommendations from the National Institute on Aging-Alzheimer's Association workgroups on diagnostic guidelines for Alzheimer's disease. *Alzheimer's Dement.* **2011**, *7*, 270–279. [CrossRef] [PubMed]
6. Pal, K.; Mukadam, N.; Petersen, I.; Cooper, C. Mild cognitive impairment and progression to dementia in people with diabetes, prediabetes and metabolic syndrome: A systematic review and meta-analysis. *Soc. Psychiatry Psychiatr. Epidemiol.* **2018**, *53*, 1149–1160. [CrossRef]
7. Gauthier, S.; Reisberg, B.; Zaudig, M.; Petersen, R.C.; Ritchie, K.; Broich, K.; Belleville, S.; Brodaty, H.; Bennett, D.; Chertkow, H. Mild cognitive impairment. *Lancet* **2006**, *367*, 1262–1270. [CrossRef]
8. Daviglus, M.L.; Bell, C.C.; Berrettini, W.; Bowen, P.E.; Connolly, E.S.; Cox, N.J.; Dunbar-Jacob, J.M.; Granieri, E.C.; Hunt, G.; McGarry, K. National Institutes of Health State-of-the-Science Conference statement: Preventing Alzheimer disease and cognitive decline. *Ann. Intern. Med.* **2010**, *153*, 176–181. [CrossRef] [PubMed]
9. Park, H.; Park, J.H.; Na, H.R.; Hiroyuki, S.; Kim, G.M.; Jung, M.K.; Kim, W.K.; Park, K.W. Combined Intervention of Physical Activity, Aerobic Exercise, and Cognitive Exercise Intervention to Prevent Cognitive Decline for Patients with Mild Cognitive Impairment: A Randomized Controlled Clinical Study. *J. Clin. Med.* **2019**, *8*, 940. [CrossRef]
10. Zucchella, C.; Sinforiani, E.; Tamburin, S.; Federico, A.; Mantovani, E.; Bernini, S.; Casale, R.; Bartolo, M. The multidisciplinary approach to Alzheimer's disease and dementia. A narrative review of non-pharmacological treatment. *Front. Neurol.* **2018**, *9*, 1058. [CrossRef] [PubMed]
11. Htut, T.Z.C.; Hiengkaew, V.; Jalayondeja, C.; Vongsirinavarat, M. Effects of physical, virtual reality-based, and brain exercise on physical, cognition, and preference in older persons: A randomized controlled trial. *Eur. Rev. Aging Phys. Act.* **2018**, *15*, 1–12. [CrossRef]
12. Optale, G.; Urgesi, C.; Busato, V.; Marin, S.; Piron, L.; Priftis, K.; Gamberini, L.; Capodieci, S.; Bordin, A. Controlling memory impairment in elderly adults using virtual reality memory training: A randomized controlled pilot study. *Neurorehabil. Neural Repair* **2010**, *24*, 348–357. [CrossRef]
13. Baus, O.; Bouchard, S. Moving from Virtual Reality Exposure-Based Therapy to Augmented Reality Exposure-Based Therapy: A Review. *Front. Hum. Neurosci.* **2014**, *8*. [CrossRef]
14. Moreno, A.; Wall, K.J.; Thangavelu, K.; Craven, L.; Ward, E.; Dissanayaka, N.N. A systematic review of the use of virtual reality and its effects on cognition in individuals with neurocognitive disorders. *Alzheimer's Dement. Transl. Res. Clin. Interv.* **2019**, *5*, 834–850. [CrossRef] [PubMed]

15. Manera, V.; Chapoulie, E.; Bourgeois, J.; Guerchouche, R.; David, R.; Ondrej, J.; Drettakis, G.; Robert, P. A feasibility study with image-based rendered virtual reality in patients with mild cognitive impairment and dementia. *PLoS ONE* **2016**, *11*, e0151487.
16. Gatica-Rojas, V.; Méndez-Rebolledo, G. Virtual reality interface devices in the reorganization of neural networks in the brain of patients with neurological diseases. *Neural Regen. Res.* **2014**, *9*, 888. [CrossRef] [PubMed]
17. Garcia-Betances, R.I.; Jiménez-Mixco, V.; Arredondo, M.T.; Cabrera-Umpiérrez, M.F. Using virtual reality for cognitive training of the elderly. *Am. J. Alzheimer's Dis. Other Demen.* **2015**, *30*, 49–54. [CrossRef]
18. Rizzo, A.S.; Kim, G.J. A SWOT analysis of the field of virtual reality rehabilitation and therapy. *Presence Teleoperators Virtual Environ.* **2005**, *14*, 119–146. [CrossRef]
19. Kim, O.; Pang, Y.; Kim, J.-H. The effectiveness of virtual reality for people with mild cognitive impairment or dementia: A meta-analysis. *BMC Psychiatry* **2019**, *19*, 219. [CrossRef]
20. Zając-Lamparska, L.; Wiłkość-Dębczyńska, M.; Wojciechowski, A.; Podhorecka, M.; Polak-Szabela, A.; Warchoł, Ł.; Kędziora-Kornatowska, K.; Araszkiewicz, A.; Izdebski, P. Effects of virtual reality-based cognitive training in older adults living without and with mild dementia: A pretest–posttest design pilot study. *BMC Res. Notes* **2019**, *12*, 776. [CrossRef]
21. Weniger, G.; Ruhleder, M.; Lange, C.; Wolf, S.; Irle, E. Egocentric and allocentric memory as assessed by virtual reality in individuals with amnestic mild cognitive impairment. *Neuropsychologia* **2011**, *49*, 518–527. [CrossRef]
22. Sayma, M.; Tuijt, R.; Cooper, C.; Walters, K. Are We There Yet? Immersive Virtual Reality to Improve Cognitive Function in Dementia and Mild Cognitive Impairment. *Gerontologist* **2019**. [CrossRef]
23. García-Betances, R.I.; Arredondo Waldmeyer, M.T.; Fico, G.; Cabrera-Umpiérrez, M.F. A succinct overview of virtual reality technology use in Alzheimer's disease. *Front. Aging Neurosci.* **2015**, *7*, 80. [PubMed]
24. Van der Hiele, K.; Vein, A.; Reijntjes, R.; Westendorp, R.; Bollen, E.; Van Buchem, M.; Van Dijk, J.; Middelkoop, H. EEG correlates in the spectrum of cognitive decline. *Clin. Neurophysiol.* **2007**, *118*, 1931–1939. [CrossRef]
25. Chandler, M.J.; Lacritz, L.; Hynan, L.; Barnard, H.; Allen, G.; Deschner, M.; Weiner, M.; Cullum, C. A total score for the CERAD neuropsychological battery. *Neurology* **2005**, *65*, 102–106. [CrossRef] [PubMed]
26. Kim, T.H.; Jhoo, J.H.; Park, J.H.; Kim, J.L.; Ryu, S.H.; Moon, S.W.; Choo, I.H.; Lee, D.W.; Yoon, J.C.; Do, Y.J. Korean version of mini mental status examination for dementia screening and its' short form. *Psychiatry Investig.* **2010**, *7*, 102. [CrossRef] [PubMed]
27. Makizako, H.; Shimada, H.; Park, H.; Doi, T.; Yoshida, D.; Uemura, K.; Tsutsumimoto, K.; Suzuki, T. Evaluation of multidimensional neurocognitive function using a tablet personal computer: Test–retest reliability and validity in community-dwelling older adults. *Geriatr. Gerontol. Int.* **2013**, *13*, 860–866. [CrossRef] [PubMed]
28. Klem, G.H.; Lüders, H.O.; Jasper, H.; Elger, C. The ten-twenty electrode system of the International Federation. *Electroencephalogr. Clin. Neurophysiol.* **1999**, *52*, 3–6.
29. Prichep, L.; John, E.; Ferris, S.; Rausch, L.; Fang, Z.; Cancro, R.; Torossian, C.; Reisberg, B. Prediction of longitudinal cognitive decline in normal elderly with subjective complaints using electrophysiological imaging. *Neurobiol. Aging* **2006**, *27*, 471–481. [CrossRef]
30. Sánchez-Moguel, S.M.; Alatorre-Cruz, G.C.; Silva-Pereyra, J.; González-Salinas, S.; Sanchez-Lopez, J.; Otero-Ojeda, G.A.; Fernández, T. Two Different Populations within the Healthy Elderly: Lack of Conflict Detection in Those at Risk of Cognitive Decline. *Front. Hum. Neurosci.* **2018**, *11*, 658. [CrossRef]
31. Van Son, D.; De Blasio, F.M.; Fogarty, J.S.; Angelidis, A.; Barry, R.J.; Putman, P. Frontal EEG theta/beta ratio during mind wandering episodes. *Biol. Psychol.* **2019**, *140*, 19–27. [CrossRef]
32. Coyle, H.; Traynor, V.; Solowij, N. Computerized and virtual reality cognitive training for individuals at high risk of cognitive decline: Systematic review of the literature. *Am. J. Geriatr. Psychiatry* **2015**, *23*, 335–359. [CrossRef]
33. Liao, Y.-Y.; Chen, I.-H.; Lin, Y.-J.; Chen, Y.; Hsu, W.-C. Effects of Virtual Reality-Based Physical and Cognitive Training on Executive Function and Dual-Task Gait Performance in Older Adults with Mild Cognitive Impairment: A Randomized Control Trial. *Front. Aging Neurosci.* **2019**, *11*, 162. [CrossRef] [PubMed]

34. Mahurin, R.K.; Velligan, D.I.; Hazleton, B.; Mark Davis, J.; Eckert, S.; Miller, A.L. Trail making test errors and executive function in schizophrenia and depression. *Clin. Neuropsychol.* **2006**, *20*, 271–288. [CrossRef] [PubMed]
35. Sánchez-Cubillo, I.; Perianez, J.; Adrover-Roig, D.; Rodriguez-Sanchez, J.; Rios-Lago, M.; Tirapu, J.; Barcelo, F. Construct validity of the Trail Making Test: Role of task-switching, working memory, inhibition/interference control, and visuomotor abilities. *J. Int. Neuropsychol. Soc.* **2009**, *15*, 438–450. [CrossRef] [PubMed]
36. Budson, A.E.; Solomon, P.R. Memory Loss, Alzheimer's disease, and dementia e-book: A practical guide for clinicians. *Elsevier Health Sci.* **2015**, 5–38.
37. Llinàs-Reglà, J.; Vilalta-Franch, J.; López-Pousa, S.; Calvó-Perxas, L.; Torrents Rodas, D.; Garre-Olmo, J. The trail making test: Association with other neuropsychological measures and normative values for adults aged 55 years and older from a Spanish-Speaking Population-based sample. *Assessment* **2017**, *24*, 183–196. [CrossRef]
38. Neri, S.G.; Cardoso, J.R.; Cruz, L.; Lima, R.M.; De Oliveira, R.J.; Iversen, M.D.; Carregaro, R.L. Do virtual reality games improve mobility skills and balance measurements in community-dwelling older adults? Systematic review and meta-analysis. *Clin. Rehabil.* **2017**, *31*, 1292–1304. [CrossRef]
39. Rodrigues-Baroni, J.M.; Nascimento, L.R.; Ada, L.; Teixeira-Salmela, L.F. Walking training associated with virtual reality-based training increases walking speed of individuals with chronic stroke: Systematic review with meta-analysis. *Braz. J. Phys. Ther.* **2014**, *18*, 502–512. [CrossRef]
40. Van Schaik, P.; Martyr, A.; Blackman, T.; Robinson, J. Involving persons with dementia in the evaluation of outdoor environments. *Cyberpsychol. Behav.* **2008**, *11*, 415–424. [CrossRef]
41. Fritz, N.E.; McCarthy, C.J.; Adamo, D.E. Handgrip strength as a means of monitoring progression of cognitive decline—A scoping review. *Ageing Res. Rev.* **2017**, *35*, 112–123. [CrossRef]
42. Sternäng, O.; Reynolds, C.A.; Finkel, D.; Ernsth-Bravell, M.; Pedersen, N.L.; Dahl Aslan, A.K. Grip strength and cognitive abilities: Associations in old age. *J. Gerontol. Ser. B Psychol. Sci. Soc. Sci.* **2016**, *71*, 841–848.
43. Vancampfort, D.; Stubbs, B.; Firth, J.; Smith, L.; Swinnen, N.; Koyanagi, A. Associations between handgrip strength and mild cognitive impairment in middle-aged and older adults in six low-and middle-income countries. *Int. J. Geriatr. Psychiatry* **2019**, *34*, 609–616. [CrossRef] [PubMed]
44. Best, J.R.; Liu-Ambrose, T.; Boudreau, R.M.; Ayonayon, H.N.; Satterfield, S.; Simonsick, E.M.; Studenski, S.; Yaffe, K.; Newman, A.B.; Rosano, C. An evaluation of the longitudinal, bidirectional associations between gait speed and cognition in older women and men. *J. Gerontol. A Biol. Sci. Med. Sci.* **2016**, *71*, 1616–1623. [CrossRef] [PubMed]
45. Buracchio, T.; Dodge, H.H.; Howieson, D.; Wasserman, D.; Kaye, J. The trajectory of gait speed preceding mild cognitive impairment. *Arch. Neurol.* **2010**, *67*, 980–986. [CrossRef] [PubMed]
46. Rasmussen, L.J.H.; Caspi, A.; Ambler, A.; Broadbent, J.M.; Cohen, H.J.; D'Arbeloff, T.; Elliott, M.; Hancox, R.J.; Harrington, H.; Hogan, S. Association of neurocognitive and physical function with gait speed in midlife. *JAMA Netw. Open* **2019**, *2*, e1913123. [CrossRef] [PubMed]
47. Sánchez, A.; Millán-Calenti, J.C.; Lorenzo-López, L.; Maseda, A. Multisensory stimulation for people with dementia: A review of the literature. *Am. J. Alzheimer's Dis. Other Demen.* **2013**, *28*, 7–14.
48. Rose, F.D.; Attree, E.A.; Brooks, B.M.; Andrews, T.K. Learning and memory in virtual environments: A role in neurorehabilitation? Questions (and occasional answers) from the University of East London. *Presence Teleoperators Virtual Environ.* **2001**, *10*, 345–358. [CrossRef]
49. Clemente, M.; Rey, B.; Rodriguez-Pujadas, A.; Breton-Lopez, J.; Barros-Loscertales, A.; Baños, R.M.; Botella, C.; Alcañiz, M.; Avila, C. A functional magnetic resonance imaging assessment of small animals' phobia using virtual reality as a stimulus. *JMIR Serious Games* **2014**, *2*, e6. [CrossRef]
50. Hikichi, H.; Kondo, K.; Takeda, T.; Kawachi, I. Social interaction and cognitive decline: Results of a 7-year community intervention. *Alzheimer's Dement. Transl. Res. Clin. Interv.* **2017**, *3*, 23–32. [CrossRef]
51. Zunzunegui, M.-V.; Alvarado, B.E.; Del Ser, T.; Otero, A. Social networks, social integration, and social engagement determine cognitive decline in community-dwelling Spanish older adults. *J. Gerontol. B Psychol. Sci. Soc. Sci.* **2003**, *58*, S93–S100. [CrossRef]

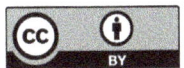

© 2020 by the authors. Licensee MDPI, Basel, Switzerland. This article is an open access article distributed under the terms and conditions of the Creative Commons Attribution (CC BY) license (http://creativecommons.org/licenses/by/4.0/).

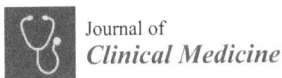

Review

Non-Immersive Virtual Reality for Rehabilitation of the Older People: A Systematic Review into Efficacy and Effectiveness

Roberta Bevilacqua [1], Elvira Maranesi [1,*], Giovanni Renato Riccardi [2], Valentina Di Donna [2], Paolo Pelliccioni [3], Riccardo Luzi [4], Fabrizia Lattanzio [1] and Giuseppe Pelliccioni [5]

1. Scientific Direction, IRCCS INRCA, 60129 Ancona, Italy; r.bevilacqua@inrca.it (R.B.); f.lattanzio@inrca.it (F.L.)
2. Clinical Unit of Physical Rehabilitation, IRCCS INRCA, 60100 Ancona, Italy; g.riccardi@inrca.it (G.R.R.); v.didonna@inrca.it (V.D.D.)
3. Eye Clinic, Polytechnic University of Marche, 60100 Ancona, Italy; paopel@hotmail.it
4. Medical Direction, IRCCS INRCA, 60100 Ancona, Italy; r.luzi@inrca.it
5. Neurology Unit, IRCCS INRCA, 60100 Ancona, Italy; g.pelliccioni@inrca.it
* Correspondence: e.maranesi@inrca.it; Tel.: +39-071-800-3163

Received: 18 September 2019; Accepted: 1 November 2019; Published: 5 November 2019

Abstract: Objective: the objective of this review is to analyze the advances in the field of rehabilitation through virtual reality, while taking into account non-immersive systems, as evidence have them shown to be highly accepted by older people, due to the lowest "cibersikness" symptomatology. Data sources: a systematic review of the literature was conducted in June 2019. The data were collected from Cochrane, Embase, Scopus, and PubMed databases, analyzing manuscripts and articles of the last 10 years. Study selection: we only included randomized controlled trials written in English aimed to study the use of the virtual reality in rehabilitation. We selected 10 studies, which were characterized by clinical heterogeneity. Data extraction: quality evaluation was performed based on the Physiotherapy Evidence Database (PEDro) scale, suggested for evidence based review of stroke rehabilitation. Of 10 studies considered, eight were randomized controlled trials and the PEDro score ranged from four to a maximum of nine. Data synthesis: VR (Virtual Reality) creates artificial environments with the possibility of a patient interaction. This kind of experience leads to the development of cognitive and motor abilities, which usually positively affect the emotional state of the patient, increasing collaboration and compliance. Some recent studies have suggested that rehabilitation treatment interventions might be useful and effective in treating motor and cognitive symptoms in different neurological disorders, including traumatic brain injury, multiple sclerosis, and progressive supranuclear palsy. Conclusions: as it is shown by the numerous studies in the field, the application of VR has a positive impact on the rehabilitation of the most predominant geriatric syndromes. The level of realism of the virtual stimuli seems to have a crucial role in the training of cognitive abilities. Future research needs to improve study design by including larger samples, longitudinal designs, long term follow-ups, and different outcome measures, including functional and quality of life indexes, to better evaluate the clinical impact of this promising technology in healthy old subjects and in neurological patients.

Keywords: virtual reality; cognitive and physical rehabilitation; oldest old person

1. Introduction

Virtual reality (VR) is a trending, widely accessible, contemporary technology of increasing utility to biomedical and health applications [1]. VR is the technological experience that allows for a full immersion in virtual spaces with which you can interact via specific wearable or using only your hand.

A key feature of all VR applications is interaction. Virtual environments (VE) are created and allow for the user to interact with not only the VE, but also with virtual objects within the environment. In some systems, the interaction might be achieved via a pointer operated by a mouse or joystick button. In other systems, a representation of the user's hand (or other body part) might be created within the environment where the virtual hand movement is generated [2].

VR ranges from non-immersive to fully immersive, depending on the degree to which the user is isolated from the physical surroundings when interacting with the virtual environment. Non-immersive virtual reality allows for interacting with the environment through mouse or joystick; immersive virtual reality, instead, uses tools that are connected to the human body in order to perform the same motor task [3,4]. Non-immersive VR systems have been studied as a therapeutic tool for improving symptoms in neurological disorders and have shown potential to promote cognitive and motor improvements even in advanced stages of different neurological diseases (e.g., stroke, Alzheimer and Parkinson disease (AD, PD), multiple sclerosis (MS), and traumatic brain injury) because of these characteristics [5–9].

The use of VR technology in rehabilitation derives from research in computational neuroscience involving motor learning mechanisms [10]. VR provides real-time visual feedback for movements, thereby increasing engagement in enjoyable rehabilitation tasks [11].

VR provides alternative rehabilitation programs with new and effective therapeutic tools that can improve the functional abilities in a wide variety of rehabilitation patients in a neurological setting, offering several features, such as goal-oriented tasks and repetition. The use of VR environments for virtual augmented exercise has recently been proposed as having the potential to increase exercise behavior in older adults [12] and it also has the potential to influence cognitive abilities in this population segment [13]. Therefore, VR represents a real opportunity for the cognitive rehabilitation of neurological patients with different neuropsychological symptoms, especially in attention, memory, problem-solving and executive dysfunction, and in behavioral impairments [7–9].

Moreover, VR training has been mostly described for the upper limb [14,15], but also for the lower limb [16], balance and walking [17,18], as well as for perceptual/cognitive skills [19].

To our knowledge, systematic reviews or meta-analyses have been undertaken to review the utility of VR technologies in a single arm of rehabilitation (i.e., motor or cognitive rehabilitation, upper or lower limb rehabilitation), focusing on a specific pathology (stroke, PD, AD, MS) [6,7,9].

Despite the growing evidence of the positive effects of VR in rehabilitation of functional and cognitive abilities, some systems still raised concerns regarding their acceptability with complex clinical populations, as, for example, the older people. In particular, during trials with immersive systems, few adverse events have been described by participants, including headache and dizziness [20]. Finally, little is known about the perceived effect of the exposure at multisensory input during a complex activity, such as treadmill walking with VR in patients during post-stroke rehabilitation to improve balance and gait ability [6,21].

The objective of this review is to analyze the advances in the field of rehabilitation through VR, while taking non-immersive systems into account, as evidence have shown to be highly accepted by older people, due to the lowest "cibersikness" symptomatology [20]. For this purpose, Randomized Controlled Trials (RCTs) were analyzed in order to investigate the effects of rehabilitation programs integrated with innovative non-immersive VR systems and suggest future clinical applications.

2. Methods

2.1. Literature Search and Study Selection

The methodology of this systematic review was based on the Preferred Reporting Items for Systematic Reviews and Meta-Analyses (PRISMA) guidelines, as the main aim of this work is mapping all the available literature in the rehabilitation with non-immersive virtual reality. A systematic review of the literature was conducted in June 2019. The data were collected from Cochrane, Embase, Scopus,

PubMed, and Science Direct databases, analyzing manuscripts and articles of the last 10 years (from June 2009 to June 2019), in order to obtain the latest evidence in the field.

Based on consultation with the multidisciplinary team, non-immersive VR studies and applications related to rehabilitation intervention were searched while using the following search terms, and the combination thereof: non-immersive, virtual reality, virtual game, rehabilitation, motor impairment, and cognitive impairment.

After the preliminary search, 26 articles resulted from PubMed, 19 from Scopus, 283 from Science Direct, 10 from Embase, and 11 from Cochrane.

The findings were analyzed and screened by four experts of the team, a bioengineer, a clinical neuropsychologist, a statistician, and a neurologist. In particular, three review authors independently reviewed titles and abstracts that were retrieved from the search in order to determine whether they met the predefined inclusion criteria. A fourth review author (a statistician) moderate any disagreement. The full text articles were subsequently analyzed.

The first screening was based on the analysis of the title and of the abstract, as well as deduplication of the findings. Another researcher confirmed the accuracy of the papers selection and screened for any possible omission. After the first step, 11 articles resulted from PubMed, two from Scopus, and 0 from Science Direct, Embase, and Cochrane.

2.2. Study Selection

We included RCTs and reviews written in English that aimed to study the use of non-immersive virtual reality in rehabilitation. Thus, we selected studies meeting the following criteria:

1. Studies conducted on adult patients aged ≥65 years
2. Studies devoted to use a non-immersive virtual reality in rehabilitation
3. Studies including upper limb rehabilitation, lower limb rehabilitation, or cognitive rehabilitation
4. Randomized clinical trials, with control group that received conventional rehabilitation therapy
5. Before-after comparison of a single group
6. Review articles

On the contrary, we excluded studies that met the following criteria:

1. Conference proceedings
2. Studies for which the full text was not found
3. Studies written in languages other than English
4. Technical papers
5. Qualitative studies

All case-report studies and case-control studies were excluded for a lack of sustainability of results, as well as works concerning the development of new technologies.

2.3. Data Collection

After the screening based on the inclusion/exclusion criteria, conducted on the full text articles, the studies were selected as follows: 0 from Scopus, 10 from PubMed, and no one from Cochrane, Science Direct and Embase, and one from other sources. The countries of the selected studies are: Spain (2), France (2), Italy (2), Israel (1), United State of America (1), Canada (2), and Brazil (1). The fact that the studies have been performed in different countries shows that the topic is of general interest. Figure 1 shows the flowchart search strategy applied.

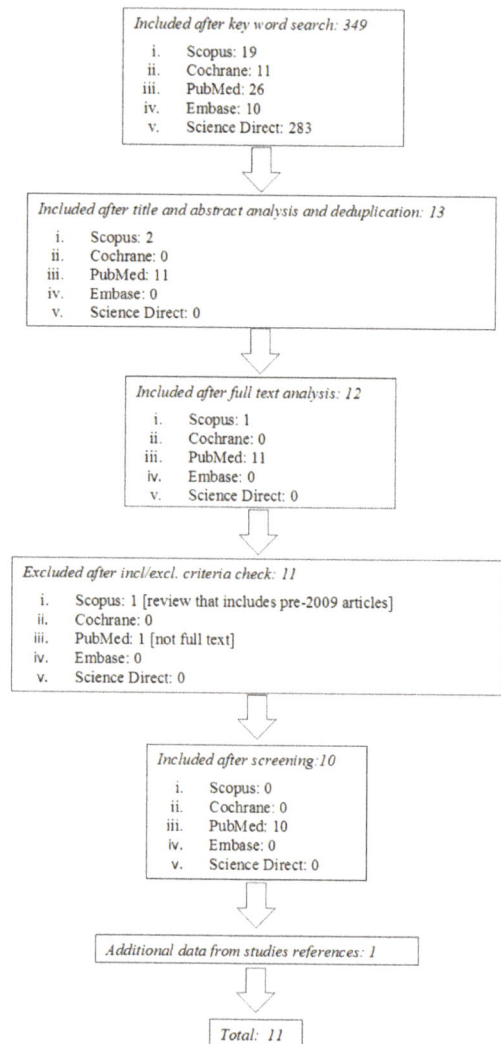

Figure 1. Flow diagram of the study selection process.

3. Results

A total of 10 papers were included. Studies are both reviews [22,23] and clinical papers [24–31].

3.1. Study Quality Evaluation

Quality evaluation was performed based on the PEDro scale and on the Cochrane's Risk of Bias (RoB) tool, suggested for evidence based review of rehabilitation while using non-immersive virtual reality [32,33]. The final score was settled when three authors reached agreement after repeated review and analysis. Of eight studies considered, five were randomized controlled trials and the PEDro score ranged from four to a maximum of nine, and the RoB score ranges from one to five (Table 1).

3.2. General Characteristics of the Study Population

All of the studies were focused on older people with a mean age of 65.2 (±9.4) years for the experimental group and 69.2 (±9.4) years in the control group. The number of participants that were involved in all the studies is 1008 ranged from 6 to 376.

To our knowledge, of the older people involved in the trials, 586 were males and 392 females.

The majority of the patients suffered from stroke ($n = 593$), followed by older people at high risk of falls, with more than two falls in six months ($n = 182$), patients with amyotrophic lateral sclerosis ($n = 30$), AD ($n = 24$), or PD ($n = 24$).

3.3. Descriptive Analysis and Outcome Measures

Table 2 shows the characteristics of the studies. The outcome could not be pooled into meta-analysis due to the following reasons. Clinical heterogeneity (Table 2) can be clearly observed from the participant, intervention, exercise mode, and outcome measures of the included studies. Diversity is seen in patient conditions and pathology, frequency, and duration of VR intervention, whether the impairment concerns the upper or the lower limb, whether the experiment conducted was pure VR (only VR) or VR mixed with traditional physical therapy or with exercise therapy, and whether the outcome measure contains follow-up.

Table 1. Scores of methodological quality assessment of the included studies.

PEDro [32]	Walker et al., 2010 [24] RCT	Turolla et al., 2013 [25] RCT	Allain et al., 2014 [26] RCT	Saposnik et al., 2016 [27] RCT	Mirelman et al., 2016 [28] RCT	Seguera-Orti et al., 2018 [29] RCT	Trevizan et al., 2018 [30] RCT	Pelosin et al., 2019 [31] RCT
Eligibility	Y	Y	Y	Y	Y	Y	Y	Y
Randomized allocation	N	N	N	Y	Y	Y	Y	Y
Concealed allocation	Z	Z	Z	Y	Y	Y	Y	Y
Baseline comparability	Y	Y	Z	Y	Y	Z	Z	Z
Blinded subject	Z	Z	Z	Z	Z	Z	Z	Z
Blinded therapists	Z	Z	Z	N	Z	Z	Z	Z
Blinded raters	Z	Z	Z	Y	Y	Y	Y	Y
Key outcomes	Y	Y	Y	Y	Y	Y	Y	Y
Intention to treat	Z	Z	Y	Y	Y	Y	Y	N
Comparison between groups	Y	Y	Y	Y	Y	Y	Y	Y
Precision and variability	Y	Y	Y	Y	Y	Y	Y	Y
	4/11	5/11	4/11	9/11	8/11	8/11	8/11	7/11
Cochrane's Risk of bias tool [33]								
Sequence generation	Z	Z	Z	Y	Y	Y	Y	Y
Allocation concealment	Z	Z	Z	Y	Y	Y	Y	Y
Blinding of participants, personnel and outcome assessors.	N N N	N N N	N N N	N N Y	N N Y	N N Y	N N Y	N N Y
Incomplete outcome data.	Z	Z	Z	Z	Z	Z	Z	N
Selective outcome reporting	Y	Y	Y	Y	Y	Y	Y	Y
Other sources of bias	N	Y	Y	Y	Y	N	N	Y
	1/8	2/8	2/8	5/8	5/8	4/8	4/8	5/8

Y: yes; N: no.

Table 2. Descriptive analysis of the included clinical studies.

	Population		Technological Devices	Intervention		Outcome
	Partecipants in Experimental Group	Partecipants in Control Group		Training Frequency	Intervention Group / Comparison Control Group	
Walker et al., 2010 [24]	6 adults within 1-year post-stroke $N = 6$, 3 F/3 M Age: 54.3 years (range 41–70 years)	-	A partial body weight-support treadmill in conjunction with a television mounted on a stand in front of the treadmill to display the VR walkthrough environment.	2 or 3 training sessions per week with partial body weight-supported treadmill with virtual reality system (total 12 training sessions). Initial training duration is 10 minutes; duration was progressed as tolerated.	-	(1) FGA scores increased by 30% (2) BBS scores improved by 10% (3) Overground walking speed increased by 38%

Table 2. Cont.

	Population		Intervention		Comparison	Outcome
	Partecipants in Experimental Group	Partecipants in Control Group	Technological Devices	Training Frequency	Intervention Group	Control Group	
Turolla et al., 2013 [25]	n = 263 post-stroke patients, 105 F/158 M Age: 60.2 ± 14.3 years	n = 113 post-stroke patients, 41 F/72 M Age: 65.4 ±12.5	The Virtual Reality Rehabilitation System (Khymeia group, Noventa padovana, Italy) includes a pc workstation connected to 3D motion-tracking system and a high-resolution LCD projector displaying the virtual scenarios on a large wall screen.	40 sessions of daily therapy provided 5 days per week, for 4 weeks.	40 sessions of daily therapy provided 5 days per week, for 4 weeks. 1 hour of conventional therapy and 1 hour of VR therapy	2 hours of conventional treatment.	Within groups: F-M UE score improved by 4% in control group, and 10% in experimental group. Between groups: significantly greater motor improvement in experimental group. Within groups: FIM scores improved in both groups. Between groups: FIM scores improved by 5% in experimental group than in control group.
Allain et al., 2014 [26]	n = 24 AD patients, 14 F/10 M Age: 76.96 ± 6.05 years	n = 32 healthy older patients, 25 F/7 M Age: 74.13 ± 5.93	The virtual environment simulated a fully texture, medium-size kitchen. In the foreground, there was a work plane with all the objects needed to prepare a cup of coffee with milk and sugar. Patients controlled the 2D cursor using a computer mouse.	1. Virtual reality: 3 sessions: 2 of training and one test session to prepare a cup of coffee in virtual condition 2. Reality: to prepare a cup of coffee	Each training sessions lasts 15 minutes	Each training sessions lasts 15 minutes	Within groups: time to complete the virtual task and MMSE score are correlated in both groups
Saposnik et al., 2016 [27]	n = 71 stroke patients, 25 F/46 M Age: 62 ± 13 years	n = 70 stroke patients, 22 F/48 M Age: 62 ± 12 years	The Nintendo Wii gaming system or recreational activities (playing cards, bingo, jenga or ball game).	10 sessions, 60 minutes each, over a 2 week period.	30 minutes of traditional rehabilitation of the upper extremity + 30 minutes of virtual reality training	60 minutes of traditional rehabilitation of the upper extremity	1. Within groups: WMFT performance time improves from baseline to the end of treatment in both groups. 2. Between groups: no differences in WMFT at the end and at 4-weeks post-intervention 3. Between groups: better performance in BBT in control group at the end of treatment.
Mirelman et al., 2016 [28]	n = 146 older people at high risk of falls (more than 2 falls in 6 months), 48 F/98 M Age: 74.2 ± 6.9 years	n = 136 older people at high risk of falls (more than 2 falls in 6 months), 52 F/84 M Age: 73.3 ± 6.4 years	The treadmill plus VR intervention included a camera for motion capture and a computer generated simulation. The virtual environments included real-life challenges with obstacles, multiple pathway and distracters.	3 times per week for 6 weeks, with each session lasting about 45 minutes	45 minutes of treadmill training with virtual reality	45 minutes of traditional treadmill training	In the 6 months after training, the incident rate was significantly lower in the treadmill training plus VR group.

Table 2. *Cont.*

	Population		Technological Devices	Intervention Training Frequency	Intervention Group	Comparison Control Group	Outcome
	Partecipants in Experimental Group	Partecipants in Control Group					
Seguera-Orti et al., 2018 [29]	$n = 9$ patients on hemodialysis, 4 F/5 M Age: 61.8 ± 13.0	$n = 9$ patients on hemodialysis, 3 F/6 M Age: 68.3 ± 15.6	The system is an adapted version of ACT (A la Caza del Tesoro), in which the subject tries to catch a series of targets by moving their leg.	16 weeks of intra-dialysis exercise program. The program lasted 4 additional weeks.	5 minutes warm-up; 30 minutes of virtual reality training.	5 minutes warm-up and strengthening exercises; 30 minute of aerobic training; 5 minutes of stretching.	1. Between groups: no significant differences in STS-60 2. Between groups: significant differences in gait speed 3. Within groups: significant improvements for STS-10, gait speed, 6 minute walking test between baseline-16 and 20 weeks, and 16–20 weeks.
Trevizan et al., 2018 [30]	$n = 30$ people with ALS, 12 F/18 M Age: 59 years (range 44–74 years)	$n = 30$ healthy people, equally matched for age and gender with experimental group	The VR environment is a 3D game in which the goal was to reach as many bubbles displayed on the computer monitor. The game was controlled by three different device system: motion tracking, finger motion and touch-screen.	Participants were randomly divided in 3 groups: motion tracking, finger motion control, touchscreen, to perform 3 task phases (acquisition, retention, transfer)			Both experimental and control group showed better performance whn using the touchscreen device in the transfer phase.
Pelosin et al., 2019 [31]	$n = 10$ PD + 7 OA 11 F/6 M Age: 73.2 ± 3.6	$n = 14$ PD + 8 OA 15 F/7 M Age: 71.9 ± 4.1	Treadmill with a non-immersive virtual reality that reacts to a virtual environment that included real-life challenges	45 minutes/session, 3 times a week for 6 weeks	To walk on a treadmill with virtual reality that included obstacles, distracters.	To walk on a treadmill without virtual reality.	Experimental group increased SAI, reduced the number of falls, improved obstacle negotiation performance.

FGA: Functional Gait Assessment. BBS: Berg Balance Scale. VR: Virtual Reality. F-M UE: Fugl-Meyer upper extremity. FIM: Functional Independence Measure. AD: Alzheimer's disease. MMSE: Mini Mental State Examination. WMFT: Wolf Motor Function Test. BBT: Box and Block Test. STS-60: sit-to-stand tests 60. ARAT: Action Research Arm Test. MMAS: Modified Modified Ashworth Scale. MAL: Motor Activity Log. FSS-7: Fatigue Severity Scale seven-item. SIPSO: Subjective Index of Physical and Social Outcome 10-item. VAS: Visual Analogue Scale. ALS: Amyotrophic Lateral Sclerosis. PD: Parkinson Disease. OA: older adults. SAI: Short-latency afferent inhibition.

3.4. Intervention Effects

Eight papers report the results of clinical trials involving a group of patients that performed a training with VR system versus a control group that performed a traditional physiotherapy training [25–29,31], or a comparison within the same group performing a VR training while using different exercise control modalities [30].

The period of VR training ranged from four to six weeks, each day of the week or three training sessions per week, while the duration of each single session with VR system ranged from 15 to 60 minutes. Only in one study [27] the duration of intervention was two weeks. Generally, all the experimental groups (EGs) in the studies have received both therapies with VR and traditional physiotherapy, while the control groups (CGs) have only received traditional physiotherapy. Two studies have a follow up after eight and 12 weeks [29] or six months [28].

The study of Walker et al. [24] reported the lowest number of subjects ($n = 6$) within one-year post-stroke. It is a before-after study and all the subjects performed training with a treadmill equipped with a VR system. All the participants made significant improvements in their ability to walk, increasing the over ground walking speed and the Berg Balance Scale (BBS) scores.

The study of Turolla et al. [25] involves 376 post-stroke patients randomized into two groups, receiving combined VR and upper limb conventional therapy or traditional therapy alone. VR rehabilitation seems more effective than conventional interventions in restoring upper limb motor impairments and motor related functional abilities.

The study of Allain et al. [26] involves 24 Alzheimer's disease patients as compared with 32 healthy elderly controls on a task designed to assess their ability to prepare a virtual cup of coffee, comparing the performance with an identical daily living task. Significant relations are found between virtual and real coffee-making scores, and between virtual score and Instrumental activities of daily living (IADL) scale, which supports the validity of the virtual reality training.

In a study of Saposnik et al. [27], 141 post-stroke patients were randomized into two groups: the first received the VR therapy and the second received recreational therapy. The results show that within each group the performance time improves from baseline to the end of treatment, whereas no differences are found between groups.

The objective of Mirelman et al. [28] was to verify whether an intervention combining treadmill training with non-immersive virtual reality (to target both cognitive aspects and mobility) would lead to fewer falls than treadmill training alone would. To do this, the authors recruited 282 older people at high risk of falls and randomized them into two groups to receive treadmill training plus VR or treadmill training alone. In the six months after training, the incident rate was significantly lower in the experimental group.

The study of Segura-Orti et al. [29] involves 18 patients on hemodialysis: nine performed 30 minutes of non-immersive virtual reality training and nine performed 30 minutes of aerobic training. Both interventions improved physical function, such as gait speed and no significant differences, were found between groups.

In the study of Trevizan et al. [30], the performance on a computer task in patients with amyotrophic lateral sclerosis while using three (motion tracking, finger motion control, or touch screen) different commonly used non-immersive devices was evaluated. The control and experimental group both showed better performance on the computer task when using the touch screen device.

Pelosin et al. [31] analyzed 39 patients with Parkinson's disease, assigned to treadmill training group or treadmill training with non-immersive virtual reality intervention group to assess cholinergic activity. The results showed that the experimental group improved obstacle negotiation performance, and reduced the number of falls as compared with control group.

4. Discussion

A review of the evidence on VR efficacy in patients affected by a neurological disease is mandatory due to the rapid development of VR programs in the last years and the increasing literature on VR application in neurological conditions, in order to enable clinicians to have an up-to-date understanding of the potential clinical beneficial effects of these techniques.

Therefore, the aim of this paper was to systematically evaluate the evidence of the effectiveness of VR compared to conventional therapies. It must be stressed that few studies summarize the current best evidence on the effectiveness, user compliance, feasibility, and safety of VR interventions for rehabilitation treatment in neurological disorders.

VR creates artificial environments with the possibility of a patient interaction. This kind of experience leads to the development of cognitive and motor abilities, which usually positively affect the emotional state of the patient, increasing collaboration and compliance.

Moreover, the VR rehabilitative treatment might be personalized according to the specific abilities and needs of the subject.

Parkinson disease is one of the most common age-related brain disorders with both dopamine-related motor symptoms and nonmotor symptoms due to other neurotransmitter circuits involvement, such as the cholinergic, noradrenergic, and serotonergic pathways.

The cognitive decline is among the most common and relevant nonmotor symptoms in PD and it affects different cognitive domains, in particular attentional, visuospatial and executive domains, and also memory. VR in the cognitive PD treatment could be useful in improving, in particular, the visuospatial and executive abilities, which represent the most compromised aspects of cognitive decline in PD patients [7].

Moreover, falls are frequent in ageing and PD patients, due to an impairment in the cholinergic-mediated gait pathway. A rehabilitation approach using treadmill training combined with non-immersive VR seems to induce changes in cortical cholinergic activity, which enables functional gait improvements and reduces the fall rate in comparison to a traditional rehabilitation method [31].

A reduction in static and dynamic balance is a major risk factor for falls also in stroke survivors [34]. In fact, the majority of the individuals with stroke who have fallen usually develop fear of falling again (88%). Fear of falling is related to balance and gait deficits [35], and it often leads to reduced physical activity and deconditioning. In fact, 44% of stroke fallers report restriction of activity after the fall. Given the very low physical activity and cardiovascular fitness levels already near the lower limit of those required for basic ADL, further activity reduction and deconditioning due to the fear of falling can easily lead to a loss of independence in individuals with stroke.

A recent review on post-stroke rehabilitation therapy [6] provided evidence for a moderate beneficial effect in balance improvement of VR combined with conventional therapy, as compared to conventional therapy alone.

More promising effects seem to be evident in the case of upper limb motor impairments in stroke rehabilitation [25], but further studies are needed on this subject. In fact, the trial described in [27] found that non-immersive VR as an add-on therapy to conventional rehabilitation was not superior to a recreational activity intervention in improving motor function, which suggested that the added intensity of training only induces early motor recovery of the upper limb, and that this can be achieved with VR or with other simple and inexpensive arm activities.

VR technology has considerable potential for detecting functional limitations in IADL performance in AD patients, beyond that of current neuropsychological measures, as shown by Allain et al. [26]. Moreover, studies were carried out to assess the effectiveness of a VR cognitive training program on cognition in mild cognitive impairment (MCI) and AD patients [36].

VR cognitive training for individuals with MCI and dementia has proven to result in improvements in the cognitive domains of attention, executive function, and visual and verbal memory. Moreover, significant reductions in depressive symptoms and anxiety were evident, with a delay in the progression of cognitive impairment [37].

Additionally, the VR format might help in training adherence, as individuals with MCI and dementia patients seem to prefer the VR format of a task over the paper version, as confirmed by a feasibility study with image-based rendered VR in patients with mild cognitive impairment and dementia [38].

Some recent studies have suggested that rehabilitation treatment interventions might be useful and effective in treating motor and cognitive symptoms in different neurological disorders, including traumatic brain injury [8], multiple sclerosis [9], and progressive supranuclear palsy [39].

Finally, VR represents an effective tool that could improve the traditional cognitive and motor rehabilitation in patients that are affected by a neurological disease. Moreover, home-based VR might offer a promising addition or alternative to existing rehabilitation programs, and a chance to provide and/or prolong the required therapy after discharge in a more accessible setting, potentially improving clinical outcomes.

Future research needs to improve the study design by including larger samples, longitudinal designs, long term follow-ups, and different outcome measures, including functional and quality of life indexes, to better evaluate the clinical impact of this promising technology in healthy old subjects and in neurological patients. In particular, the next challenge for the research on VR and rehabilitation can be summarized in the following questions:

1. Does an innovative intervention enriched with VR provide a significant improvement in mobility, compared to traditional physiotherapy?
2. Is the intervention cost-effective for the health management systems?

To answer to these questions, it is crucial to understand how to improve the rehabilitation path of older people, through multidisciplinary multicomponent and person-centered intervention, integrated with VR.

The evidence reported in the paper are in line with the aims that were expressed by the National Plan for Health Research, whose priorities are defined in accordance with the indications contained in the regulation of the European Parliament and of the Council on the establishment of the "Health for growth" program, which pursues as a goal the achievement of a strong potential for economic growth thanks to the improvement of the state of health, through the facilitation of innovation in health care, the improvement of skills and information on specific diseases, and the identification of good practices for effective prevention [40]. In line with what has been expressed, the role of health technology assessment is of crucial importance. In this perspective, the available services must necessarily be enriched with adequate equipment of proven efficacy, as the promising sector of VR, to be able to advance at both the methodological and assistance level.

5. Conclusions

As it is shown by the numerous studies in the field, the application of VR has a positive impact on the rehabilitation of the most predominant geriatric syndromes. The level of realism of the virtual stimuli seems to have a crucial role in the training of the cognitive abilities. Nevertheless, semi-immersive or non-immersive VR systems have the advantage of being more accepted by the users, as they experienced less cybersickness after the training. Moreover, the integration of these devices in the health management systems are still lacking despite the evidence and the peculiarity of VR technologies with different level of immersivity. A tentative explanation can be found, not only in the cost of technology that seems to be more affordable in the recent years, but, most of all, in the absence of a standardized protocol and procedure, to harmonize traditional rehabilitation therapies and innovative VR systems. For this reason, it will be necessary to improve the research in the field, adopting RCTs study design as well as indicators of health technology assessment, to understand the effectiveness and efficacy also in terms of optimization of the clinical pathways. In addition, as VR systems can be easily adopted at home, it can be considered to be useful for the continuity of care.

Author Contributions: Study concept and design: E.M., R.B.; Acquisition of data (Literature search and Study Selection): E.M., R.B.; Analysis and interpretation of data (literature): E.M., R.B.; Drafting of the manuscript: E.M., R.B., V.D.D., G.R.R., G.P.; Critical revision of the manuscript for important intellectual content: F.L., L.R., P.P.

Conflicts of Interest: The authors declare no conflict of interest.

Abbreviations

VR	Virtual Reality
AD	Alzheimer disease
PD	Parkinson disease
MS	Multiple sclerosis
RCTs	Randomized Controlled Trials
EGs	experimental groups
CGs	control groups
BBS	Berg Balance Scale
IADL	Instrumental activities of daily living
MCI	Mild cognitive impairment

References

1. Torner, J.; Skouras, S.; Molinuevo, J.L.; Gispert, J.D.; Alpiste, F.; Molinuevo, J.L. Multipurpose Virtual Reality Environment for Biomedical and Health Applications. *IEEE Trans. Neural Syst. Rehabil. Eng.* **2019**, *27*, 1511–1520. [CrossRef] [PubMed]
2. Sveistrup, H. Motor rehabilitation using virtual reality. *J. Neuroeng. Rehabil.* **2004**, *1*, 1–10. [CrossRef] [PubMed]
3. Henderson, A.; Korner-Bitensky, N.; Levin, M. Virtual reality in stroke rehabilitation: A systematic review of its effectiveness for upper limb motor recovery. *Top. Stroke Rehabil.* **2007**, *14*, 52–61. [CrossRef] [PubMed]
4. Piron, L.; Turolla, A.; Agostini, M.; Zucconi, C.S.; Ventura, L.; Tonin, P.; Dam, M. Motor Learning Principles for Rehabilitation: A Pilot Randomized Controlled Study in Poststroke Patients. *Neurorehabil. Neural Repair* **2010**, *6*, 501–508. [CrossRef] [PubMed]
5. Perrochon, A.; Borel, B.; Istrate, D.; Compagnat, M.; Daviet, J.C. Exercise-based games interventions at home in individuals with a neurological disease: A systematic review and meta-analysis. *Ann. Phys. Rehabil. Med.* **2019**, *62*, 366–378. [CrossRef] [PubMed]
6. Mohammadi, R.; Semnani, A.V.; Mirmohammadkhani, M.; Grampurohit, N. Effects of Virtual Reality Compared to Conventional Therapy on Balance Poststroke: A Systematic Review and Meta-Analysis. *J. Stroke Cerebrovasc. Dis.* **2019**, *28*, 1787–1798. [CrossRef] [PubMed]
7. Maggio, M.G.; De Cola, M.C.; Latella, D.; Maresca, G.; Finocchiaro, C.; La Rosa, G.; Cimino, V.; Sorbera, C.; Bramanti, P.; De Luca, R.; et al. What about the Role of Virtual Reality in Parkinson Disease's Cognitive Rehabilitation? Preliminary Findings from a Randomized Clinical Trial. *J. Geriatr. Psychiatry Neurol.* **2018**, *31*, 312–318. [CrossRef]
8. Alashram, A.R.; Annino, G.; Padua, E.; Romagnoli, C.; Mercuri, N.B. Cognitive rehabilitation post traumatic brain injury: A systematic review for emerging use of virtual reality technology. *J. Clin. Neurosci.* **2019**, *66*, 209–219. [CrossRef]
9. Maggio, M.G.; Russo, M.; Cuzzola, M.F.; Destro, M.; La Rosa, G.; Molonia, F.; Bramanti, P.; Lombardo, G.; De Luca, R.; Calabrò, R.S. Virtual reality in multiple sclerosis rehabilitation: A review on cognitive and motor outcomes. *J. Clin. Neurosci.* **2019**, *65*, 106–111. [CrossRef]
10. Freeman, D.; Reeve, S.; Robinson, A.; Ehlers, A.; Clark, D.; Spanlang, B.; Slater, M. Virtual reality in the assessment, understanding, and treatment of mental health disorders. *Psychol. Med.* **2017**, *47*, 2393–2400. [CrossRef]
11. Ahn, S.; Hwang, S. Virtual rehabilitation of upper extremity function and independence for stoke: A meta-analysis. *J. Exerc. Rehabil.* **2019**, *15*, 358–369. [CrossRef] [PubMed]
12. Van Schaik, P.; Blake, J.; Pernet, F.; Spears, I.; Fencott, C. Virtual augmented exercise gaming for older adults. *Cyberpsychol. Behav.* **2008**, *11*, 103–106. [CrossRef] [PubMed]
13. Zelinski, E.M.; Reyes, R. Cognitive benefits of computer games for older adults. *Gerontechnology* **2009**, *8*, 220–235. [CrossRef] [PubMed]
14. Patel, J.; Fluet, G.; Qiu, Q.; Yarossi, M.; Merians, A.; Tunik, E.; Adamovich, S. Intensive virtual reality and robotic based upper limb training compared to usual care, and associated cortical reorganization, in the acute and early sub-acute periods post-stroke: A feasibility study. *J. Neuroeng. Rehabil.* **2019**, *16*, 92. [CrossRef]

15. Lee, S.H.; Jung, H.Y.; Yun, S.J.; Oh, B.M.; Seo, H.G. Upper Extremity Rehabilitation Using Fully Immersive Virtual Reality Games with a Head Mount Display: A Feasibility Study. *PM R.* **2019**. [CrossRef]
16. Dos Santos, L.F.; Christ, O.; Mate, K.; Schmidt, H.; Krüger, J.; Dohle, C. Movement visualisation in virtual reality rehabilitation of the lower limb: A systematic review. *Biomed. Eng. Online* **2016**, *15* (Suppl. 3), 144.
17. Ku, J.; Kim, Y.J.; Cho, S.; Lim, T.; Lee, H.S.; Kang, Y.J. Three-Dimensional Augmented Reality System for Balance and Mobility Rehabilitation in the Elderly: A Randomized Controlled Trial. *Cyberpsychol. Behav. Soc. Netw.* **2019**, *22*, 132–141. [CrossRef]
18. Vogt, S.; Skjæret-Maroni, N.; Neuhaus, D.; Baumeister, J. Virtual reality interventions for balance prevention and rehabilitation after musculoskeletal lower limb impairments in young up to middle-aged adults: A comprehensive review on used technology, balance outcome measures and observed effects. *Int. J. Med. Inform.* **2019**, *126*, 46–58. [CrossRef]
19. Törnbom, K.; Danielsson, A. Experiences of treadmill walking with non-immersive virtual reality after stroke or acquired brain injury—A qualitative study. *PLoS ONE* **2018**, *13*, e0209214. [CrossRef]
20. An, C.M.; Park, Y.H. The effects of semi-immersive virtual reality therapy on standing balance and upright mobility function in individuals with chronic incomplete spinal cord injury: A preliminary study. *J. Spinal. Cord Med.* **2018**, *41*, 223–229. [CrossRef]
21. Darekar, A.; McFadyen, B.J.; Lamontagne, A.; Fung, J. Efficacy of virtual reality-based intervention on balance and mobility disorders post-stroke: A scoping review. *J. Neuroeng. Rehabil.* **2015**, *12*, 46. [CrossRef] [PubMed]
22. García-Betances, R.I.; Arredondo Waldmeyer, M.T.; Fico, G.; Cabrera-Umpiérrez, M.F. A succinct overview of virtual reality technology use in Alzheimer's disease. *Front. Aging Neurosci.* **2015**, *7*, 80. [PubMed]
23. Palacios-Navarro, G.; Albiol-Pérez, S.; García-Magariño García, I. Effects of sensory cueing in virtual motor rehabilitation. A review. *J. Biomed. Inform.* **2016**, *60*, 49–57. [CrossRef]
24. Walker, M.L.; Ringleb, S.I.; Maihafer, G.C.; Walker, R.; Crouch, J.R.; Van Lunen, B.; Morrison, S. Virtual Reality–Enhanced Partial Body Weight–Supported Treadmill Training Poststroke: Feasibility and Effectiveness in 6 Subjects. *Arch. Phys. Med. Rehabil.* **2010**, *91*, 115–122. [CrossRef] [PubMed]
25. Turolla, A.; Dam, M.; Ventura, L.; Tonin, P.; Agostini, M.; Zucconi, C.; Kiper, P.; Cagnin, A.; Piron, L. Virtual reality for the rehabilitation of the upper limb motor function after stroke: A prospective controlled trial. *J. Neuroeng. Rehabil.* **2013**, *10*, 85. [CrossRef]
26. Allain, P.; Foloppe, D.A.; Besnard, J.; Yamaguchi, T.; Etcharry-Bouyx, F.; Le Gall, D.; Nolin, P.; Richard, P. Detecting everyday action deficits in Alzheimer's disease using a nonimmersive virtual reality kitchen. *J. Int. Neuropsychol. Soc.* **2014**, *20*, 468–477. [CrossRef]
27. Saposnik, G.; Cohen, L.G.; Mamdani, M.; Pooyania, S.; Ploughman, M.; Cheung, D.; Shaw, J.; Hall, J.; Nord, P.; Dukelow, S.; et al. Efficacy and safety of non-immersive virtual reality exercising in stroke rehabilitation (EVREST): A randomised, multicentre, single-blind, controlled trial. *Lancet Neurol.* **2016**, *15*, 1019–1027. [CrossRef]
28. Mirelman, A.; Rochester, L.; Maidan, I.; Del Din, S.; Alcock, L.; Nieuwhof, F.; Rikkert, M.O.; Bloem, B.R.; Pelosin, E.; Avanzino, L.; et al. Addition of a non-immersive virtual reality component to treadmill training to reduce fall risk in older adults (V-TIME): A randomised controlled trial. *Lancet* **2016**, *388*, 1170–1182. [CrossRef]
29. Segura-Ortí, E.; Pérez-Domínguez, B.; Ortega-Pérez de Villar, L.; Meléndez-Oliva, E.; Martínez-Gramage, J.; García-Maset, R.; Gil-Gómez, J.A. Virtual reality exercise intradialysis to improve physical function: A feasibility randomized trial. *Scand. J. Med. Sci. Sports* **2019**, *29*, 89–94. [CrossRef]
30. Trevizan, I.L.; Silva, T.D.; Dawes, H.; Massetti, T.; Crocetta, T.B.; Favero, F.M.; Oliveira, A.S.B.; de Araújo, L.V.; Santos, A.C.C.; de Abreu, L.C.; et al. Efficacy of different interaction devices using non-immersive virtual tasks in individuals with Amyotrophic Lateral Sclerosis: A cross-sectional randomized trial. *BMC Neurol.* **2018**, *18*, 209. [CrossRef]
31. Pelosin, E.; Cerulli, C.; Ogliastro, C.; Lagravinese, G.; Mori, L.; Bonassi, G.; Mirelman, A.; Hausdorff, J.M.; Abbruzzese, G.; Marchese, R.; et al. A multimodal training modulates short-afferent inhibition and improves complex walking in a cohort of faller older adults with an increased prevalence of Parkinson's disease. *J. Gerontol. A Biol. Sci. Med. Sci.* **2019**. [CrossRef] [PubMed]
32. Maher, C.G.; Sherrington, C.; Herbert, R.D.; Moseley, A.M.; Elkins, M. Reliability of the PEDro scale for rating quality of randomized controlled trials. *Phys. Ther.* **2003**, *83*, 713–721. [PubMed]

33. Doniger, G.M.; Beeri, M.S.; Bahar-Fuchs, A.; Gottlieb, A.; Tkachov, A.; Kenan, H.; Livny, A.; Bahat, Y.; Sharon, H.; Ben-Gal, O.; et al. Virtual reality-based cognitive-motor training for middle-aged adults at high Alzheimer's disease risk: A randomized controlled trial. *Alzh. Dement. (N. Y.)* **2018**, *4*, 118–129. [CrossRef] [PubMed]
34. Savović, J.; Weeks, L.; Sterne, J.A.C.; Turner, L.; Altman, D.G.; Moher, D.; Higgins, J.P.T. Evaluation of the Cochrane Collaboration's tool for assessing the risk of bias in randomized trials: Focus groups, online survey, proposed recommendations and their implementation. *Syst. Rev.* **2014**, *3*, 37. [CrossRef] [PubMed]
35. Weerdesteyn, V.; de Niet, M.; van Duijnhoven, H.J.R.; Geurts, A.C.H. Falls in individuals with stroke. *JRRD* **2008**, *45*, 1195–1214. [CrossRef]
36. Botner, E.M.; Miller, W.C.; Eng, J.J. Measurement properties of the Activities-specific Balance Confidence Scale among individuals with stroke. *Disabil. Rehabil.* **2005**, *27*, 156–163. [CrossRef]
37. Coyle, H.; Traynor, V.; Solowij, N. Computerized and virtual reality cognitive training for individuals at high risk of cognitive decline: Systematic review of the literature. *Am. J. Geriatr. Psychiatry* **2015**, *23*, 335–359. [CrossRef]
38. Manera, V.; Chapoulie, E.; Bourgeois, J.; Guerchouche, R.; David, R.; Ondrej, J.; Drettakis, G.; Robert, P. A feasibility study with image-based rendered virtual reality in patients with mild cognitive impairment and dementia. *PLoS ONE* **2016**, *11*, e0151487. [CrossRef]
39. Maggio, M.G.; Maresca, G.; Scarcella, I.; Latella, D.; De Domenico, C.; Destro, M.; De Luca, R.; Calabro, R.S. Virtual reality-based cognitive rehabilitation in progressive supranuclear palsy. *Psychogeriatr. Soc.* **2019**. [CrossRef]
40. Regulation (EU) No 282/2014 of the European Parliament and of the Councilof 11 March 2014 on the Establishment of a Third Programme for the Union's Action in the Field of Health (2014–2020) and Repealing Decision No 1350/2007/EC. Available online: https://eur-lex.europa.eu/legal-content/EN/TXT/PDF/?uri=CELEX:32014R0282&from=EN (accessed on 23 October 2019).

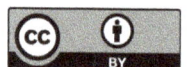

© 2019 by the authors. Licensee MDPI, Basel, Switzerland. This article is an open access article distributed under the terms and conditions of the Creative Commons Attribution (CC BY) license (http://creativecommons.org/licenses/by/4.0/).

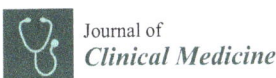

Review

Neurorehabilitation of Spatial Memory Using Virtual Environments: A Systematic Review

Jessica Isbely Montana [1,*], Cosimo Tuena [2], Silvia Serino [3], Pietro Cipresso [2,4] and Giuseppe Riva [2,4]

1. Department of Human Sciences for Education, University of Milano-Bicocca, Piazza dell'Ateneo Nuovo 1, 20126 Milano, Italy
2. ATN-P Lab, Department of Psychology, IRCSS Auxologico Italiano, Via Magnasco 2, 20149 Milano, Italy; cosimotuena@gmail.com (C.T.); p.cipresso@auxologico.it (P.C.); giuseppe.riva@unicatt.it (G.R.)
3. MySpace Lab, Department of Clinical Neurosciences, University Hospital Lausanne-CHUV, CH-1011 Lausanne, Switzerland; silvia.serino@chuv.ch
4. Department of Psychology, Catholic University of the Sacred Heart, Largo Gemelli,1, 20100 Milan, Italy
* Correspondence: jessica.montana@unimib.it; Tel.: +39-345-605-5281

Received: 29 July 2019; Accepted: 19 September 2019; Published: 20 September 2019

Abstract: In recent years, virtual reality (VR) technologies have become widely used in clinical settings because they offer impressive opportunities for neurorehabilitation of different cognitive deficits. Specifically, virtual environments (VEs) have ideal characteristics for navigational training aimed at rehabilitating spatial memory. A systematic search, following PRISMA guidelines, was carried out to explore the current scenario in neurorehabilitation of spatial memory using virtual reality. The literature on this topic was queried, 5048 papers were screened, and 16 studies were included, covering patients presenting different neuropsychological diseases. Our findings highlight the potential of the navigational task in virtual environments (VEs) for enhancing navigation and orientation abilities in patients with spatial memory disorders. The results are promising and suggest that VR training can facilitate neurorehabilitation, promoting brain plasticity processes. An overview of how VR-based training has been implemented is crucial for using these tools in clinical settings. Hence, in the current manuscript, we have critically debated the structure and the length of training protocols, as well as a different type of exploration through VR devices with different degrees of immersion. Furthermore, we analyzed and highlighted the crucial role played by the selection of the assessment tools.

Keywords: navigation; neurorehabilitation; spatial memory; systematic review; virtual environment; virtual reality

1. Introduction

Virtual reality (VR) is a computer application by which humans interact with computer-generated environments in a way that simulates real life and involves various senses [1] and gives the user an experience of being "immersed" in the VR [2,3]. The experience created in VR depends on output tools (visual, aural, and haptic) that immerse the user in the virtual environments (VEs), input tools (trackers, gloves, or mice) that continually track the position and movements of the users, and the human interaction [4,5]. The degree of physical stimulation impacting on the sensory systems and the sensitivity of the system to motor inputs characterize the immersion experience. The product of immersion is *presence*, defined as the psychological sensation of "being there" in the VE instead of the physical and real environment [1,2,6] or as the "feeling of being in a world that exists outside the self" [4,7–10]. The most commonly used forms of sensory stimulation in VR systems are visual displays. A virtual camera controls the viewpoint from which the subject experiences the computer-generated image. The user's perspective changes according to where he is looking; therefore, it is indispensable to track their location by an incorporated, highly sensitive head and body tracking systems. Sensors monitor the subject's position to provide an egocentric reference frame for the simulation. The images can be delivered either by a head-mounted display (HMD) or by a computer monitor or projection screen. HMDs may be more immersive but can induce cybersickness in vulnerable subjects, whose symptoms are a headache, eye strain, nausea, or, in extreme cases, vomiting [11,12]. In this sense, display screens, semi-immersive systems, are generally more comfortable to use. Auditory and haptic stimulations are often combined with a visual display and are increasingly able to provide a strong sense of physical contact with the VE [13]. In less immersive systems, the input is retrieved from standard joystick controllers, mouse, and keyboard. These control devices are easy to use and naturalistic interfaces that simulate real-world interactions are largely used [1]. The use of VR in neurorehabilitation has grown in a meaningful way, and experimental evidence suggests that this technology could have a positive impact on functional recovery in neuropsychological disorders [8,14]. It is a fascinating tool in neurorehabilitation for its peculiarities. First, the possibility of creating tailor-made training that has the value of highlighting how each rehabilitation process must be individualized, addressing the recovery of the patient's specific disorder and adaptation request [1]. The active involvement that this tool can generate in the subjects is due to the possibility of creating new and appealing environments without forgetting the valuable immediate and concrete feedback that comes to the person. The movement accomplished can be reproduced by the avatar within the VR and this is crucial feedback for the patient [15–18]. VR also offers the opportunity for controlled, ecological, and secure testing environments with different degrees of immersion and interaction [1,19]. Thus, an increasing number of cognitive rehabilitation programs have started using VE to simulate daily activities, such as shopping, traveling [20], or exploring a city [21].

The literature shows that virtual reality is an acceptable and promising therapeutic tool for several pathological fields [13], such as mental health disorders in patients with post-traumatic stress disorder, anxiety and depression [22,23], or eating disorders [14,24,25] and in neuropsychological deficits, for instance, in patients with traumatic brain injury (TBI) [26]. Interesting are the results in which VR has been shown to have potential for improving the assessment and treatment of TBI and dementia [27–29], even in cases where the probabilities of recovery appear low [30]. It has been demonstrated as a successful tool in spatial memory and navigational abilities, particularly in Alzheimer's disease (AD) and in mild cognitive impairment (MCI) [13,31,32].

Spatial memory is reflected in a person's navigation and orientation abilities, fundamental requirements for moving in the surrounding environment. The ability to reach landmarks efficiently depends upon the ability to form, retain, and utilize a cognitive representation of the environment [33]. Human navigation involves several cognitive functions and processes. It can be based on self-motion cues and static environmental cues. The tracking of a person's position and orientation is based on self-motion cues, motor efferences, and vestibular and proprioceptive feedback [34]. Environmental cues are based on landmarks and extended boundaries that can provide one's position and orientation relative to the environment. Self-motion and static environmental cues can inform allocentric and egocentric reference frames [35,36]. Allocentric representation is independent of the position of the navigator and does not change with the navigator through space. An egocentric frame, however, involves the representation of locations based on the subject's viewpoint [37]. The self-reference system uses self-motion cues to update body location and face direction relative to an allocentric, orientation-free, immediately available, object-to-object map [38].

Spatial memory problems, such as forgetting the orientation and the position of objects or getting lost, are often a result of hippocampal damage in humans [32,37,39,40]. The consequence of these representations can be dissociated in terms of behavioral and developmental elements, and, finally, of their neural bases. Thus, the hippocampus and medial temporal lobe offer allocentric environmental representations, whereas the parietal lobe egocentric representations and the retrosplenial cortex and parieto-occipital sulcus allow both types of representation to interact with each other [37,39,41,42].

In human navigation, the role of the hippocampus and associated mesial temporal lobe structures has been widely demonstrated [37]. Meanwhile, differential activity in the hippocampus and caudate correspond to the acquisition and expression of information about locations derived from environmental boundaries or landmarks, respectively [43]. Changes in the navigation network may be a result of cognitive decline and can manifest in impaired spatial navigation [35].

In conclusion, the environments recreated using VR technology represent a context through which the user has the opportunity to experience real-life scenarios and increase their abilities and experience new adaptation strategies [13]. In [44], it is suggested that patients are able to transfer information about the environment acquired from VE to real life. They suggest that mental representations of space in VE are rather like those implicated in the navigation of the real world. Concerning the growing interest in VR and high potential applications in neurorehabilitation, it is necessary to examine the treatment procedures and the results obtained so far. According to these premises, we aimed at providing a systematic review of the experiments in the field of spatial memory neurorehabilitation to comprehend if VR navigational training, compared to treatment as usual, is effective in improving navigational abilities. The specific objectives of the present work are two-fold. First, to provide an overview of which apparatus are available for neurorehabilitation and understanding how these VR training regimes have been implemented in clinical settings. We analyzed different types of software and procedures for implementing the training. Finally, in light of the cognitive and neural theories of spatial processing, we attempted to compare different VR navigational training used and analyzed which is more useful.

2. Method

2.1. Search Methodology

Preferred Reporting Items for Systematic Reviews and Meta-Analysis (PRISMA) guidelines were followed [45]. Two high-profile databases (PubMed and Web of Science) were used to perform the computer-based research on the 6 July 2019. According to PICO format, we defined the question (following the identification of problem, intervention, comparison group, and outcome) as "In spatial memory disorder, is VR navigational training, compared to treatment as usual, effective in improving navigation abilities?". We then proceeded with the definition of keywords for the search strategy. The string used to carry out the search strategy was virtual-realit* OR virtual-environment* AND neurorehabilitation OR rehabilitation OR training OR stimulation OR navigation OR learning OR abilit* OR memor* AND spatial OR space.

From the search of both databases, we obtained 5048 articles, excluding duplicates. Title and abstract screening was carried out, and 24 articles passed to the full-text screening phase. Eight studies were excluded with reasons as follow: Not Controlled trial (= 1); Results of neuropsychological outcome for spatial memory not reported (= 3); Qualitative/descriptive study (= 2); Not neuropsychological rehabilitation for spatial memory (= 2).

2.2. Inclusion Criteria

The review considered randomized control trials, nonrandomized control trials, intervention studies, and case-control studies in clinical patient populations with an overt spatial memory disorder. Studies on rehabilitation's programs of navigation abilities with virtual reality (VR) devices in different population of patients (such as mild cognitive impairment (MCI), Alzheimer's disease (AD), traumatic brain injury (TBI), multiple sclerosis (MS), stroke, cerebral palsy, epilepsy, incomplete cervical vertebro-spinal trauma, topographical disorientation disorders and neglect) were included. We only included studies in the English language and which satisfied strict criteria for eligibility for the review (research studies, clinical patient population, VR training, spatial memory disorders, rehabilitation programs). The qualitative component also considered the type of VR navigational training and methodological design. We excluded articles which lacked necessary information for review in the full-text or the abstract. Reviews, meeting abstracts, proceedings, notes, case reports, letters to the editor, assessment protocols, editorials, and other editorial materials were also excluded. Retrospective studies were not included because the area of interest requires performing experiments.

2.3. Risk of Bias Assessment

To assess the risk of bias, the reviewers followed the methods recommended by The Cochrane Collaboration Risk of Bias Tool [46] and the STROBE Statement [47]. Two reviewers (J.M. and C.T.) independently assessed the risk of bias of each included study against key criteria: random sequence generation, allocation concealment, blinding of participants, personnel, and outcomes, incomplete outcome data, selective outcome reporting, and other sources of bias. The following judgments were used: low risk, high risk, or unclear (either lack of information or uncertainty over the potential for bias). Disagreements were resolved through consensus, and a third author was consulted to resolve disagreements if necessary. In particular, the selected studies followed strict criteria in the methods, including presenting critical elements of study design, clearly defining all outcomes, describing the setting and relevant dates, including periods of recruitment and exposure, giving sources of data and details of methods of assessment (measurement).

2.4. PRISMA Flow Diagram

PRISMA guidelines were strictly followed; all titles and abstracts were screened according to the abovementioned inclusion criteria after removing the duplicates. Full texts of eligible articles were retrieved and assessed by two reviewers (J.M. and C.T.) for individual selection of papers to reduce the risk of bias and resolving disagreements through consensus as explained in Section 2.1. See Figure 1 for the paper selection procedure.

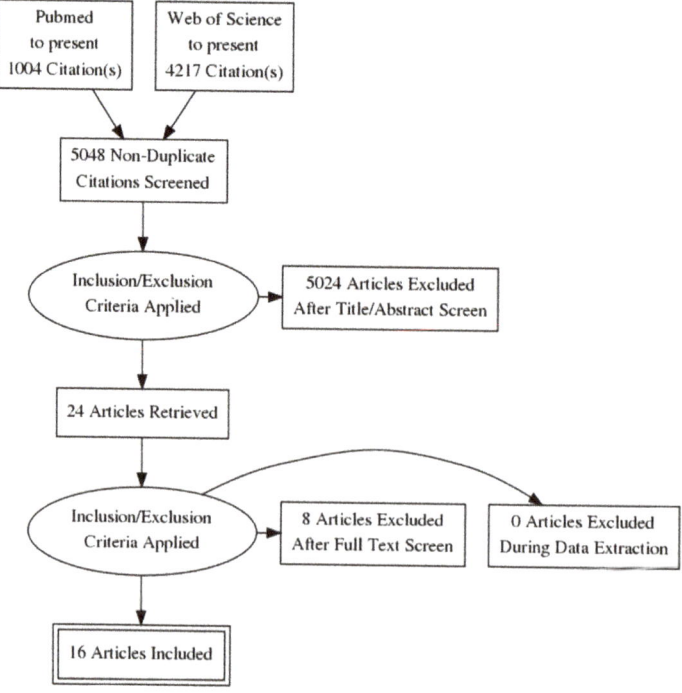

Figure 1. PRISMA flow diagram.

3. Results

Sixteen studies were analyzed to test the usefulness of rehabilitative interventions using virtual reality (VR) systems. However, growing interest in VR has led researchers to question how the characteristics of VR equipment and different aspects of the training tasks could influence the treatment outcomes, with particular regard to the results that reflect on the patient's daily life in an ecological way. In our review, we aim at giving more awareness to the researchers and at guiding them in the selection of the most appropriate VR device to use. Considering the studies mentioned in this analysis, it could be possible to understand which is the most suitable program for the treatment of spatial memory disorders, in terms of the type of apparatus used and the training method. Furthermore, it is essential to understand which kind of patient will benefit from the intervention. To satisfy our aims and to facilitate the understanding, we considered the following clusters: (1) Authors; (2) Year; (3) Sample (N); (4) Sample characteristics; (5) Mean age; (6) VR Task; (7) Virtual Apparatus; (8) Neuropsychological assessment; (9) Primary Outcomes. Results are reported in Table 1.

Table 1. Papers included in the PRISMA systematic review. MMSE—Mini-Mental State Assessment; MoCA—Montreal Cognitive Assessment; ACE—Addenbrooke's Cognitive Examination; ADAS—Alzheimer's Disease Assessment Scale; WAIS-III—Weschler Adult Intelligent Scale; RAVLT—Rey Auditory verbal Learning Test; RBMT—Rivermead Behavioural Memory Test; CBTT—Corsi Block-Tapping Test; DART—Dutch Version of Reading Test; BIT—Behavioural Inattention Test; FIM—Functional Independence Measure; FAB—Frontal Assessment Battery; AM—attentive Matrices; TMT A- B- A/B—Trial Making Test; BIT—Behavioural Inattention Test; WMS IV—Wechsler memory scale; WTAR—Wechsler Scale of adult Reading; VOSP—Visual Object and Space Perception Battery; CFMT—Cambridge Face Memory Test; CFPT—Cambridge Face Perception Test; BRLD—Bergen Left-Right Discrimination Test; ROCF—Rey-Osterrieth Complex Figure Test; RWT—Regensburg Verbal Fluency Test; VLMT—German adaptation of the Rey Verbal Learning Test; LPS 50+—The Achievement Measure System 50+; LVT—Visual Pursuit Test.

	Authors	Year	Sample (N)	Sample Characteristics	Mean Age (SD or Range)	VR Task	VR Apparatus	Pre- and Post- Assessment	Primary Outcomes
1	Pugnetti et al. [48]	1998	30	Experimental Group (EG) 15 MS patients. Control Group (CG) 15 healthy controls.	EG active condition mean age = 39.1; Standard Deviation (SD) =11.1/passive condition mean age = 37.7; SD = 8.1. CG active condition mean age = 35.8; SD = 9.4/passive condition mean age = 35.4; SD = 12.2	The aim was to explore the VE of a house, composed of four rooms and corridors, in search of an object.	Nonimmersive Virtual Reality (Superscape Software, version 4).	ROF, CBTI, Raven's matrices IQ.	Spatial memory improved in the active subject (MS and healthy) suggesting that direct interaction with the environment can enhance navigation ability.
2	Akhutina et al. [49]	2003	EXP 1. 21 EXP 2. 45	EXP 1. EG/CG 21 patients with a diagnosis of cerebral palsy. EXP 2. EG/CG 45 patients with a diagnosis of cerebral palsy.	EXP 1. EG 12 (range 7–14) CG 9 (range 7–14) EXP 2. EG 23 (range 7–14) CG 22 (range 7–14)	The aim in each version of the task (drawn, real or virtual) was to move through a maze to reach a tree.	Non immersive environments IBM-PC and a mouse (Super Scape VRT 3-D Software) displayed on a 40.630 cm monitor.	EXP1. computer versions of the Koos Block Design Test, and a Clown Assembly Test. Decentration of Viewpoint Test, and Directional Pointing to a Hidden Object Test. EXP 2. Additional measures: Raven Progressive Matrices; The Benton Judgment of Line Orientation Test; The arrows subtest of the Nepsy; The Roads Test.	The studies have demonstrated that the general spatial abilities of a group of children with motor disabilities can be enhanced using a battery of training tasks that demand the use of various spatial skills. The battery included VEs that provided the children with navigational spatial experience, of a kind that most would rarely (if ever) experience in the course of their daily lives.

Table 1. Cont.

	Authors	Year	Sample (N)	Sample Characteristics	Mean Age (SD or Range)	VR Task	VR Apparatus	Pre- and Post- Assessment	Primary Outcomes
3	Caglio et al. [6]	2012	1	TBI patient with hemorrhagic contusions in the bilateral frontal, temporal and parietal lobes.	24 (male)	The aim was to explore part of a virtual town (London) from a ground-level perspective.	Nonimmersive Virtual Reality (Midtown Madness 2 videogame).	Corsi Block-Tapping Test, Corsi Supra-Span Test, Backward digit span, RAVLT, TMT A-B, Phonemic fluency, ADAS, RBMT.	Improvement in immediate verbal learning, immediate and delayed spatial learning and everyday-spatial memory persisted at follow-ups.
4	Grewe et al. [20]	2013	24	EG 5 patients with focal epilepsy (2 right temporo-parietal; 1 right hippocampal; 1 bilateral temporal; 1 bilateral occipital periventricular). CG 19 healthy participants	EG mean age = 35.04, SD = 8.08; CG mean age = 23; SD = 3.45	The aim was to navigate into a virtual medium-sized supermarket, modeled according to a real standard supermarket, in search of a specific list of objects.	OctaVis, semi-immersive Virtual Reality device.	ROF	The supermarket training provided preliminary evidence of effectiveness, but significant improvement was not found. A strong limitation was due to the small sample size.

Table 1. Cont.

	Authors	Year	Sample (N)	Sample Characteristics	Mean Age (SD or Range)	VR Task	VR Apparatus	Pre- and Post- Assessment	Primary Outcomes
5	Kober et al. [51]	2013	23	EG 23 patients: 3 right and 1 arteria cerebri media stroke, 1 basal ganglia and thalamus stroke, 1 right arteria cerebri media, 1 basal ganglia stroke, 1 right fronto-parietal stroke, 2 right aneurysm and subsequent infarct (arteria cerebri posterior and arteria communicans with parietal infarct), 1 arteria cerebri media hemorrhage, 1 TBI (left hippocampus and pons). CG 11 healthy participants	EG mean age = 66.09; SD = 3.30 CG mean age = 66.18; SD = 2.97	The aim was a route-finding in a district of the real-world town of Graz, Austria.	Nonimmersive Virtual Reality.	Four spatial tests before and after the five VR training sessions: the Benton Test, the LPS 50+, the LVT, and the CBTI.	Route finding ability in the VR task increased over the five training sessions. Moreover, both groups improved different aspects of spatial abilities after VR training in comparison to the spatial performance before VR training.

Table 1. *Cont*.

	Authors	Year	Sample (N)	Sample Characteristics	Mean Age (SD or Range)	VR Task	VR Apparatus	Pre- and Post- Assessment	Primary Outcomes
6	Grewe et al. [52]	2014	33	EG 14 patients with focal epilepsy (frontal = 3, temporal = 8, central = 2, parietal = 1). CG 19 healthy participants	EG mean age = 31.29; SD = 9.44; 8 males. CG mean age = 31.21; SD = 14.26; 4 males	The aim was to navigate into a virtual medium-sized supermarket, modeled according to a real standard supermarket, in search of a specific list of objects.	OctaVis, semi-immersive Virtual Reality device.	BRLD-A, BRLD-B; ROCF copy, ROCF immediate and delayed recall; RWT Total Score; Digit Span Forward and Backward; VLMT immediate recallB, VLMT total learningB Trials, VLMT loss after InterferenceB, VLMT loss after delayB.	Spatial navigation and memory performance (n° of correct products, movements trajectories, time) significantly increased in the course of the 8-day training. Due to the small sample sizes in the subgroups, it could not be established the effects of different sites of epileptic foci.
7	Claessen et al. [53]	2015	6	6 stroke patients with left (N = 3), right (N = 2) and bilateral (N = 1) supratentorial stroke. No control group.	mean age = 57; SD = 8.9; 2 males	The aim was a route-finding in the Virtual Tübingen town.	Nonimmersive Virtual Reality with a joystick (Virtual Tübingen).	CBTt, TMT A-B, WAIS-III, DART, Virtual Tübingen Test (Scene recognition, Route continuation/sequence/ order/progression/ distance, Pointing to start/to end, Map drawing/recognition).	Navigation abilities clearly improved in one patient, partially in four cases. For other cases, were successful in adopting an alternative navigation strategy and improved on most of the trained abilities. VR was judged as highly feasible by the patients.
8	Faria et al. [54]	2016	18	EG 9 stroke patients. CG 9 stroke patients	EG mean age = 58 – 71; male = 44%. CG mean age = 53; male = 44%	The aim was to navigate in order to accomplish some common ADL´s (in a supermarket, a post office, a bank, and a pharmacy) in a virtual city with streets, sidewalks, commercial buildings, parks and moving cars.	Nonimmersive Virtual Reality with a joystick (Reh@City).	ACE, TMT A-B, Picture Arrangement Test, SIS 3.0.	VR group improved in attention, visuospatial abilities, memory, executive functions, emotion, global cognition, and overall recovery. Between comparisons showed training effect on global cognition, executive functions and attention for VR group.

Table 1. Cont.

	Authors	Year	Sample (N)	Sample Characteristics	Mean Age (SD or Range)	VR Task	VR Apparatus	Pre- and Post- Assessment	Primary Outcomes
9	White & Moussavi [55]	2016	1	MCI patient with probable development of AD	74 (male)	The aim was to navigate into a virtual building in search of specific targets.	Immersive Virtual Reality system with Head-mounted Display and joypad.	MoCA, VRN task (Byagowi & Moussavi, 2012), navigation diary.	The patient improved navigation during the sessions assessed with the VRN task and as reported with the wife's diary.
10	Bate et al. [56]	2017	1	Patient with developmental prosopagnosia with concurrent topographical disorientation	58 (female)	The aim was to navigate in a virtual city, (containing six landmarks such as cinema, restaurant, pub, hotel, pharmacy, and florist) and recall the position of each landmark on a top-view map of the city.	Nonimmersive Virtual Reality with the keypad.	WAIS-III, WMS-IV, Wisconsin Card Sorting Test, CBTT, Rey's complex figures, Picture Naming, WTAR, VOSP. Face processing tasks: CFMT, famous faces, CFPT, Ekman 60, navigational assessment: Benton, Santa Barbara Sense of direction Scale, Memory of building, 'O clock task, route map.	Following the last session of treatment, the patient was able to form a cognitive map faster than the first one and the performance in the retrieval task was improved. A similar performance was observed at the one-week follow-up session.

Table 1. *Cont.*

	Authors	Year	Sample (N)	Sample Characteristics	Mean Age (SD or Range)	VR Task	VR Apparatus	Pre- and Post- Assessment	Primary Outcomes
11	De La Torre-Luque et al. [57]	2017	20	20 patients with a neurological diagnosis included cerebral palsy (20%), intellectual development disorder (20%) and both disorders (55%); TBI (5%).	mean age= 34.35, SD= 10.2; 13 males and 7 females.	The aim was to move through the virtual environment, and then through the equivalent real-life one and to find the same two rooms for both environments.	Semi-immersive Virtual Reality with a joystick and a mouse. A Mitsubishi® projector (model XL8U), projecting onto a × 1.5-m screen.	For the assessment of cognitive visuospatial planning and orientation, 2 tests: Porteus Maze Test; Mindscape's Brain Trainer® 2 Maze Stair Test.	Both groups improved in a similar way, though we can say that the best results in the virtual and the real building and generalization goals were due to virtual training. Firstly, a reduction in errors and time needed to locate the objectives in the virtual building was found after the training, so as to point out that the active navigational training showed changes. In addition, the participants had better scores in the posttest and generalization tasks in the real environment and when using maps of the building, and these tasks were not directly trained.
12	De Luca et al. [58]	2017	1	Neglect patient (subarachnoid hemorrhage, right fronto-temporal-parietal region).	57	The aim was to move in the virtual environment and manipulate specific objects, in order to realize specific associations.	Semi-immersive VR (BTs Nirvana PC System connected to a projector or a big screen).	MMSE; BIT; line crossing and bisection, letter and star cancellation, map navigation, card, and coin sorting, drawing and copying tests, phone dialing, menu and article reading, telling and setting the time.	The training enhanced spatial cognition, visual search, and attention. In addition, with standard cognitive treatment was observed a nearly complete recovery of Unilateral Spatial Neglect.

Table 1. Cont.

	Authors	Year	Sample (N)	Sample Characteristics	Mean Age (SD or Range)	VR Task	VR Apparatus	Pre- and Post- Assessment	Primary Outcomes
13	Serino et al. [21]	2017	28	EG 10 patients with AD. 8 healthy participants. CG 10 patients with AD	EG patients mean age = 86.60; SD = 6.13; 1male. healthy mean age = 86.62; SD = 6.19; 4 males. CG patients mean age = 88.7; SD = 3.59; 2 males	The aim was to navigate inside the virtual environment, to discover one, two or three hidden objects (i.e., a bottle of milk, a plant in a vase and a trunk) to retrieve their positions in the last phase.	Nonimmersive VR (NeuroVR software).	MMSE, Phonemic fluency, Categorical fluency, FAB, Attentional Matrices Test, Digit span test, Corsi Block-Tapping Test, Corsi Supra-Span Test.	The training enhanced spatial learning in the VR group-AD compared to control group-AD and VR healthy group improved executive functions compared to VR group-AD.
14	De Luca et al. [59]	2018	12	EG 6 post-stroke patients. CG 6 post-stroke patients	EG/CG mean age = 40; SD = 14	The aim was to move in the virtual environment and manipulate specific objects, in order to realize specific associations.	Semi-immersive VR (BTs Nirvana PC System connected to a projector or a big screen).	MoCA, FIM, FAB, AM, TMT A, TMT B, TMT A/B.	VR can be useful in potentiating the cognitive recovery in post-stroke chronic phase. It improved visuospatial and attention in the experimental group.

Table 1. *Cont.*

	Authors	Year	Sample (N)	Sample Characteristics	Mean Age (SD or Range)	VR Task	VR Apparatus	Pre- and Post- Assessment	Primary Outcomes
15	Maresca et al. [6]	2018	1	A right-handed patient affected by incomplete cervical vertebro-spinal trauma, presented with a moderate tetraparesis, mainly involving the left side.	60 (male)	The aim was to move in the virtual environment and manipulate specific objects, and to realize specific associations.	A nonimmersive virtual reality rehabilitation system (VRRS) by Khymeia, interacting with a touch screen or a magnetic tracking sensor.	MoCA, AM, TMT, digit span, RAVLI, RAVLR, Wigl's sorting test, Raven's colored matrices, VFI, SFI, HRS-D, HRS-A.	The combined approach using VRRS demonstrated a significant improvement in different cognitive domains as spatial abilities, executive functions, selective attention, and memory abilities.
16	Mrakic-Sposta et al. [61]	2018	10	EG 5 MCI patients with compromise visuospatial abilities. CG 5 MCI patients with compromise visuospatial abilities	EG/CG aged > 65 years; 4 males and 6 females	The aim was to navigate and to orientate inside three virtual environments (ride a bike in a park, crossroads in a city and shopping in a supermarket).	Semi-immersive scenarios with a finger touch projector and a PlayStation controller and cycle-ergometer, a Wearable smart garment (heart rate)	MMSE; RAVLT-I and RAVLT-D; ROCFI; AM; TMT-A and TMT-B; FAB; VFI.	The presented results suggest that the adopted training protocol was able to affect MMSE tasks and to increase the global cognition levels of MCI patients.

Analysis of results in spatial navigation rehabilitation programs was carried out starting from the outcomes of 16 studies, taking into consideration the patient population, the VR apparatus (immersive/semi- or nonimmersive) and the type of training used. We analyzed clinical, methodological, and technical outcomes to cast research and clinical applications of VR in the context of VR navigational training. The results were argued in response to the following three questions.

3.1. Which Virtual Apparatus Is Recommended for Spatial Memory Rehabilitation?

3.1.1. Type of Device and Controllers During Navigation

Among all the studies reviewed, the only one that used an immersive virtual reality (VR) system with a head-mounted display HMD Oculus Rift DK2, using the Unity 5 game engine, and a joypad is described in [39] (see Table 1 for an overview of VR equipment). Several studies [20,52,57–59,61], used semi-immersive systems: the previous one used OctaVis, a circle of eight screens in which the participant can freely rotate on a fixed chair and interact with a joystick; while [58,59] used a BTs Nirvana PC System connected to a projector or a big screen and to an infrared sensor for movements; in [61], a finger touch projector was used and the scenarios were developed using Unity 3D. In order to increase the user's presence in the VE, attention was paid to elements such as the visual flow synchronized with the cycling velocity in real-time, realistic 3D sound, perception of the wind through the movement of trees; [57] used a projector on a big screen (2 × 1.5 m) and a viewing height of 1.8 m. Virtual Scene Designer was used to create the scenarios. The advantage conferred by the semi-immersive system is that it allows sensorial isolation, but it presents fewer signs of cybersickness. Even this system demonstrates the generalizability of VR measures by correlations with subjective estimations of cognitive abilities and real-life shopping performance [52]. Immersive and semi-immersive systems have proved to be useful tools in navigational training for improving spatial cognition and attention processes [55,58].

Nine further studies reviewed used nonimmersive systems. In [50] the rehabilitation training was based on a navigational task, exploring part of a virtual town (London) from a ground-level perspective, using a computer videogame driving simulator (Midtown Madness 2, Microsoft Game Studios). Other studies have used nonimmersive VR training on a computer with joystick or keypad to navigate the city, using Unity 3D software—Reh@city [54,56]—on a standard IBM-PC computer and in an environment developed with the Super Scape VRT-3D construction package [49]; or a specific software developed by authors—Virtual Tübingen [53]. Other studies used Superscape software version 4 and NeuroVR. NeuroVR is a free VR-platform for customizing a large number of predeveloped virtual environments [9,21,48,62]. One study [51] created a simulation of the real-world town of Graz (Austria) using Instantreality software, a high-performance Mixed-Reality framework that provides a comprehensive set of features to support classic virtual reality [63]. Another study [60] used a certified medical device with high customization capacity, the virtual reality rehabilitation system (VRSS), which comprises a central hub connected to specialized peripheral devices, such as magnetic sensors for movements, which is fully synchronized and integrated with the system. Also, the rehabilitation programs that used a nonimmersive system showed promising enhancement of different cognitive abilities through spatial and navigational training [21,48,50–53,58].

3.1.2. VR Spatial Navigation

The usefulness of VR navigational tasks in rehabilitation programs for spatial memory has been highlighted. Promising results have been demonstrated with the use of navigation tasks on simple display screens of a computer (nonimmersive devices). However, better performance can be achieved through immersive rather than semi-immersive systems by using head-mounted displays. This is explained by the greater sense of presence [4,8], with integrated systems that record the user's movement and take advantage of up to six degrees of freedom, and providing feedback to the user about their performance [15]. Since navigation in virtual environments can trigger the same brain mechanisms as navigation in the real world, spatial "presence" can be generated [64].

3.2. Which Virtual Training Method Is Suitable for Spatial Memory Rehabilitation?

The studies included in the current review are all focused on the rehabilitation of spatial memory and navigation abilities in different neurologic patients, including mild cognitive impairment (MCI), Alzheimer's disease (AD), traumatic brain injury (TBI), multiple sclerosis (MS), stroke, cerebral palsy, epilepsy, incomplete cervical vertebro-spinal trauma, prosopagnosia with topographical disorientation disorders, and neglect. all patients have used virtual reality (VR) devices in different rehabilitation programs, and nobody had any difficulty in following the training. Overall, the emerging outcomes are positive, and they present improvements to different degrees. All of the mentioned studies had a control group [20,21,48,49,51,52,54,57,59,61] except one [53]. Five of them reported results of single case studies [50,55,56,58,60]. Virtual rehabilitation enables clinicians to control the specific features of the virtual environment, enabling tailoring of the challenge to suit individual patient needs [65]. The characteristics of virtual training (detailed in the following paragraphs) that are crucially important are the overall duration of the training, the frequency, the intensity of each session, and, last but not least, the time elapsed since the damage [57]. Additionally, some studies have already demonstrated that the use of a map as a navigational aid improved the performance of users performing complex navigational tasks [66]. Furthermore, the presence of a small-scale interactive aerial view facilitated the retrieval of stored spatial layout and an arrow or salient landmarks, giving more comprehensive information about the egocentric heading in environment, were effective in supporting the navigation [67,68]. Also, findings in the studies examined underline the importance of using active navigation protocols to promote the neurorehabilitation of spatial memory [62,67], and that the degree of the visual similarities between the virtual world and the real one boosts the transfer of learning between contexts [57].

3.2.1. VR Training Duration

The protocol duration turned out to be an important variable for rehabilitation training outcomes (details are visible in Table 2). The training proposed by [50,60] was the most intensive. The first regime consisted of 15 sessions of 90 min each, amounting to 22.5 h. The second regime consisted of three weekly sessions of 60 min for a total of 36 treatments. The improvements are visible after a certain period of time, as evidenced by two-month and one-year follow-ups [50]. One study [55] proposed 21 sessions of 45 min each, amounting to 15.75 h, and [61] proposed 18 sessions lasting 40–45 min each for a total of 13.5 h. In these studies, the patients showed substantial improvement in navigation ability. Another study [59] conducted 20 sessions for stroke patients in which an intensive and long training program was essential for obtaining substantial improvements. Other rehabilitation programs, which lasted between eight to 15 sessions, showed an improvement in long-term spatial memory after VR-based training [21,52,57]. Transference of improvements from the VR-based training to more general aspects of spatial cognition was observed [21]. Interesting results are also connected with high frequency and intensity of sessions [21,50,52,55,58,59] rather than low-intensity training regimes [49]. A protocol lasting less than four hours returns vulnerable outcomes [20,51,53,54,56,62]. For example, one study [53] based on four sessions of 1 h each was only able to significantly improve one patient's performance.

Table 2. Training characteristics.

	Authors	Type of Training	Single Session Duration (min)	Repetitions	Frequency/Period	Total Hours
1	Pugnetti et al. (1998)	Navigational training with active and passive conditions + recall landmarks	30	1		30 min
2	Akhutina et al. (2003)	Navigational task	30–60	6–8	within a month	3–8 h
3	Caglio et al. (2012)	Navigational training	90	15	3 times a week for 5 weeks	22.5 h
4	Grewe et al. (2013)	Navigational training + free recall of objects list and positions (at last session)	20	8	daily	2.6 h
5	Kober et al. (2013)	Navigational training + recall up to maximal three different routes	20	6	-	2 h
6	Grewe et al.	Navigational training + free recall of objects list and positions (at last session) + real-life performance	30	8	Every 1–3 days within 2 weeks	4 h
7	Claessen et al. (2015)	Navigational training	60	4	-	4 h
8	Faria et al. (2016)	Navigational training	20	12	4–6 weeks	4 h
9	White & Moussavi (2016)	Navigational training	45	21	3 times a week for 7 weeks	15.75 h
10	Bate et al. (2017)	Navigational training + recall landmarks	60–70	7	Every 3–4 days	7–8 h
11	De La Torre Luque et al. (2017)	Navigational training	20	15	daily	5 h
12	De Luca et al. (2017)	Navigational training + association of object position	45	20	5 times a week for 1 month	15 h
13	Serino et al. (2017)	Navigational training + recall object positions	30	10	3 times a week for 3–4 weeks	5 h
14	De Luca et al. (2018)	Navigational training + association of object position	45	24	3 times a week for 8 weeks	18 h
15	Maresca et al. (2018)	Navigational training	60	36	3 times a week for 12 weeks	36 h
16	Mrakic et al (2018)	Navigational training	45	18	3 times a week for 6 weeks	13.5 h

3.2.2. Time Elapsed Since Damage

Another important variable is the time elapsed from the brain injury to the starting point of cognitive rehabilitation. One study [54] found an overall recovery and showed a positive training effect on global cognitive functions in post-stroke patients which started the treatment within 7 months from the stroke. A long-distance from the traumatic event, instead, does not promise good results, as happened in patients who started an average of 43 months after stroke [53]. A short interval was also important in other disorders. One study [50] have gained promising results with a single traumatic brain injury (TBI) patient that began the training within 1 year. The shorter the period between the traumatic event and the beginning of treatment, the higher the probability of achieving a better outcome [50,52,54].

3.2.3. Training Procedure

A detailed description of the different procedures is outlined below. In one study [50], the patient was given the instruction "You must cut down poles and trees that you find all along the way", with the aim of inducing the participant to explore the virtual town, avoiding passing the same roads twice. The spatial memory task was implicit, while the explicit task was a simple game, which entertained the participant. The participant did not have access to a city map during the task.

One study [53] used training divided into implicit (free exploration) and explicit tasks (following specific routes). During the sessions, the patients were encouraged to practice the instructed navigational strategy learned in a previous psycho-educational phase. The participants had access to a city map during the task. Two studies [54,56] used implicit tasks. In the first study, the participant was guided by instructions such as "Go to the supermarket". Visual feedback elements (time and point counters) were used to reward successful actions. The participant had access to a mini-map in the lower half of the screen and/or a guidance arrow. In the second study, the participant was asked to follow three routes, differing in length, as quickly and as accurately as possible. In the next learning phase, the patient was required to create a mental representation of the city, incorporating the spatial location of six landmarks. In the retrieval phase, he was required to navigate via the city in order to reach a location as quickly as possible and using the shortest route possible.

In [55], the participant was instructed to enter a building and find the correct window, which had been previously shown from an external view of the building. Two studies [21,51] used specific tasks with encoding and retrieval phases. In the first study, the neuropsychologist asked participants to find and memorize the position of hidden objects within the virtual city. Then, they were asked to retrieve the position of the objects identified before, starting from another point of the city. Participants had access to a city map during the task. In the second study, the participant had to learn a route by following verbal instructions and subsequently had to recall the correct directions. In two studies [48,57], the participants received explicit instructions to explore and memorize a route in the virtual environment (VE) during the research of an object. Subsequently, in the first study, they were asked to draw the layout of the VE, and in the second study they had to move through the equivalent real-life environment. Also, in [49], the participants were asked to move through a maze to reach a tree. In the first and second versions, the plan of the maze was visible, and the target always remained visible. In the third version, the target tree could be seen only from a short distance when not hidden by the maze walls. In [20,52], the participants had to memorize an auditory shopping list of 20 items as an implicit spatial memory task and subsequently buy all the items remembered in a VR supermarket. In the second study, the same authors presented a new interfering list with 20 distractor items during the training.

Three studies [58–60] included a series of exercises involving different cognitive functions. The participants were asked to remember the positions and the name of elements observed or to program movements to manipulate specific objects and to realize specific associations with dynamic interaction in VE. In [61], three scenarios were used, in which patients had to navigate freely to accomplish the task explicitly requested, for example, purchasing five items form a supermarket. The spatial memory task was explicit, and only in the last version was no aid was given for completing the task. In conclusion, independently from the simulation, the outcomes showed that VR training enhanced spatial memory abilities in the clinical population.

3.2.4. Visual Cues

In terms of guide elements which facilitate the patient during the training, different cues have been included in some of the tasks, such as maps [21,53,54], guidance arrows [54], and lists of objects. In particular, [54] employed a method of fading cues, decreasing assistance (DA), in which the training continues with all the cues until correct performance is achieved on three consecutive sessions and then they are gradually removed. Furthermore, in [21], the number of objects to be memorized depended on the level reached by each participant; if the patient was not able to locate the first object, the other ones were not presented. The task presented to the participant was guided in some cases by explicit navigational instructions [21,53,56] that needed to be followed to memorize the route.

3.3. Which Assessment Method Is Best for Spatial Memory?

3.3.1. Spatial Memory Outcomes

In clinical practice, the most common neuropsychological test for the evaluation of short and long-term spatial memory, given its psychometric characteristics, is the Supraspan Corsi Test. In these studies, the Supraspan Corsi Test has proved to be adequately sensitive and has indicated a significant improvement in spatial memory [50], with a medium effect size $r = 0.474$ and $p = 0.03$ [21]. Another ecological spatial memory assessment tests, Route delayed recall (RBMT), has generated desirable changes (0/5 to 4/5) that persisted at 2-month and 1-year follow-ups (respectively 4/5 and 5/5) [50]. One study [53] has shown that the virtual reality (VR) system is a sensitive assessment tool for the same cognitive function (Virtual Tübingen Test). They found that one patient improved in nine out of the 10 virtual navigation subtasks. To assess spatial navigation and memory performance in the VR supermarket, [52] analyzed the enhancements in "number of correctly bought products", "number of the correct products relative to distance", and "number of the correct products relative to time". Other authors asked the participant to form a cognitive map of the VE, and active participants showed significantly better performance [48] and were quicker [56] than the control group. A similar performance pattern was observed at the one-week follow-up session. VR neurorehabilitation programs for spatial memory can also provide a positive effect on other cognitive domains. By using specific-domain assessments, it is possible to observe if a transference of improvements occurs from VR-based training to more general aspects of spatial cognition. Following the treatment, however, general enhancement of cognitive functions occurs and is reflected in several assessment tests. The Rey Auditory Verbal Learning Test (RAVLT) has shown significant improvement in the immediate recall that persists at 1-year follow-up [50]. A considerable improvement can be observed in screening tests, such as in Addenbrooke's Cognitive Examination (ACE) ($r = 0.85$, $p = 0.011$), particularly in visuospatial ($r = 0.80$, $p = 0.017$), attention ($r = 0.79$, $p = 0.018$), and memory ($r = 0.79$, $p = 0.017$) domains and in the Mini-Mental State Examination (MMSE) ($r = 0.75$, $p = 0.025$) [54]. Montreal Cognitive Assessment (MoCA) results significantly improved in the experimental group after treatment in visuospatial and attention domains [59]. However, [55] did not observe consistent changes in MoCA. However, after the training, the participant was able to complete the VRN Building navigational task correctly, and the effects persisted at 5- and 28-week follow-ups. Improvements in navigational abilities have also been confirmed in daily life as recorded in wives' diaries. In [51], the patient group showed significantly higher scores in the Achievement Measure System LSP 50+, a German standardized intelligence test developed for older people between 50 and 90 years, and in the Benton Visual Retention Test, which assesses visual perception and visual memory. Also, in the Visual Pursuit Test (LVT) for visual orientation assessment, the authors observed a significant result [51]. De La-Torre [57] showed the existence of a main effect between the targets and the average errors committed to locate them within the virtual building (F adjusted $(1.37, 28.01) = 8.55$, $p < 0.01$; η^2 partial $= 0.32$, observed potency $= 0.87$).

One study [52] to analyze changes following treatment made correlations between VR measures and cognitive performances in the patient group. They observed that the mean number of correct products per time across all learning trials was correlated with higher performance on the Bergen Right-Left Discrimination Test (BRLD-B) to assess mental rotation. The percentile of the Digit Span Forward for short-term verbal memory was significantly correlated with the number of correctly bought products in the last learning trial on day 6 and number of correct products on the free recall trial after interference on day 7. The mean number of correct products per time and per distance across all learning trials were correlated with better performance on, respectively, the delayed free recall and immediate and delayed free recall of the Rey-Osterrieth Complex Figure (ROCF) for the assessment of visuo-construction, planning, and long term visual memory. A significant improvement was also observed in ROF [48]. In [56], the patients' face recognition performance significantly improved as measure by the Cambridge Face Memory Test (CFMT) following training. The effects persisted at one-week and 6-month follow-ups.

3.3.2. Traditional and Virtual Assessment

Results of the current review support the idea that virtual reality-based training improves orientation and navigation abilities in different neuropsychological disorders. Although the efficacy of treatment needs to be critically analyzed using a scientifically validated method, for this reason, the use of validated measures with adequate psychometric properties is fundamental. Over the past decade, evidence-based clinical guidelines have become a significant feature of healthcare services to improve the quality of care [69]. Indeed, among the studies analyzed, those that used specific-domain assessments (Corsi Supraspan, Virtual Tübingen, Route delayed recall RBMT, cognitive maps, or variables extracted from the supermarket task) were more able to demonstrate clear and significant results after the spatial memory rehabilitation training [21,48,50,53,56], highlighting the crucial role played by the selection of the assessment tools. In addition to the traditional paper-and-pencil tests used, new virtual assessment measures also emerged in the analyzed studies. These last have shown that the virtual reality (VR) system could be a sensitive assessment tool for detecting spatial memory improvements. Therefore, it is urgent to find more scientific evidence regarding the psychometric validity of these new measuring instruments, particularly concerning navigation abilities.

4. Discussion

In the current review, we provided initial, positive results concerning the effect of virtual reality (VR) training on spatial memory rehabilitation, highlighting the potential of navigational tasks in virtual environments (VEs) to enhance navigation and orientation abilities in patients with spatial memory disorders. The rapid development and diffusion of VR technologies are amending the accessibility landscape of VR technology for the average consumer. Lower-cost VR systems such as the Oculus Rift, Go, Quest, and the HTC Vive are already issued on the market and have significantly reduced the cost barrier of VR hardware. Even lower-cost options are currently available using a smartphone, for example, Gear VR is compatible with specific Samsung phones, and both Google Cardboard and Google Daydream can be used with several smartphones. Although the review underlined encouraging results, current research in this topic has some limitations that researchers need to overcome. The current work is meant to provide methodological solutions for future studies.

As the first result of the review, we have found clear improvements in spatial memory through the application of navigational tasks in VR. Both immersive and nonimmersive VR systems have shown appropriate enhancements for navigation and orientation abilities, underling the power of the navigational tasks proposed. Furthermore, the results have shown a transference of improvements from VR-based training to more general aspects of spatial cognition. However, the mode of exploration influences the spatial learning of a new environment. The active exploration has an essential role in the acquisition of spatial knowledge and it is characterized by five components: motor orders that determine the path of locomotion, proprioceptive and vestibular information for self-motion, allocation of attention to navigation-related features of the environment, and cognitive decisions about the direction during navigation and mental manipulation of spatial information [70]. If immersive systems are able to target all these components, nonimmersive systems do not allow the activation of the idiothetic and motor systems, even if input devices require motor planning and execution. In this review, only one study [55] used an immersive virtual reality system with the Oculus Rift DK2 head-mounted display and a joypad. Instead, other studies [20,52,58,59] used semi-immersive systems: the first one used OctaVis, a circle of eight screens in which the participants can freely rotate on a fixed chair and interact with a joystick; the latter used the BTs Nirvana PC system connected to a projector or a big screen and an infrared sensor for movements. The recent availability of lower-cost options for immersive VR may change the situation soon, allowing more protocols that fully support active exploration.

Another important element for the rehabilitation program is the structure and length of the training protocol. Some studies have already demonstrated that the use of visual cueing, such as a map as a navigational aid, improved the performance of users performing complex navigational tasks [66] and in patients with Alzheimer's disease or mild cognitive impairment [70]. The presence of an interactive aerial view facilitated the retrieval of stored spatial layout and arrows or salient landmarks, giving more comprehensive information about the egocentric heading in the environment, were effective in supporting the navigation [67,68]. Also, the current review underlined the importance of cues in the tasks, such as maps, guidance arrows, methods of fading cues, and instructions (explicit or implicit), to support the patient during the training [21,53,54]. It has been demonstrated that a large visual arrow supports the neurorehabilitation of spatial memory due to the cognitive synchronization between the allocentric viewpoint-independent representation (including object-to-object information) and the allocentric viewpoint-dependent representation (i.e., comprising information about the current egocentric heading in the environment), as suggested by the "mental frame syncing hypothesis" [32,71]. Furthermore, the duration of the protocol [50,60] and time elapsed since damage onset are also key factors [50,52,54]. The analysis of these studies showed that a short duration—less than four hours—is insufficient to provide consistent changes. Concerning the distance from onset, the shorter the period between the traumatic event and the beginning of treatment, the higher the probability of better outcomes.

The rehabilitation programs analyzed all focused on spatial memory and navigation abilities in different neurologic patients, including mild cognitive impairment (MCI), Alzheimer's disease (AD), traumatic brain injury (TBI), stroke, epilepsy, prosopagnosia with topographical disorientation disorders, and neglect. An important aspect to keep in mind is the clear characterization of the sample of patients to whom the therapeutic procedure is provided. The severity and the qualitative characteristics of the mnestic deficit are extremely variable from subject to subject. Furthermore, memory disorders rarely occur in an isolated form, and are often accompanied by an impairment of other cognitive functions, such as attention, language, reasoning. In this view, the most effective protocols are the ones that target a specific pathology.

The difficulty in finding homogeneous groups of patients is the reason why most of the experimental studies reported in the literature are based on the treatment of a single patient or a tiny group of patients. However, to monitor the improvements due to the treatment, the presence of an adequate control group is necessary to ensure that the observed improvement is not due to spontaneous recovery nor is the result of generic cognitive stimulation. In this view, the most reliable control condition is the repeated evaluation of the same patients receiving the experimental treatment, for example, through cross-over trials [72]. Another possible approach is the involvement of patients who, in the immediately preceding period, were followed in the absence of therapy or using another type of cognitive treatment. Moreover, the studies that used domain-specific assessments (Corsi Supraspan, Virtual Tübingen, Route delayed recall RBMT, cognitive maps, or variables extracted from the supermarket) were more able to demonstrate clear and significant results after the spatial memory rehabilitation training [21,48,50,53,56], highlighting the crucial role played by the selection of the assessment tools. Among the tests used (Corsi Supraspan, Virtual Tübingen, Route delayed recall RBMT), only the Virtual Tübingen can investigate the several aspects (scene recognition, route continuation/sequence/order/progression/distance, pointing to start/to end, map drawing recognition) involved in navigation. Thus, the scarcity of tools for spatial memory assessment is evident, particularly concerning navigation abilities.

This review was subject to certain limitations. Extensive literature research was performed to deliver these findings; however, only two databased were queried. A second limitation of this review may be the selection of the keywords in the search strategy. In order to provide a considerable quantity of studies in the field, the authors decided to use wider keywords. However, the inclusion criteria reduced the focus to only studies according to the objectives of the review. A final limitation may be the fact that the discussion on duration and intensity of VR navigational training cannot draw firm conclusions due to the heterogeneity of interventions. Moreover, the difficulty of finding a homogeneous group of patients is the reason why most of the experimental studies reported in the literature are based on the treatment of a single patient or a tiny group of patients. Because our findings are positive, we hope that the literature could soon be enriched with clinical trials investigating VR's effectiveness in more specific and larger clinical populations.

5. Conclusions

In conclusion, the results of this systematic review demonstrate that all studies, although to varying degrees, suggest that patients improved their spatial memory following treatment. This result highlights the potential of navigational tasks performed in virtual environments (VEs) for enhancing navigation and orientation abilities in patients with spatial memory disorders. In neuroscience, researchers have long faced the challenge of conducting ecologically valid measurements of experimental variables while maintaining strict experimental control over visual displays. Virtual reality (VR) systems enable the researchers to design and consequently control dynamic, realistic, and immersive environments, while closely monitoring behavioral and physiological responses during experimentation [1,73]. In this view, VR systems offer impressive opportunities as an ecological tool which is currently available for neuropsychologists to assess and enhance spatial memory, particularly navigation and orientation abilities using the "affordances" [74] offered to the patients in the virtual environment. One of the significant advantages of VR is the high degree of experimental control that is afforded to investigate the cognitive and behavioral components that are involved in spatial navigation [75]. VR training can facilitate neurorehabilitation, promoting brain plasticity processes through complex mechanisms related to the reactivation of brain neurotransmitter capacities, maximizing the results compared to those obtained by conventional treatment [66,76]. Monitoring EEG activities of the patients could be a suitable practice to assess the biomarkers of neuroplasticity and to measure rehabilitation progress [67,77]. The results are promising; hence, we encourage researchers to develop new spatial memory VR-based protocols for neurorehabilitation. However, more research is required to validate and support this result.

Funding: This work is supported in part by the Italian funded project "High-end and Low-End Virtual Reality Systems for the Rehabilitation of Frailty in the Elderly" (PE-2013-02355948) and by the research project Tecnologia Positiva e Healthy Aging (Positive Technology and Healthy Aging) (Grant D.3.2., 2014).

Conflicts of Interest: The authors declare no conflict of interest.

References

1. Bohil, C.J.; Alicea, B.; Biocca, F.A. Virtual reality in neuroscience research and therapy. *Nat. Rev. Neurosci.* **2011**, *12*, 752–762. [CrossRef] [PubMed]
2. Steuer, J. Defining Virtual Reality: Characteristics Determining Telepresence. *J. Commun.* **1992**, *42*, 73–94. [CrossRef]
3. Sanchez-Vives, M.V.; Slater, M. Opinion: From presence to consciousness through virtual reality. *Nat. Rev. Neurosci.* **2005**, *6*, 332–339. [CrossRef] [PubMed]

4. Riva, G. From Virtual to Real Body. *J. Cyberther. Rehabil.* **2008**, *1*, 7–22.
5. Riva, G.; Baños, R.M.; Botella, C.; Mantovani, F.; Gaggioli, A. Transforming Experience: The Potential of Augmented Reality and Virtual Reality for Enhancing Personal and Clinical Change. *Front. Psychol.* **2016**, *7*, 164. [CrossRef] [PubMed]
6. Slater, M. Place illusion and plausibility can lead to realistic behaviour in immersive virtual environments. *Philos. Trans. R. Soc. B Boil. Sci.* **2009**, *364*, 3549–3557. [CrossRef] [PubMed]
7. Riva, G.; Waterworth, J.A.; Waterworth, E.L. The Layers of Presence: A Bio-cultural Approach to Understanding Presence in Natural and Mediated Environments. *CyberPsychol. Behav.* **2004**, *7*, 402–416. [CrossRef] [PubMed]
8. Riva, G.; Castelnuovo, G.; Mantovani, F. Transformation of flow in rehabilitation: The role of advanced communication technologies. *Behav. Res. Methods* **2006**, *38*, 237–244. [CrossRef] [PubMed]
9. Riva, G.; Gaggioli, A.; Villani, D.; Preziosa, A.; Morganti, F.; Corsi, R.; Faletti, G.; Vezzadini, L. NeuroVR: An open source virtual reality platform for clinical psychology and behavioral neurosciences. *Stud. Health Technol. Inform.* **2007**, *125*, 394–399.
10. Witmer, B.G.; Singer, M.J. Measuring Presence in Virtual Environments: A Presence. *Presence* **1998**, *7*, 225–241. [CrossRef]
11. Laviola, J.J. A discussion of cybersickness in virtual environments. *ACM SIGCHI Bull.* **2000**, *32*, 47–56. [CrossRef]
12. Pot-kolder, R.; Veling, W.; Counotte, J.; van der Gaag, M. Anxiety Partially Mediates Cybersickness Symptoms in Immersive Virtual Reality Environments. *Cyberpsychol. Behav. Soc. Netw.* **2017**, *21*, 187–193. [CrossRef] [PubMed]
13. Gatica-Rojas, V.; Méndez-Rebolledo, G. Virtual reality interface devices in the reorganization of neural networks in the brain of patients with neurological diseases. *Neural Regen. Res.* **2014**, *9*, 888–896. [CrossRef] [PubMed]
14. Riva, G.; Dakanalis, A.; Gaggioli, A. From body dissatisfaction to obesity: How virtual reality may improve obesity prevention and treatment in adolescents. *Stud. Health Technol. Inform.* **2011**, *184*, 356–362.
15. Slater, M.; Sanchez-Vives, M.V. Enhancing Our Lives with Immersive Virtual Reality. *Front. Robot. AI* **2016**, *3*, 1–47. [CrossRef]
16. Slater, M. Grand Challenges in Virtual Environments. *Front. Robot. AI* **2014**, *1*, 1–4. [CrossRef]
17. Slater, M.; Spanlang, B.; Corominas, D. Simulating virtual environments within virtual environments as the basis for a psychophysics of presence. *ACM Trans. Grapghics* **2010**, *29*, 1–9. [CrossRef]
18. Slater, M.; Marcos, D.P.; Ehrsson, H.H.; Sanchez-Vives, M.V. Inducing Illusory Ownership of a Virtual Body. *Front. Mol. Neurosci.* **2009**, *3*, 214–220. [CrossRef] [PubMed]
19. Serino, S.; Baglio, F.; Rossetto, F.; Realdon, O.; Cipresso, P.; Parsons, T.D.; Cappellini, G.; Mantovani, F.; De Leo, G.; Nemni, R.; et al. Picture Interpretation Test (PIT) 360°: An Innovative Measure of Executive Functions. *Sci. Rep.* **2017**, *7*, 16000. [CrossRef]
20. Grewe, P.; Kohsik, A.; Flentge, D.; Dyck, E.; Botsch, M.; Winter, Y.; Markowitsch, H.J.; Bien, C.G.; Piefke, M. Learning real-life cognitive abilities in a novel 360 degrees -virtual reality supermarket: A neuropsychological study of healthy participants and patients with epilepsy. *J. Neuroeng. Rehabil.* **2013**, *10*, 42. [CrossRef]
21. Serino, S.; Pedroli, E.; Tuena, C.; De Leo, G.; Stramba-Badiale, M.; Goulene, K.; Mariotti, N.G.; Riva, G. A novel virtual reality-based training protocol for the enhancement of the 'mental frame syncing' in individuals with Alzheimer's disease: A development-of-concept trial. *Front. Aging Neurosci.* **2017**, *9*, 1–12. [CrossRef] [PubMed]
22. Mishkind, M.C.; Norr, A.M.; Katz, A.C.; Reger, G.M. Review of Virtual Reality Treatment in Psychiatry: Evidence Versus Current Diffusion and Use. *Curr. Psychiatry Rep.* **2017**, *19*, 80. [CrossRef] [PubMed]
23. Zeng, N.; Pope, Z.; Lee, J.E.; Gao, Z. Virtual Reality Exercise for Anxiety and Depression: A Preliminary Review of Current Research in an Emerging Field. *J. Clin. Med.* **2018**, *7*, 42. [CrossRef] [PubMed]
24. Ferrer-García, M.; Gutiérrez-Maldonado, J.; Pla-Sanjuanelo, J.; Vilalta-Abella, F.; Riva, G.; Clerici, M.; Ribas-Sabaté, J.; Andreu-Gracia, A.; Fernandez-Aranda, F.; Forcano, L.; et al. A Randomised Controlled Comparison of Second-Level Treatment Approaches for Treatment-Resistant Adults with Bulimia Nervosa and Binge Eating Disorder: Assessing the Benefits of Virtual Reality Cue Exposure Therapy. *Eur. Eat. Disord. Rev.* **2017**, *25*, 479–490. [CrossRef] [PubMed]

25. Clus, D.; Larsen, M.E.; Lemey, C.; Berrouiguet, S. The Use of Virtual Reality in Patients with Eating Disorders: Systematic Review. *J. Med. Internet Res.* **2018**, *20*, 1–9. [CrossRef] [PubMed]
26. Spreij, L.A.; Visser-Meily, J.M.A.; Van Heugten, C.M.; Nijboer, T.C.W. Novel insights into the rehabilitation of memory post acquired brain injury: A systematic review. *Front. Hum. Neurosci.* **2014**, *8*, 1–19. [CrossRef] [PubMed]
27. Valladares-Rodriguez, S.; Perez-Rodriguez, R.; Facal, D.; Fernandez-Iglesias, M.J.; Anido-Rifon, L.; Mouriño-Garcia, M. Design process and preliminary psychometric study of a video game to detect cognitive impairment in senior adults. *PeerJ* **2017**, *5*, 1–35. [CrossRef] [PubMed]
28. Schedlbauer, A.M.; Copara, M.S.; Watrous, A.J.; Ekstrom, A.D. Multiple interacting brain areas underlie successful spatiotemporal memory retrieval in humans. *Sci. Rep.* **2014**, *4*, 6431. [CrossRef]
29. Carrieri, M.; Petracca, A.; Lancia, S.; Moro, S.B.; Brigadoi, S.; Spezialetti, M.; Ferrari, M.; Placidi, G.; Quaresima, V. Prefrontal Cortex Activation Upon a Demanding Virtual Hand-Controlled Task: A New Frontier for Neuroergonomics. *Front. Hum. Neurosci.* **2016**, *10*, 1–13. [CrossRef]
30. Zanier, E.R.; Zoerle, T.; Di Lernia, D.; Riva, G. Virtual Reality for Traumatic Brain Injury. *Front. Neurol.* **2018**, *9*, 1–4. [CrossRef]
31. Colombo, D.; Serino, S.; Tuena, C.; Pedroli, E.; Dakanalis, A.; Cipresso, P.; Riva, G. Egocentric and allocentric spatial reference frames in aging: A systematic review. *Neurosci. Biobehav. Rev.* **2017**, *80*, 605–621. [CrossRef] [PubMed]
32. Serino, S.; Riva, G. Getting lost in Alzheimer's disease: A break in the mental frame syncing. *Med. Hypotheses* **2013**, *80*, 416–421. [CrossRef] [PubMed]
33. Allison, S.L.; Fagan, A.M.; Morris, J.C.; Head, D. Spatial Navigation in Preclinical Alzheimer's Disease. *J. Alzheimers Dis.* **2016**, *52*, 77–90. [CrossRef] [PubMed]
34. Kuehn, E.; Perez-Lopez, M.B.; Diersch, N.; Döhler, J.; Wolbers, T.; Riemer, M. Embodiment in the aging mind. *Neurosci. Biobehav. Rev.* **2018**, *86*, 207–225. [CrossRef] [PubMed]
35. Lester, A.W.; Moffat, S.D.; Wiener, J.M.; Barnes, C.A.; Wolbers, T. The Aging Navigational System. *Neuron* **2017**, *95*, 1019–1035. [CrossRef] [PubMed]
36. E Cullen, K.; Taube, J.S. Our sense of direction: Progress, controversies and challenges. *Nat. Neurosci.* **2017**, *20*, 1465–1473. [CrossRef]
37. Bird, C.M.; Burgess, N. The hippocampus and memory: Insights from spatial processing. *Nat. Rev. Neurosci.* **2008**, *9*, 182–194. [CrossRef] [PubMed]
38. Holmes, M.C.; Sholl, M.J. Allocentric Coding of Object-to-Object Relations in Overlearned and Novel Environments. *J. Exp. Psychol. Learn. Mem. Cogn.* **2005**, *31*, 1069–1087. [CrossRef]
39. Hartley, T.; Lever, C.; Burgess, N.; O'Keefe, J. Space in the brain: How the hippocampal formation supports spatial cognition. *Philos. Trans. R. Soc. B Biol. Sci.* **2013**, *369*, 20120510. [CrossRef]
40. Burgess, N. Spatial cognition and the brain. *Ann. N. Y. Acad. Sci.* **2008**, *1124*, 77–97. [CrossRef]
41. D'Esposito, M.; Aguirre, G.K. Topographical disorientation: A synthesis and taxonomy. *Brain* **1999**, *122*, 1613–1628.
42. Vann, S.D.; Aggleton, J.P.; Maguire, E.A. What does the retrosplenial cortex do? *Nat. Rev. Neurosci.* **2009**, *10*, 792–802. [CrossRef] [PubMed]
43. Doeller, C.F.; King, J.A.; Burgess, N. Parallel striatal and hippocampal systems for landmarks and boundaries in spatial memory. *Proc. Natl. Acad. Sci. USA* **2008**, *105*, 5915–5920. [CrossRef] [PubMed]
44. Borrego, A.; Latorre, J.; Llorens, R.; Alcañiz, M.; Noé, E. Feasibility of a walking virtual reality system for rehabilitation: Objective and subjective parameters. *J. Neuroeng. Rehabil.* **2016**, *13*, 68. [CrossRef] [PubMed]
45. Moher, D.; Liberati, A.; Tetzlaff, J.; Altman, D.G.; Grp, P. Preferred Reporting Items for Systematic Reviews and Meta-Analyses: The PRISMA Statement (Reprinted from Annals of Internal Medicine). *Phys. Ther.* **2009**, *89*, 873–880. [PubMed]
46. Higgins, J.; Green, S. *Cochrane Handbook for Systematic Reviews of Interventions*; Version 5; The Cochrane Collaboration: London, UK, 2011.
47. Von Elm, E.; Altman, D.G.; Egger, M.; Pocock, S.J.; Gøtzsche, P.C.; Vandenbroucke, J.P. The Strengthening the Reporting of Observational Studies in Epidemiology (STROBE) Statement: Guidelines for reporting observational studies. *Lancet* **2007**, *370*, 1453–1457. [CrossRef]

48. Pugnetti, L.; Mendozzi, L.; Brooks, B.; Attree, E.; Barbieri, E.; Alpini, D.; Motta, A.; Rose, D. Active versus passive exploration of virtual environments modulates spatial memory in MS patients: A yoked control study. *Ital. J. Neurol. Sci.* **1998**, *19*, S424–S430. [CrossRef]
49. Akhutina, T.; Foreman, N.; Krichevets, A.; Matikka, L.; Närhi, V.; Pylaeva, N.; Vahakuopus, J. Improving spatial functioning in children with cerebral palsy using computerized and traditional game tasks. *Disabil. Rehabil.* **2003**, *25*, 1361–1371. [CrossRef]
50. Caglio, M.; Latini-Corazzini, L.; D'Agata, F.; Cauda, F.; Sacco, K.; Monteverdi, S.; Zettin, M.; Duca, S.; Geminiani, G. Virtual navigation for memory rehabilitation in a traumatic brain injured patient. *Neurocase (Psychology Press)* **2012**, *18*, 123–131. [CrossRef]
51. Kober, S.E.; Wood, G.; Hofer, D.; Kreuzig, W.; Kiefer, M.; Neuper, C. Virtual reality in neurologic rehabilitation of spatial disorientation. *J. Neuroeng. Rehabil.* **2013**, *10*, 1–13. [CrossRef]
52. Grewe, P.; Lahr, D.; Kohsik, A.; Dyck, E.; Markowitsch, H.; Bien, C.; Botsch, M.; Piefke, M. Real-life memory and spatial navigation in patients with focal epilepsy: Ecological validity of a virtual reality supermarket task. *Epilepsy Behav.* **2014**, *31*, 57–66. [CrossRef] [PubMed]
53. Claessen, M.H.G.; van der Ham, I.J.M.; Jagersma, E.; Visser-Meily, J.M.A. Navigation strategy training using virtual reality in six chronic stroke patients: A novel and explorative approach to the rehabilitation of navigation impairment. *Neuropsychol. Rehabil.* **2016**, *26*, 822–846. [CrossRef] [PubMed]
54. Faria, A.L.; Andrade, A.; Soares, L.; I Badia, S.B. Benefits of virtual reality based cognitive rehabilitation through simulated activities of daily living: A randomized controlled trial with stroke patients. *J. Neuroeng. Rehabil.* **2016**, *13*, 1–12. [CrossRef] [PubMed]
55. White, P.J.; Moussavi, Z. Neuro-Cognitive Treatment for an Alzheimer's Patient using a Virtual Reality Navigational Environment. *J. Exp. Neurosci.* **2016**, *10*, 129–135. [CrossRef] [PubMed]
56. Bate, S.; Adams, A.; Bennetts, R.; Line, H. Developmental prosopagnosia with concurrent topographical difficulties: A case report and virtual reality training programme. *Neuropsychol. Rehabil.* **2017**, *29*, 1–23. [CrossRef]
57. De La Torre-Luque, A.; Valero-Aguayo, L.; De La Rubia-Cuestas, E.J. Visuospatial Orientation Learning through Virtual Reality for People with Severe Disability. *Int. J. Disabil. Dev. Educ.* **2017**, *64*, 420–435. [CrossRef]
58. De Luca, R.; Buono, V.L.; Leo, A.; Russo, M.; Aragona, B.; Leonardi, S.; Buda, A.; Naro, A.; Calabrò, R.S. Use of virtual reality in improving poststroke neglect: Promising neuropsychological and neurophysiological findings from a case study. *Appl. Neuropsychol.* **2017**, *26*, 1–5. [CrossRef]
59. De Luca, R.; Russo, M.; Naro, A.; Tomasello, P.; Leonardi, S.; Santamaria, F.; Desireè, L.; Bramanti, A.; Silvestri, G.; Bramanti, P.; et al. Effects of virtual reality-based training with BTs-Nirvana on functional recovery in stroke patients: Preliminary considerations. *Int. J. Neurosci.* **2018**, *7454*, 1–6. [CrossRef]
60. Maresca, G.; Maggio, M.G.; Buda, A.; la Rosa, G. A novel use of virtual reality in the treatment of cognitive and motor de fi cit in spinal cord injury. *Medicine (Baltimore)* **2018**, *97*, e13559. [CrossRef]
61. Mrakic-Sposta, S.; Di Santo, S.G.; Franchini, F.; Arlati, S.; Zangiacomi, A.; Greci, L.; Moretti, S.; Jesuthasan, N.; Marzorati, M.; Rizzo, G.; et al. Effects of Combined Physical and Cognitive Virtual Reality-Based Training on Cognitive Impairment and Oxidative Stress in MCI Patients: A Pilot Study. *Front. Aging Neurosci.* **2018**, *10*, 1–11. [CrossRef]
62. Cipresso, P.; Serino, S.; Riva, G. Psychometric assessment and behavioral experiments using a free virtual reality platform and computational science. *BMC Med. Inform. Decis. Mak.* **2016**, *16*, 1–11. [CrossRef] [PubMed]
63. Behr, J.; Bockholt, U.; Fellner, D. Instantreality—A Framework for Industrial Augmented and Virtual Reality Applications. In *Virtual Reality & Augmented Reality in Industry*; Ma, D., Fan, X., Gausemeier, J., Grafe, M., Eds.; Springer: Berlin/Heidelberg, Germany, 2011.
64. Brotons-Mas, J.R.; O'Mara, S.; Sanchez-Vives, M.V. Neural processing of spatial information: What we know about place cells and what know about place cells and what they can tell us about presence. *Presence Teleoperators Virtual Environ.* **2006**, *15*, 485–499. [CrossRef]
65. De Luca, R.; Portaro, S.; Le Cause, M.; De Domenico, C.; Maggio, M.G.; Ferrera, M.C.; Giuffrè, G.; Bramanti, A.; Calabrò, R.S. Cognitive rehabilitation using immersive virtual reality at young age: A case report on traumatic brain injury. *Appl. Neuropsychol. Child* **2019**, 1–6. [CrossRef] [PubMed]

66. Darken, R.P.; Sibert, J.L. Navigating Large Virtual Spaces. *Int. J. Hum-Comput. Interact.* **1996**, *8*, 49–72. [CrossRef]
67. Serino, S.; Mestre, D.; Mallet, P.; Pergandi, J.; Cipresso, P.; Riva, G. *Don't Get Lost in Translation: The Role of Egocentric Heading in Spatial Orientation*; Elsevier: Amsterdam, The Netherlands, 2015.
68. Cogné, M.; Auriacombe, S.; Vasa, L.; Tison, F.; Klinger, É.; Sauzeon, H.; Joseph, P.-A.; N'kaoua, B. Are visual cues helpful for virtual spatial navigation and spatial memory in patients with mild cognitive impairment or Alzheimer's disease? *Neuropsychology* **2018**, *32*, 385–400.
69. Flores-Mateo, G.; Argimon, J.M. Evidence based practice in postgraduate healthcare education: A systematic review. *BMC Health Serv. Res.* **2007**, *7*, 1–8. [CrossRef] [PubMed]
70. Chrastil, E.R.; Warren, W.H. Active and passive contributions to spatial learning. *Psychon. Bull. Rev.* **2012**, *19*, 1–23. [CrossRef]
71. Serino, S.; Riva, G. What is the role of spatial processing in the decline of episodic memory in Alzheimer's disease? The 'mental frame syncing' hypothesis. *Front. Aging Neurosci.* **2014**, *6*, 1–7. [CrossRef]
72. Senn, S. *Cross-over Trials in Clinical Research*; John Wiley & Sons, Ltd: Hoboken, NJ, USA, 2002.
73. Loomis, J.M.; Blascovich, J.J.; Beall, A.C. Immersive virtual environment technology as a basic research tool in psychology. *Behav. Res. Methods Instrum. Comput.* **1999**, *31*, 557–564. [CrossRef]
74. Gibson, J.J. The Theory of Affordances. In *The Ecological Approach to Visual Perception*; Routledge: Abingdon, UK, 1979.
75. Meade, M.E.; Meade, J.G.; Fernandes, M.A. Active Navigation in Virtual Environments Benefits Spatial Memory in Older Adults. *Brain Sci.* **2019**, *9*, 47. [CrossRef]
76. Maggio, M.G.; Maresca, G.; De Luca, R.; Stagnitti, M.C.; Porcari, B.; Ferrera, M.C.; Galletti, F.; Casella, C.; Manuli, A.; Calabrò, R.S. The Growing Use of Virtual Reality in Cognitive Rehabilitation: Fact, Fake or Vision? A Scoping Review. *J. Natl. Med. Assoc.* **2019**. [CrossRef] [PubMed]
77. Wen, D.; Lan, X.; Zhou, Y.; Li, G.; Hsu, S.-H.; Jung, T.-P. The Study of Evaluation and Rehabilitation of Patients with Different Cognitive Impairment Phases Based on Virtual Reality and EEG. *Front. Aging Neurosci.* **2018**, *10*, 1–6. [CrossRef] [PubMed]

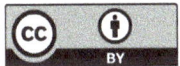

© 2019 by the authors. Licensee MDPI, Basel, Switzerland. This article is an open access article distributed under the terms and conditions of the Creative Commons Attribution (CC BY) license (http://creativecommons.org/licenses/by/4.0/).

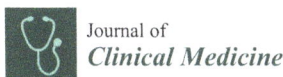

Article

A Computational Approach for the Assessment of Executive Functions in Patients with Obsessive–Compulsive Disorder

Elisa Pedroli [1,2,*], Filippo La Paglia [3], Pietro Cipresso [1,4], Caterina La Cascia [3], Giuseppe Riva [1,4] and Daniele La Barbera [3]

1. Applied Technology for Neuro-Psychology Lab, IRCCS Istituto Auxologico Italiano, Via Magnasco 2, 20149 Milano, Italy; Pietro.Cipresso@unicatt.it (P.C.); giuseppe.riva@unicatt.it (G.R.)
2. Faculty of Psychology, eCampus University, Via Isimbardi, 10, 22060 Novedrate, Italy
3. Department of Experimental Biomedicine and Clinical Neuroscience, University of Palermo, Piazza Marina, 61, 90133 Palermo, Italy; filippo.lapaglia@unipa.it (F.L.P.); erika.lacascia@unipa.it (C.L.C.); daniele.labarbera@unipa.it (D.L.B.)
4. Psychology Department, Catholic University of Milan, Largo Gemelli 1, 20123 Milan, Italy
* Correspondence: e.pedroli@auxologico.it; Tel.: +39-02-61911-2892

Received: 16 October 2019; Accepted: 12 November 2019; Published: 14 November 2019

Abstract: Previous studies on obsessive–compulsive disorder (OCD) showed impairments in executive domains, particularly in cognitive inhibition. In this perspective, the use of virtual reality showed huge potential in the assessment of executive functions; however, unfortunately, to date, no study on the assessment of these patients took advantage of the use of virtual environments. One of the main problems faced within assessment protocols is the use of a limited number of variables and tools when tailoring a personalized program. The main aim of this study was to provide a heuristic decision tree for the future development of tailored assessment protocols. To this purpose, we conducted a study that involved 58 participants (29 OCD patients and 29 controls) to collect both classic neuropsychological data and precise data based on a validated protocol in virtual reality for the assessment of executive functions, namely, the VMET (virtual multiple errands test). In order to provide clear indications for working on executive functions with these patients, we carried out a cross-validation based on three learning algorithms and computationally defined two decision trees. We found that, by using three neuropsychological tests and two VMET scores, it was possible to discriminate OCD patients from controls, opening a novel scenario for future assessment protocols based on virtual reality and computational techniques.

Keywords: Obsessive–compulsive disorders; virtual reality; multiple errands test; cognitive assessment; executive functions; computational models; decision tree; cross-validation

1. Introduction

According to the Diagnostic and Statistical Manual of Mental Disorders, Fifth Edition (DSM-5) [1], patients with obsessive–compulsive disorder (OCD) usually show obsessions and/or compulsions that reduce quality of life because of interference with daily routines, as well as work, social, or family life. This disorder affects about 2% of the population, and the World Health Organization highlighted that OCD is one of the 20 causes of disability in subjects within the 15–44 age range [2]. Moreover, OCD patients show dysfunctions in executive domains, particularly in cognitive inhibition [3], probably caused by a serotoninergic and dopaminergic dysfunction [4]. A deficit in executive functions may give problems when responding to both internal and external requirements, by inhibiting the ability to manage and orient the necessary cognitive resources. Specifically, the term "executive function" indicates a complex domain that includes a large number of cognitive processes and behavioral capabilities such as problem-solving, planning, sequencing, ability to sustain attention, resisting interference, utilizing feedback, cognitive inhibition, multitasking, cognitive flexibility, etc. [5–7]. Despite this abnormality, research on neuropsychological impairments in OCD produced unclear results [8]. Analyzing this specific syndrome, we can find some symptoms strongly related to dysexecutive deficits, such as checking behaviors. It is important to understand which one has a causal role in OCD and which one is a consequence of the syndrome [9]. Some articles showed deficits in planning abilities and nonverbal memory, while other studies reported deficits in cognitive flexibility and inhibition, and others displayed no neuropsychological deficits [10–14]. There are many possible explanations, e.g., differences in the methodology, in the instruments used, or in the characteristics of the samples. Specifically, the diversity of tools used during the assessment phase is related to an unsolved debate: the difference between paper-and-pencil and ecological tests [15]. Classic tasks in a classic setting analyze single aspects of complex domains and request simple responses to single events. Conversely, tasks in naturalistic settings may analyze cognitive functions in a complete way, requiring complex answers and, sometimes, the inhibition of inappropriate or irrelevant actions within several subtasks [6]. Therefore, it is critical to increase the ecological validity of a neuropsychological battery, especially for a complex cognitive domain such as an executive function. The assessment procedure has to become more sensitive to different aspects of patient behavior reflecting real-life situations [16]. However, it is too difficult to create a feasible assessment of executive functions during real-life situations because of implementation problems and the difficulty in involving patients in the procedure [17].

Virtual reality (VR) represents a valid solution to address the problems of classical assessment protocols. VR is a new technology that allows users to actively interact in a computer-generated tridimensional environment that simulates the real world [18]. This technology allows subjects to explore and manage several situations inspired by daily experiences using real correspondent behaviors in a more controlled, safe, and low-cost setting than real-life situations [19]. In the last few years, VR was applied for the assessment and rehabilitation of several psychological diseases such as post-traumatic stress disorder [20–22], anxiety [23,24], and eating disorders [25], as well as for neuropsychological domains such as neglect [26,27], executive functions [28,29], decision-making [30], spatial memory and orientation [31–33], and cognitive rehabilitation of schizophrenia [34].

In the current study, we proposed a computational approach based on classification learning algorithms to discriminate OCD patients from a control group. There were many studies that highlighted the usefulness of a VR-based approach for the assessment of executive functions in OCD patients [35–37]. These patients showed a specific pattern of symptoms that could be easily detected with the use of VR or an integrated assessment. Our purpose was to provide a heuristic decision tree for a more precise but simple diagnosis, giving evidence-based indications for a possible rehabilitation protocol using virtual reality tailored to these patients. The assessment of the OCD disorder was based on a clinical interview, integrated with a questionnaire, as well as neuropsychological assessment in rare cases. This last aspect is important because it may highlight a particular pattern of functioning in OCD patients [38]. We tried providing indications of the most useful assessment tools for the analysis of these specific aspects.

2. Materials and Methods

2.1. Participants

The 58 participants consisted of 29 OCD patients (mean age: 33.07; SD: 9.91), diagnosed by a clinical psychologist or psychiatrist as meeting the DSM-5 [1] criteria for OCD, and 29 healthy and partially matched controls (mean age: 40.48; SD: 15.59). The mean value for years of education (y.o.e.) of patients was 12.03 (SD: 3.2) and that for the healthy control group was 12.03 (SD: 3.2). In the OCD group, there were 14 females and 15 males, and, in the healthy control group, there were 14 females and 15 males. In Table 1, the descriptive statistics of both groups are presented. In Table 2, a comparison between age and y.o.e. and between the cognitive level of control and patient groups is presented. According to the results, the two groups were matched for both age and y.o.e. but not for cognitive level. The general exclusion criteria were as follows: (1) presence of sensory and/or motor limitation; (2) presence of deficit in general cognitive level (Mini Mental State Examination <19); (3) deficit in perception (Street Test <2.25); (4) deficit in language comprehension (Token Test <26.5); (5) anxiety (State Trait Anxiety Inventory - STAI >40); (6) depression (Beck Depression Inventory >16). We did not control the level of OCD symptoms with quantitative methods; however, all patients were currently undergoing treatment and, according to a clinician, in partial remission. Furthermore, OCD patients with comorbidities and healthy controls with any psychiatric diagnosis were excluded. The subjects involved were treated with both drugs and psychotherapy according to the standard. All participants were experienced with the use of personal computers (PCs) and came from the hospital's area. Participants were asked not to drink caffeine or alcohol and not to smoke prior to the experimental test to avoid any effects of these substances on test execution and performance.

Table 1. Descriptive statistics of the two groups. SE—standard error; y.o.e.—years of education; MMSE—Mini Mental State Examination.

	Group	N	Mean	SD	SE
Age	1	29	33.07	9.906	1.840
	2	29	40.48	15.588	2.895
y.o.e.	1	29	12.03	3.201	0.594
	2	29	12.03	3.029	0.563
MMSE	1	29	26.56	2.675	0.497
	2	29	28.53	1.028	0.191

Table 2. Independent sample Mann–Whitney U test.

	W	p
Age	312.5	0.094
y.o.e.	425.5	0.936
MMSE	194.0	<0.001

2.2. Ethics Statement

The study was approved by the scientific review board of the "U.O. di Psichiatria dell'Azienda Universitaria Ospedaliera Policlinico 'Paolo Giaccone' di Palermo", in accordance with the Declaration of Helsinki. All participants gave written informed consent to the experimental procedure according to the rules of the scientific review board. All participant data were stored in encrypted and password protected files, following the criteria to protect personal health information [39].

2.3. Protocol

Participants were selected from the outpatient Unit of Psychiatry of Palermo University Hospital. The subject who met the experimental criteria were contacted, and a meeting was scheduled at the University Hospital. The experimental session was held by a specialized psychiatrist of the University of Palermo. At the beginning of the session, the examiner explained the general goals of the clinical protocol and the procedures to be used, and discussed the patient's doubts and concerns. During the experimental session, two parts were planned: the classical neuropsychological assessment and the VR-based assessment. The presentation order was counterbalanced; half of the patients started the assessment with the VR test, and the other half started with the classic neuropsychological battery. Before the VR-based assessment, patients were trained for the use of a joypad within a virtual environment.

2.4. Neuropsychological Battery

To understand the cognitive profile of the participants, a complete neuropsychological battery was administered. A Mini Mental State Evaluation (MMSE) [40] was administered to assess the general cognitive level. To assess verbal memory, the Digit Span (Digit S) Test [41] was used to assess short-term memory, the Short Story Recall Test and the Paired-Associate Learning Test (PALT) [42] were used to assess long-term memory, and the Corsi Span (Corsi S) and the Corsi Block Task (Corsi BT) [41] were used for the assessment of short- and long-term spatial memory. For analysis of the executive domain, several tests were used: the Frontal Assessment Battery (FAB) [43], a general battery to assess frontal lobe functions, the Trail Making Test (TMT, forms A, B, and B-A) [44] for the assessment of selective attention, and the Tower of London (TOL) Test [45] for the assessment of planning abilities. Also, a Phonemic Fluency (PF) Test and a Semantic Fluency (SF) Test [46] were used. All scores of the tests were corrected for age, education level, and gender where appropriate.

2.5. VMET

The assessment protocol was created with NeuroVR (Version 2.0, Istituto Auxologico Italiano, Milan, Italy), a free software where the user can modify a pre-existing virtual environment by selecting contents from a database of objects (both two- and three-dimensional (2D and 3D)) and videos [47], expanded with NeuroVirtual 3D [48]. The scene was visualized in the player using non-immersive displays. The task took place in a virtual supermarket shown on a laptop screen, and the patient had to use a joypad to move around the environment. All users were trained for virtual reality use in another smaller shop, specifically designed for training purposes. In the virtual supermarket, all products were organized in categories such as beverages, fruits and vegetables, breakfast foods, hygiene products, frozen foods, garden products, and animal products.

2.6. VMET Scoring

Before starting the task, the participants received a shopping list, a sheet with the rules, a map of the supermarket, information about the supermarket (opening and closing times, products on sale, etc.), a pen, and a wristwatch. The examiner read and explained all the information relative to the subject in order to guarantee complete understanding. The VMET test was composed of four main tasks. The first involved purchasing six items (e.g., one product on sale). The second involved asking the examiner information about one item to be purchased. The third involved writing the shopping list 5 min after beginning the test. The fourth involved responding to some questions at the end of the virtual session by using the given materials (e.g., the closing time of the virtual supermarket). The rules that the patients had to follow to complete the task were as follows: (1) they had to execute all the proposed tasks; (2) they could execute all tasks in any order; (3) they could not go to a place unless it was a part of a task; (4) they could not pass through the same passage more than once; (5) they could not buy more than two items per category (looking at the chart); (6) they had to take as little time as possible to complete the exercise; (7) they could not talk to the researcher unless this was a part of the task; (8) they had to go to their "shopping cart" 5 min after the beginning of the task and make a list of all their products. After the explanation of the material, the clinician measured the time, stopping it when the participant said they finished the task. During the assessment, the examiner recorded all the participant's behaviors in the virtual environment according to a predefined form. To better understand the patient's work, the following items were recorded [49]: task failures (total and partial), inefficiencies, strategies, rule breaks, and interpretation failures. When a subtask was not totally completed, a task failure occurred, and the scoring range for total errors was from 11 (all 11 subtasks were correctly done) to 33 (all 11 subtasks were incorrectly done). To calculate the scoring for each task, the scale ranged from 1–3 (1 = the task was performed correctly; 2 = the participant performed part of the task; 3 = the participant totally omitted the task). An inefficiency was deemed a behavior that could prevent the correct execution of the tasks, such as not grouping similar tasks when possible. The general scoring range was from eight (several inefficiencies) to 32 (no inefficiencies), and the scoring scale for each inefficiency was from 1–4 (1 = always; 2 = more than once; 3 = once; 4 = never). To analyze the strategies, 13 behaviors that facilitated carrying out the tasks were evaluated, such as accurate planning before starting a specific subtask. The scoring scale for each strategy was from 1–4 (1 = always; 2 = more than once; 3 = once; 4 = never), and the total score ranged from 13 (good strategies) to 52 (no strategies). A rule break occurred when patients violated one or more of the eight rules listed (e.g., talking with the examiner when not necessary). The scoring scale for each rule break was from 1–4 (1 = always; 2 = more than once; 3 = once; 4 = never) and the total score ranged from eight (a large number of rule breaks) to 32 (no rule breaks). Finally, an interpretation failure occurred when the requirements of particular tasks were misunderstood, for example, when a participant thought that the subtasks all had to be done in the order presented on the information sheet. The general score ranged from three (a large number of interpretation failures) to six (no interpretation failures), and the score for each interpretation failure ranged from 1–2 (1 = yes; 2 = no). Furthermore, for every subtask, we analyzed the following variables: (1) sustained attention; (2) maintaining the correct sequence of the task; (3) remembering the instructions; (4) divided attention; (5) correct organization of the materials; (6) self-corrections; (7) absence of perseverations. The general score ranged from seven (no errors) to 14 (a large number of errors), and the score for each interpretation failure ranged from 1–2 (1 = yes; 2 = no). According to the analysis prosed by Cipresso and colleagues [35], we analyzed three subtasks that they recognized as particularly crucial in the OCD patients' performance: (1) "going to the shopping chart after 5 min"; (2) "buying two products instead of just one"; (3) "going into a specific place and asking the examiner what to buy". These tasks represented a break during the normal task execution because they required a different, confusing, or stopping behavior, which required attention and the elaboration of different information at the same time. These tasks represented a "break in time", a "break in choice", and a "break in social rules", respectively.

2.7. Data Analysis

Data were analyzed with the aid of the statistical software STATA MP-Parallel Edition (Release 14.0, StataCorp LP, College Station, Texas) Orange (Version 3.3.5, Universitas Labacensis, Ljubljana and Portorož, Slovenia) with Python (Version 3.4, Python Software Foundation, Beaverton, OR, USA), JASP (Version 0.7.1.4, University of Amsterdam, Nieuwe Achtergracht, Amsterdam, The Netherlands) [50]. Comparisons between patients and controls were done by using a series of independent sample *t*-tests. To classify data, we used the following approaches [51,52]:

- Logistic regression classification algorithm with ridge regularization;
- Random forest classification using an ensemble of decision trees;
- Support vector machine (SVM), to map inputs to higher-dimensional feature spaces that best separated different classes.

Specifications about the algorithms used for computational data analyses can be found in the seminal article recently published by Zhou and colleagues (https://bmcmedinformdecismak.biomedcentral.com/track/pdf/10.1186/s12911-019-0890-0)

3. Results

Table 3 shows the results of OCD patients compared with normative data. The results showed intact cognitive levels in these patients.

Tables 4 and 5 report the sample descriptive statistics for the neuropsychological battery and the VMET scores, respectively. Table 6 indicates the independent sample *t*-tests comparing OCD patients with controls, for both the executive function domain and the other cognitive domains. On the other hand, Table 7 reports the independent sample *t*-tests for the VMET scoring.

Table 3. Neuropsychological battery in obsessive–compulsive disorder (OCD) patients compared to deficit level in normative sample.

Test	Mean	Standard Deviation	Normative Data
MMSE	26.56	2.68	>18
Frontal Assessment Battery (FAB)	14.97	1.4	>13.5
Trail Making Task A (TMTA)	63.07	23.58	<93
Trail Making Task B (TMTB)	191.93	112.04	<282
Trail Making Task B-A (TMTBA)	129.93	100.27	<186
Phonemic Fluency (PF)	27.38	9.42	>16
Semantic Fluency (SF)	33.69	8.43	>24
Tower of London (TOL)	22.72 [a]	5.45	Not available
Digit Span (Digit S)	5.28	1.09	>3.5
Paired-Associate Learning Test (PALT)	10.84	4.04	>6
Corsi Span (Corsi S)	4.51	0.78	>3.5
Short Story	12.62	5.24	>7.5
Corsi Block Task (Corsi BT)	16.09	8.21	>5.5

[a] Normally considered non-pathological level.

Table 4. Classical neuropsychological battery descriptive statistics (Group 1: OCD patients; Group 2: controls).

Test	Group	N	Mean	SD	SE
MMSE	1	29	26.565	2.675	0.497
	2	29	28.532	1.028	0.191
FAB	1	29	14.965	1.403	0.261
	2	20	16.274	0.849	0.190
TMTA	1	29	63.069	23.584	4.379
	2	29	37.632	15.624	2.901
TMTB	1	29	191.310	112.041	20.806
	2	29	95.448	46.144	8.569
TMTBA	1	29	129.931	100.269	18.619
	2	29	58.616	45.439	8.438
PF	1	29	27.379	9.420	1.749
	2	29	41.138	11.192	2.078
SF	1	29	33.690	8.431	1.566
	2	29	48.172	10.275	1.908
TOL	1	29	22.724	5.450	1.012
	2	29	28.448	3.582	0.665
Digit S	1	29	5.284	1.087	0.202
	2	29	6.010	0.847	0.157
PALT	1	29	10.845	4.036	0.749
	2	20	13.072	4.759	1.064
Corsi S	1	29	4.508	0.778	0.144
	2	29	6.345	2.660	0.494
Short Story	1	29	12.621	5.242	0.973
	2	29	14.491	4.454	0.827
Corsi BT	1	29	16.091	8.208	1.524
	2	29	21.239	5.843	1.085

Table 5. Virtual multiple errands test (VMET) descriptive analysis.

VMET	Group	N	Mean	SD	SE
Errors	1	29	17.276	2.840	0.527
	2	29	13.897	1.633	0.303
Break in time	1	29	13.379	2.821	0.524
	2	29	11.655	2.844	0.528
Break in choice	1	29	9.655	1.951	0.362
	2	29	8.379	0.979	0.182
Break in social rules	1	29	10.517	2.181	0.405
	2	29	8.793	1.544	0.287
Inefficiencies	1	29	22.552	4.733	0.879
	2	29	24.379	6.439	1.196
Rule break	1	29	21.172	3.733	0.693
	2	29	22.897	5.453	1.013
Strategies	1	29	36.414	7.238	1.344
	2	29	31.793	6.298	1.170
Interpretation failures	1	29	5.207	0.940	0.175
	2	29	5.241	0.872	0.162
Time	1	29	649.448	320.076	59.437
	2	29	595.759	266.793	49.542
Sustained attention	1	29	8.345	1.610	0.299
	2	29	7.759	0.830	0.154
Sequence	1	29	8.241	1.640	0.305
	2	29	7.828	0.805	0.149
Instructions	1	29	8.276	1.623	0.301
	2	29	7.517	0.634	0.118
Divided attention	1	29	10.448	2.667	0.495
	2	29	8.276	1.556	0.289
Organization	1	29	10.483	3.158	0.586
	2	29	8.000	1.282	0.238
Self-corrections	1	29	9.241	1.902	0.353
	2	29	7.759	0.786	0.146
Perseverations	1	29	8.724	1.830	0.340
	2	29	7.414	0.682	0.127

Clearly, both the neuropsychological battery and the VMET scores were able to differentiate patients from healthy controls; however, the mean scores of the neuropsychological battery for both patients and healthy controls were situated in the normal range (Table 3). Because of this fact, it is important to define classification models able to identify mutual information among the variables to make predictions based on a limited number of tests in a clinical setting. To pursue this aim, we ran three different learning algorithms for a cross-validation based on logistic regression, random forest, and support vector machine. Two different models were built: one based on classical neuropsychological tests for executive functions (FAB, TMTA, TMTB, TMTBA, TOL, PF, and SF) and the other one by also adding the previously defined VMET scores. Results of the two cross-validations can be seen in Table 8.

Table 6. Independent sample *t*-Test comparing OCD patients vs. controls for neuropsychological battery. df—degrees of freedom.

Test	t	df	p	Mean Difference	SE Difference	Cohen's d
Executive Function Domain↓						
FAB	−4.061	46.36	<0.001	−1.309	0.322	−1.082
TMTA	4.842	48.61	<0.001	25.437	5.253	1.272
TMTB	4.260	37.23	<0.001	95.862	22.501	1.119
TMTBA	3.489	39.04	0.001	71.315	20.442	0.916
PF	−5.065	54.42	<0.001	−13.759	2.717	−1.330
SF	−5.868	53.94	<0.001	−14.483	2.468	−1.541
TOL	−4.726	48.38	<0.001	−5.724	1.211	−1.241
Other Cognitive Domains↓						
MMSE	−3.696	36.10	<0.001	−1.967	0.532	−0.971
Digit S	−2.836	52.84	0.006	−0.726	0.256	−0.745
PALT	−1.712	36.44	0.095	−2.228	1.301	−0.513
Corsi S	−3.568	32.75	0.001	−1.837	0.515	−0.937
Short Story	−1.465	54.58	0.149	−1.871	1.277	−0.385
Corsi BT	−2.752	50.58	0.008	−5.149	1.871	−0.723

Note. For all tests, variances of groups were not assumed equal.

Table 7. Independent sample *t*-test for VMET index.

VMET	t	df	p	Mean Difference	SE Difference	Cohen's d
Errors	5.555	56.00	<0.001	3.379	0.608	1.459
Break in time	2.318	56.00	0.024	1.724	0.744	0.609
Break in choice	3.148	56.00	0.003	1.276	0.405	0.827
Break in social rules	3.474	56.00	<0.001	1.724	0.496	0.912
Inefficiencies	−1.232	56.00	0.223	−1.828	1.484	−0.323
Rule break	−1.405	56.00	0.166	−1.724	1.227	−0.369
Strategies	2.593	56.00	0.012	4.621	1.782	0.681
Interpretation failures	−0.145	56.00	0.885	−0.034	0.238	−0.038
Time	−0.033	56.00	0.974	−2.117	64.666	−0.009
Sustained attention	1.743	56.00	0.087	0.586	0.336	0.458
Sequence	1.220	56.00	0.228	0.414	0.339	0.320
Instructions	2.344	56.00	0.023	0.759	0.324	0.616
Divided attention	3.789	56.00	<0.001	2.172	0.573	0.995
Organization	3.923	56.00	<0.001	2.483	0.633	1.030
Self-corrections	3.879	56.00	<0.001	1.483	0.382	1.019
Perseverations	3.613	56.00	<0.001	1.310	0.363	0.949

Note. For all tests, variances of groups were assumed equal.

Table 8. Classification table. Three learning algorithms were compared, namely, logistic regression (LogReg), random forest, and support vector machine (SVM). In the first analysis (Panel A), the classifications were run referring to the classic neuropsychological test used for executive functions. In the second analysis (Panel B), VMET scores were added to the classic test for the classification learning algorithm [53–55].

Panel A: Classification with classic neuropsychological test for executive functions.					
Features:	FAB, TMTA, TMTB, TMTBA, TOL, PF, SF				
Sampling type:	Stratified 10-fold cross-validation				
Target class:	Average over classes				

Method	AUC	CA	F1	Precision	Recall
LogReg	0.742	0.741	0.746	0.733	0.759
Random forest	0.817	0.810	0.800	0.846	0.759
SVM	0.783	0.776	0.787	0.750	0.828

Table 8. *Cont.*

Panel B: Classification with classic neuropsychological test for executive functions and the VMET.					
Features	*FAB, TMTB, TMTA, TMTBA, TOL, PF, SF, ERRORS, break in time, break in choice, break in social rules, inefficiencies, rule break, strategies, interpretation failures, sustained attention, sequence, instructions, divided attention, organization, self-corrections, perseverations*				
Sampling type	Stratified 10-fold cross-validation				
Target class	Average over classes				
Method	AUC	CA	F1	Precision	Recall
LogReg	0.700	0.707	0.702	0.714	0.690
Random forest	0.850	0.845	0.852	0.812	0.897
SVM	0.775	0.776	0.772	0.786	0.759

AUC (area under the receiver operating characteristic (ROC) curve) is the area under the classic receiver operating characteristic curve. CA (classification accuracy) represents the proportion of examples correctly classified. F1 represents the weighted harmonic average of precision and recall (see below). Precision represents the proportion of true positives among all instances classified as positive. In our case, this was the proportion of OCD patients correctly identified as patients and not controls. Recall represents the proportion of true positives among the positive instances in our data, i.e., the number of OCD patients diagnosed as patients instead of controls.

Finally, a classification tree for both models was built based on feature selection, choosing entropy as a measure of homogeneity [56–58] for split selection (Figures 1 and 2). Small circles indicate the ratio of classifications reported inside the rectangle in terms of percentage of correctness in recognizing the specific characteristics. The colors indicate classification as one of the two groups: blue for OCD patients, red for control participants.

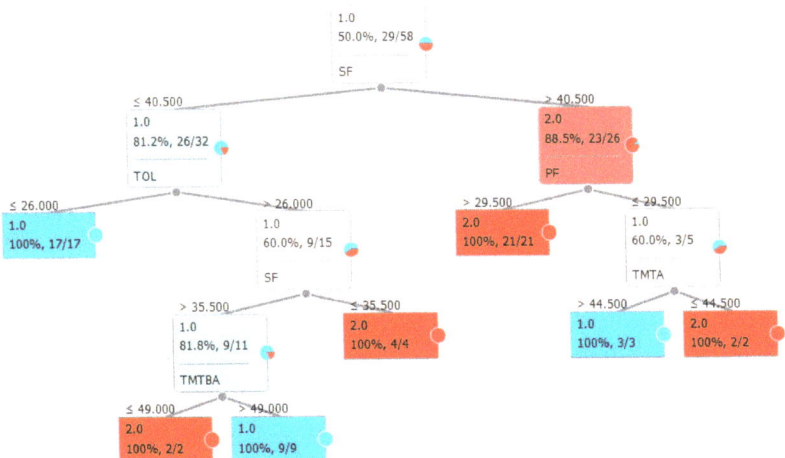

Figure 1. Classification tree using classic neuropsychological test for executive functions.

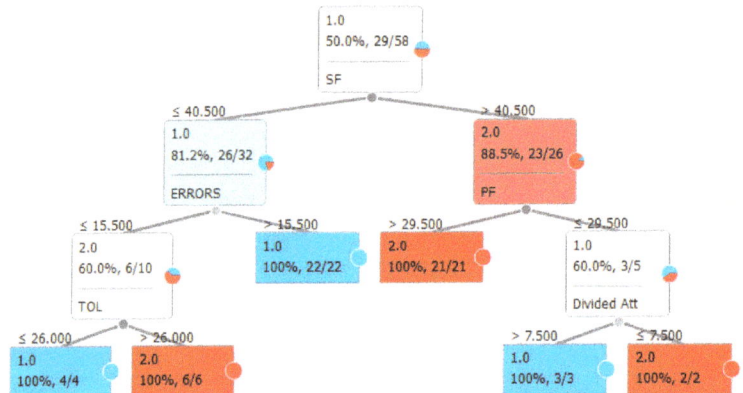

Figure 2. Classification tree using the classic test for executive functions and the virtual multiple errands test (VMET).

4. Discussion

The general aim of this study was twofold. Firstly, we investigated executive functions in OCD patients and controls. To this purpose, we used the virtual version of the multiple errands test and a classic neuropsychological battery. On the other hand, our purpose was to find a method to discriminate the two groups in a better way. Indeed, the goal was scaled on the minimal number of variables possible to pursue an ecological assessment of executive functions with these patients. VMET was demonstrated to be effective in the assessment of several patients, such as for OCD [35], Parkinson's disease [28], and stroke [49]; however, previous studies focused on single scores, such as time, total and partial errors, inefficiencies, and others. In this study, we exploited the multivariate nature of the VMET for the assessment of a particular patient sample (i.e., OCD), where dysfunction is slightly higher than or equal to a normative sample. Thus, this aim shed new light on using multidimensional scaling for understanding the deficits of executive functions.

The results showed a clear difference between OCD patients and the control group, particularly in executive functions, as highlighted in Table 4 for the classic neuropsychological test and Table 5 for most of the VMET scores. However, the complexity of a complete neuropsychological battery with the complete execution of VMET hindered the assessment of these patients. With this limitation in mind, we used computational techniques, which are also used in VR settings [59], to advance our knowledge based on consistent and relevant data from the sample presented. The first strategy was to understand the classification ability within the sample with a supervised machine learning approach. The results showed precision levels between 71.4% and 84.6%, making us confident of the goodness of fit of the model to data. This result is important since, on the one hand, it allowed discriminating OCD patients from healthy subjects (see Table 6, where results are all related to such a domain). On the other hand, at the clinical level, we need to reduce complexity and, consequently, the number of used tests. To this purpose, we opted for a visual classification tree to provide clear indications (based on data) of heuristic choice (Figures 1 and 2). The main and most encouraging result was that, by using both the classic neuropsychological battery and the VMET scores, we obtained a tree based on only five variables (Figure 2), two of which are VMET-based and, not surprisingly, particularly related to OCD patients (errors and divided attention).

Even if the tree based on classic neuropsychological battery (Figure 1) could provide a useful tool for patient evaluation, it does not represent a simple tool to be used for the assessment of executive functions as a whole. On the other hand, the tree based on semantic and phonemic fluency, as well as the TOL and the two VMET scores (Figure 2), can be very useful as a shortened model for the assessment of executive functions in OCD patients.

During the assessment process of OCD, the clinician has many variables to take into account, and deficits of executive function could be one of them. A method which provides clinicians with a simple and complete indication of the best assessment process may have great impact on the clinical process and on rehabilitation.

In clinical neuropsychological assessment, there is always the necessity of integrating different types of information, such as psychometric and ecological data [60,61] in order to better understand the patient's cognitive functioning. VMET is able to play a crucial role in integrating classical neuropsychological tests with ecological settings, especially for executive function assessment in different type of patients.

Making a guided diagnosis for a specific cognitive domain in a specific target of patients is an important goal for both the assessment and the rehabilitation process because it could be able, on one hand, to reduce the time and effort expended by patients and clinicians. On the other hand, a virtual rehabilitation program developed for a targeting assessment would potentially be more personalized and efficient.

This study also had some limitations that could be overcome in future studies. Firstly, the sample size was limited; in a future study, an accurate sample size calculation could be done. Also, adding a clinical control group could be interesting in order to understand the potential of our algorithm for differential diagnosis.

According to our algorithm, the important test for discrimination between OCD patients and controls are fluency, both semantic and phonological, Tower of London, and VMET. This setting would require a minimum amount of time and reduced effort for the clinician during the assessment procedure.

Author Contributions: E.P. wrote the first version of the article. F.L.P. and C.L.C. recruited controls and patients and executed the clinical tests and the experimental protocol. P.C. and E.P. carried out the statistical and computational analyses and wrote the results. G.R. and D.L.B. supervised the scientific and clinical aspects of the study. All authors revised and approved the final version of the manuscript.

Funding: This research received no external funding.

Conflicts of Interest: The authors declare no conflicts of interest.

References

1. APA. *Diagnostic and Statistical Manual of Mental Disorders-DSM-5*; American Psychiatric Publishing: Arlington, VA, USA, 2013.
2. Garfinkel, P.E.; Goldbloom, D.S. Mental health-getting beyond stigma and categories. *Bull. World Health Organ.* **2000**, *78*, 503. [PubMed]
3. Muller, J.; Roberts, J.E. Memory and attention in Obsessive-Compulsive Disorder: A review. *J. Anxiety Disord.* **2005**, *19*, 1–28. [CrossRef] [PubMed]
4. Morein-Zamir, S.; Craig, K.J.; Ersche, K.D.; Abbott, S.; Muller, U.; Fineberg, N.A.; Bullmore, E.T.; Sahakian, B.J.; Robbins, T.W. Impaired visuospatial associative memory and attention in obsessive compulsive disorder but no evidence for differential dopaminergic modulation. *Psychopharmacology* **2010**, *212*, 357–367. [CrossRef] [PubMed]
5. Burgess, P.W.; Veitch, E.; De Lacy Costello, A.; Shallice, T. The cognitive and neuroanatomical correlates of multitasking. *Neuropsychologia* **2000**, *38*, 848–863. [CrossRef]
6. Chan, R.C.; Shum, D.; Toulopoulou, T.; Chen, E.Y. Assessment of executive functions: Review of instruments and identification of critical issues. *Arch. Clin. Neuropsychol.* **2008**, *23*, 201–216. [CrossRef]
7. Grafman, J.; Litvan, I. Importance of deficits in executive functions. *Lancet* **1999**, *354*, 1921–1923. [CrossRef]
8. Abramovitch, A.; Dar, R.; Schweiger, A.; Hermesh, H. Neuropsychological Impairments and Their Association with Obsessive-Compulsive Symptom Severity in Obsessive-Compulsive Disorder. *Arch. Clin. Neuropsychol.* **2011**, *26*, 364–376. [CrossRef]
9. Lader, M. Current Controversies in the Anxiety Disorders. *BMJ* **1996**, *312*, 984. [CrossRef]
10. Shin, N.Y.; Kang, D.H.; Choi, J.S.; Jung, M.H.; Jang, J.H.; Kwon, J.S. Do organizational strategies mediate nonverbal memory impairment in drug-naïve patients with obsessive-compulsive disorder? *Neuropsychology* **2010**, *24*, 527. [CrossRef]

11. Moritz, S.; Kloss, M.; Von Eckstaedt, F.V.; Jelinek, L. Comparable performance of patients with obsessive–compulsive disorder (OCD) and healthy controls for verbal and nonverbal memory accuracy and confidence: Time to forget the forgetfulness hypothesis of OCD? *Psychiatry Res.* **2009**, *166*, 247–253. [CrossRef]
12. Abramovitch, A.; Abramowitz, J.S.; Mittelman, A. The neuropsychology of adult obsessive–compulsive disorder: A meta-analysis. *Clin. Psychol. Rev.* **2013**, *33*, 1163–1171. [CrossRef] [PubMed]
13. Pauls, D.L.; Abramovitch, A.; Rauch, S.L.; Geller, D.A. Obsessive-compulsive disorder: An integrative genetic and neurobiological perspective. *Nat. Rev. Neurosci.* **2014**, *15*, 410–424. [CrossRef] [PubMed]
14. Penades, R.; Catalan, R.; Rubia, K.; Andres, S.; Salamero, M.; Gasto, C. Impaired response inhibition in obsessive compulsive disorder. *Eur. Psychiatry* **2007**, *22*, 404–410. [CrossRef] [PubMed]
15. Sbordone, R.J.; Purisch, A.D. Hazards of blind analysis of neuropsychological test data in assessing cognitive disability: The role of confounding factors. *Neurorehabilitation* **1996**, *7*, 15–26. [CrossRef]
16. Burgess, N. Spatial memory: How egocentric and allocentric combine. *Trends Cogn. Sci.* **2006**, *10*, 551–557. [CrossRef] [PubMed]
17. Rand, D.; Rukan, S.B.A.; Weiss, P.L.; Katz, N. Validation of the Virtual MET as an assessment tool for executive functions. *Neuropsychol. Rehabil.* **2009**, *19*, 583–602. [CrossRef]
18. Schultheis, M.T.; Himelstein, J.; Rizzo, A.A. Virtual reality and neuropsychology: Upgrading the current tools. *J. Head Trauma Rehabil.* **2002**, *17*, 378–394. [CrossRef]
19. Riva, G. Virtual reality in psychotherapy: Review. *Cyberpsychol. Behav.* **2005**, *8*, 220–230. [CrossRef]
20. Difede, J.; Hoffman, H.G. Virtual reality exposure therapy for World Trade Center post-traumatic stress disorder: A case report. *Cyberpsychol. Behav.* **2002**, *5*, 529–535. [CrossRef]
21. Serino, S.; Triberti, S.; Villani, D.; Cipresso, P.; Gaggioli, A.; Riva, G. Toward a validation of cyber-interventions for stress disorders based on stress inoculation training: A systematic review. *Virtual Real.* **2014**, *18*, 73–87. [CrossRef]
22. Villani, D.; Grassi, A.; Cognetta, C.; Cipresso, P.; Toniolo, D.; Riva, G. The effects of a mobile stress management protocol on nurses working with cancer patients: A preliminary controlled study. *Stud. Health Technol. Inform.* **2012**, *173*, 524–528. [PubMed]
23. Safir, M.P.; Wallach, H.S.; Bar-Zvi, M. Virtual reality cognitive-behavior therapy for public speaking anxiety: One-year follow-up. *Behav. Modif.* **2011**. [CrossRef] [PubMed]
24. Repetto, C.; Gaggioli, A.; Pallavicini, F.; Cipresso, P.; Raspelli, S.; Riva, G. Virtual reality and mobile phones in the treatment of generalized anxiety disorders: A phase-2 clinical trial. *Pers. Ubiquitous Comput.* **2013**, *17*, 253–260. [CrossRef]
25. Serino, S.; Dakanalis, A.; Gaudio, S.; Carrà, G.; Cipresso, P.; Clerici, M.; Riva, G. Out of body, out of space: Impaired reference frame processing in eating disorders. *Psychiatry Res.* **2015**, *230*, 732–734. [CrossRef]
26. Pedroli, E.; Serino, S.; Cipresso, P.; Pallavicini, F.; Riva, G. Assessment and rehabilitation of neglect using virtual reality: A systematic review. *Front. Behav. Neuroscience.* **2015**, *9*, 226. [CrossRef]
27. Cipresso, P.; Pedroli, E.; Serino, S.; Semonella, M.; Tuena, C.; Colombo, D.; Pallavicini, F.; Riva, G. Assessment of Unilateral Spatial Neglect using a free mobile application for Italian clinicians. *Front. Psychol.* **2018**, *9*. [CrossRef]
28. Cipresso, P.; Albani, G.; Serino, S.; Pedroli, E.; Pallavicini, F.; Mauro, A.; Riva, G. Virtual multiple errands test (VMET): A virtual reality-based tool to detect early executive functions deficit in Parkinson's disease. *Frontiers in Behavioral Neuroscience.* **2014**, *8*, 405. [CrossRef]
29. Raspelli, S.; Pallavicini, F.; Carelli, L.; Morganti, F.; Poletti, B.; Corra, B.; Silani, V.; Riva, G. Validation of a Neuro Virtual Reality-based version of the Multiple Errands Test for the assessment of executive functions. *Stud. Health Technol. Inform.* **2010**, *167*, 92–97.
30. La Paglia, F.; La Cascia, C.; Rizzo, R.; Riva, G.; La Barbera, D. Decision Making and Cognitive Behavioral Flexibility in a OCD Sample: A Study in a Virtual Environment. *Stud. Health Technol. Inform.* **2016**, *219*, 53–57.
31. Serino, S.; Pedroli, E.; Keizer, A.; Triberti, S.; Dakanalis, A.; Pallavicini, F.; Chirico, A.; Riva, G. Virtual Reality Body Swapping: A Tool for Modifying the Allocentric Memory of the Body. *Cyberpsychol. Behav. Soc. Netw.* **2016**, *19*, 127–133. [CrossRef]
32. Serino, S.; Mestre, D.; Mallet, P.; Pergandi, J.M.; Cipresso, P.; Riva, G. Do not get lost in translation: The role of egocentric heading in spatial orientation. *Neurosci. Lett.* **2015**, *602*, 84–88. [CrossRef] [PubMed]

33. Ferrucci, R.; Serino, S.; Ruggiero, F.; Repetto, C.; Colombo, D.; Pedroli, E.; Marceglia, S.; Riva, G.; Priori, A. Cerebellar Transcranial Direct Current Stimulation (tDCS), Leaves Virtual Navigation Performance Unchanged. *Front. Neurosci.* **2019**, *13*. [CrossRef] [PubMed]
34. La Paglia, F.; La Cascia, C.; Rizzo, R.; Sideli, L.; Francomano, A.; La Barbera, D. Cognitive rehabilitation of schizophrenia through NeuroVR training. *Stud. Health Technol. Inform.* **2013**, *191*, 158–162. [PubMed]
35. Cipresso, P.; La Paglia, F.; La Cascia, C.; Riva, G.; Albani, G.; La Barbera, D. Break in volition: A virtual reality study in patients with obsessive-compulsive disorder. *Exp. Brain Res.* **2013**, *229*, 443–449. [CrossRef]
36. La Paglia, F.; La Cascia, C.; Rizzo, R.; Cangialosi, F.; Sanna, M.; Riva, G.; La Barbera, D. Cognitive assessment of OCD patients: NeuroVR vs neuropsychological test. *Stud. Health Technol. Inform.* **2014**, *199*, 40–44.
37. Van Bennekom, M.J.; Kasanmoentalib, M.S.; de Koning, P.P.; Denys, D. A virtual reality game to assess obsessive-compulsive disorder. *Cyberpsychol. Behav. Soc. Netw.* **2017**, *20*, 718–722. [CrossRef]
38. Bragdon, L.B.; Gibb, B.E.; Coles, M.E. Does neuropsychological performance in OCD relate to different symptoms? A meta-analysis comparing the symmetry and obsessing dimensions. *Depress. Anxiety* **2018**, *35*, 761–774. [CrossRef]
39. El Emam, K.; Moreau, K.; Jonker, E. How Strong are Passwords Used to Protect Personal Health Information in Clinical Trials? *J. Med. Internet Res.* **2011**, *13*, 13–22. [CrossRef]
40. Magni, E.; Binetti, G.; Bianchetti, A.; Rozzini, R.; Trabucchi, M. Mini-Mental State Examination: A normative study in Italian elderly population. *Eur. J. Neurol.* **1996**, *3*, 198–202. [CrossRef]
41. Monaco, M.; Costa, A.; Caltagirone, C.; Carlesimo, G.A. Forward and backward span for verbal and visuo-spatial data: Standardization and normative data from an Italian adult population. *Neurol. Sci.* **2012**, *34*, 749–754. [CrossRef]
42. Novelli, G.; Papagno, C.; Capitani, E.; Laiacona, M. Tre test clinici di memoria verbale a lungo termine: Taratura su soggetti normali. *Arch. Psicol. Neurol. Psichiatr.* **1986**, *47*, 278–296.
43. Appollonio, I.; Leone, M.; Isella, V.; Piamarta, F.; Consoli, T.; Villa, M.L.; Forapani, E.; Russo, A.; Nichelli, P. The Frontal Assessment Battery (FAB): Normative values in an Italian population sample. *Neurol. Sci.* **2005**, *26*, 108–116. [CrossRef] [PubMed]
44. Amodio, P.; Wenin, H.; Del Piccolo, F.; Mapelli, D.; Montagnese, S.; Pellegrini, A.; Musto, C.; Gatta, A.; Umiltà, C. Variability of trail making test, symbol digit test and line trait test in normal people. A normative study taking into account age-dependent decline and sociobiological variables. *Aging Clin. Exp. Res.* **2002**, *14*, 117–131. [CrossRef]
45. Allamanno, N.; Della Sala, S.; Laiacona, M.; Pasetti, C.; Spinnler, H. Problem solving ability in aging and dementia: Normative data on a non-verbal test. *Ital. J. Neurol. Sci.* **1987**, *8*, 111–119. [CrossRef]
46. Novelli, G.; Papagno, C.; Capitani, E.; Laiacona, M. Tre test clinici di ricerca e produzione lessicale. Taratura su sogetti normali. *Arch. Psicol. Neurol. Psichiatr.* **1986**, *47*, 477–506.
47. Riva, G.; Gaggioli, A.; Grassi, A.; Raspelli, S.; Cipresso, P.; Pallavicini, F.; Vigna, C.; Gagliati, A.; Gasco, S.; Donvito, G. NeuroVR 2-a free virtual reality platform for the assessment and treatment in behavioral health care. *Stud. Health Technol. Inform.* **2011**, *163*, 493–495.
48. Cipresso, P.; Serino, S.; Riva, G. Psychometric assessment and behavioral experiments using a free virtual reality platform and computational science. *BMC Med. Inform. Decis. Mak.* **2016**, *16*(1), 37. [CrossRef]
49. Raspelli, S.; Pallavicini, F.; Carelli, L.; Morganti, F.; Pedroli, E.; Cipresso, P.; Poletti, B.; Corra, B.; Sangalli, D.; Silani, V.; et al. Validating the Neuro VR-based virtual version of the Multiple Errands Test: Preliminary results. *Presence Teleoper. Virtual Environ.* **2012**, *21*, 31–42. [CrossRef]
50. Love, J.; Selker, R.; Marsman, M.; Jamil, T.; Dropmann, D.; Verhagen, A.J.; Wagenmakers, E.J. *JASP (Version 0.7.1.4)[Computer Software]*; JASP Project: Amsterdam, The Netherlands, 2015; Available online: https://jasp-stats.org (accessed on 16 October 2019).
51. Caruana, R.; Niculescu-Mizil, A. An empirical comparison of supervised learning algorithms. In Proceedings of the ACM 23rd International Conference on Machine Learning, Pittsburgh, PA, USA, 25 June 2006.
52. Suthaharan, S. Supervised Learning Algorithms. In *Machine Learning Models and Algorithms for Big Data Classification*; Springer: Berlin, Germany, 2016; pp. 183–206.
53. Wang, S.; Li, D.; Petrick, N.; Sahiner, B.; Linguraru, M.G.; Summers, R.M. Optimizing area under the ROC curve using semi-supervised learning. *Pattern Recognit.* **2015**, *48*, 276–287. [CrossRef]

54. Kotsiantis, S.B.; Zaharakis, I.; Pintelas, P. Supervised Machine Learning: A Review of Classification Techniques. 2007. Available online: https://datajobs.com/data-science-repo/Supervised-Learning-[SB-Kotsiantis].pdfURL (accessed on 16 October 2019).
55. Davis, J.; Goadrich, M. The relationship between Precision-Recall and ROC curves. In Proceedings of the ACM 23rd International Conference on Machine Learning, Pittsburgh, PA, USA, 25 June 2006.
56. Quinlan, J.R. Induction of decision trees. *Mach. Learn.* **1986**, *1*, 81–106. [CrossRef]
57. Wagacha, P.W. Induction of Decision Trees. *Foundations of Learning and Adaptive Systems.* 2003. Available online: https://www.researchgate.net/profile/Peter_Wagacha/publication/283569199_Instance_Based_Learning/links/563f951808ae34e98c4e723a/Instance-Based-Learning.pdfURL (accessed on 16 October 2019).
58. Sheth, N.; Deshpande, A. A Review of Splitting Criteria for Decision Tree Induction. *Fuzzy Syst.* **2015**, *7*, 1–4.
59. Cipresso, P. Modeling behavior dynamics using computational psychometrics within virtual worlds. *Front. Psychol.* **2015**, *6*, 1725. [CrossRef] [PubMed]
60. Macniven, J.A. *Neuropsychological Formulation: A Clinical Casebook*; Springer: Berlin, Germany, 2015.
61. Savage, G. Cognitive Neuropsychological Formulation. In *Neuropsychological Formulation*; Springer: Berlin, Germany, 2016; pp. 221–239.

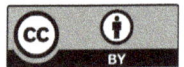

© 2019 by the authors. Licensee MDPI, Basel, Switzerland. This article is an open access article distributed under the terms and conditions of the Creative Commons Attribution (CC BY) license (http://creativecommons.org/licenses/by/4.0/).

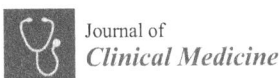

Review

Virtual Enactment Effect on Memory in Young and Aged Populations: A Systematic Review

Cosimo Tuena [1,*], Silvia Serino [2], Léo Dutriaux [3], Giuseppe Riva [1,4] and Pascale Piolino [5,6,7]

1. Applied Technology for Neuro-Psychology Lab, IRCCS Istituto Auxologico Italiano, 20149 Milan, Italy
2. MySpace Lab, Department of Clinical Neurosciences, University Hospital Lausanne (CHUV), CH-1011 Lausanne, Switzerland; silvia.serino@chuv.ch
3. Institute of Neuroscience and Psychology, University of Glasgow, Glasgow G12 8QB, UK; leo.dutriaux@glasgow.ac.uk
4. Department of Psychology, Catholic University of the Sacred Heart, 20123 Milan, Italy; giuseppe.riva@unicatt.it
5. Memory and Cognition Laboratory, Institute of Psychology, Paris Descartes University, Sorbonne Paris Cité, 92774 Boulogne-Billancourt, France; pascale.piolino@parisdescartes.fr
6. INSERM UMR S894, Center for Psychiatry and Neurosciences, 75014 Paris, France
7. Institut Universitaire de France (IUF), 75231 Paris, France
* Correspondence: cosimotuena@gmail.com; Tel.: +39-02-619112726

Received: 4 April 2019; Accepted: 2 May 2019; Published: 7 May 2019

Abstract: Background: Spatial cognition is a critical aspect of episodic memory, as it provides the scaffold for events and enables successful retrieval. Virtual enactment (sensorimotor and cognitive interaction) by means of input devices within virtual environments provides an excellent opportunity to enhance encoding and to support memory retrieval with useful traces in the brain compared to passive observation. Methods: We conducted a systematic review with Preferred Reporting Items for Systematic Reviews and Meta-Analysis (PRISMA) guidelines concerning the virtual enactment effect on spatial and episodic memory in young and aged populations. We aim at giving guidelines for virtual enactment studies, especially in the context of aging, where spatial and episodic memory decline. Results: Our findings reveal a positive effect on spatial and episodic memory in the young population and promising outcomes in aging. Several cognitive factors (e.g., executive function, decision-making, and visual components) mediate memory performances. Findings should be taken into account for future interventions in aging. Conclusions: The present review sheds light on the key role of the sensorimotor and cognitive systems for memory rehabilitation by means of a more ecological tool such as virtual reality and stresses the importance of the body for cognition, endorsing the view of an embodied mind.

Keywords: spatial memory; episodic memory; virtual reality; enactment; memory rehabilitation; embodied cognition; aging

1. Introduction

When we think of an event, we commonly see with our mind's eye where this event occurred and what temporal, perceptual, and affective details were associated with it; indeed, this spatial scaffold influences the specificity, richness, and vividness of events we retrieve from the memory [1]. When not defined in its schematic representation of the topography, this ability is considered as the ability to visualize the detailed spatial context (e.g., street, room, park) of specific episodes [2]. In its topographical definition, spatial memory [3] is a complex ability devoted to the encoding and storage of different types of information from our surroundings for successful orientation and navigation. Spatial information is represented and used in our brain with two frames of reference [4]:

egocentric (self-to-object) and allocentric (object-to-object), respectively located in the parietal and medial temporal regions with the retrosplenial cortex, playing a critical role in switching between these representations [5]. Spatial information can be divided into survey (e.g., maps, wayfinding, and pointing task), route (e.g., dynamic sequencing of landmarks), and landmark knowledge (e.g., landmark recognition) [6]. Survey knowledge refers to an allocentric map of the spatial layout, whereas route and landmark knowledge are based on an egocentric representation of the space.

On the other hand, episodic memory is a neurocognitive system that allows people to remember the *what*, *where*, and *when* of a personally experienced event [7]. Binding [8–10] is a key feature of this system; it is the process that binds the *what* with the other contextual features (i.e., *when*, *where*, and *details* such as perceptual and affective details). These elements are crucial for the so-called "autonoetic consciousness", or the feeling of mentally travelling back to the spatiotemporal and phenomenal features of the experienced event [7,11,12].

The hippocampus is known to play a crucial role in spatial cognition [4,13,14], episodic memory [15,16], and recognition [17]; this structure binds cognitive, bodily and emotional information [18–20] and connects to cortical representations facilitating the retrieval of episodes [21]. In particular, according to Nadel and colleagues [13,22] the hippocampus provides the allocentric spatial scaffold for episodes binding neocortical representations of the event (i.e., Multiple Trace Theory). The link between spatial cognition and episodic memory is also highlighted by the fact that egocentric spatial updating with self-motion cues (i.e., path integration of dynamic bodily signals) plays a critical role during retrieval (recall and recognition) of dynamically encoded scenes [23], confirming the role of egocentric information in manipulating and translating allocentric long-term representations of events [24,25]. Despite the crucial role of medial temporal lobes during encoding, storage, and retrieval [26], the parietal and frontal lobes have been also identified as a crucial substrate of episodic memory, absolving different declarative memory functions such as encoding, retrieval, storage, and monitoring [27–30] (for a meta-analysis of navigation and episodic memory brain network, see [31]).

Recent insights from philosophy, psychology, and neuroscience have drawn attention to the essential role of the body in cognition [32,33]. The framework known as the "embodied cognition" theory provided a fresh and innovative way to conceptualize the relationship between these two long-debated components of human psychology. Indeed, psychological processes are influenced by body morphology and sensorimotor systems [34]. There is growing interest and evidence on how the body affects several cognitive domains, including memory [35,36]. However, the concept of memory can be expanded to take into account the whole body as crucial in encoding, storage, and retrieval [37]. These assumptions have great relevance in the context of normal and pathological aging, where physiological changes modify regions of the brain involved in memory formation, leaving primary cortices spared [38–40].

Indeed, sensorimotor involvement may leave traces that are useful for memory retrieval [41–43], and encoding strategies are among the most effective methods to enhance memory [8]. The encoding specificity principle states that recollection is facilitated when an overlap occurs between the elements of the retrieval context and those of the encoding context [44]. Retrieval is possible thanks to a cue, and a memory trace is mediated by the same cognitive operations that occurred during encoding [45]. From a neuroanatomical point of view, there is growing theoretical and empirical evidence indicating how retrieval may be considered an overlapping process [46,47] that reactivates the same brain regions at encoding [21,48,49], including primary cortices [50–52].

Interestingly, active navigation in virtual environments (VEs) by means of input tools can be considered a form of enactment able to enhance spatial [41] and episodic [8] performance. According to Wilson and colleagues [53], active navigation in VEs can be divided into physical activity (motor control) and psychological activity (decision-making). More precisely, the manipulation of spatial information is not the only process involved in navigation; rather, motor commands, proprioceptive information, vestibular information, decision-making, and allocation of attentional resources are all also essential parts of what is called "active spatial learning" in everyday life, whereas passive navigation involves visual information only [6]. We define the virtual enactment effect as the effect provided by one or more of these components on memory retrieval compared to the virtual passive observation of the environment. Virtual reality (VR) allows individuals to interact with the environment thanks to multimodal stimulation, providing a rich embodied experience [54] that can be used to enhance memory in elders [55]. Indeed, technological devices (e.g., joysticks or 3D visors) require the subject to process psychological information, as well as idiothetic (i.e., motor commands, proprioception, and vestibular information) and allothetic information (e.g., landmarks and boundaries). The aim of this work is to review the potential of the virtual enactment effect (i.e., the role of active components of virtual navigation compared to passive observation) in order to contribute to a better understanding of its beneficial effect on spatial and episodic memory. This contribution will provide research and clinical guidelines for future studies within the context of VR memory rehabilitation and enhancement. In order to provide a complete overview of the results, we will cluster findings according to spatial memory (survey and route and landmark knowledge; respectively allocentric and egocentric frames) and episodic memory tasks (episodic features, such as *what*, *where*, *when*, *details*, and binding; episodic functioning, like learning, forgetting, and strategic processing; and item recognition).

2. Method

Preferred Reporting Items for Systematic Reviews and Meta-Analysis (PRISMA) guidelines were followed [56].

2.1. Search Strategy

Two high-profile databases (PubMed and Web of Science) were used to perform the computer-based research on the 25 January 2019. The string used to carry out the search (Title/Abstract for PubMed and Topic for Web of Science) was as follows: ("active" OR "enactment") AND ("spatial memory" OR "spatial knowledge" OR "episodic memory") AND ("virtual reality" OR "environment*"). The search resulted in 647 articles for Web of Science and 94 for PubMed (total of 741). We made a first selection by reading titles and abstracts after removing duplicates. Four papers were identified through other sources. A total of 35 manuscripts were chosen for full-text screening. This procedure resulted in 31 experimental studies. See the flow diagram (Figure 1) for the paper selection procedure.

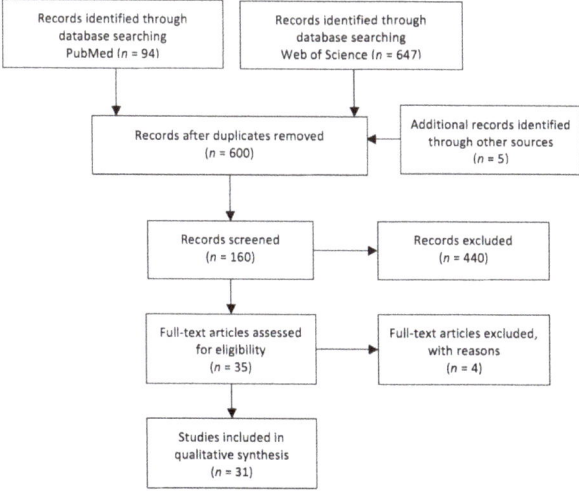

Figure 1. PRISMA flow chart.

2.2. Selection Criteria

Studies on the role of active navigation and enactment on spatial and episodic memory in young and aged populations (healthy and pathological) were included. We also included studies in languages other than English and excluded studies which did not follow our aims (non-age-related diseases, developmental studies, active- or passive-only conditions, active vs. passive conditions not related to the context of active navigation and action). We excluded articles for which the full text was not available or for which the abstract lacked basic information for review. Reviews, meeting abstracts, notes, case reports, letters to the editor, research protocols, patents, editorials and other editorial materials were also excluded. Five studies [57–61] did not appear during our search but were in line with our inclusion criteria; therefore, they were added to the included studies.

2.3. Quality Assessment and Data Abstraction

PRISMA guidelines were strictly followed; search results found by the first author (C.T.) were shared with the review authors for individual selection of papers in order to reduce the risk of bias, and disagreements were resolved through consensus. The data extracted from each included study were as follows: reference, year, sample(s), conditions, design (for the navigation condition), virtual apparatus, memory assessment, and primary outcomes.

3. Results

Several studies have been conducted to assess the role of active navigation in human memory. However, the growing interest in virtual reality (VR) has led researchers to question how the different aspects of navigation interact with the virtual environment. In particular, sensorimotor involvement, which is known for its positive effect on memory enhancement, seems to be one of the most investigated virtual enactment form. In our review, we aim at discovering whether this beneficial effect could also be observed when the subjects interact with technology devices.

To satisfy our aim, six clusters will be discussed: (1) the target population; (2) virtual apparatus; (3) conditions manipulated during navigation; (4) memory tasks; (5) the role of action and its effects on memory; and (6) cognitive domains underlying active navigation and memory performances. A synthesis of the results is reported in Table 1. Nine studies in Table 1 are reported with each sub-experiment; among these, only the experiments (e.g., Exp. 1, Exp. 2) that aim specifically at studying spatial or episodic memory appear in the table.

Table 1. Summary of the included studies. VE: virtual environment; HMD: head-mounted display; VR: virtual reality; OA: older adults; YA: young adults; aMCI: amnestic mild cognitive impairment; AD: Alzheimer's disease; HNC: high navigation control; IC: itinerary control; LNC: low navigation control; Exp.: experiment; //: same as above; 1A: first trial apartment; 2A: second trial apartment; B: third trial apartment.

Ref.	Sample (s)	Conditions	Design (Navigation)	Virtual Apparatus	Memory Assessment	Primary Outcomes
[62]	48 YA (age range: 21–38; 24 males)	Effect of active (no decisional level) vs. passive (prerecorded travel) vs. snapshot exploration (static condition) on scene recognition and memory of displacements. Intentional encoding.	Within	Non-immersive (CaTS driving simulator); input device: joystick.	Scene recognition (route snapshots); Pointing toward the origin test using the joystick; drawing test (shape of the path).	Path shape task benefitted from active condition, whereas recognition and pointing task were not affected by the exploring conditions.
[41] Exp. 1	30 YA (mean age = 27.1; 14 males)	Effect of active vs. passive (recorded navigation) navigation on spatial memory. No intentional encoding. Participants could freely navigate the apartment.	Between (yoked)	Non-immersive; input device: joystick; house apartment navigation.	Spatial layout test (spatial layout drawing of the VE); recall test (location and objects name on VE map).	Active group showed better spatial layout scores. No effect on recall test.
[41] Exp. 2	40 YA (mean age = 26; 18 males)	Effect of active vs. passive (recorded navigation) navigation on spatial memory. No intentional encoding. Participants could freely navigate the apartment.	//	Non-immersive; input device: joystick; house apartment navigation.	Spatial layout test (spatial layout drawing of the VE); recognition task (objects); object location test.	Spatial layout recall replicated for active condition. No effect on other tasks.
[63]	30 YA (age range = 18–30) and 30 OA (age range = 58–72)	Role of active vs. passive (pre-recorded video) motor exploration on spatial memory and wayfinding. Intentional encoding. No decision-making.	Between	Non-immersive; input device: joystick; virtual replica of Bordeaux.	Wayfinding task (replication of the path; use of spatial representation, errors and stops were calculated); spatial memory task (map drawing + picture classification; route and survey representations).	Active condition worsened survey knowledge (spatial map) in both groups, led to better wayfinding scores in YA and worsened in OA. Executive functions have a crucial role during active navigation.
[64] Exp. 1	22 undergraduates (14 males)	Exploring the role of motion control (VE tour) vs. passive condition (VE tour) on spatial learning. Intentional encoding (learning phase before test phase). Navigation instructions were given.	Between	Non-immersive; input device: keyboard; VE of a research lab.	Spatial learning test (indicate position and direction of egocentric pictures on a lab map; object location test).	View positioning test was better for active participants, no significant difference between the conditions was observed for object location task. Active navigation contributes partially to survey representation.
[64] Exp. 2	80 undergraduates (49 males)	Exploring the role of optical flow (action with object in active condition) vs. passive navigation vs. static condition on spatial learning between active. Intentional encoding (learning phase before test phase). Navigation instructions were given.	//	Non-immersive; input device: keyboard; VE of a research lab.	Spatial learning test (indicate position and direction of egocentric pictures on a lab map; object location test).	Active participants performed better in object locations task and passive condition performed better than static condition. No difference among the conditions was observed for the first task.
[65] Exp. 1	82 university students (age range: 19–33; 43 males)	Effect of intentional vs. incidental encoding vs. active vs. passive navigation (observing the participant navigating) on spatial memory. Auditory route instructions were given (no decision-making).	Between (yoked)	Non-immersive; input devices: keyboard and mouse; virtual city.	Spatial memory test (landmark recognition task, pointing task and path-sketching, route navigation task; respectively, landmark, survey and route knowledge).	Active navigation led to better landmark and route knowledge performances. No effect on survey knowledge. No effect of encoding.

Table 1. Cont.

Ref.	Sample (s)	Conditions	Design (Navigation)	Virtual Apparatus	Memory Assessment	Primary Outcomes
[65] Exp. 2	88 university students (age range: 18–33; 10 males)	Effect of movement (active navigation vs. passive) vs. instruction control (instructing vs. listening vs. instruction specificity (landmark information vs. layout information) on spatial memory. Navigation instructions were written (no decision-making).	//	Non-immersive; input devices: keyboard and mouse; apartment with rooms.	Spatial memory test (landmark recognition task, tour integration task, route navigation task).	Landmark knowledge, tour integration and route knowledge benefited from self-contained condition. Effect on performance was mediate by instruction specificity and control in the latest task.
[65] Exp. 3	102 students (age range: 19–41; 21 males)	Effect of active vs. passive navigation vs. decision-making (map) vs. less decision-making (map with suggested path) vs. no-map condition on spatial memory. Participants were asked to find the shortest possible route.	//	Non-immersive; input devices: keyboard and mouse; apartment with rooms.	Spatial memory test (landmark recognition task and tour integration task; route navigation task).	Active navigation led to better landmark recognition performance. Decision-making helped participants in observed movement condition and less decision-making worsened route knowledge.
[66]	24 undergraduates (age range: 18–21; 7 males)	Effect of active free navigation (with decision-making) vs. passive on object-memory. Intentional encoding.	Between (yoked)	Non-immersive; input device: keyboard; virtual city.	Object task (locate objects) and recognition task.	No difference between the two conditions in the tasks.
[53] Exp. 1	72 undergraduates (age range: 18–27; 22 males)	Effect of psychological activity (decision-making vs. no decision-making on directions) and physical activity (motor control vs. no motor control on keyboard) vs. control group on spatial performance. No intentional encoding (explore VE).	Between	Non-immersive; input device: keyboard; virtual city.	Orientation task (direction test + map drawing).	No difference was observed between the conditions manipulated.
[53] Exp. 2	36 undergraduates (age range: 18–42)	Effect of active exploration vs. passive observation of navigation vs. control (no exploration of VE) on wayfinding. No intentional encoding (explore VE).	Between	Non-immersive; input device: keyboard; virtual arena.	Wayfinding task.	No difference was observed between the conditions manipulated.
[67]	18 YA (age range: 20–39; 9 males)	Effect of active (with decision-making) vs. passive dynamic (recorded video) vs. passive static (slide-like scenes) free exploration on spatial layout performances. Intentional encoding.	Within	Non-immersive; input device: joystick; virtual arena with cubes.	Target location test (8 trials; score, time, orientation and verbal or drawing description of the strategies used to reach a given target were calculated).	Active participants performed better than the two passive conditions in the task (scores, time, verbal and layout descriptions but no orientation task). Active motor behaviour with active perception is crucial to extract invariants in the VE.
[68]	30 YA (age range = 18–25) and 30 OA (age range = 60–81)	Active (with decision-making) vs. passive (computer-guided tour) free navigation effects on memory for everyday objects. Intentional encoding.	Between	Non-immersive; input devices: keyboard and mouse; VR-based Human Objects Memories from Everyday Scenes (HOMES).	Free recall and recognition (learning, proactive interference, semantic clustering, recognition hits, and false recognitions). VE 1A followed by free recall task + VE 2A followed by recognition task.	Active navigation had a beneficial effect on recognition hits only, in both YA and OA compared with passive mode. Active mode reduced false recognitions in YA but increased these in OA. Active navigation enhanced memory in older adults when is not demanding.

Table 1. Cont.

Ref.	Sample (s)	Conditions	Design (Navigation)	Virtual Apparatus	Memory Assessment	Primary Outcomes
[69]	44 students (mean age = 21.94, SD = 2.13; 21 males)	Active (with decision-making) vs. passive (computer-guided tour) free navigation effects on memory for everyday objects. Intentional encoding.	Between	Non-immersive; input devices: keyboard and mouse; VR-based HOMES.	Free recall and recognition (learning, proactive interference, semantic clustering, recognition hits, and false recognitions). VE 1A followed by free recall task + VE 2A followed by free recall task + VE B followed by recognition task.	Active navigation led to better recognition hits performances compared to passive condition. Active participants had less source-based false recognitions compared with passive participants. Active navigation was useful to enrich visuomotor details of episodic memory traces but had no effect on semantic relational processing.
[9] Exp. 3	41 participants (age range: 18–34, 12 males)	Active vs. passive (recorded actions; no motor response) selection affects memory for object. Intentional encoding. Instructions.	Between	Non-immersive; input device: keyboard; WWW (what–where–when) variation built with Second Life arena.	Object name cued recall (full episodic recall: *what* + *where* + *when*; non-episodic: *where* + *what* or *where* + *what* or *what* only).	Active condition reduced distractor encoding compared to the passive viewing of the action of the avatar.
[43]	72 Psychology students (mean age = 22.23, SD = 3.94; 36 males)	Interaction condition (motor trace in memory, no decision on itinerary) vs. planning condition (no control of the vehicle; decisional level) vs. passive (recorded video). Intentional encoding.	Between	Non-immersive; input devices: steering wheel and pedals; virtual city.	Free recall of elements; visuospatial memory test (draw map + locate elements); visuospatial cued recall (locate elements on a prepared map); recognition test (elements, locations and navigation directions after seeing the elements).	Interaction enhanced memory recall, in particular spatial memory recall (no effect on influence on visuospatial cued recall or recognition); however, interaction worsened elements recognition compared with passive condition; planning condition boosted visuospatial recalls. Both interaction and planning had an effect on episodic memory.
[70]	21 healthy OA (4 males), 15 aMCI (7 males) and 15 AD (2 males)	Active vs. passive (recorded video) encoding influences episodic memory. Intentional encoding. Predetermined route.	Between	Non-immersive; input devices: steering wheel and pedals; two virtual cities.	Immediate free recall (*what*, *details*, *when*, egocentric *where*, allocentric *where*, binding); recognition (elements, spatial and temporal relations between elements; remember/know paradigm); delayed free recall (same as immediate free recall).	Active exploration led in OA, aMCI, and AD groups to better recall of elements, allocentric spatial information and binding. Procedural skills and self-involvement may be crucial for episodic performances in aMCI and AD patients.
[71]	113 psychology students (mean age = 21.57, SD = 2.99) and 45 OA	Effect of active vs. passive navigation and intentional vs. incidental encoding on episodic memory. Intentional encoding. Predetermined route.	Between	Non-immersive; input devices: steering wheel and pedals; virtual city.	Free recall (*what*, verbal *where*, visuospatial *where*, *when*, *details*); recognition test (elements).	Encoding conditions affect differently episodic features in YA and OA. However, any effect due to sensorimotor implication emerged in the study.
[8]	64 YA and 64 OA (32 males)	HNC (real-life driving conditions) vs. LNC (only pedals; no enactment associated with direction) vs. IC (verbal instructions without driving; decisional level only) vs. passive (no driving no decision) effect on episodic memory performance. Intentional encoding.	Between	Non-immersive; input devices: steering wheel and pedals; virtual city.	Immediate free recall (*what* and *details*; binding: *what* + *where* + *when*; remember/know paradigm) visuospatial recall test (*what*, *where*, *when* on real map); delayed free recall test (*what*, *details*, *where*, and *when*); recognition test (elements).	Binding, regardless of age-groups, was enhanced by LNC and IC; HNC and passive conditions did not help episodic memory performance in both groups. Interestingly, Remember responses were boosted in older adults by IC condition. Active condition may be helpful when do not overload cognitive resources.
[72]	90 students (average age of 20; 45 males)	Passive VE (recorded route) vs. active VE vs. real environment (navigate the environment with instructions) and immediate vs. 48-h recall. Predetermined route.	Between	Non-immersive; input device: joystick; virtual replica of the Bordeaux area.	Immediate or 48-h recall task: real world wayfinding (replication of the real route), freehand sketch (directional changes) and photograph classification (picture in chronological order).	Transfer and sketch task are efficient after 48 h of retention and it is efficient for the two paper-pencil tasks. Active navigation led to benefits in wayfinding task, irrespective of the delay retention.

Table 1. Cont.

Ref.	Sample (s)	Conditions	Design (Navigation)	Virtual Apparatus	Memory Assessment	Primary Outcomes
[73]	59 YA (age range: 19–29; 19 males)	Effect of active vs. passive free exploration on object recognition in VEs.	Between	Immersive; input device: keyboard; virtual rooms with objects.	Recognition task (objects).	Active navigation led to higher hit and lower miss responses than the passive condition. Active navigation has an important role in landmark recognition.
[74] Exp. 1	32 YA (age range: 18–34; 16 males)	Active vs. passive free navigation with four trials with different virtual maze.	Between	Non-immersive with static navigation; input devices: keyboard and mouse; virtual maze.	"Active" test: number of moves and time.	Navigational knowledge is represented regardless the kind of exploration condition.
[58]	20 male students (age range: 20–26)	Active (self-governed) vs. passive (avatar-guided) free exploration. Four exploring sessions. Intentional encoding.	Between	Immersive (HMD); input device: joystick; virtual school.	Wayfinding task (short route to starting point); pointing task (orienting to the starting point); sketch-map (local accuracy or survey-type organization).	Self-governed explorers were better in completing the wayfinding task. Sketch-map accuracy was similar in both groups, whereas self-governed group had better survey-type organization. No differences were shown in pointing task. Self-governed participants organize their knowledge in survey mode.
[75]	34 YA (age range: 18–38; 7 males)	Active vs. passive (passenger condition) condition. Participants were before divided in driver and non-drivers. Intentional encoding and decision-making.	Between	Non-immersive: input devices: steering wheel and pedals; virtual city.	Survey knowledge: pointing error scores (street-level view) and map placement error scores (bird's eye view); route knowledge: route scores (shortest route).	Driver had better route scores during active navigation compared with drivers in passive and non-driver in active conditions. Drivers showed better map scores (no condition effect). Active navigators do not learn more spatial layout knowledge and dual task effect may affect scores in non-drivers.
[59]	54 students (9 males)	Active vs. passive (passenger condition). Three exposures (3, 10, or 15 times). No intentional encoding. Predetermined path.	Between (yoked)	Non-immersive: input devices: steering wheel and pedals; virtual city.	Survey knowledge (map sketch drawing and map rates' score), route knowledge (travel directions) and landmark knowledge (landmarks recall).	Passengers recalled more landmarks across exposure conditions. Survey errors reduced between 5 and 15 times in both conditions. Exposure led to better map reliability especially for the passive condition. Attentional resources could have led to worst performance in active drivers.
[76] Exp. 3	41 undergraduates (age range: 18–24; 20 males)	VE active vs. VE passive (watch experimenter navigation) vs. VE + line (active with path to follow; no free exploration) vs. control (no VE training; real-world wayfinding).	Between	Non-immersive. Input device: keyboard; virtual replica of an office.	Real world transfer task (balloons wayfinding times and errors from virtual to real places); training task (wayfinding time and errors in VE conditions).	Times for active condition were lower compared with control condition and active and VE + line led to fewer errors than control condition. Virtual real transfer occurs thanks to virtual interaction.

Table 1. Cont.

Ref.	Sample (s)	Conditions	Design (Navigation)	Virtual Apparatus	Memory Assessment	Primary Outcomes
[50]	64 students (average age of 20; 32 males)	Ground vs. areal point of view and active vs. passive navigation. Predetermined route	Between	Non-immersive; input device: joystick; virtual replica of the Bordeaux area.	Real-world wayfinding task (replication of the real route; error scores); sketch-drawing task (directional changes; errors and omissions scores) and scene-sorting task (errors).	Active navigation boosted sketch-mapping task and worsened wayfinding and picture-sorting scores. Grounded-level condition improved performance in wayfinding and picture-sorting tasks, whereas aerial-level in sketch-mapping task. Active navigation and grounded-level interaction had a positive effect in the wayfinding and picture-sorting tasks, whereas passive and aerial-level condition improved sketch-mapping scores. Egocentric information and motor information create a correct perception-action coupling.
[77]	64 students (average age of 20; 32 males)	Detailed vs. undetailed visual fidelity and active vs. passive navigation. Predetermined route.	Between	Non-immersive; input device: joystick; virtual replica of the Bordeaux area.	Real-world wayfinding task (replication of the real route; errors and hesitations scores), sketch-mapping task (directional changes; errors and omissions scores), and scene-sorting task (errors).	Results highlighted better performance for each spatial task in both active and detailed condition. Interaction effect (active and detailed) led to better scores for sketch task and active condition combined with undetailed VE worsened scene-sorting task. Perceptual-motor information is crucial in spatial knowledge. Visual fidelity has positive effect for allocentric representation but not for route knowledge.
[78] Exp. 1 & 2	28 students (age range: 18–23; 9 males)	Active exploration (experiment 1) vs. passive exploration (experiment 2; video of active exploration). Predetermined route of familiar environment.	Between	Non-immersive; input device: keyboard; university building.	Orientation test trials of external cues from four virtual rooms (internal visited and unvisited, external visited and unvisited).	There is no difference in the two conditions.
[78] Exp. 3	54 visitors (mean age = 17.55, SD = 1.14; 19 males)	Active exploration vs. passive exploration. Predetermined route of unfamiliar environment.	Between	Non-immersive; input device: keyboard; university building.	Orientation test trials of external cues from four virtual rooms (internal visited and unvisited, external visited and unvisited).	No effect of unfamiliarity for active participants. Passive participants had greater error for the internal unvisited room. Active exploration enhances survey knowledge for unfamiliar environments.
[79]	60 adults (mean age = 25.2, SD = 4.5; males 49)	Active exploration vs. passive exploration (video of passive exploration) and immersive vs. computer screen. Predetermined rout of Gowanus canal. Intentional encoding. An allocentric map of the canal was provided in all conditions.	Within	Immersive (Emotiv EPOC headset) and non-immersive; input device: mouse and headset gyroscope; Gowanus Canal.	Elements recognition task	No difference between the two navigation conditions. However, active navigation with the mouse has higher level of engagement.

Table 1. Cont.

Ref.	Sample (s)	Conditions	Design (Navigation)	Virtual Apparatus	Memory Assessment	Primary Outcomes
[80] Exp. 1 and 2		3D active exploration (Exp. 1) vs. 2D passive snapshots presentation (Exp. 2). Free exploration and intentional encoding.	Between	Immersive (nVisor SX111) and non-immersive; input device: Wiimote; virtual apartment.	Search trials of geometric and contextual objects.	Search task improved in both conditions but in the immersive condition initial fixations and time spent in the incorrect rooms and better selection of the correct room indicate higher use of memory.
[83]	28 YA (mean age = 25.6, SD = 5.4; 17 males)	Active navigation vs. passive navigation (video). Immediate (intentional encoding) and 24 h delayed (naïve) recall. Participants could freely navigate the environment.	Between	Non-immersive; input device: keyboard and mouse; virtual city.	Immediate and delayed free recall of semantically linked images of 3D objects placed in the town.	No effect of navigation types on spatial memory.
[57]	14 YA (mean age = 22, SD = 2.08; 7 males)	Full condition (full control over the navigation) vs. medium condition (participants move but do not control pre-recorded navigation) vs. low condition (watch pre-recorded navigation).	Within	Immersive (Oculus Rift DK2); input device: Kinect for legs and arms movement detection; virtual city.	Immediate free recall (*what*, egocentric *where*, *details*, *when*, *binding*) and item recognition (source memory, remember/know/guess paradigm), egocentric, allocentric and temporal recognition.	Any significance was found among the conditions. However, the full and medium (virtual embodiment) conditions were more immersive than the passive one.
[82]	16 students (females = 16)	Active navigation vs. passive (watching the navigation of the active participant). Free exploration.	Between (yoked)	Non-immersive (46-inch touchscreen monitor); input device: joystick; virtual rooms	Immediate memory recognition for objects manipulated in each room).	Both passive and active navigation had a significant negative effect on memory of object, with active navigation having a greater effect compared to passive.
[61]	22 YA (mean age = 19.71, SD = 2.19; females = 11) and 22 OA (mean age = 74.55, SD = 7.82; females = 10)	Active navigation vs. passive. Free exploration.	Within (yoked)	Immersive (cardboard) mobile application (input device: button headset and head movements); VE (city, park, mall)	Encoding-Retrieval route overlap accuracy	Active encoding leads to better spatial memory in OA; accuracy is predicted by age, active exploration and visuospatial abilities.

290

3.1. What Populations Have Been Included?

From our systematic search, it emerged that the majority of the experiments included healthy participants, mainly young adults (YA), but also older adults (OA). Studies focused on spatial domain; however, a cluster of seven studies investigated episodic memory and its subcomponents in healthy populations (YA and OA). Nevertheless, age ranges varied across the studies for YA and OA, and for the "student" samples the age information was vague. Importantly, in six studies no gender information [53,63,68,71] or matching [58,82] were reported. Only one study recruited clinical populations of Alzheimer's disease (AD) pathology: 15 AD patients and 15 amnestic mild cognitive impairment (aMCI) patients compared to 21 healthy OA were included in the study of Plancher and colleagues [70] to assess the effect of active and passive virtual navigation on episodic performance. A synthesis of populations (YA, OA, AD, and aMCI), with mean age and standard deviation and number of males/females, is reported in Table 1.

3.2. What Virtual Apparatus Have Been Used?

For the purposes of our review, it is essential to summarize the apparatus been used in each experiment. Ecological virtual environments (VEs) have been used to assess the virtual enactment effect regardless of the domain (spatial or episodic memory); specifically, cities or apartments were used to evaluate the effect of active interaction (e.g., input device interaction)—namely, the "virtual enactment effect"—on memory recall, while four experiments [9,53,67,74] used basic virtual scenarios with poor ecological validity (e.g., virtual arenas). Concerning the input devices, researchers mainly used joysticks and keyboards to navigate the VEs, whereas five studies used a steering wheel and pedals to control a virtual car. The use of these controllers is linked to the type of immersion; indeed, the vast majority of the experiments' apparatus were non-immersive (PC screen or projectors). Only six experiments [57,58,61,73,79,80] used head-mounted display (HMD) to assess the role of active navigation on spatial performances and only one study used immersive virtual reality to assess the effect of full body involvement during encoding on episodic retrieval.

3.3. What are the Navigation Conditions in the Included Studies?

In the following paragraph, studies will be discussed in terms of navigation condition, degree of decision-making, and type of encoding. Active navigation studies used classic dynamic navigation, whereas non-dynamic navigation (e.g., snapshots or teleporting) were added as the comparison condition [62,67,80]. The former might be more suitable compared to static navigation if we consider the role of constant mapping provided by the hippocampus (i.e., place cells) in building the map of the environment [83]. Passive navigation in the studies included in the review consisted of a yoked condition or pre-recorded navigations. Navigational decision-making, or free exploration, is another crucial aspect of active navigation and spatial knowledge [84]; however, in 17 experiments [9,59–65,70–72,77–79], researchers gave a predetermined route or instructions to follow. Moreover, decision-making is a crucial aspect of the virtual enactment effect when older participants are involved in active navigation [8] due to overload on the frontal lobes and the executive functions capacity on memory encoding [68], which are known to decline with aging [85]. Indeed, Jebara and colleagues [8] found that navigational decision-making, intended as a form of virtual enactment effect, is more effective in OA compared to the active motor condition due to executive function overload at encoding [8,63,68]. Another aspect to consider is the point of view (areal vs. egocentric). The egocentric point of view along combined with the active motor condition improves allocentric and egocentric memory, whereas the areal point of view with passive navigation improves allocentric memory only [60]. Graphic realism when building VEs should take into account the fact that a detailed environment positively affects memory performances [77]. Other elements that neuroscientists in the field of VR and memory should consider are the type of encoding (incidental vs. intentional); although the authors of [62] showed no effect of encoding, in our review intentional encoding leads to better performance across the populations and the type of memory assessed [8,9,43,58,59,67–70,75,80]. Crucially, only one study [72] compared active VR vs. passive VR vs. real-world navigation, with real-world navigation and active VR leading to better spatial recall, in this order, compared to passive VR. Lastly, from a methodological point of view, researchers are encouraged to evaluate the consequences of using between or within condition. In our review, the majority of the studies included between navigation conditions, while only five studies [57,61,62,67,79] used within conditions. Researchers should consider strengths and weaknesses of within and between designs with potential biases in the light of the objectives of their study [86], as explained in the discussion paragraph.

3.4. How Has Memory Performance Been Measured?

Several VEs (cities, rooms, mazes, and arenas) were used in the reviewed experiments in order to test two main memory clusters: spatial memory and episodic memory (event and object memory). The evaluation included for spatial memory tasks involved survey knowledge (maps, pointing and wayfinding tasks), route knowledge (chronological order tasks), and item recognition/recall for landmark knowledge (see Table 1 for a summary of these tasks).

To investigate the role of active navigation in episodic memory, six studies used a similar navigation paradigm in a virtual city in which events occurred [10,43,57,70,71]. Participants were tested on events encountered, landmarks and spatial layout of the cities. These paradigms aim at assessing *what*, *where* (egocentric and allocentric), *when*, *details*, and binding among elements in ecological VEs with free recall, delayed recall, and recognition. Laurent et al. [9] studied the different components of episodic memory; a variation of the WWW (*what–when–where*) task was used in order to study the binding of contextual aspects to objects. Finally, Sauzéon and colleagues [68,69] used free recall (learning, proactive interference, semantic clustering based on the California Verbal Learning Test (CVLT) [87]) and a recognition task (recognition hits and false recognitions); object recognition memory was also used to assess event memory in Pettijohn and Radvansky [82]. Interestingly, Pacheco and Verschure [81] assessed their samples on an immediate and delayed free recall task of images semantically associated with an object they found in the virtual town. For a summary of these tasks, see Table 1.

3.5. Do "Virtual" Actions Have a "Real" Effect on Spatial and Episodic Memory?

In the following subsection, memory performance will be clustered by the different components taken into consideration in the included study of the review: spatial memory, episodic memory, and recognition memory of both spatial and episodic studies (Figure 2). The Primary Outcomes column in Table 1 provides in detail the virtual enactment effect on each task/measure. Using the correct task to target specific sub-components is crucial for the researchers; we suggest future research to put effort into designing and conceptualizing the task and test method to tap memory processes. In the present review, we found a general positive effect of virtual enactment in young adults for spatial memory; however, further studies need to assess this in older adults as spatial enhancement in OA is controversial [61,63]. In particular for spatial scores in aging, active navigation involving an overloading task during encoding affected retrieval [63]; decision-making in active navigation appeared to be more suitable in this sample [8].

Similarly, experiments investigating episodic memory showed initial support for a virtual enactment effect in young adults (Figure 2); although findings are few, encouraging results come from studies of neurodegenerative conditions that may benefit from virtual enactment, whereas non-spatial features of episodic memory are influenced by demanding tasks during encoding (Figure 2). These findings could also confirm the embodied nature of episodic memory as a cognitive and bodily experience [18,20,35,88–90].

Initial recognition scores in spatial and memory performance results are controversial and need further investigation. Although past research on enactment showed a positive effect on recognition memory [91], recognition scores in spatial and memory performance results are controversial. A possible explanation for this could be that recognition occurs in the brain at different degrees [92,93] such as visual recognition, guessing (Guess responses), familiarity (Know responses), and source recognition and recollection (Remember responses); the latter, with source memory, is thought to be related to recollective aspects of episodic memory linked with autonoesis and full detailed recall. As a consequence, it is important to adopt a recognition paradigm that is able to grasp perceptual and sensory elements of the memory traces at retrieval.

No effect was found in these spatial studies [53,66,74,78,79], and on episodic memory scores (*what*, verbal *where*, visuospatial *where*, *when*, and *details* in the works of Plancher et al. [71] and Tuena and colleagues [57]), or on object recognition memory in the work of Pacheco and Verschure [81]. Finally, although results are encouraging, some studies showed passive enhancement (see Figure 2); therefore, results of the review are preliminary, and future studies need to deepen the virtual enactment effect in order to confirm the enhancing effect from which different populations might benefit.

It is well known that active navigation promotes better learning performance [6]. We found confirmations of how the body shapes memories and how it can be used as a medium to enhance learning by means of input tools as an extension of previous research on the enactment effect with ecological scenarios and items [42,88,94,95].

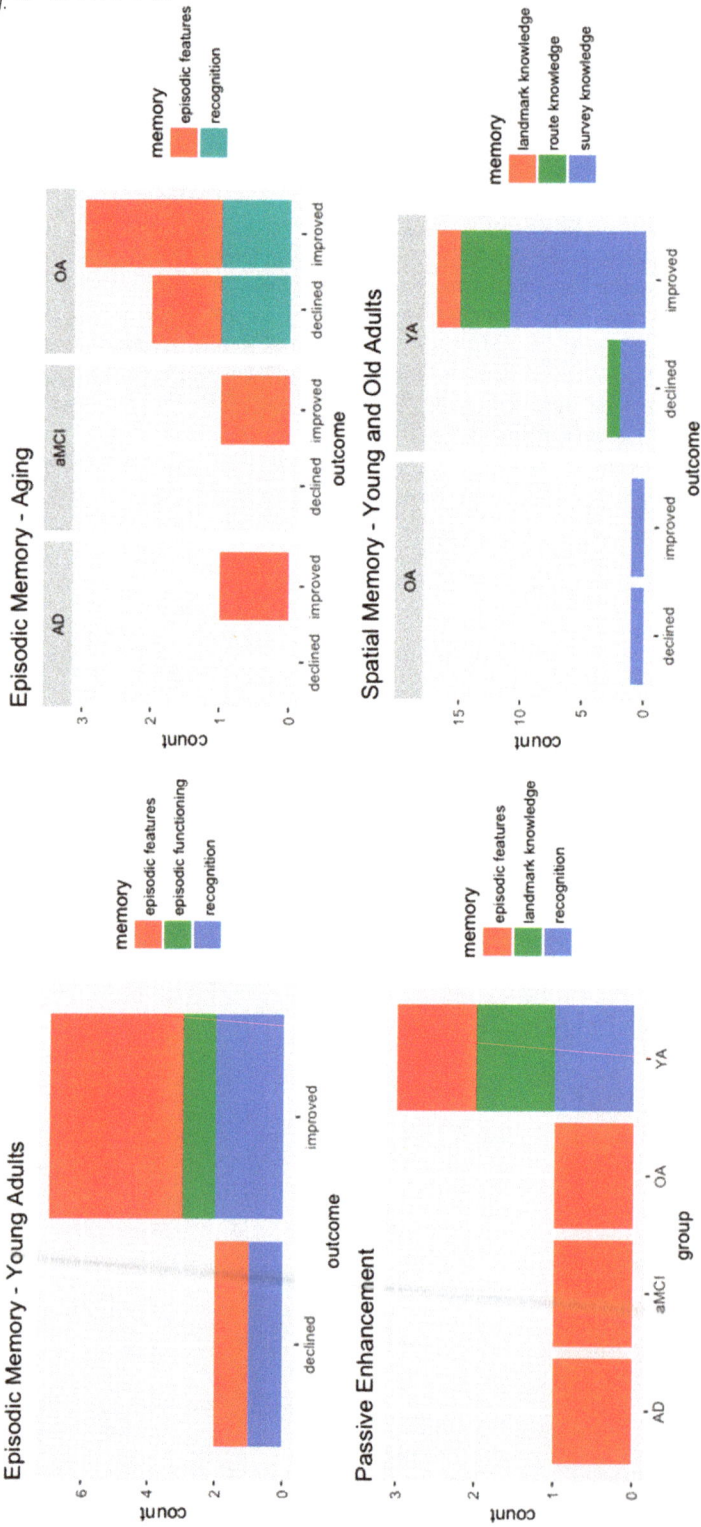

Figure 2. Summary of virtual enactment effect and passive enhancement in the samples. YA: young adults; OA: older adults; aMCI: amnestic mild cognitive impairment; AD: Alzheimer's disease.

3.6. What Are the Cognitive Factors Mediating Active Navigation and Memory Performance?

Among the included studies, cognitive factors underlying navigation have been studied in the same healthy population [74], whereas neuropsychological factors were used to evaluate the effect of active navigation on memory in YA vs. OA [8,63]. In particular, visuospatial abilities and especially executive function seem to be crucial for spatial memory [63,74] and for episodic memory functioning [68] and features [70,71]; in particular, executive function and attention appear to influence performance [8,69].

Cutmore et al. [74] conducted four experiments in order to evaluate the effect of gender, visuospatial abilities, cognitive style, and cerebral asymmetry during static active navigation (teleporting). Males showed faster results in finding the exit of the virtual maze compared with females, while both groups benefited from a landmark cue condition (landmark associated with a room). Moreover, males were more accurate; in this case, a compass cue condition (compass heading cue) led to better performance compared to a landmark condition. Visuospatial abilities were evaluated with the Wechsler Adult Intelligence Scale—Revised (WAIS-R) [96]. The high visuospatial group was better at Euclidean (survey knowledge) distance estimation compared with the low group. Participants' cognitive styles (verbal-sequential vs. visuospatial) were evaluated with the same test. The visuospatial group showed better navigation performance; moreover, this effect was shown for static navigation when compared with verbal-sequential participants. The visuospatial group was also better in navigating the maze backward. Finally, Cutmore and colleagues [74] used electroencephalography to observe cerebral asymmetry: the verbal-sequential group showed a greater right hemisphere activation (effort computing spatial problem solving) compared with the visuospatial group. However, only females were recruited for the last three experiments, since a gender effect was found in the second experiment. The authors wanted to evaluate whether navigation is related to superior spatial skills in a sample of females, but von Stülpnagel [88] found that sense of orientation abilities affected false alarms and route navigation performance regardless of gender.

Taillade et al. [63] found that YA were better than OA in terms of executive function, visuospatial abilities, and memory. In particular, wayfinding tasks (survey knowledge) seemed to be affected by executive function. Jebara et al. [8] correlated the binding scores with age and neuropsychological tests. An effect of age was found in all the navigation conditions. Binding score was significantly correlated with visual memory and working memory in high navigation control (HNC; motor trace and decision-making), low navigation control (LNC; motor trace only), and itinerary condition (IC; decision-making only) conditions. Shifting (executive function) negatively affected the VR binding scores for LNC and HNC but not for the passive condition and IC. When controlling for age, the scores in HNC were still significantly affected by executive function. Verbal memory correlated positively only with the IC condition. Similarly, Sauzéon and colleagues found a positive correlation between recognition hits and episodic memory (CVLT [87]) and executive function (mental rotation and Stroop color-word task; [97,98]) in the active but not the passive navigation condition. Total false recognitions (source-based and gist-based) were correlated with episodic memory and executive function tests. An age effect on false recognition was also found. In particular, executive function, after partial correlation between age and false recognitions, contributed to recognition performance under the active navigation condition [68].

It is also worth reporting that cognitive differences among the populations emerged in terms of gender, age and pathology. Plancher and colleagues [70] found differences among individuals with AD, aMCI, and OA in their episodic memory task. The same performance pattern (AD < aMCI < OA) emerged for *what*, *details*, egocentric and allocentric *where*, and recognition. AD and aMCI individuals had less recollection compared to controls. AD patients' binding was lower than that of aMCI patients and OA, whereas aMCI patients had a delayed recall deficit compared to OA. *When* scores were lower for the AD group compared with the aMCI group and OA, while AD and aMCI individuals presented a difference between immediate and delayed recall. Moreover, the authors found better *what* recognition in OA, aMCI, and AD compared to other episodic recognitions. Plancher and colleagues found that

AD and aMCI patients had worse recognition than OA; similarly, OA performed better in terms of recollection rates than aMCI and AD.

Tasks revealed an age effect in different studies [8,61,63,71,80] as well as a gender effect [43,65,80]. The findings of Jebara and co-authors [8] revealed an age effect for *what* (immediate and delayed), binding (immediate and delayed), visuospatial recall, and recognition total score. An age effect on spatial memory and recognition was found by other studies. Sauzéon and co-authors [68] showed that OA have worse learning, proactive interference, and false recognition compared with YA. Taillade and colleagues [63] found that YA fared better in a wayfinding task than OA, but this pattern did not emerge for spatial memory tasks. An age effect emerged in the first study of Plancher and colleagues [71]. Young participants were better compared to OA in terms of verbal and visuospatial *where*, *when*, and *details*. Moreover, findings showed a main effect of intentional encoding for *what*, verbal *where*, visuospatial *where*, *when*, and *details*. In an active navigation condition, OA had better *what* recall in incidental encoding, while YA had better recognition, *when*, verbal *where*, and visuospatial *where* on intentional encoding compared with OA. Finally, Plancher and co-authors [56] found that women performed better (statistical tendency) on the recognition task, whereas men had better scores for the cued visuospatial task. No effect of condition emerged. Von Stülpnagel and Steffens [65] showed that women had more false alarms than men, who were faster in a route navigation task; moreover, women revealed a lower sense of orientation and computer experience than men. Findings of Dalgarno et al. [64] were not affected by gender. Lastly, recall decreased with age [68] for both immediate and delayed recall [6]. Taillade et al. [63] highlighted an age effect for a wayfinding task but not for a spatial memory task. Recognitions decreased with age [8], but the same was not found by Sauzéon and co-authors [68], who showed more false recognition for OA.

The following neuropsychological tests were correlated with memory tasks [71]. Trail Making Test (TMT) A and B [99] was used to evaluate executive functions and attention in OA and was negatively correlated with *what* and *where* and sustained attention scores were associated with *where* responses; lastly, the Cognitive Difficulties Scale [70,71] was significantly associated with episodic scores in normal and pathological aging.

Von Stülpnagel and Steffens [65] found different interactions with the movement (self-contained vs. observed) condition. In the second experiment, providing layout and landmark information along with self-contained movement led to better route knowledge (tour integration task), whereas for the route navigation task better scores were obtained when self-contained movements were associated with reading instructions. In the last of their experiments, recognition performance was enhanced when any allocentric map was given, whereas the tour integration task benefited by a map with path to follow and not by self-contained condition. Finally, in the route navigation, the map with a path to follow worsened the scores, whereas the active map helped participants in the observed movement condition. Farrell and colleagues [76], in their first experiment, found that active navigation with or without an allocentric map led to better virtual to real world transfer of spatial knowledge compared to control (real-world wayfinding) and this is true also for active virtual exploration with a path to follow (no decision-making). In their second experiment, virtual exploration with the map did not lead to better transfer compared to the allocentric map studying condition without real or virtual exploration.

Other relevant effects that interact with cognition are reported. In particular, dynamic active navigation generally led to better results, as noted by three studies [62,67,80]; however contradictory (path shape but not orientation and recognition; [62]) were also reported. Some authors [62,64,80] have highlighted the importance of optic flow for spatial learning in VE. Visual fidelity is also crucial for both survey and route knowledge [77], and the first-person perspective of the virtual environment boosted wayfinding and route knowledge, whereas an aerial-view improved allocentric representation [60]. Three-dimensional virtual reality seems to stimulate memory due to higher body involvement but also reduced energy consumption [74]; however, Palermo and co-authors [79] found that immersive interaction with a gyroscope, although reported as interesting, could be frustrating and showed a minor degree of engagement compared to classic active interaction with a mouse. Finally, a trial effect emerged confirming the positive effect of repetition on performance (e.g., [59]). Interestingly, exposure times led to better survey representation for passive participants, as noted by Sandamas and Foreman [59]. Wallet et al. [72] found better delayed recall, but not Pacheco and Verschure [81], in their 24-h delayed recall, for active participants after 48 h for spatial memory. Similarly, Jebara et al. [6] found YA, but not OA, had better delayed (20-min) as compared to immediate recall for episodic recall (item information and binding). No effect of condition emerged in the latter study. With regard to expertise, Sandamas and Foreman [75] found that drivers, regardless of the navigation condition, were better in the map task (survey knowledge). Moreover, different studies aimed at balancing driving [6,43,75] and technology experience (e.g., [60,65]), since these could influence the performance.

In addition to age, gender, skills, and cognitive functioning, it is crucial for neuropsychology research to consider the roles of consolidation, repetition, and dynamic changes in order to build effective and ergonomic training for memory rehabilitation and enhancement.

4. Discussion

In the present review, we provided initial positive results concerning the virtual enactment effect on spatial and episodic memory performance, highlighting the embodied potential of virtual reality (VR). For each of the questions presented (see Section 3 subsection headings), we provided theoretical and practical solutions to guide future studies within the context of the virtual enactment effect and its use in aging. To summarize, the virtual enactment effect on memory is: (1) present in the young population; (2) possible in aging but needs further investigation; (3) mediated by neurocognitive factors, especially in aging; and (4) dependent on the use of technological devices and their interaction characteristics.

In general, we suggest that future research should aim at designing experiments for older people and pathological aging, in both spatial and episodic memory in order to test the virtual enactment effect. Moreover, we encourage further research on episodic memory involving young participants to consolidate or extend the findings we reported in this systematic review. Innovative cognitive rehabilitative systems are needed to slow down or prevent memory decline in neurodegenerative conditions, and VR provides a powerful tool to stimulate brain plasticity in Alzheimer's disease and aging [100,101].

We highly recommend that researchers take into account these elements and consider the use of immersive apparatus by means of head-mounted display (HMD). The main limits of non-immersive studies reported in the review are that they do not grasp the full experience of active navigation, since they do not involve bodily-based (e.g., idiothetic) components [6], and the motor traces used while using controllers might be too weak to have an impact on memory traces [71]. Therefore, researchers should consider the use of a HMD. For instance, with an HMD it is possible to walk around a small area with trackers detecting movements and interact with the scenario with controllers. Moreover, VR enables the user to experience an "egocentric space" [102], which is a critical aspect of spatial processing as it occurs in everyday life [4]. Researchers should not forget the role of interaction (e.g., intentions and actions) on the sense of presence, which is considered to impact more on presence rather than graphic realism [103]. Another critical aspect of memory performance is the type of encoding of virtual scenarios. In real-life situations, episodic memory encoding occurs non-intentionally [10], whereas with spatial learning a certain amount of information is encoded incidentally and with procedural memory [104,105]. However, when planning interventions that exploit the virtual enactment effect, clinicians and neuroscientists are encouraged to design instructions according to the sample; for instance, aging is known to affect incidental rather than intentional encoding, with attentional and executive components playing a critical role in encoding and storage in the former [106]. Lastly, from a methodological point of view, we encourage the use of within-interaction conditions: first, within-subject studies have greater statistical power compared to between-subjects designs; second, they allow the researcher to control variables (e.g., gender) that may affect memory performance (e.g., gender effect on spatial memory [80]), thus providing balanced groups; finally, within-subject designs permit the researcher to assess source memory by asking the participants to recall the context in which an event occurred (see [57]). However, within-subjects studies might overload or confound memory traces if the tasks are too complex or numerous. Researchers should consider the strengths and weaknesses of within and between subjects designs with potential biases in light of the objectives of their studies [86].

Assessment of performance is a critical aspect of research and clinical practice in order to evaluate and analyse what the researcher really wants to achieve. We highly recommend defining tasks based on strong theoretical and empirical considerations when assessing the complexity of memory within the context of virtual enactment. In the context of spatial memory, we suggest using egocentric and allocentric measures to tap spatial cognition features [4]; this can be achieved using landmarks, boundaries and maps with paper-and-pencil, computerized or VR tasks. However, in the present review, this is especially true when the spatial layout is considered within the context of episodic memory (e.g., [8,57]). When research focused on schematic/topographical representation [2], papers mainly used spatial levels of knowledge of the space (survey, route and landmark); therefore, we applied these levels to the cluster spatial task (Figure 2). Nevertheless, recent discoveries in cognitive neuroscience and clinical neuropsychology support the crucial role of spatial frames of reference in representing the space [5,14,83]; moreover, survey knowledge and landmark knowledge resemble, respectively, allocentric and egocentric representation, whereas route knowledge appears to be related to procedural memory due to landmark-based navigation [105,107]. For episodic memory, we strongly encourage the paradigms that tap the elements described by Tulving [7] as central aspects of this type of memory (i.e., event, spatiotemporal details, and emotional and perceptual details). The advent of VR enables neuroscientists to study in an ecological, standardized, and realistic way a complex function such as episodic memory [8,108].

Concerning the virtual enactment effect on spatial memory, the young population reported more positive outcomes on survey knowledge compared to route and landmark knowledge; nevertheless, findings in general are promising. Young adults and both the healthy and pathological aged population showed improvements on episodic item memory, spatial context and binding. However, further studies need to evaluate this effect on aging and neurodegenerative disorders in the domains of both spatial and episodic memory. It might be of interest to deepen our understanding of in which situations passive enhancement is present and why (Figure 2). Moreover, we suggest that future studies include real-world navigation conditions; while all of the studies had a passive control condition, only one [72] used a real-world control condition. Finally concerning mediating factors, although visuospatial abilities are crucial for spatial memory [74], executive functions have a great impact on spatial and episodic performances, and this is especially true for older people [8,63,68]. Other variables such as age, gender, expertise (e.g., videogames, driving), dynamic navigation, virtual realism, and delayed testing influence memory performance.

Findings are promising in the light of memory decline in aging. An age-dependent decrease is normally observed in these crucial cognitive domains [109], and the decline in spatial and episodic memory is accompanied by neural changes in the medial temporal lobe, hippocampus and prefrontal cortex in the aged population [110–112]. Aging is accompanied by spatial memory decline [113]. Indeed, Colombo and colleagues [114] recently shown that older people have specific allocentric impairments and difficulty in switching between the egocentric and the allocentric frame of reference; the translation from the allocentric to the egocentric frame of reference is possible thanks to the activity of the retrosplenial cortex, which converts neural representations of the medial temporal lobe to parietal and vice versa [5,115].

In particular, spatiotemporal details, along with associative (i.e., medial temporal binding processes) and strategic (i.e., frontal monitoring during encoding and retrieval) information, decline with aging [8]. Aging is also accompanied by differences in the encoding and retrieval of episodic memories [10,11]. Piolino and colleagues [11] showed that this was particularly true for autobiographical events in recent periods, with more responses (less spatiotemporal information, details, familiarity and third-person perspective) associated with reduced autonoesis for older adults (OA) compared to young adults (YA).

Memory impairments due to medial temporal lobe degeneration are classic features of Alzheimer's disease (AD) [116], mild cognitive impairment (MCI) [117], and amnestic mild cognitive impairment (aMCI) [118], which are considered part of the prodromal stage of dementia and in particular AD [119]. Deactivation and decreased functional connectivity of the default mode network is shown in healthy aging, MCI, and AD [120–122]. Retrosplenial cortex hypoactivity occurs in both AD and MCI and may explain episodic and navigation deficits in these patients [5]. Spatial disorientation in AD and aMCI is thought to be the result of degenerative processes taking place in the hippocampus and in deficient spatial frame synchronization [123]. Indeed, early markers of AD can be the switching abilities in aMCI and AD individuals [124]: allocentric impairments are present in aMCI and AD patients and moreover a deficit in the switch from egocentric to allocentric was found in these groups. Concerning episodic memory, these neurological conditions lead to deficits in the spatiotemporal and binding components of episodic recall [70], as well as autonoetic consciousness [125,126].

Finally, the present findings stress the essential role of the body in cognition, and memory in particular, as claimed by embodied cognition researchers. The virtual enactment effect could be used to study how the different levels of active and passive virtual navigation contribute to spatial and episodic performance and could potentially be used as a way to enhance memory in aging.

Author Contributions: Conceptualization: C.T., S.S. and P.P.; methodology: C.T., L.D. and S.S.; writing—review and editing: C.T., S.S., L.D., G.R.; supervision: P.P.; funding acquisition: G.R.

Funding: This work was partially supported by the Italian funded project "High-end and Low-End Virtual Reality Systems for the Rehabilitation of Frailty in the Elderly" (PE-2013-02355948).

Conflicts of Interest: The authors declare that no competing interests exist.

References

1. Robin, J. Spatial scaffold effects in event memory and imagination. *Wiley Interdiscip. Rev. Cogn. Sci.* **2018**, *9*, e1462. [CrossRef] [PubMed]
2. Moscovitch, M.; Rosenbaum, R.S.; Gilboa, A.; Addis, D.R.; Westmacott, R.; Grady, C.; McAndrews, M.P.; Levine, L.; Black, S.; Winocur, G.; et al. Functional neuroanatomy of remote episodic, semantic and spatial memory: A unified account based on multiple trace theory. *J. Anat.* **2005**, *207*, 35–66. [CrossRef] [PubMed]
3. American Psychological Association. *APA Dictionary of Psychology*; American Psychological Association: Washington, DC, USA, 2007.
4. Burgess, N. Spatial cognition and the brain. *Ann. N. Y. Acad. Sci.* **2008**, *1124*, 77–97. [CrossRef]
5. Vann, S.D.; Aggleton, J.P.; Maguire, E.A. What does the retrosplenial cortex do? *Nat. Rev. Neurosci.* **2009**, *10*, 792–802. [CrossRef] [PubMed]
6. Chrastil, E.R.; Warren, W.H. Active and passive contributions to spatial learning. *Psychon. Bull. Rev.* **2012**, *19*, 1–23. [CrossRef] [PubMed]
7. Tulving, E. Episodic Memory: From Mind to Brain. *Annu. Rev. Psychol.* **2002**, *53*, 1–25. [PubMed]
8. Jebara, N.; Orriols, E.; Zaoui, M.; Berthoz, A.; Piolino, P. Effects of enactment in episodic memory: A pilot virtual reality study with young and elderly adults. *Front. Aging Neurosci.* **2014**, *6*, 338. [CrossRef] [PubMed]
9. Laurent, X.; Ensslin, A.; Marí-Beffa, P. An Action to an Object Does Not Improve Its Episodic Encoding but Removes Distraction. *J. Exp. Psychol. Hum. Percept. Perform.* **2016**, *42*, 494–507.
10. Plancher, G.; Gyselinck, V.; Nicolas, S.; Piolino, P. Age effect on components of episodic memory and feature binding: A virtual reality study. *Neuropsychology* **2010**, *24*, 379–390. [CrossRef] [PubMed]
11. Piolino, P.; Desgranges, B.; Clarys, D.; Guillery-Girard, B.; Taconnat, L.; Isingrini, M.; Eustache, F. Autobiographical memory, autonoetic consciousness, and self-perspective in aging. *Psychol. Aging* **2006**, *21*, 510–525. [CrossRef] [PubMed]
12. Prebble, S.C.; Addis, D.R.; Tippett, L.J. Autobiographical memory and sense of self. *Psychol. Bull.* **2013**, *139*, 815–840. [CrossRef]
13. O'Keefe, L.; Nadel, J. *The Hippocampus as a Cognitive Map*; Clarendon Press: Oxford, UK, 1978.

14. Hartley, T.; Lever, C.; Burgess, N.; O'Keefe, J. Space in the brain: How the hippocampal formation supports spatial cognition. *Philos. Trans. R. Soc. Lond. B Biol. Sci.* **2014**, *369*, 20120510. [CrossRef] [PubMed]
15. Burgess, N.; Maguire, E.A.; O'Keefe, J. The human hippocampus and spatial and episodic memory. *Neuron* **2002**, *35*, 625–641. [CrossRef]
16. Kühn, S.; Gallinat, J. Segregating cognitive functions within hippocampal formation: A quantitative meta-analysis on spatial navigation and episodic memory. *Hum. Brain Mapp.* **2014**, *35*, 1129–1142. [CrossRef] [PubMed]
17. Manus, J.R.; Hopkins, R.O.; Reed, J.M.; Kitchener, E.G.; Squire, L.R. Recognition memory and the human hippocampus. *Neuron* **2003**, *37*, 171–180. [CrossRef]
18. Bergouignan, L.; Nyberg, L.; Ehrsson, H.H. Out-of-body–induced hippocampal amnesia. *Proc. Natl. Acad. Sci. USA* **2014**, *111*, 4421–4426. [CrossRef]
19. Eichenbaum, H. Time cells in the hippocampus: A new dimension for mapping memories. *Nat. Rev. Neruosci.* **2014**, *15*, 732–744. [CrossRef]
20. Glenberg, A.M.; Hayes, J. Contribution of embodiment to solving the riddle of infantile amnesia. *Front. Psychol.* **2016**, *7*, 10. [CrossRef] [PubMed]
21. Ritchey, M.; Wing, E.A.; Labar, K.S.; Cabeza, R. Neural Similarity Between Encoding and Retrieval is Related to Memory Via Hippocampal Interactions. *Cereb. Cortex* **2012**, *23*, 2818–2828. [CrossRef] [PubMed]
22. Nadel, L.; Winocur, G.; Ryan, L.; Moscovitch, M. Systems consolidation and hippocampus: Two views. *Debates Neurosci.* **2007**, *1*, 55–66. [CrossRef]
23. Gomez, A.; Rousset, S.; Baciu, M. Egocentric-updating during navigation facilitates episodic memory retrieval. *Acta Psychol.* **2009**, *132*, 221–227. [CrossRef]
24. Burgess, N. The hippocampus, space, and view points in episodic memory. *Q. J. Exp. Psychol.* **2002**, *55A*, 1057–1080. [CrossRef]
25. Gomez, A.; Rousset, S.; Charnallet, A. Spatial deficits in an amnesic patient with hippocampal damage: Questioning the multiple trace theory. *Hippocampus* **2012**, *22*, 1313–1324. [CrossRef]
26. Tromp, D.; Dufour, A.; Lithfous, S.; Pebayle, T.; Després, O. Episodic memory in normal aging and Alzheimer disease: Insights from imaging and behavioral studies. *Ageing Res. Rev.* **2015**, *24*, 232–262. [CrossRef] [PubMed]
27. Wheeler, M.A.; Stuss, D.T.; Tulving, E. Toward a theory of episodic memory: The frontal lobes and autonoetic consciousness. *Psychol. Bull.* **1997**, *121*, 331–354. [CrossRef] [PubMed]
28. Habib, R.; Nyberg, L.; Tulving, E. Hemispheric asymmetries of memory: The HERA model revisited. *Trends Cogn. Sci.* **2003**, *7*, 241–245. [CrossRef]
29. Lepage, M.; Ghaffar, O.; Nyberg, L.; Tulving, E. Prefrontal cortex and episodic memory retrieval mode. *Proc. Natl. Acad. Sci. USA* **2000**, *97*, 506–511. [CrossRef]
30. Burgess, N.; Maguire, E.A.; Spiers, H.J.; O'Keefe, J. A temporoparietal and prefrontal network for retrieving the spatial context of lifelike events. *Neuroimage* **2001**, *14*, 439–453. [CrossRef] [PubMed]
31. Spreng, R.N.; Mar, R.A.; Kim, A.S.N. The Common Neural Basis of Autobiographical Memory, Prospection, Navigation, Theory of Mind, and the Default Mode: A Quantitative Meta-analysis. *J. Cogn. Neurosci.* **2008**, *21*, 489–510. [CrossRef]
32. Clark, A. An embodied cognitive science? *Trends Cogn. Sci.* **1999**, *3*, 345–351. [CrossRef]
33. Wilson, M. Six views of embodied cognition. *Psychon. Bull. Rev.* **2002**, *9*, 625–636. [CrossRef] [PubMed]
34. Glenberg, A.M. Embodiment as a unifying perspective for psychology. *Wiley Interdiscip. Rev. Cogn. Sci.* **2010**, *1*, 586–596. [CrossRef] [PubMed]
35. Dijkstra, K.; Post, L. Mechanisms of embodiment. *Front. Psychol.* **2015**, *6*, 1525. [CrossRef] [PubMed]
36. Vallet, G.T. Embodied cognition of aging. *Front. Psychol.* **2015**, *6*, 463. [CrossRef]
37. Spackman, J.S.; Yanchar, S.C. Embodied Cognition, Representationalism, and Mechanism: A Review and Analysis. *J. Theory Soc. Behav.* **2014**, *44*, 46–79. [CrossRef]
38. Braak, H.; Braak, E. Neuropathological stageing of Alzheimer-related changes. *Acta Neuropathol.* **1991**, *82*, 239–259. [CrossRef]
39. Fjell, A.M.; Westlye, L.T.; Amlien, I.; Espeseth, T.; Reinvang, I.; Raz, N.; Agartz, I.; Salat, D.H.; Greve, D.N.; Fischl, B.; et al. High consistency of regional cortical thinning in aging across multiple samples. *Cereb. Cortex* **2009**, *19*, 2001–2012. [CrossRef]

40. Braak, H.; Braak, E. Staging of alzheimer's disease-related neurofibrillary changes. *Neurobiol. Aging* **1995**, *16*, 271–278. [CrossRef]
41. Brooks, B.M.; Attree, E.A.; Rose, F.D.; Clifford, B.R.; Leadbetter, A.G. The Specificity of Memory Enhancement During Interaction with a Virtual Environment. *Memory* **1999**, *7*, 65–78. [CrossRef]
42. Engelkamp, J. *Memory for Actions*; Psychology Press/Taylor & Francis: London, UK, 1998.
43. Plancher, G.; Barra, J.; Orriols, E.; Piolino, P. The influence of action on episodic memory: A virtual reality study. *Q. J. Exp. Psychol.* **2013**, *66*, 895–909. [CrossRef]
44. Tulving, E. Ecphoric process in episodic memory. *Philos. Trans. R. Soc. Lond. B* **1983**, *1110*, 361–370. [CrossRef]
45. Rugg, M.D.; Wilding, E.L. Retrieval processing and episodic memory. *Trends Cogn. Sci.* **2000**, *4*, 108–115. [CrossRef]
46. Kent, C.; Lamberts, K. The encoding-retrieval relationship: Retrieval as mental simulation. *Trends Cogn. Sci.* **2008**, *12*, 92–98. [CrossRef]
47. Meyer, K.; Damasio, A. Convergence and divergence in a neural architecture for recognition and memory. *Trends Neurosci.* **2009**, *32*, 376–382. [CrossRef]
48. Johnson, J.D.; Price, M.H.; Leiker, E.K. Episodic retrieval involves early and sustained effects of reactivating information from encoding. *Neuroimage* **2015**, *106*, 300–310. [CrossRef] [PubMed]
49. Rugg, M.D.; Johnson, J.D.; Park, H.; Uncapher, M.R. Encoding-retrieval overlap in human episodic memory: A functional neuroimaging perspective. *Prog. Brain Res.* **2008**, *169*, 339–352. [PubMed]
50. Danker, J.F.; Anderson, J.R. The ghosts of brain states past: Remembering reactivates the brain regions engaged during encoding. *Psychol. Bull.* **2010**, *136*, 87–102. [CrossRef] [PubMed]
51. Nyberg, L.; Habib, R.; McIntosh, A.R.; Tulving, E. Reactivation of encoding-related brain activity during memory retrieval. *Proc. Natl. Acad. Sci. USA* **2000**, *97*, 11120–11124. [CrossRef]
52. Wheeler, M.; Petersen, S.; Buckner, R. Memory's Echo: Vivid Remembering Reactivates Sensory-Specific Cortex. *Proc. Natl. Acad. Sci. USA* **2000**, *97*, 11125–11129. [CrossRef]
53. Wilson, P.N.; Foreman, N.; Gillett, R.; Stanton, D. Active Versus Passive Processing of Spatial Information in a Computer- Simulated Environment. *Ecol. Psychol.* **1997**, *9*, 37–41. [CrossRef]
54. Riva, G. From virtual to real body: Virtual reality as embodied technology. *J. Cyber Ther. Rehabil.* **2008**, *1*, 7–22.
55. Repetto, C.; Serino, S.; Macedonia, M.; Riva, G. Virtual Reality as an Embodied Tool to Enhance Episodic Memory in Elderly. *Front. Psychol.* **2016**, *7*, 1839. [CrossRef]
56. Moher, D.; Liberati, A.; Tetzlaff, J.; Altman, D.G.; Grp, P. Preferred Reporting Items for Systematic Reviews and Meta-Analyses: The PRISMA Statement (Reprinted from Annals of Internal Medicine). *Phys. Ther.* **2009**, *89*, 873–880.
57. Tuena, C.; Serino, S.; Gaston-Bellegarde, A.; Orriols, E.; Makowski, D.; Riva, G.; Piolino, P. How virtual embodiment affects episodic memory functioning: A proof-of-concept study. *Annu. Rev. Cyberther. Telemed.* **2017**, *15*, 98–103.
58. Carassa, A.; Geminiani, G.; Morganti, F.; Varotto, D. Active and passive spatial learning in a complex virtual environment: The effect of effcient exploration. *Cogn. Process.* **2002**, *3*, 65–81.
59. Sandamas, G.; Foreman, N. Drawing maps and remembering landmarks after driving in a virtual small town environment. *J. Maps* **2007**, *3*, 35–45. [CrossRef]
60. Wallet, G.; Sauzéon, H.; Larrue, F.; N'Kaoua, B. Virtual/real transfer in a large-scale environment: Impact of active navigation as a function of the viewpoint displacement effect and recall tasks. *Adv. Hum. Comput. Interact.* **2013**, *2013*, 8. [CrossRef]
61. Meade, M.E.; Meade, J.G.; Sauzéon, H.; Fernandes, M.A. Active Navigation in Virtual Environments Benefits Spatial Memory in Older Adults. *Brain Sci.* **2019**, *9*, 47. [CrossRef]
62. Gaunet, F.; Vidal, M.; Kemeny, A.; Berthoz, A. Active, passive and snapshot exploration in a virtual environment: Influence on scene memory, reorientation and path memory. *Cogn. Brain Res.* **2001**, *11*, 409–420. [CrossRef]
63. Taillade, M.; Sauzéon, H.; Pala, P.A.; Déjos, M.; Larrue, F.; Gross, C.; N'Kaoua, B. Age-Related Wayfinding Differences in Real Large-Scale Environments: Detrimental Motor Control Effects during Spatial Learning Are Mediated by Executive Decline? *PLoS ONE* **2013**, *8*, e67193. [CrossRef]
64. Dalgarno, B.; Bennett, S.; Harper, B. The Importance of Active Exploration, Optical Flow, and Task Alignment for Spatial Learning in Desktop 3D Environments. *Hum. Comput. Interact.* **2010**, *25*, 25–66. [CrossRef]

65. von Stülpnagel, R.; Steffens, M.C. Active route learning in virtual environments: Disentangling movement control from intention, instruction specificity, and navigation control. *Psychol. Res.* **2013**, *77*, 555–574. [CrossRef]
66. Wilson, P.N. Active exploration of a virtual environment does not promote orientation or memory for objects. *Environ. Behav.* **1999**, *31*, 752–763. [CrossRef]
67. Peruch, P.; Vercher, J.; Gauthier, G.M. Acquisition of Spatial Knowledge Through Visual Exploration of Simulated Environments. *Ecol. Psychol.* **1995**, *7*, 1–20. [CrossRef]
68. Sauzéon, H.; N'Kaoua, B.; Arvind Pala, P.; Taillade, M.; Guitton, P. Age and active navigation effects on episodic memory: A virtual reality study. *Br. J. Psychol.* **2016**, *107*, 72–94. [CrossRef]
69. Sauzéon, H.; Pala, P.A.; Larrue, F.; Wallet, G.; Déjos, M.; Zheng, X.; Guitton, P.; N'Kaoua, B. The use of Virtual Reality for episodic memory assessment: Effects of active navigation. *Exp. Psychol.* **2012**, *59*, 99–108. [CrossRef]
70. Plancher, G.; Tirard, A.; Gyselinck, V.; Nicolas, S.; Piolino, P. Using virtual reality to characterize episodic memory profiles in amnestic mild cognitive impairment and Alzheimer's disease: Influence of active and passive encoding. *Neuropsychologia* **2012**, *50*, 592–602. [CrossRef]
71. Plancher, G.; Nicolas, S.; Piolino, P. Apport de la réalité virtuelle en neuropsychologie de la mémoire: Étude dans le vieillissement. *Psychol. Neuropsychiatr. Vieil.* **2008**, *6*, 7–22.
72. Wallet, G.; Sauzéon, H.; Rodrigues, J.; Larrue, F.; N'Kaoua, B. Virtual/real transfer of spatial learning: Impact of activity according to the retention delay. *Stud. Health Technol. Inform.* **2010**, *154*, 145–149.
73. Hahm, J.; Lee, K.; Lim, S.-L.; Kim, S.-Y.; Kim, H.-T.; Lee, J.-H. Effects of active navigation on object recognition in virtual environments. *CyberPsychol. Behav.* **2007**, *10*, 305–308. [CrossRef]
74. Cutmore, T.R.H.; Hine, T.J.; Maberly, K.J.; Langford, N.M.; Hawgood, G. Cognitive and gender factors influencing navigation in a virtual environment. *Int. J. Hum. Comput. Stud.* **2000**, *53*, 223–249. [CrossRef]
75. Sandamas, G.; Foreman, N. Active Versus Passive Acquisition of Spatial Knowledge While Controlling a Vehicle in a Virtual Urban Space in Drivers and Non-Drivers. *SAGE Open* **2015**, *5*, 2158244015595443. [CrossRef]
76. Farrell, M.J.; Arnold, P.; Pettifer, S.; Adams, J.; Graham, T.; MacManamon, M. Transfer of route learning from virtual to real environments. *J. Exp. Psychol. Appl.* **2003**, *9*, 219–227. [CrossRef]
77. Wallet, G.; Sauzéon, H.; Pala, P.A.; Larrue, F.; Zheng, X.; N'Kaoua, B. Virtual/real transfer of spatial knowledge: Benefit from visual fidelity provided in a virtual environment and impact of active navigation. *Cyberpsychol. Behav. Soc. Netw.* **2011**, *14*, 417–423. [CrossRef]
78. Allison, C.; Redhead, E.S. Factors in fluencing orientation within a nested virtual environment: External cues, active exploration and familiarity. *J. Environ. Psychol.* **2017**, *51*, 158–167. [CrossRef]
79. Palermo, E.; Laut, J.; Nov, O.; Cappa, P.; Porfiri, M. Spatial memory training in a citizen science context. *Comput. Hum. Behav.* **2017**, *73*, 38–46. [CrossRef]
80. Liu, I.; Levy, R.M.; Barton, J.J.S.; Iaria, G. Age and gender differences in various topographical orientation strategies. *Brain Res.* **2011**, *1410*, 112–119. [CrossRef]
81. Pacheco, D.; Verschure, P.F.M.J. Long-term spatial clustering in free recall. *Memory* **2018**, *26*, 798–806. [CrossRef]
82. Pettijohn, K.A.; Radvansky, G.A. Walking through doorways causes forgetting: Active and passive interaction. *J. Cogn. Psychol.* **2018**, *30*, 771–777. [CrossRef]
83. Barry, C.; Burgess, N. Neural Mechanisms of Self-Location. *Curr. Biol.* **2014**, *24*, R330–R339. [CrossRef]
84. Chrastil, E.R.; Warren, W.H. Active and Passive Spatial Learning in Human Navigation: Acquisition of Graph Knowledg. *J. Exp. Psychol. Learn. Mem. Cogn.* **2015**, *41*, 1162–1178. [CrossRef]
85. Greenwood, P.M. The frontal aging hypothesis evaluated. *J. Int. Neuropsychol. Soc.* **2000**, *6*, 705–726. [CrossRef]
86. Charness, G.; Gneezy, U.; Kuhn, M.A. Experimental methods: Between-subject and within-subject design. *J. Econ. Behav. Organ.* **2012**, *81*, 1–8. [CrossRef]
87. Delis, D.C.; Kramer, J.H.; Kaplan, E.; Thompkins, B.A.O. *CVLT: California Verbal Learning Test-Adult Version: Manual*; Psychological Corporation: London, UK, 1987.
88. Madan, C.R.; Singhal, A. Using actions to enhance memory: Effects of enactment, gestures, and exercise on human memory. *Front. Psychol.* **2012**, *3*, 507. [CrossRef]

89. Dijkstra, K.; Kaschak, M.P.; Zwaan, R.A. Body posture facilitates retrieval of autobiographical memories. *Cognition* **2007**, *102*, 139–149. [CrossRef]
90. Guterstam, A.; Bjornsdotter, M.; Bergouignan, L.; Gentile, G.; Li, T.-Q.; Ehrsson, H.H. Decoding illusory self-location from activity in the human hippocampus. *Front. Hum. Neurosci.* **2015**, *9*, 412. [CrossRef]
91. Steffens, M.C.; Von Stülpnagel, R.; Schult, J.C. Memory Recall After 'Learning by Doing' and 'Learning by Viewing': Boundary Conditions of an Enactment Benefit. *Front. Psychol.* **2015**, *6*, 1907. [CrossRef]
92. Potter, M.C. Recognition and memory for briefly presented scenes. *Front. Psychol.* **2012**, *3*, 32. [CrossRef]
93. Migo, E.M.; Mayes, A.R.; Montaldi, D. Measuring recollection and familiarity: Improving the remember/know procedure. *Conscious. Cogn.* **2012**, *21*, 1435–1455. [CrossRef]
94. Nyberg, L.; Persson, J.; Nilsson, L.G. Individual differences in memory enhancement by encoding enactment: Relationships to adult age and biological factors. *Neurosci. Biobehav. Rev.* **2002**, *26*, 835–839. [CrossRef]
95. Zimmer, H.D.; Cohen, R.L. *Memory for Action: A Distinct Form of Episodic Memory?* Oxford University Press: Oxford, UK, 2001.
96. Wechsler, D. *WAIS-R Manual: Wechsler Adult Intelligence Scale-Revised*; Psychological Corporation: London, UK, 1981.
97. Stroop, J.R. Studies of interference in serial verbal reactions. *J. Exp. Psychol.* **1935**, *18*, 643. [CrossRef]
98. Vandenberg, S.G.; Kuse, A.R. Mental rotations, a group test of three-dimensional spatial visualization. *Percept. Mot. Skills* **1978**, *47*, 599–604. [CrossRef]
99. Reitan, R.M. Validity of the Trail Making Test as an indicator of organic brain damage. *Percept. Mot. Skills* **1958**, *8*, 271–276. [CrossRef]
100. García-Betances, R.I.; Arredondo Waldmeyer, M.T.; Fico, G.; Cabrera-Umpiérrez, M.F. A succinct overview of virtual reality technology use in Alzheimer's disease. *Front. Aging Neurosci.* **2015**, *7*, 80.
101. Serino, S.; Pedroli, E.; Tuena, C.; Leo, G.D.; Stramba-Badiale, M.; Goulene, K.; Mariotti, N.G.; Riva, G. A Novel Virtual Reality-Based Training Protocol for the Enhancement of the 'Mental Frame Syncing' in Individuals with Alzheimer's Disease: A Development-of-Concept Trial. Serino, Silvia et al. "A Novel Virtual Reality-Based Training Protocol for the Enhancement of the "Mental Frame Syncing" in Individuals with Alzheimer's Disease: A Development-of-Concept Trial.". *Front. Aging Neurosci.* **2017**, *9*, 240.
102. Serino, S.; Riva, G. Getting lost in Alzheimer's disease: A break in the mental frame syncing. *Med. Hypotheses* **2013**, *80*, 416–421. [CrossRef]
103. Triberti, S.; Riva, G. Being present in action: A theoretical model about the 'interlocking' between intentions and environmental affordances. *Front. Psychol.* **2016**, *6*, 2052. [CrossRef]
104. Münzer, S.; Zimmer, H.D.; Schwalm, M.; Baus, J.; Aslan, I. Computer-assisted navigation and the acquisition of route and survey knowledge. *J. Environ. Psychol.* **2006**, *26*, 300–308. [CrossRef]
105. Doeller, C.F.; King, J.A.; Burgess, N. Parallel striatal and hippocampal systems for landmarks and boundaries in spatial memory. *Proc. Natl. Acad. Sci. USA* **2008**, *105*, 5915–5920. [CrossRef]
106. Kontaxopoulou, D.; Beratis, I.N.; Fragkiadaki, S.; Pavlou, D.; Yannis, G.; Economou, A.; Papanicolaou, A.C.; Papageorgiou, S.G. Incidental and Intentional Memory: Their Relation with Attention and Executive Functions. *Arch. Clin. Neuropsychol.* **2017**, *32*, 19–532. [CrossRef]
107. Guderian, S.; Dzieciol, A.M.; Gadian, D.G.; Jentschke, S.; Doeller, C.F.; Burgess, N.; Mishkin, M.; Vargha-Khadem, F. Hippocampal Volume Reduction in Humans Predicts Impaired Allocentric Spatial Memory in Virtual-Reality Navigation. *J. Neurosci.* **2015**, *35*, 14123–14131. [CrossRef]
108. Serino, S.; Repetto, C. New Trends in Episodic Memory Assessment: Immersive 360 Ecological Videos. *Front. Psychol.* **2018**, *9*, 1878. [CrossRef]
109. Salthouse, T.A. When does age-related cognitive decline begin? *Neurobiol. Aging* **2009**, *30*, 507–514. [CrossRef]
110. Hedden, T.; Gabrieli, J.D.E. Insights into the ageing mind: A view from cognitive neuroscience. *Nat. Rev. Neurosci.* **2004**, *5*, 87–96. [CrossRef]
111. Kinugawa, K.; Schumm, S.; Pollina, M.; Depre, M.; Jungbluth, C.; Doulazmi, M.; Mariani, J. Aging-related episodic memory decline: Are emotions the key? *Front. Behav. Neurosci.* **2013**, *7*, 2. [CrossRef]
112. Robitsek, R.J.; Fortin, N.J.; Koh, M.T.; Gallagher, M.; Eichenbaum, H. Cognitive Aging: A Common Decline of Episodic Recollection and Spatial Memory in Rats. *J. Neurosci.* **2008**, *28*, 8945–8954. [CrossRef]
113. Wolbers, T.; Dudchenko, P.A.; Wood, E.R. Spatial memory—A unique window into healthy and pathological aging. *Front. Aging Neurosci.* **2014**, *6*, 35. [CrossRef]

114. Colombo, D.; Serino, S.; Tuena, C.; Pedroli, E.; Dakanalis, A.; Cipresso, P.; Riva, G. Egocentric and allocentric spatial reference frames in aging: A systematic review. *Neurosci. Biobehav. Rev.* **2017**, *80*, 605–621. [CrossRef]
115. Alexander, A.S.; Nitz, D.A. Retrosplenial cortex maps the conjunction of internal and external spaces. *Nat. Neurosci.* **2015**, *18*, 1143–1151. [CrossRef]
116. Dubois, B.; Feldman, H.H.; Jacova, C.; DeKosky, S.T.; Barberger-Gateau, P.; Cummings, J.; Delacourte, A.; Galasko, D.; Gauthier, S.; Jicha, G.; et al. Research criteria for the diagnosis of Alzheimer's disease: Revising the NINCDS-ADRDA criteria. *Lancet Neurol.* **2007**, *6*, 734–746. [CrossRef]
117. Nordahl, C.W.; Ranganath, C.; Yonelinas, A.P.; DeCarli, C.; Reed, B.R.; Jagust, W.J. Different mechanisms of episodic memory failure in mild cognitive impairment. *Neuropsychologia* **2005**, *43*, 1688–1697. [CrossRef] [PubMed]
118. Dunn, C.J.; Duffy, S.L.; Hickie, I.B.; Lagopoulos, J.; Lewis, S.J.; Naismith, S.L.; Shine, J.M. Deficits in episodic memory retrieval reveal impaired default mode network connectivity in amnestic mild cognitive impairment. *NeuroImage Clin.* **2014**, *4*, 473–480. [CrossRef] [PubMed]
119. Petersen, R.C.; Doody, R.; Kurz, A.; Mohs, R.C.; Morris, J.C.; Rabins, P.V.; Ritchie, K.; Rossor, M.; Thal, L.; Winblad, B. Current Concepts in Mild Cognitive Impairment. *Arch. Neurol.* **2011**, *58*, 1985–1992. [CrossRef]
120. Hafkemeijer, A.; van der Grond, J.; Rombouts, S.A.R.B. Imaging the default mode network in aging and dementia. *Biochim. Biophys. Acta Mol. Basis Dis.* **2012**, *1822*, 431–441. [CrossRef]
121. Buckner, R.L.; Snyder, A.Z.; Shannon, B.J.; LaRossa, G.; Sachs, R.; Fotenos, A.F.; Sheline, Y.I.; Klunk, W.E.; Mathis, C.A.; Morris, J.C.; et al. Molecular, Structural, and Functional Characterization of Alzheimer's Disease: Evidence for a Relationship between Default Activity, Amyloid, and Memory. *J. Neurosci.* **2005**, *25*, 7709–7717. [CrossRef] [PubMed]
122. Buckner, R.L.; Andrews-Hanna, J.R.; Schacter, D.L. The brain's default network: Anatomy, function, and relevance to disease. *Ann. N. Y. Acad. Sci.* **2008**, *1124*, 1–38. [CrossRef] [PubMed]
123. Serino, S.; Morganti, F.; Di Stefano, F.; Riva, G. Detecting early egocentric and allocentric impairments deficits in Alzheimer's disease: An experimental study with virtual reality. *Front. Aging Neurosci.* **2015**, *7*, 88. [CrossRef]
124. Ruggiero, G.; Iavarone, A.; Iachini, T. Allocentric to egocentric spatial switching: Impairment in amci and Alzheimer's disease patients? *Curr. Alzheimer Res.* **2018**, *15*, 229–236. [CrossRef]
125. Piolino, P.; Desgranges, B.; Belliard, S.; Matuszewski, V.; Lalevée, C.; De La Sayette, V.; Eustache, F. Autobiographical memory and autonoetic consciousness: Triple dissociation in neurodegenerative diseases. *Brain* **2003**, *126*, 2203–2219. [CrossRef]
126. Rauchs, G.; Piolino, P.; Mézenge, F.; Landeau, B.; Lalevée, C.; Pélerin, A.; Viader, F.; De La Sayette, V.; Eustache, F.; Desgranges, B. Autonoetic consciousness in Alzheimer's disease: Neuropsychological and PET findings using an episodic learning and recognition task. *Neurobiol. Aging* **2007**, *28*, 1410–1420. [CrossRef]

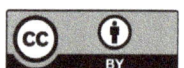

© 2019 by the authors. Licensee MDPI, Basel, Switzerland. This article is an open access article distributed under the terms and conditions of the Creative Commons Attribution (CC BY) license (http://creativecommons.org/licenses/by/4.0/).

MDPI
St. Alban-Anlage 66
4052 Basel
Switzerland
Tel. +41 61 683 77 34
Fax +41 61 302 89 18
www.mdpi.com

Journal of Clinical Medicine Editorial Office
E-mail: jcm@mdpi.com
www.mdpi.com/journal/jcm